# Computed Tomography in Intracranial Tumors

## Differential Diagnosis and Clinical Aspects

Edited by
E. Kazner · S. Wende · Th. Grumme
W. Lanksch · O. Stochdorph

Authors
G.B. Bradač · U. Büll · R. Fahlbusch · Th. Grumme
E. Kazner · K. Kretzschmar · W. Lanksch · W. Meese
J. Schramm · H. Steinhoff · O. Stochdorph · S. Wende

With 693 Figures

Springer-Verlag
Berlin Heidelberg New York 1982

Translator: Dr. F.C. DOUGHERTY, Berlin
Translation of the German edition
Computertomographie intrakranieller Tumoren aus klinischer Sicht
© by Springer-Verlag Berlin Heidelberg 1981

ISBN-13:978-3-642-96655-2 e-ISBN-13:978-3-642-96653-8
DOI: 10.1007/978-3-642-96653-8

Library of Congress Cataloging in Publication Data. Computertomographie intrakranieller Tumoren aus klinischer Sicht. English. Computed tomography in intracranial tumors. Translation of: Computertomographie intrakranieller Tumoren aus klinischer Sicht. Bibliography: p. Includes index. 1. Brain–Tumors–Diagnosis. 2. Tomography. 3. Brain–Tumors. I. Kazner, Ekkehard. II. Bradač, G.B., 1939-. [DNLM: 1. Brain neoplasms–Radiography. 2. Orbital neoplasms–Radiography. 3. Tomography, X-ray computed. 4. Brain–Radiography. WL 358 C738]. RC280.B7C5713. 616.99'28107572. 82-5706.

Softcover reprint of the hardcover 1st edition 1982


2122/3130-543210

# Preface

The current book represents a distillation of the experience gained in diagnosis of intracranial tumors with computed X-ray tomography at the University Hospitals of Berlin, Mainz, and München. To what purpose? Standard radiological techniques such as pneumoencephalography with lumbar puncture and cerebral arteriography with puncture of the common carotid artery are invasive procedures which entail a certain amount of risk as well as discomfort for the patient. Furthermore, diagnoses made with these procedures rely primarily on indirect signs of an intracranial space-occupying lesion – such as displacement of the air-filled ventricles or of normal cerebral vessels. Only a few types of tumor are demonstrated directly with these techniques.

In contrast, computed tomography demonstrates the pathology directly in almost all cases, and this with a minimum of risk and discomfort. In addition, normal intracranial structures are demonstrated, so that the tumor's effect on its surroundings can be evaluated.

Today, almost a decade after HOUNSFIELD's revolutionary invention, diagnosis of brain tumors without computed tomography is almost unthinkable, if not in fact irresponsible.

Computed tomography is an integral part of preoperative diagnostics. The tumor is clearly demonstrated, accurately located, and often defined as to histological type. In addition, it is usually possible to decide whether the tumor is operable or not. As a result, unnecessary and risky operations can be avoided – in cases where the tumor proves to be larger than expected and in which vital centers are involved, for example. Computed tomography is also ideally suited for postoperative follow-up, for planning adjunctive radiation therapy, and for determining the success of irradiation or other conservative treatment. The enormous cost of computed tomography is justified only by improved diagnostic accuracy and, concurrently, elimination of costs for other diagnostic procedures. Computed tomography is capable of detecting up to 98% of brain tumors and is far more accurate than any other single diagnostic technique. Even histological diagnoses can be predicted with an accuracy approaching 90% in certain types of tumor.

Cost-benefit analysis has shown conclusively that computed tomography has resulted in a considerable reduction in overall cost, since diagnosis may be performed on an outpatient basis in many cases, since average time in hospital is reduced, and since other expensive procedures may be eliminated. The three CT study groups at the University Hospitals of Berlin, Mainz, and München examined over 40000 patients in the period from 1975 to the middle of 1980. This includes 3750 patients with brain tumors and over 600 patients with orbital lesions. Extensive experience in the use of computed tomography as well as the opportunity to compare CT findings with surgical results and neuropathological studies are summarized in this book. It is intended to help clinicians and general practitioners in determining the location and type of tumor, using CT findings together with the clinical data and the results of supplementary diagnostic techniques.

The editors conceived the project in 1975 with the intention of developing the most comprehensive experience possible in the appearance of brain tumors in computed tomography. Regular meetings allowed a continuous interchange of experience as well as analysis of problem cases. As a result all three study groups developed a comparable level of knowledge, which provided a common standard for evaluation of CT findings. This allowed the presentation of the collected experience in a genuine cooperative study by neuroradiologists, neurosurgeons, and neuropathologists.

The study was initiated with the help of the Volkswagenwerk Foundation, the Ludwig-Maximilians-Universität München, the Senat of Berlin, the Freie Universität Berlin, the Deutsche Forschungsgemeinschaft, and the Johannes-Gutenberg-Universität Mainz. The generous financial support from these institutions made possible the purchase of computed tomography systems with which fundamental knowledge in CT diagnosis of intracranial lesions could be developed.

We should like to thank the many general practitioners and participating institutions who referred their patients to us for diagnostic procedures and provided us with the clinical data in these cases. The following listing presents in alphabetical order the department heads at various institutions who, with their colleagues, lent valuable support to our efforts:

Freie Universität Berlin: Prof. Dr. J. CERVÓS-NAVARRO, Dept. of Neuropathology; Prof. Dr. H.J. EBERLEIN, Dept. of Anesthesiology; Prof. Dr. R. FELIX, Radiology Dept.; Prof. Dr. W. GIRKE, Neurology Dept.; Prof. Dr. F. HANEFELD, Dept. of Pediatrics; Prof. Dr. D. JANZ, Neurology Dept.; Prof. Dr. E. KASTENBAUER, Dept. of Otorhinolaryngology; Prof. Dr. W. SCHWAB, formerly Dept. of Otorhinolaryngology; Prof. Dr. J. WOLLENSAK, Dept. of Ophthalmology; Prof. Dr. R. WÜLLENWEBER, formerly Dept. of Neurosurgery.

Johannes-Gutenberg-Universität Mainz: Prof. Dr. R. FREY †, Dept. of Anesthesiology; Prof. Dr. J. HELMS, Dept. of Otorhinolaryngology; Prof. Dr. H.-CH. HOPF, Neurology Dept.; Prof. Dr. A. NOVER, Dept. of Ophthalmology; Prof. Dr. J.M. SCHRÖDER, Dept. of Neuropathology; Prof. Dr. K. SCHÜRMANN, Dept. of Neurosurgery; Prof. Dr. J. SPRANGER, Dept. of Pediatrics.

Ludwig-Maximilians-Universität München: Prof. Dr. K. BETKE, Dept. of Pediatrics; Prof. Dr. R. ENZENBACH, Dept. of Neuroanesthesiology; Prof. Dr. J. LISSNER, Dept. of Radiology; Prof. Dr. O. LUND, Dept. of Ophthalmology; Prof. Dr. F. MARGUTH, Dept. of Neurosurgery; Prof. Dr. H. NAUMANN, Dept. of Otorhinolaryngology; Prof. Dr. A. SCHRADER, Neurology Dept.

We should like to express our particular thanks to all participating physicians and technicians who performed the great majority of CT studies presented here.

Mrs. ILKA FÖRSTER and Mrs. BRIGITTE GRAEF were of invaluable help in preparing the manuscript. Graphics and photography were provided by Mr. M. TIDNAM.

We are grateful to Dr. h.c. H. GÖTZE, Mr. W. BERGSTEDT, and the employees of Springer-Verlag for their cooperation and effort in the excellent layout and production of the book.

Finally, the editors E. KAZNER and W. LANKSCH would like to express their appreciation and special thanks to Prof. Dr. F. MARGUTH, Director of the Neurosurgical Dept., Klinikum Großhadern, Ludwig-Maximilians-Universität München, for his unflagging support of their efforts over the years.

Berlin, Mainz, München

E. KAZNER, S. WENDE, TH. GRUMME,
W. LANKSCH, O. STOCHDORPH

# Contents

# List of Authors


Prof. Dr. med. Gianni B. Bradač
Abteilung für Röntgendiagnostik – Neuroradiologie im Klinikum Steglitz der Freien Universität Berlin, Hindenburgdamm 30, 1000 Berlin 45

Prof. Dr. med. Udalrich Büll
Leiter der Nuklearmedizinischen Abteilung der Radiologischen Klinik im Klinikum Großhadern der Ludwig-Maximilians-Universität, Marchioninistr. 15, 8000 München 70

Prof. Dr. med. Rudolf Fahlbusch
Neurochirurgische Klinik im Klinikum Großhadern der Ludwig-Maximilians-Universität, Marchioninistr. 15, 8000 München 70

Prof. Dr. med. Thomas Grumme
Oberarzt der Neurochirurgischen Abteilung im Klinikum Charlottenburg der Freien Universität Berlin, Spandauer Damm 130, 1000 Berlin 19

Prof. Dr. med. Ekkehard Kazner
Leiter der Abteilung für Neurochirurgie im Klinikum Charlottenburg der Freien Universität Berlin, Spandauer Damm 130, 1000 Berlin 19

Dr. med. Konrad Kretzschmar
Oberarzt der Abteilung für Neuroradiologie, Johannes-Gutenberg-Universität, Langenbeckstr. 1, 6500 Mainz

Priv. Doz. Dr. med. Wolfgang Lanksch
Oberarzt an der Neurochirurgischen Klinik im Klinikum Großhadern der Ludwig-Maximilians-Universität, Marchioninistr. 15, 8000 München 70

Dr. med. Wolfang Meese
Neurochirurgische Abteilung im Klinikum Charlottenburg der Freien Universität Berlin, Spandauer Damm 130, 1000 Berlin 19

Priv. Doz. Dr. med. Johannes Schramm
Oberarzt der Neurochirurgischen Abteilung im Klinikum Steglitz der Freien Universität Berlin, Hindenburgdamm 30, 1000 Berlin 45

Dr. med. Harald Steinhoff
Oberarzt der Radiologischen Klinik im Klinikum Großhadern der Ludwig-Maximilians-Universität, Marchioninistr. 15, 8000 München 70

Prof. Dr. med. Otto Stochdorph
Vorstand des Instituts für Neuropathologie der Ludwig-Maximilians-Universität München, Thalkirchner Str. 36, 8000 München 2

Prof. Dr. med. Sigurd Wende
Vorstand der Abteilung für Neuroradiologie, Johannes-Gutenberg-Universität, Langenbeckstr. 1, 6500 Mainz

# A. Introduction

Neurological examination was the only means for detecting and localizing brain tumors until well into the twentieth century. Neuroradiological diagnosis was introduced by DANDY in 1918, when he injected *air into the ventricles* by direct puncture of a fontanelle or through a burrhole. In 1919, he also reported demonstration of the ventricular system after introducing air by lumbar puncture.

MONIZ reported on *cerebral angiography* in 1927. This was the first method which allowed direct visualization of brain tumors, through demonstration of their pathological vessels. BERGER developed *electroencephalography* for diagnosis of intracranial lesions in 1928, and the technique is still of major importance, especially where functional disorders of the brain are concerned. *Radioactive isotopes* were first used in the diagnosis of brain tumors in 1948 (MOORE; SELVERSTONE and SOLOMON).

In 1955 LEKSELL introduced *echoencephalography,* which permits exact measurement of displacement of intracranial midline structures and ventricular width with a relatively simple technical procedure.

A new era in the diagnosis of intracranial space-occupying lesions opened in 1972, when GODFREY NEWBOLD HOUNSFIELD presented first results with *computed tomography,* which he had developed for the British Company EMI. The era of WILHELM KONRAD RÖNTGEN gave way to the HOUNSFIELD era. G.N. HOUNSFIELD and ALLAN M. CORMACK received the Nobel Prize in Medicine for their revolutionary development of RÖNTGEN'S technique in 1979.

Despite its substantial cost, computed tomography became *the* standard procedure for demonstration of intracranial tumors within a very few years. The systems have been continually improved, and the end of this development is not yet in sight. However, experience in the past few years has shown that improvements in resolution have not changed the fundamentals of brain tumor diagnosis with CT. Differences in density between tumor and normal brain tissue before and after administration of contrast media still constitute the basis of CT diagnosis. This also pertains to demonstration of ventricular dilatation, brain edema, displacement of normal structures, and intracranial hematomas of various etiologies. Improvements in density resolution and spatial resolution have resulted in a considerable refinement of tumor diagnosis, especially in delineation of adjacent normal structures and in demonstration of the internal composition of the tumor itself.

Further technical improvements have allowed studies of the skull in multiple planes. New software permits rapid analysis and visual demonstration in multiplanar reconstructions based on the data obtained during standard examinations. It is to be expected that further progress in the development of dynamic computed tomography will contribute to the differential diagnosis of brain tumors.

# B. Classification of Intracranial Tumors

## 1. History and Problems in Classification

L. Bruns (1914) stated in Krause's "General Neurosurgery" that brain tumors included all neoplasms growing within the cranial cavity and that these might be divided into three groups: (1) genuine tumors, (2) granulomatous lesions, and (3) parasites. Current use of the term "brain tumor" is more precise and limited to the first of L. Bruns' categories. Even so, brain tumors represent a large and inhomogeneous group. The comparison and evaluation of such a diverse set of observations is only possible after making a systematic classification of pertinent data.

There are many possible criteria for classification: according to age and sex of the patient, location and clinical aspects, naked-eye and microscopic appearance. Microscopic findings provide a generally valid principle for the classification of tumors of all tissues of the body according to histogenetic derivation. This should not be equated with cytogenetic derivation. Form and structure of individual tumor cells are related to the tissue from which the tumor arises. However, the formula "*Omnis cellula e cellula eiusdem generis* (every cell derives from a cell of the same general type)" does not imply "*e cellula eiusdem speciei* (from a cell of the same specific type)." A tumor cell closely resembling a normal cell is not necessarily the offspring of a fully differentiated cell of this type but may be derived from a primitive and pluripotential stem cell.

Grouping according to the tissue of origin provides a fundamental basis for classification of intracranial tumors. The germ-layer theory ("neuro-ectodermal tumors") has become obsolete in human embryology and need not be taken into further account. Histogenetic classification is, to a certain degree, topographic as well since the tissues of origin are related to anatomical structures. However, the location of the tissue should not be confused with the structure. A tumor located within the meninges is not necessarily a meningioma in the histogenetic sense.

The largest group among the intracranial tumors derives from the tissues of the brain itself, i.e., from that portion of the central nervous system which is located within the skull. (Division of the CNS into brain and spinal cord is a linguistic convention; it results from the simplified conception of the body as composed of head, torso, and extremities.) In this restricted sense, brain tumors are defined according to derivation from any tissue located within the meninges.

As with any other organ, brain tissue is made up from parenchymal tissue and mesenchymal stroma with blood vessels. Chief components of the parenchymal elements are the nerve cells or neurons. A nerve cell consists of a perikaryon (with the nucleus) and of an axon (efferent) and dendrites (afferent). Gray matter is composed primarily of nerve cell bodies and the so-called neuropil made up of tangled masses of dendrites permeated by axons. White matter consists chiefly of bundles of axons.

The neuronal population of the CNS receives its main input from the nerve cells of the afferent ganglionic system (spinal ganglia and their intracranial counterparts) and the olfactory sensory neurons and has as its effectors the muscle fibers with end plates and the neurons of the efferent ganglionic system, the autonomic nervous system.

The chief nonexcitable cells of the CNS are the glial cell types. There are two basic classes, the macroglia derived from the neural plate, and the microglia from mesenchymal components. The macroglia comprises astrocytes which serve as all-purpose cells, and oligodendrocytes which provide myelin sheaths. The astrocytes may be subdivided into protoplasmatic and fibrillary forms, which are defined by

WOLFF (1980) as "adaptive forms related to differentiation and reaction." Nerve cells of the CNS retain only a limited capacity for DNA synthesis and persist in the postmitotic phase. It is therefore the glial cells which are the primary substrate for the development of tumors within the CNS.

Neuroglial cells were first identified by VIRCHOW in 1862 and designated *"Nervenkitt"* or "nerve glue." He also named the tumors originating from the "interstitial material" gliomas, which he considered to be "partial hyperplasias." Later on (1864/65) he subclassified these tumors on the basis of secondary characteristics into "soft and hard, or – more accurately – into cellular or medullary, fibrous, and telangiectatic gliomas." He regarded tumors with some areas resembling mucus-producing tissue as transitional types between gliomas and myxogliomas with looser meshwork. "If the number of cells increases, the tissue becomes more compact, and one finds a true medullary glioma which may develop into medullary sarcoma. ... Such transitions between myxoma, glioma, and sarcoma may occur within a single tumor. In fact, the largest, fist-sized tumors of this type which I have found in the occipital lobes, belonged to this mixed form." In VIRCHOW's terminology "sarcoma" denotes any tumor with excessive cellularity. He states that, on the one hand, one can distinuguish fibromas, lipomas, chondromas, myxomas, osteoid chondromas, gliomas, etc. as opposed to the general term "sarcomas," but that, on the other hand, the term "sarcoma" should be retained as a special designation for tumors which originate in connective tissue but show a general histological type rather than a strict analogy to normal tissue types.

VIRCHOW described the gliomas as soft, hard, telangiectatic, etc. but noted in addition that there is no sharp dividing line between most gliomas and normal brain tissue. In 1878 RINDFLEISCH wrote that "one of the most striking characteristics of the glioma leads me to substitute the term 'gliomatous degeneration of the brain structures' for the name glioma. If one inspects a glioma in situ, one can almost always recognize the part of the brain – the thalamus, the striate body, the anterior portion of the centre of VIEUSSENS, or a portion of the cortex – which has been transformed into a glioma. The shape of these structures remains intact while the histological characteristics of normal tissue have disappeared entirely and been replaced by glioma. Simple round-shaped, nodular gliomas do not occur, and it may be difficult to trace the outlines of gliomas since they resemble the structures which they replace both in texture and in color, and since there is only a very gradual transition from tumor to adjacent normal tissue."

The indefinable extent of a typical glioma results from the fact that these tumors do not originate as a single and circumscribed group of cells, as is the case in metastasis. "Observations of the early stages of tumor development in man demonstrates that tumors originate in a field or several closely related fields of cells which fuse in the course of time" (EDER 1977). Of particular significance for gliomas is WILLIS' hypothesis that the initial stage of tumor development is characterized by *"spreading neoplastic change"* and is followed by a second stage of cell proliferation. There is often a reciprocal relation between the extent of the initial *"field of origin"* and the rate of proliferation in the secondary phase. The glial tumor is more sharply delineated when proliferation is excessive. At the other end of the scale one finds so-called gliomatosis, in which the *"field of origin"* extends through large areas of the brain, while tumor cellularity is only slightly higher than normal. Proliferation may start at several points within a single large *"field of origin,"* giving the impression of multifocal growth since the tissue between centers of proliferation appears normal.

Delayed tumor growth in adjacent tissue should not be equated with infiltration. Tumor cells do not advance into the tangle of axons and dendrites; proliferation merely takes place in larger areas of tissue. The intrinsic tendency of the local tissue to proliferate is significant. This explains why the molecular layer overlying seemingly normal cortical structures may show proliferation and extension into the leptomeninges in a tumor primarily involving the subcortical white matter. Even when a manifest tumor has been resected in toto, delayed proliferation in the surrounding area may simulate tumor recurrence.

After VIRCHOW had introduced the concept of glial cells in 1864/1865, attention soon turned to the finer structure of the tissue and led to the classification of different glial cell forms.

In WEIGERT'S stain fibrous glia appeared as a type of connective tissue. Later on, silver impregnation after GOLGI (1894) demonstrated "long-branched" cells and "short-branched" cells (v. KOELLIKER 1896), for which STROEBE (1895) introduced the common term of astrocytes. DEL RIO-HORTEGA (1921) identified oligodendroglial cells or oligodendrocytes as part of R. Y. CAJAL'S "third element" (1913) (the other two elements of the brain tissue being neurons and astrocytes).

Where the brain tissue texture is determined by the presence of nerve cell bodies and neurites – *neuronal* tissue – the glial component is chiefly made up of astrocytes and oligodendrocytes. This is different with paraneuronal tissue where nerve cell bodies and neurites are not the principal component. *Paraneuronal* tissue structures include the glial layer and ependyma of the ventricle walls, the choroid plexuses, and the other circumventricular organs (HOFER 1965), such as the posterior lobe of the pituitary body, the vascular organ of the terminal lamina, the subfornical organ, the subcommissural organ, the pineal body, and the area postrema. The subpial layer of the cortex represents a transition between neuronal and paraneuronal structures. The understanding of the special nature of circumventricular organs is relatively new. The older tumor classification systems and more recent systems derived from them do not make allowance, in their terminology, for the existence of these special cell forms.

Cerebral and cerebellar gliomas develop chiefly in the gray and white substances, less frequently in the ependymal "organ" (LEONHARDT 1980) and other paraneuronal structures. In 1894, GOLGI stated that gliomas consist of "branched cells similar to those found in large numbers in all parts of the CNS." As late as 1922 KAUFMANN made the cautious statement that some gliomas contain large numbers of the so-called spider cells, or astrocytes with long processes, and that gliomas with a large proportion of such cells are termed astromas or astrocytomas. The term astroma had been proposed by v. LENHOSSEK in 1895. In 1924, BAILEY and HILLER identified oligodendrogliomas. Tumors originating from ependyma had been reported earlier.

Progress in neurosurgery promoted interest in the question whether histological findings in gliomas might be clinically relevant. Simple classification according to cellularity does not allow accurate prognosis *subsequent to resection*. Gliomas with predominant differentiation into oligodendrocytes, a long previous history, and extended postoperative survival may demonstrate higher cell density than moderately anaplastic gliomas of chiefly astrocytic differentiation with a definitely less favorable prognosis.

BAILEY and CUSHING (1926) proposed a system of embryogenetic classification in which deficient differentiation of rapidly proliferating tumor cells was interpreted as immaturity rather than as anaplasia. The authors developed a number of pedigrees starting from primitive and highly proliferative progenitor cells. Contradictions resulting from this basic approach – such as naming a cerebellar tumor of adolescence generally associated with an excellent prognosis a spongioblastoma after a very immature cell type – as well as an excessive number of differentiation stages led to a decline in the use of embryogenetic terms and the original hypothesis. However, this implied abandoning a basic premise of embryogenetic classification, namely that incompletely differentiated cells might continue to differentiate and produce variegated cell types. Instead, it was assumed that each cell type was rigidly preformed. The reduction to fewer glioma types of presumably exact delimitation – astrocytoma, oligodendroglioma, ependymoma, and glioblastoma multiforme – resulted in a simplification of the complicated version proposed by BAILEY and CUSHING. Glioblastoma multiforme was considered a *distinct and separate tumor entity* and the "true cancer of the brain" (ZÜLCH 1956).

However, it is unlikely that fully differentiated astrocytes regain a capacity for uninhibited proliferation. The rather slow cell turnover in the glial cell population as well as any reactive proliferation are maintained primarily – and this is probably true for neoplastic proliferation as well – by a stem cell resembling oligodendroglial cells or so-called resting microglia, as shown by studies with $H^3$-thymidine (BUNGE et al. 1962; KLEIHUES and SCHULTZE 1968). Cell division in partly differentiated cell lines may result in two different cell types, one cell maturing into an astrocyte and the other into an oligodendrocyte (NIESSING 1980).

Clearly distinguishing among the various glial cell forms is not always possible in normal tissue, and experience shows that gliomas with pure cell lines hardly ever occur. It is much more common that a tumor contains a variety of different cell types, none of which conforms in every respect to the ideal form of one of the differentiated glial cell types. In some cases the tumor cells in question approach one of the differentiated glial cell forms to some degree and give the impression of incompletely differentiated cells such as "myelination glia." Other tumors demonstrate a pepper-and-salt mixture of cells with resemblance to various differentiated glial cells. A third group contains several cell populations, with the result that one microscopic field shows astrocytic forms and an adjacent field oligodendrocytic forms. The first of these patterns probably represents incomplete differentiation, the second may result from bivalent cell division, and the third pattern expresses proliferation of individual tumor cell clones.

As a result, even relatively well-differentiated gliomas do not correspond, as a rule, exactly to a single glial cell type and are best classified according to the principle "*A potiori fit denominatio* (designation according to prevailing part)." This principle necessarily entails a subjective element which works against exact quantification. In addition gliomas may show – just as other tumors – a degree of anaplasia proportional to the degree of proliferation.

Most tumor cells have an obvious deficit in differentiation. The total amount of these deficits defines the degree of tissue anaplasia, which may increase in subsequent tumor cell generations. However, anaplasia or dedifferentiation is always a tissue quality and does not apply to single cells.

Bailey and Cushing (1926) had already recognized that glioblastoma multiforme might in fact be derived from protoplasmatic astrocytes. Kernohan et al. (1949) concluded from their observations at the Mayo Clinic that glioblastoma multiforme represents, in a number of cases, the maximal dedifferentiation of an astrocytoma (or ependymoma) and proposed that the term glioblastoma be dropped. Willis had arrived at the same conclusion in 1948. Two years later, Ringertz (1950) developed a classification system similar to that proposed by Henschen in 1934, in which glioblastomas are not recognized as a separate tumor entity but rather as extremely dedifferentiated variants of the various types of gliomas. Ackerman and Rosai (1974) suggested an even more simplified classification into astrocytoma, malignant astrocytoma, oligodendroglioma, ependymoma, and undifferentiated glioma. They argued against the continued use of the term glioblastoma on the grounds that "it implies an origin from (or at least a relationship with) the embryonal glioblast which probably does not exist, and it conveys the impression of a specific tumor type when it simply represents the undifferentiated form of all types of gliomas."

Using squamous cell carcinomas of the lip as a model, Broders (1926) has shown that with some tumors the degree of anaplasia and the clinical course correspond to a certain extent. In such cases cytological and histological characteristics may be useful parameters in establishing prognosis. Grading systems such as that proposed by Broders usually run from 1 to 4, depending on the presence of one quantifiable characteristic in up to 25%, 50%, 75%, or 100% of cells, tumor cell groups, high-power fields, etc.

Kernohan et al. (1949) applied this principle to the spectrum of tumors in the astrocytoma-glioblastoma group and the ependymomas and assigned them to four grades. In practice the pathologist attempts to establish whether the histological findings at hand suggest either long or short postoperative survival, and then estimates the higher or lower probability for this expectation. Choosing twice between alternatives results in four grades. Ringertz (1950) preferred categorization in three grades with favorable, questionable, and unfavorable

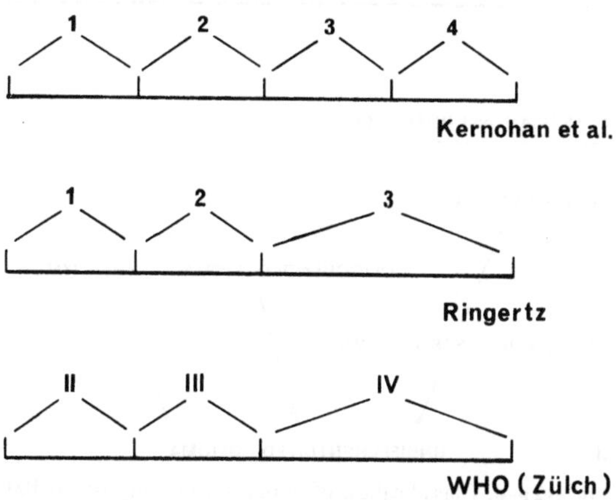


**Fig. B1.** Classification of anaplasia and prognosis of gliomas in grades

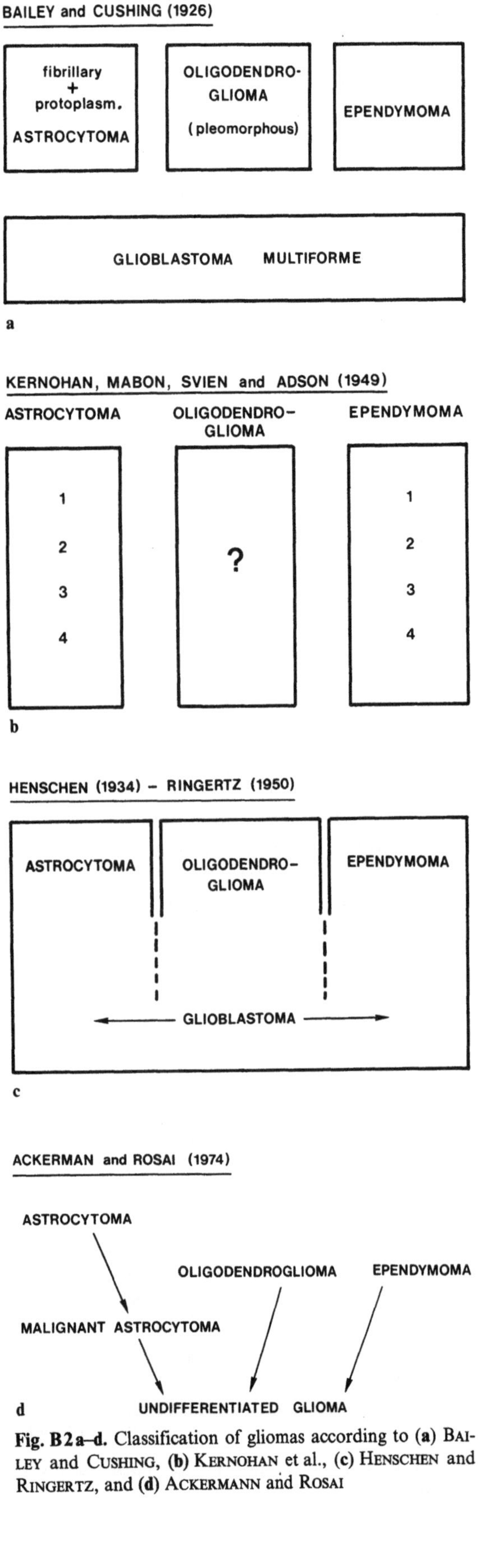


**Fig. B2a–d.** Classification of gliomas according to (**a**) BAILEY and CUSHING, (**b**) KERNOHAN et al., (**c**) HENSCHEN and RINGERTZ, and (**d**) ACKERMANN and ROSAI

prognosis, and was supported by HENSCHEN (1955), who found this system less complicated but nevertheless histologically and clinically adequate. HENSCHEN's arguments are in turn supported by our own observations. Grade 3 in the latter system comprises both grades 3 *and* 4 in the four-grade classification (cf. Fig. B1).

One can systematize the chief groups of gliomas on a two-dimensional system with glial cell forms on one axis and degree of anaplasia on the other. This allows graphic demonstration of the various classification systems (cf. Fig. B2a–d). In the proposal supported by RINGERTZ and HENSCHEN (Fig. B2c) the relation of tumor type to individual glial cell form is precise in low degrees of anaplasia but becomes less distinct with increasing anaplasia. The presumedly clear differentiation between degrees of anaplasia or between cell types used in the other systems is symbolized by sharp outlines in Fig. B2.

Classification in degrees of malignancy is practicable and relevant only within a single tumor type or group of closely related tumors such as the glial tumors. It is unfortunate that the WHO classification promoted and edited by ZÜLCH (1979) uses an entirely different set of criteria but retains the term "grading". In this system, clinical experience is the basis for comparison of totally unrelated tumors without regard for the average range of anaplasia observed within a given tumor type. For example, medulloblastomas are assigned to "grade" IV, although most pathologists agree that there are virtually no prognostically relevant differences in degree of anaplasia among medulloblastomas. This means that categorization of medulloblastomas in grades 1–3 is impracticable. Similarly, some tumors are classified in "grades" I and III without a "grade" II form. Fully differentiated astrocytomas and oligodendrogliomas are assigned to "grade" II. This means that there are only two higher categories amounting to three degrees of anaplasia for the astrocytoma-glioblastoma group and the oligodendroglioma-glioblastoma group, just as in RINGERTZ' classification, but designated II–IV instead of 1–3.

It is possible that the WHO classification will lead to a good deal of confusion. For example, readers of an article on CT findings in grade 2 glioma may fail to recognize whether the tumor in question is thought to be a moder-

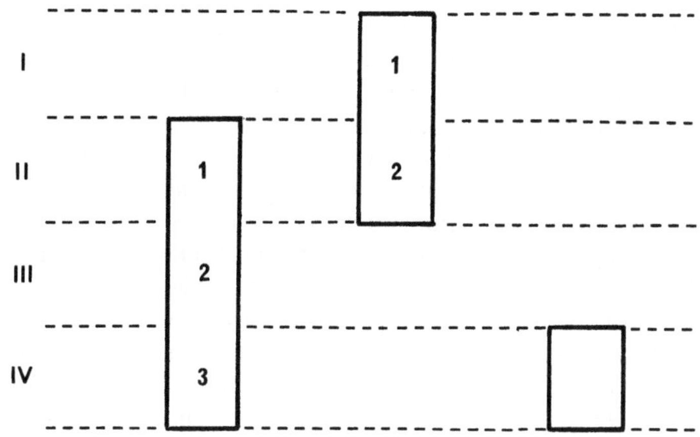


**Fig. B3.** Degree of anaplasia (arabic numerals) and classification of prognosis (roman numerals). Left, astrocytoma and glioblastoma; middle, pilocytic astrocytoma; right, medulloblastoma

ately anaplastic glioma (under the previous system) or a "grade" II lesion devoid of anaplastic characteristics or proliferative tendency. Previous differences between the three-grade and the four-grade systems were not problematical since grade 3 in the one system included grades 3 and 4 in the other.

The WHO classification is also open to question in another respect. It lists astrocytic and oligodendrocytic gliomas separately, ependymomas and tumors of the choroid plexuses jointly, followed by tumors of the pineal body and nerve cell tumors. The following chapter treats glioblastomas and medulloblastomas jointly although these are entirely different tumor entities of quite different age groups, without any histological relationship. This disrupts the astrocytoma-glioblastoma group.

The *I*nternational *C*lassification of *D*iseases for *O*ncolocy – ICD-O – is a useful guide to statistics. Synonyms in the classification of tumors – often scientific opinions in disguise – are included there in generous numbers. In the ICD-O code number the fourth place is usually available for subclassification of tumor entities.

# 2. Types of Intracranial Tumors

In a classification of intracranial tumors based on histogenesis, autochthonous brain tumors are listed first, with tumors of the brain tissue itself preceding tumors of the choroid plexuses, pineal body, and posterior lobe of the pituitary. Among the tumors of the brain proper, glial cell tumors have precedence over tumors of the ependymal "organ" which originate from modified glial cells, tumors developing from nerve cell forms, medulloblastomas – derived from a pluripotential matrix – and tumors originating within the mesenchymal brain stroma around the blood vessels.

Differentiation of tumor cells to astrocytic cell forms produces typical **astrocytomas.** There are astrocytes of the *protoplasmatic* short-branched and *fibrillary* long-branched type. The latter are found in both gray and white matter tumor areas as opposed to normal fibrillary astrocytes found chiefly in the white matter. Fibrillary astrocytes may be a reactive modification as found in nontumorous isomorphic gliosis. A *gemistocyte* has a cell body resembling that of a protoplasmatic astrocyte but carries glial fibers like a fibrillary astrocyte, again perhaps as a reactive modification. Low cell density, absence of mitotic figures, and a quiescent histological aspect are indicative of low-grade malignancy – grade 1 in the systems proposed by Kernohan and Ringertz, "grade" II in the WHO classification. **Anaplastic astrocytomas** (grade 2 after Kernohan and Ringertz, WHO "grade" III) show greater cell density, a higher rate of mitosis, disordered vascular structure, and disruption of the blood-brain barrier. This results in increased permeability for contrast media, for example.

**Oligodendrogliomas** are characterized by relatively high cellularity and a typical honeycomb appearance – round-shaped nuclei surrounded by clear cytoplasm and sharp cell boundaries – the result of regressive changes. Calcified droplets of protein are found throughout the tissue and embedded in the capillary walls. Areas with lower cellularity often show *"croissance périneuronale"* (SCHERER 1936), i.e., an increase in the number of satellite cells around the nerve cell bodies, as well as proliferation in the superficial layer of the cortex. BAILEY and BUCY (1929) have described variations in cell size and transitions to astrocytic forms. A cytological diagnosis of anaplastic oligodendroglioma is difficult if not impossible, especially in low-grade malignancy (KERNOHAN 1971). Areas with obviously malignant features such as seen in grade 3 oligodendroglioma (RINGERTZ), grade 3 and 4 (KERNOHAN) and WHO "grade" IV or oligodendrocytic glioblastoma, within a tumor with otherwise regular histological structures suggest a diagnosis of anaplastic oligodendroglioma.

Classification as either astrocytoma or oligodendroglioma is difficult both in tumors with less malignant histological features but also less differentiated (indifferent) cell forms, and in tumors containing a mixture of differentiated astrocytic and oligodendrocytic cell forms or adjacent fields of either type. For statistical purposes, the first pattern may be listed under either heading. COOPER (1935) suggested the term oligo-astrocytoma for the second pattern. It is, however, used by some authors for the third pattern as is the designation *"mixed glioma."* Again, gliomas almost never demonstrate a pure culture of a single cell type. Most of the so-called **gliomatoses** involve growth of indifferent cell forms in extensive *"fields of origin"* with a limited proliferation rate. Just as VIRCHOW (1864/65) retained the term "sarcoma" for undifferentiated connective-tissue neoplasms as opposed to fibromas, lipomas, etc., use of the term **"glioblastoma"** for certain glial tumors may be justifiable, despite the well-founded criticisms of ACKERMAN and ROSAI (1974). Correct usage requires that the designation be understood in the sense of extreme anaplasia in any glial tumor type and *not* in the sense of an independent tumor entity. Histological features of these tumors include variegation and loss of differentiation at the same time. Upon increasing dedifferentiation, astrocytic, oligodendrocytic, and ependymal tumor types resemble each other not only in histology but in clinical behaviour as well. Extremely subtle discrimination then tends to lose clinical relevance. Some glial tumors seem to develop in phases and may change in appearance from one phase to the next. Histological findings in a recurrence of the tumor may be identical to those obtained in the first specimen, but progressive loss of differentiation may also be observed. An uncharacteristically long history of a tumor with the macroscopic appearance of glioblastoma may be clarified by identification of an oligodendrocytic glioblastoma (RINGERTZ' grade 3 oligodendroglioma; KERNOHAN'S grades 3 and 4, WHO "grade" IV), which suggests a long period of growth through successive stages of dedifferentiation. It is not always possible to identify an extremely anaplastic tumor as to its origin since gliomas with indifferent cells and mixed gliomas may finally appear as glioblastomas.

Close interaction between glial cells, especially astrocytes, and vascular structures is evident in the proliferation of these structures in glioblastomas, especially in the vicinity of necroses. In some cases mesenchymal proliferation exceeds neoplastic glial cell proliferation. Such tumors are called *mixed glioblastoma* and *fibrosarcoma* (RUBINSTEIN 1972) or, all together, **gliosarcomas.** Proliferation of connective tissue fibers is most common in tumors with large numbers of astrocytic giant cells but may also occur in well-differentiated glial tumors with low cellularity (FRIEDE 1978). "Monstrocellular sarcoma" (ZÜLCH) apparently designates an inhomogeneous group including **giant cell glioblastomas** and other tumor types.

Research in recent years has resulted in the definition of an additional glial cell type which originates in the ependymal "organ" and is termed tanycyte. There are a variety of forms ranging from typical ependymal cells to "unipolar" and "bipolar" cells and astrocytes. They are part of the ependymal tissue layer and of the circumventricular organs which arise in or near the midline (LEONHARDT 1980). They appear to be less differentiated than avarage astrocytes. Tumors made up from cells of this type of differentiation comprise a spectrum of cell forms ranging from ependymal cells to tanycytes and so-called piloid astrocytes. They were so named by PENFIELD due to the presence of fascicles of delicate glial fibers such as those found with isomorphic gliosis (FRIEDE and POLLAK 1978). BAILEY and CUSHING (1926, 1930) had referred to such tumors as spongioblastomas and fibrillary astrocytomas. BERGSTRAND (1932) called them embryonal gliocytomas. The

WHO classification defines them as **pilocytic astrocytomas** in reference to PENFIELD's term. KUHLENDAHL and STOCHDORPH (1968) suggested the term BERGSTRAND tumors, and JELLINGER (1977) spoke of tanycytomas, referring to their origin, as did WEINDL et al. (1975). These tumors account for approximately 90% of cerebellar tumors in adolescents and comprise 10% of low-grade cerebral astrocytomas found in several large series (RINGERTZ and NORDENSTAM 1951). Other locations include the walls of the third ventricle including the lamina terminalis as well as the median eminence, the chiasm, and the proximal segments of the optic nerves.

The ependyma lining the ventricle walls assumes a somewhat special position, since glial tissue elements predominate over nerve cell elements, although it is an intrinsic part of the cerebral hemispheres. Nerve cells are present in the form of so-called CSF contact neurons but do not govern tissue structure. The CSF space is derived from the amniotic cavity as a result of upfolding and fusion of the margins of the neural plate. In the choroid plexus area the CSF space is lined by a structure possessing both an epithelium and a basal membrane. At all other locations the superficial layer is not an epithelium but rather a continuous transition to the tissue beneath just as a crust forms the surface on the bread. The ventricle wall forms the primary matrix, in the ontogenetic sense. **Cerebral ependymomas** of younger age groups (ZÜLCH 1956, 1958) are embryonal tumors of this matrix. They are highly cellular, show many mitotic figures, and demonstrate various degrees of differentiation. Cytological criteria suggest classification as ependymoblastoma in the young and as ependymal glioblastoma in adults. In contrast to most other glial cell tumor groups, **ependymomas of the fourth ventricle** demonstrate exophytic growth, and their histological characteristics make them resemble hyperplasias of the ependymal cell layer. The *"subependymal glomerate astrocytomas – subependymomas"* first depicted by RIBBERT in 1909 also demonstrate exophytic growth while representing hyperplasia of the glial layer rather than of the ependymal cells. Their clinical relevance is restricted to occurrence at narrow points in the CSF pathways such as the interventricular foramen. **Subependymal giant cell astrocytomas,** which occur in association with tuberous sclerosis in most cases, also originate in the glial layer of the ependyma. Again, their clinical relevance is restricted to possible obstruction of CSF flow as is also the case with ependymomas of the foramen of Monro with oligodendrocytic character as described by ZÜLCH (1956).

Glial cells of the ependymal layer often interact closely with the blood vessels and may be attached to the vessel wall by a conical footplate, similar to astrocytes of the gray matter and the white matter. Perivascular coronas are especially prominent in subependymal giant cell astrocytomas and may resemble findings in slightly dedifferentiated astrocytomas, termed **astroblastomas,** and in ependymomas. RUSSELL and RUBINSTEIN (1977) report that these cell extensions are finer in ependymoma than in astroblastoma. BAILEY (1932) reported bodies resembling diplosomes – "blepharoplasten" – in astroblastomas as well as in ependymomas. RUSSELL and RUBINSTEIN suggested that astroblastomas might be a separate tumor entity rather than a less-differentiated form of astrocytoma.

Normal nerve cells of the mature brain persist in a postmitotic stage, and **nerve cell tumors** always suggest dysplastic origin. These neoplasms might also be termed gangliogliomas, since proliferation is hardly ever confined to the nerve cell population. Terminology analogous to that used in ganglion cell tumors of the peripheral nervous tissue results in the classification of less-differentiated specimens as partly differentiated gangliogliomas, ganglioneuroblastomas, and neuroblastomas. Nodules of dysplastic nerve cells in the hypothalamic region are commonly designated hamartomas, though they are in fact ectopic tissue and hence more properly called choristomas. A unique cerebellar neoplasm, variously termed gangliocytoma, purkinjeoma, or LHERMITTE-DUCLOS tumor (1920), demonstrates giant nerve cells as large as Purkinje cells in the granular layer of the cerebellar cortex together with expansion of the gyri with space-occupying effect.

**Medulloblastomas** are tumors with pronounced embryonal character. Their matrix is composed of pluripotential cells and is obviously related to the tissues of the circumventricular organs. As a result, a variety of shades of differentiation may be found, from neuroblastoma to single rather well-differentiated nerve cells. One may encounter characteristics of astrocytic, oligodendrocytic, and tanycytic glial cell forms as well as ependymal differentiation ("ependymal medulloblastoma"). Occasional findings of striated muscle ("myomedulloblastoma") and of rosettes suggest relation to the matrix of the pineal body, where tumors resembling medulloblastoma also occur. The strong mesenchymal component of the area postrema is repeated in the pattern of so-called desmoplastic medulloblastomas. These are possibly anaplastic versions of hemangioblastoma and sometimes feature highly vascular areas. They occur both in children and in adults and display somewhat special clinical aspects and courses. Some authors have called them circumscribed arachnoidal sarcomas or *cerebellar sarcomas* rather than medulloblastomas.

Lymphoproliferative and myeloproliferative processes affect the brain more frequently than generally presumed. Most primary **malignant lymphomas** of the brain are of immunocytic or lymphoblastic type (JELLINGER and RADASZKIEWICZ 1976). Another form including Hodgkin's disease may also occur in the brain in cases of systemic lymphoma. Secondary spread of **leukemic** conditions may take place either through metastasis or through direct extension from meningeal foci.

Intracranial fibrous **histiocytomas** are rare tumors. Pleomorphic fibrous xanthoma with gliofibrillary protein demonstrated by immunohistochemistry is still a matter of controversy, and it is as yet unclear whether there is xanthomatous transformation of astrocytes or GFAP uptake in stromal cells (KEPES et al. 1979). Some giant cell tumors (**"monstrocellular sarcomas"**), especially those with lipid storage, might be "xanthoastrocytomas" (KEPES 1979), if not pleomorphic malignant fibrous histiocytomas. **Histiocytosis X** (comprising Hand-Schueller-Christian's disease, eosinophilic granuloma, and Abt-Letterer-Siwe's disease) affects the hypothalamus in some cases.

Differentiation between immunoblastic variants of non-Hodgkin lymphoma and microglial tumors is another as yet unsettled question. Since DEL RIO-HORTEGA (1921) eliminated oligodendroglia from R. Y CAJAL'S "third element," glial stem cells ("resting microglia") and adapted macrophages ("progressive microglia") with close relations to histiocytes were left in the group of microglial cell forms. RUBINSTEIN (1972) suggested the term **reticulum cell sarcoma/microglioma** as a way round the problem.

The choroid plexuses develop where the neural tube differentiates into a single-layered epithelium and are the only true neuroepithelial structures. Hypertrophy leads to the development of **plexus papillomas,** which may produce hydrocephalus in children. Rare plexus adenomas with mucus production (RUBINSTEIN 1972) might represent metaplastic transition to tissue of the subcommissural organ. Malignant plexus papillomas or plexus carcinomas are extremely rare. The dissemination of plexus papilloma throughout the CSF pathways is not equivalent to metastasis in the usual sense.

Tumors originating in the tissue of the pineal body are termed **"pine(al)ocytomas"** or **"pine(al)oblastomas,"** depending on their degree of dedifferentiation. Since glial nodules are a normal component of the pineal body of adults, the pineal tumors properly include astrocytomas, sometimes with giant cell forms (SCHMINCKE 1930) and even with nerve cells. Germ-cell tumors of the pineal body were designated "anisomorphic" pinealomas in the older literature (cf. below).

Pilocytic astrocytomas are found in the wall of the third ventricle and in the median eminence. The pituitary stalk may contain cell groups similar to those of granular-cell tumors of Schwann-cell origin in peripheral nerves etc. These tumors are most often incidental findings and rarely produce space-occupying effects. STERNBERG (1921) and PRIESEL (1922) considered them ectopic structures and designated them as **choristomas.** Although the term provides no information as to histogenesis, the name is still in use. A metabolic resemblance between the sheath cells of peripheral nerve fibers and the cells of this circumventricular organ is suggested by the similar appearance of peripheral and pituitary granular-cell tumors.

**Suprasellar germinomas** are germ-cell tumors which differ from their pineal counterparts only in location. The older literature referred to them as ectopic pinealomas.

The leptomeningeal tumors are the most important neoplasms originating in the external CSF spaces and the choroid plexus stroma. Their cells differentiate to arachnothelial elements, the basic shape appearing as a flat disc. Time-lapse studies in tissue cultures show characteristic circular movement of single cells which is imparted to adjacent cells and leads to laminated structures, often with central hyaline degeneration and calcium salt deposition. Stacks of these cells cut in a perpendicular or oblique direction have often been interpreted as spindle-shaped cells similar to fibroblasts, although there are no cross sections of bundles. **Meningiomas** rarely show mitotic activity. Loss of laminated structures and stacking coupled with increased mitotic activity suggest increased proliferation tendency (grade 2), which attains clinical relevance only after incomplete resection. Further loss of differentiation implies the classification as a **meningeal sarcoma** (grade 3). Highly vascular meningiomas may occur as well as tumors with sharply defined cell borders resulting from lipid deposits.

**Hemangiopericytomas,** which occur in the meninges as in other parts of the body, should be differentiated from vascular meningiomas. The former are rarely benign and have a strong tendency to recur and metastasize. Designation of these tumors and of supratentorial hemangioblastomas (cf. below) as "angioblastic meningiomas" substitutes a simple topographical classification for a histogenetic one.

Scheithauer and Rubinstein (1976) have redefined the so-called chondroblastic meningiomas as meningeal mesenchymal chondrosarcomas, and have thus eliminated them from the category of meningiomas.

The melanocytes of the pia mater are yet another component of the meningeal tissue. They may proliferate and develop into leptomeningeal melanosis without space-occupying effects, or into circumscribed **meningeal melanomas,** sometimes of malignant quality with metastasis to other parts of the body.

**Fibromas** may develop in the dura mater. Rare tumors in the pia mater with histological characteristics similar to the so-called soft fibromas have also been reported. – A neurothelial cell population located between the arachnothelial layer and the innermost layer of the dura mater was described by Andres in 1967. These cells are fragile and prone to autolysis, and their disappearance may simulate the existence of a subdural space. They proliferate in order to reabsorb hemorrhage and may develop into the granulation tissue of so-called pachymeningiosis haemorrhagica interna. These cells may also proliferate into tumors resembling endotheliomas or histiocytomas.

Outside the central nervous system, the processes of nerve cells are sheathed by a population of cells which differ from the neuroglia. The Schwann sheath-cells of uniaxonal fibers and the Remak sheath-cells of multiaxonal fibers are related to the perineural cells which envelop the fascicles. Tumors of these sheath-cell populations are neurofibromas and **neurinomas,** the latter also termed schwannomas, neurilemomas, or neurolemmomas. **Neurofibromas** are characterized by subperineural accumulation of mucoid material which might be related to basal membranes and by proliferating sheath cells, while proliferation alone characterizes schwannomas. Nerve roots are similar to fascicles but lack a perineurium, so that mucoid material does not accumulate but disappears into the CSF. That is why nerve root tumors in neurofibromatosis always take the appearance of neurinomas rather than of neurofibromas. Proliferation of the sheath cells promotes outgrowth of collateral axons, so that schwannomas temporarily adopt the quality of true neuromas as defined by Virchow (1864/65).

**Adenomas of the anterior pituitary lobe** may have, in some cases, space-occupying effects. Simplistic classification as chromophobic, eosinophilic, and basophilic has been gradually replaced by designation according to the substance produced (ACTH, Prolactin, or GH, for example) and the storage phase.

Although angiomas have not been included among the tumors in this book, **hemangioblastomas** must be taken into consideration. They most often occur in the cerebellum, much less frequently at supratentorial locations, then chiefly at the sphenoid plane (Earle 1980). Terminology of these tumors is still controversial, so that the designation "Lindau tumor" may serve. Recent demonstration of GFAP in stroma cells (Kepes 1979) has rekindled discussion of the origin of these cells and their lipid inclusions. Desmoplastic medulloblastomas may demonstrate unmistakable similarities to hemangioblastoma. Multiple occurrence is possible and may simulate recurrence. Mesenchymal tumors among the so-called monstrocellular sarcomas are related to the vascular stroma and should not be classified together with angiomas.

The brain's complex development naturally implies the possibility of **dysplastic growth** with foci eventually qualifying as tumors. Some of these observations involve ectopic growth while others such as hamartomas demonstrate anomalous overgrowth of a tissue component.

Circumscribed foci with tissue characteristics similar to those of glioma but without actual proliferation and space-occupying effects are most often found in the temporal lobe, where they may be associated with seizures. These **hamartomas** produce a wide variety of appearances and may resemble low-grade forms of any type of brain-tissue neoplasms including ganglioglioma or may imitate reactive gliosis. A mosaic pattern including areas of astrocytic, oligodendrocytic or other forms of differentiation is not uncommon. It is as yet undecided whether these hamartomas are arrested gliomas or hyperplastic regeneration secondary to encephalitic or circulatory damage sustained in the perinatal period, similar to keloid formation in scars of the skin.

Small nests of squamous epithelium with or without keratinization or small epithelial cysts are frequently found in the pars intermedia of the hypophysis of the adult. **Craniopharyngeomas** in children and adolescents or even in older age groups show a similar tendency to ectopic differentiation of epithelial structures of the stomatodeum.

Cysts lined with mucus-secreting epithelium with yellow pigment granules are found in the tela choroidea near the interventricular foramen. They contain colloid material of remarkable CT density. The epithelium of these **colloid cysts** resembles the nonneuronal components of the olfactory field. The cysts probably do not develop from the neural tube and should not be called neuroepithelial cysts.

**Endodermal cysts** lined with an epithelium suggestive of that of the alimentary tract are another intrameningeal ectopy. They occur chiefly in the spinal canal.

Meningeal **lipomas** are yet another ectopic dysplasia. Their lobules of adipose tissue probably result from the pluripotentiality of primitive mesenchyma.

**Dermoid** and **epidermoid cysts** arise from ectopic differentiation of skin structures within the meninges with or without dermal appendages. They grow chiefly through accumulation of desquamated keratinized epithelium. Their growth is extremely slow and may attain incredible dimensions before causing damage due to space-occupying effects.

Intracranial **germ-cell tumors,** i.e., teratomas and germinomas, are obvious ectopies of developmental origin. **Teratomas** are chiefly found in the pineal region (craniopagus without an organizer?), less frequently in the suprasellar region. **Embryonal carcinomas** are endodermal structures reminiscent of the yolk sack and are of more simplified histology than teratomas. **Choriocarcinoma** imitates trophoblast structures. **Germinomas** are akin to seminomas of the testis and to dysgerminoma of the ovary. They lack embryogenetic traits. Their rather uniform cell population, sometimes with giant cells, evokes a lymphocytic tissue reaction, sometimes of granulomatous and even tuberculoid appearance with giant cells of Langhans type. Like teratomas, germinomas arise chiefly in the pineal and less frequently in the suprasellar region. These suprasellar germinomas are called ectopic pinealomas in the older literature due to the then prevailing interpretation of pineal germinomas as pinealomas.

**Tuberous sclerosis** is a dysplastic disease entity manifesting itself in brain, heart, kidneys, lung, and skin without any regard for germlayer schemes. The lesions of the cerebral cortex may be classified as quiescent foci of hyperplasia. Typical subependymal giant cell "astrocytomas" arise in the ventricle wall.

Tumors originating in skeletal elements of the skull include **osteomas, osteogenic sarcomas, chondromas, chondromyxoid fibromas,** and lesions such as those found in **fibrous dysplasia. Chordomas** possess the histological characteristics of the chorda dorsalis. They are not particularly rare. They may pose problems in differential diagnosis as so-called **chondroid chordomas.**

Intracranial extension is a secondary feature of tumors of any tissue origin which grow primarily outside the cranial cavity and reach the intracranial space by local invasive growth. **Adenoid-cystic carcinomas** arise from glands of the mucous membranes of the paranasal sinuses and were formerly known as cylindromas. **Aesthesioneuroblastomas** develop from the olfactory neuronal population, i.e., from a neuronal population independent from either neural tube or neural crest. They encroach upon the cranial cavity starting from the upper nasal cavity. Juvenile **rhabdomyosarcomas** of the orbit or the ear region may take similiar courses.

Tumors of the glomus tympanicum and glomus jugulare are other examples of extension into the cranial cavity from a primarily extracranial location. They arise from peripheral nerve structures which are related to peripheral ganglia in a way similar to the relationship between circumventricular organs and neuronal structures. They are termed paraganglia and either produce neurohormones as does the adrenal medulla, or serve as sensory organs. Tumors originating from them are designated as **chemodectomas** or **paragangliomas.**

While tumors of intracranial origin may be considered primary tumors, **metastases** are secondary tumors within the brain. Bronchial carcinomas, hypernephroid renal carcinomas, and malignant melanomas are the major sources of hematogenous spread to the brain. Some metastases acquire space-occupying significance by causing perifocal edema. Others are restricted to mere volume-replacing growth if there is no edema. Metastatic sarcomas are decidedly less frequent than metastatic carcinomas or malignant melanomas. Some carcinomas achieve tertiary involvement of the brain. Gastric carcinoma, for example, may metastasize to the cranial vault, trigger local pachymeningitic reaction, infiltrate the meninges, and ultimately produce meningeal carcinosis with intracerebral foci.

# C. Technique of CT Examination

## 1. Computed Tomography Systems

The three study groups used the same CT systems during the investigation period: the EMI Mark I head scanner from 1975 until June 1977 and the EMI CT 1010 head scanner from the middle of 1977, with the Diagnostic Enhancement Package since March 1980. Special studies of the base of the skull were performed with an EMI CT 5005 body scanner (Department of Radiology, Klinikum Steglitz, Free University of Berlin).

The majority of CT studies was performed with normal resolution, and higher density resolution or higher spatial resolution was employed when necessary. Slice thicknesses were 13 mm or 10 mm with 120 kV and 33 mA, and 8 mm or 5 mm with 140 kV and 28 mA.

## 2. Procedure in CT Examination

In the *standard examination* CT slices are aligned parallel to the orbitomeatal line. The head is inclined 15° for studies of the cerebellar region and retroflected 20° for examination of the basal portions of the temporal lobe and the orbits.

*Coronary projections* require different positioning of the head, since the opening of the gantry is only 24 cm and since the gantry cannot be tilted. These studies are performed in the prone position with the head reclined as far as possible.

In order to reduce *artifacts* to a minimum, the patient has to be as immobile as possible, which sometimes requires general anaesthesia. However, some artifacts are unavoidable, especially in the region between the petrous bones and near the base of the skull. Artifacts due to dental fillings may disturb coronal scans.

Since artifacts due to *metal clips* reduce the diagnostic value of follow-up studies after neurosurgical procedures, we have modified our techniques since 1975, so that metal clips are used only in treatment of aneurysms and large arteriovenous malformations.

We routinely perform *a precontrast study* from the base of the skull to the crown in all cases. In our experience, it is advantageous to obtain a complete series of slices, even when *contrast media* are used, in order to demonstrate multiple lesions that might otherwise go undetected. Overlapping slices are made in the region of an intracranial space-occupying lesion. The contrast-enhanced scan is recorded immediately after administration of the contrast medium.

## 3. Analysis of CT Pictures

Both the analog picture and the digital printout from specific regions of interest are analyzed with the help of special computer programs. The latter contain statistical procedures for calculation of density values in the region of interest and for development of histograms with data from these areas. Frequent determinations of the zero point of the system using a phantom are a prerequisite for accurate analysis of absorption characteristics. (See page 19ff.)

## 4. Intravenous Contrast Enhancement

Experience has shown that exact analysis of CT scans and an accurate diagnosis of the type of lesion require both precontrast and postcontrast studies. A large proportion of primary isodense brain tumors, which make up almost 15% of all neoplasms in our series, may escape CT detection when contrast enhancement is not employed. This was the case in 6% of all patients with intracranial tumors in our collective. Improved delineation of a brain tumor in relation to perifocal edema and normal brain structures is an additional advantage of contrast enhancement. This is especially true in cases of glioblastoma and metastases. Furthermore, changes in density of the tumor after application of contrast media provide important information indispensable for the differential diagnosis of the lesion. Contrast enhancement is decisive in the differentiation of vascular processes and brain tumors. However, indiscriminate use of contrast media in all cases would result in an unacceptable increase in the complication rate. *A precontrast study should be obtained in all cases, since the indication for contrast enhancement is derived from the results of the former,* as we shall discuss later. In addition, there are lesions – such as brain infarction with disruption of the blood-brain barrier in the early and late phase – which become isodense after contrast application. These processes would escape detection if a precontrast study were not available for comparison. In some cases it would be impossible to differentiate among intracerebral hematoma, calcification, and a tumor with marked uptake of contrast medium.

The total *applied dose of iodine* was related to body weight and ranged from 20 to 30 g in adults, administered as a bolus injection of a 60–66% contrast medium solution. We have recently begun to administer 30 g iodine as a continuous i.v. infusion in adults. Children receive a much smaller dose of iodine, usually 1 ml of a 60% solution per kilogram body weight. The following contrast media have proved suitable for CT studies: Angiografin, Conray 60, Rayvist, Telebrix 300 B, and Urografin 60.

## Risks Associated with the Application of Contrast Media

Administration of contrast media is always accompanied by a certain degree of risk, since individual reactions are unpredictable and cannot be excluded by exposition tests. All patients must be questioned about a history of allergy and previous exposure to contrast media, though a negative history does not exclude the possibility of an idiosyncratic reaction.

We do not wish to deal with *mild to moderate reactions* on the skin and mucous membranes or with symptoms related to the cardiovascular, respiratory, autonomic, and central nervous systems. These reactions, which are probably due to release of biogenic amines such as histamine as well as to activation of complement pathways and the coagulation system, appear in 80% of cases within the first 5 min following injection and can usually be effectively countered by qualified medical personnel.

*The physician performing the studies must be present at all times.* We should like to cite ELKE and FERSTL (1974), who said "every physician who routinely administers contrast media must be prepared to institute necessary therapy without delay in a case of allergic reaction to contrast media."

There have been a number of reports in recent years on renal damage related to contrast application in CT studies. We should like to deal with this problem in greater detail.

Both radiologists and urologists make *routine contrast studies* in patients with signs of *pathological renal function.* Increased serum creatinine concentrations are often disregarded when urographic studies are performed on outpatients. Indeed, the dose of contrast medium is usually increased in these patients in order to obtain better radiological results. First reports of renal damage due to contrast media came from BERGMAN et al. in their article "Acute renal failure after drip infusion pyelography" in 1968. A number of authors subsequently reported similar phenomena following pyelography, angiography, and computed tomography with contrast enhancement. Most reports concerned reversible disorders of renal function, but a number of fatalities related to intractable renal failure has also been reported (PILLAY et al. 1970; DUDZINSKI et al. 1971; MYERS and WITTEN 1971; BARSHAY et al. 1973; ELKE and FERSTL 1974; KLEINKNECHT et al. 1974; PORT et al. 1974; DIAZ-BUXO et al. 1975; ANSARI and BALDWIN 1976; BEREZIN 1977; HANAWAY and BLACK 1977; KAMDAI et al. 1977; ALEXANDER et al. 1978; BALTZER 1978; CARVALLO et al. 1978; SHAFI et al. 1978; SWARTZ et al. 1978; WAGONER 1978; WARREN et al. 1978; WEINRAUCH et al. 1978; VAN ZEE et al. 1978; PIERACH 1979; MAURER 1980).

Which patients are at risk of a disorder of renal function due to contrast media?

What are the signs of this disorder?

What are its causes?

How can such disorders and reactions be prevented?

Patients with the *following medical disorders* are at *particular risk of renal failure* when contrast media are administered: *renal insufficiency, type I diabetes mellitus, hypertension, vascular disease, and dehydration.* A combination of these factors potentiates the risk to the patient.

Both *large single doses of contrast medium* and *repeated doses over a period of several days* can lead to severe reversible or irreversible renal disorders in patients with only slightly compromised renal function.

The disorder of renal function may take the form of *oliguria* or an *increase in serum creatinine.* Oliguria usually develops within 12–24 h of contrast application, and the disorder resolves within 8–10 days in most cases.

A temporary reduction in renal function often goes unnoticed by both patient and physician. Careful observation of each patient with attention to signs of renal disorder is necessary in order to detect the minor complication.

Serum creatinine values may increase to 6 or 8 mg/dl and more, which indicates severe renal dysfunction that may even require dialysis. DIAZ-BUXO et al. (1975) and WEINRAUCH et al. (1978) reported on patients suffering renal failure after contrast application who required dialysis or renal transplantation. MEEKER (1978) reported a fatality in the case of a 67-year-old diabetic patient who had undergone a CT study with contrast enhancement.

The *causes of disorders in renal function following contrast application* have not been fully clarified. Possible explanations include changes in blood flow within the kidney, an increase in blood viscosity with a resultant decrease in renal circulation, precipitation of protein in the renal tubules and an antigen-antibody reaction. The most likely cause is a direct toxic effect of the contrast medium on the kidneys, since histological studies have revealed interstitial inflammation and edema as well as acute necrosis in the proximal and distal tubules (ANSARI and BALDWIN 1976).

*How can renal disorders associated with contrast application be avoided?*

The physician ordering a CT study must provide the physician performing the examination with more than a simple instruction and a preliminary diagnosis. Relevant data from the history, the physical examination, and laboratory data as well as the specific purpose of the study must be communicated to the physician performing the examination. The latter has the responsibility for informing himself in detail about his patient and is not justified in assuming that adequate preliminary investigations have been performed. The examining physician is also responsible for estimating the risk and potential benefit of a CT study with contrast enhancement in the particular case.

Studies which involve little or no risk to the patient, such as skull films and electroencephalograms, should be performed first. CT studies with contrast enhancement do not belong at the beginning of a diagnostic series; the indication for this procedure derives from the history, the physical examination, and the results of noninvasive studies including the precontrast CT study.

*Fluid and electrolyte imbalances* must be detected and corrected, as well as possible, before contrast media are administered. It may be necessary to force fluids prior to the examination, and adequate fluid intake must be assured for at least 12 h following a contrast study.

The physician performing CT studies is obliged to inform the patient's attending physician of possible disorders of renal function due to contrast administration and to recommend appropriate measures. In patients at risk, urine output and serum creatinine values must be monitored daily for the first few days after CT studies. When contrast studies are necessary in a patient with severe renal disease and diabetes or a vascular disorder, provision must be made for possible dialysis therapy in the first 3 days after administration of contrast media. Contrast studies are contraindicated in patients with serum creatinine values higher than 4.5 mg/dl.

*Thyrotoxicosis following administration of iodine* is a further problem. It is well known that administration of iodine may provoke thyrotoxicosis in patients with latent hyperthyroidism. This is true not only of contrast media but of all other medications and disinfectants containing iodine. Thyroid disease must be excluded by history. *Patients with manifest thyroid disease must not receive iodine.*

At present a diagnosis of plasmocytoma is not an absolute contraindication to contrast studies. However, adequate fluid intake of up to 2 liters is necessary before contrast media are administered.

Reports in the literature vary on the dosage of contrast media in CT studies. In our experience 30 g iodine are adequate for a CT examination (see page 15). Reports in the American literature suggest an average dose of 40 g iodine, while some authors report administering up to 80 g iodine without complications (PALING 1978; DAVIS et al. 1979; HAYMAN et al. 1979, 1980). The use of high doses of contrast medium was first reported by ETHIER et al. (1975) and KRAMER et al. (1975), who claimed that large doses allowed better demonstration of cerebral lesions. For example, they found that multiple metastases, which would have gone undetected with smaller doses of contrast media, could be demonstrated reliably.

DAVIS (1979) emphasized that doses of 80 g iodine are not permissible in patients with serum creatinine values higher than 1.5 mg/dl or with signs of dehydration. These authors maintain that there are no differences in the frequency, severity, and duration of renal disorders between patients receiving 40 g and those receiving 80 g iodine. HAYMAN et al. (1980) recommend high doses of iodine (80 g) with delayed CT studies (1 h) for demonstration of lesions with minimal disruption of the blood-brain barrier which would otherwise escape detection in the CT scan.

In our experience, *higher doses of iodine do not result in a significant improvement in diagnosis of cerebral lesions.* It is true that tumors and, more particularly, metastases are more clearly delineated in some cases when 80 g iodine are administered. However, these lesions are also clearly demonstrated with 40 g iodine, and we believe that there is little advantage to be derived from demonstration of ten intracerebral metastases rather than only five.

Administration of large doses of iodine may increase the complication rate, but it certainly increases the cost. It should also be noted that large doses of contrast media may be followed by major disruption of fluid and electrolyte balance, especially in elderly patients and infants.

In summary, the risk associated with large doses of iodine outweighs the benefits and is therefore not justified as a routine procedure in our opinion.

# 5. Intrathecal Administration of Contrast Media

GREITZ and HINDMARSH (1974) introduced computerized cisternography with water-soluble contrast media. The application of metrizamide (Amipaque) by the lumbar route may be useful for CT diagnosis in selected cases. For example, it may be necessary to demonstrate communication between a cystic lesion and the CSF spaces, as in cases of cysts in the suprasellar region or in differentiation between an arachnoid cyst and a large cisterna magna. The same procedure is necessary for demonstration of a space-occupying lesion with the same density as CSF – epidermoid cyst, for example – in the cisternal regions. We use water-soluble contrast media for demonstration of the intracranial CSF spaces and delineation of tumors extending into the basal cisterns (sella region, cerebellopontine angle) only in rare cases, since this procedure may be accompanied by a number of side effects (see below) and because other procedures are better suited to this purpose (see Chapt. D 3. Neurinomas, p. 258).

*Adequate demonstration of the cisterns in the CT scan* requires 5–8 ml isotonic metrizamide solution containing 170 mg iodine/ml. Positioning the patient with the pelvis slightly elevated and the head inclined for 3–6 h after intrathecal administration of contrast medium results in adequate filling of all cisterns (SPRUNG and GRUMME 1979). Intrathecal administration of metrizamide may be associated with headache, vomiting, and vertigo. Elderly patients may suffer from confusion and disorientation (SCHMIDT 1980).

# D. Computed Tomography in Brain Tumors

## Collective

Craniocerebral injury and brain tumor are the two most important indications for CT studies. There is unanimous agreement that computed tomography is unequalled in its diagnostic accuracy in demonstration of intracranial tumors. Our own experience is based on observations in 3,750 patients with brain tumors or cerebral metastases who were studied in the period from December 1974 to March 1980 (Table 1). Initial CT studies demonstrated the intracranial tumor or tumors in 3,589 cases (95.7%). Several CT examinations were necessary for diagnosis of a brain tumor in 112 patients (3.0%). Other diagnostic procedures or postmortem studies revealed a brain tumor which had not been demonstrated with CT studies in 49 cases (1.3%) (Table 1). In the majority of the latter, the tumor was a small lesion near the base of the skull – acoustic neurinoma less than 15 mm in diameter or meningioma, for example – and almost all of these patients were examined with the earlier EMI Mark I scanner. Some patients from the earliest part of our series had small tumors high in the parietal lobe. They were not demonstrated because studies were not performed at all levels up to and including the

**Table 1.** CT findings in 3,750 patients with brain tumors

| Histological diagnosis | Number of patients | X-ray absorption values of tumor tissue as compared to normal brain tissue in precontrast CT studies | | | | Failure to demonstrate the tumor in precontrast CT studies | Failure to demonstrate the tumor in CT studies either precontrast or postcontrast |
|---|---|---|---|---|---|---|---|
| | | Hypodense | Isodense | Hyperdense | Mixed density | | |
| Astrocytoma | 153 | 150 | 1 | – | 2 | – | – |
| Anaplastic astrocytoma | 157 | 52 | 20 | 30 | 55 | 5 | – |
| Oligodendroglioma | 174 | 45 | 8 | 24 | 97 | – | – |
| Glioblastoma | 711 | 65 | 80 | 61 | 505 | 16 | 2 |
| Pilocytic astrocytoma | 112 | 35 | 22 | 17 | 38 | 5 | – |
| Ependymoma | 54 | 7 | 5 | 22 | 20 | 1 | – |
| Medulloblastoma | 67 | 3 | 7 | 43 | 14 | 3 | 1 |
| Malignant lymphoma, sarcoma | 26 | 9 | 9 | 27 | 17 | 1 | – |
| Plexus papilloma | 14 | – | 3 | 9 | 2 | 1 | – |
| Meningioma | 602 | 5 | 85 | 441 | 59 | 40 | 12* |
| Neurinoma | 196 | 16 | 111 | 33 | 18 | 79 | 18* |
| Pituitary adenoma | 377 | 16 | 66 | 248 | 47 | 20 | 1 |
| Hemangioblastoma | 41 | 27 | 3 | 5 | 6 | 2 | – |
| Craniopharyngioma | 81 | 11 | 5 | 30 | 35 | 4 | 1 |
| Epidermoid, dermoid, teratoma | 36 | 25 | 1 | 1 | 9 | 1 | – |
| Other brain tumors | 192 | 48 | 21 | 93 | 30 | 11 | 4 |
| Intracranial metastases | 575 | 97 | 99 | 194 | 184 | 17 | 5* |
| Brain tumors of unknown histological type | 146 | 33 | 25 | 53 | 35 | 17 | 5* |
| Total | 3,750 | 644 | 571 | 1,331 | 1,173 | 223 | 49** |
| Percent | 100 | 17.2 | 15.2 | 35.5 | 31.3 | 6.0 | 1.3 |

vertex. Histological classification of the tumor was possible in 3,604 cases; in the remaining 146 patients inoperability or other reasons prevented histological examination of tumor material.

Table 1 summarizes the most important histological diagnoses and CT findings. The large number of brain tumors may be explained by the fact that the three CT study groups are affiliated with neurosurgical departments. Some tumors, such as pituitary adenomas, are overrepresented as a result of the special activities of individual neurosurgical teams in the three participating clinics. Close cooperation with local tumor centers resulted in an unexpectedly high percentage of patients with intracranial metastases.

## Criteria for Evaluation of Computed Tomograms

The *absorption characteristics of tumor tissue* in the plain CT scan were determined and compared to the gray shade of normal brain tissue in the analog picture. This suggested a classification in four groups.

1. *Tumors which appear brighter than adjacent, nonedematous brain tissue in the analog picture* as a result of **higher** absorption values. These processes are designated **hyperdense.**
2. *Tumors which appear darker than normal brain tissue in the analog picture* **as a result of lower** density are described as **hypodense.**
3. *Tumors with the same gray shade as normal brain tissue in the analog picture* demonstrate the same X-ray absorption values and are defined as **isodense.**
4. *Tumors which contain portions with different radiation absorption characteristics* do not demonstrate uniform gray tone and are described as **mixed density** lesions.

Evaluation of an *increase in density following administration of contrast media* was performed with reference to the analog picture in the plain CT scan. A visible increase in brightness was required as evidence of contrast uptake in the tumor. Changes in radiation absorp-

| Postcontrast studies | Contrast uptake in the tumor | | Demonstration of perifocal edema | | | | Comments |
|---|---|---|---|---|---|---|---|
| | Positive | Negative | Total | Grade I | Grade II | Grade III | |
| 140 | 2* | 138 | 3 | 2 | 1 | – | * Gemistocytic astrocytoma |
| 143 | 117 | 26 | 196 | 51 | 47 | 8 | |
| 163 | 75 | 88 | 66 | 38 | 25 | 3 | |
| 695 | 671 | 24 | 652 | 160 | 376 | 116 | |
| 106 | 87 | 19 | 28 | 26 | 2 | – | |
| 49 | 41 | 8 | 23 | 14 | 6 | 3 | |
| 60 | 56 | 4 | 31 | 28 | 3 | – | |
| 56 | 54 | 2 | 45 | 20 | 22 | 3 | |
| 13 | 13 | – | 6 | 4 | 1 | 1 | |
| 546 | 531 | 15 | 369 | 147 | 181 | 41 | * 12 tumors near the base; very small or wrong CT slice |
| 194 | 173 | 21 | 53 | 47 | 5 | 1 | * 18 tumors smaller than 15 mm in diameter |
| 358 | 343 | 15 | 5 | 5 | – | – | |
| 40 | 21 | 19 | 10 | 9 | 1 | – | |
| 66 | 45 | 21 | 1 | 1 | – | – | |
| 28 | 4 | 24 | 2 | 2 | – | – | |
| 158 | 102 | 56 | 38 | 15 | 17 | 6 | |
| 540 | 510 | 30 | 500 | 172 | 253 | 75 | * 1 × false CT slice |
| 128 | 94 | 34 | 32 | 18 | 13 | 1 | * Three isodense pontine tumors among these five negative cases |
| 3,483 | 2,939 | 544 | 1,970 | 759 | 953 | 258 | ** Total amounts only to 99.2% since some tumors were not demonstrated or not scanned in the right plane |
| 100 | 84.4 | 15.6 | 52.5 | 20.2 | 25.4 | 6.9 | |

tion of 1–4 HU in tumor tissue was not considered positive, since normal brain tissue demonstrates this degree of change after contrast enhancement, and the difference in gray values between tumor and normal brain tissue necessarily remained unchanged in these cases. Table 1 contains data on the frequency and extent of *perifocal edema* in various tumors. We proposed the following classification in an earlier publication (KAZNER et al. 1975).

**Grade I edema –** a margin of edema measuring up to 2 cm around a tumor

**Grade II edema –** a region of edema extending more than 2 cm from the border of a tumor and encompassing up to one half of a cerebral hemisphere

**Grade III edema –** tumor edema extending to more than one half of a cerebral hemisphere

The same classification applies to edema in the cerebellum. Frequency of brain edema with each histological entity is summarized in the figure at the beginning of each section dealing with a particular tumor.

## Type-Specific Diagnosis with CT

The possibility of making a histological diagnosis from the CT scan is a matter of controversy. One should recall KRICHEFF's remark that *"everything can look like everything."* Even the most common tumors such as meningioma, glioblastoma, and pituitary adenoma, which usually have a characteristic appearance in the CT scan, may provide major difficulties in differential diagnosis in individual cases. However, when both the history and clinical data are also considered, a diagnosis of histological type is possible in more than 80% of cases. In our series, diagnosis was correct in 84% of meningiomas, 83% of glioblastomas, and more than 90% of pituitary adenomas. Metastases were correctly identified in about 80% of cases, and the history provided useful information in these patients. Even rare brain tumors which make up less than 2% of the total were correctly identified in 56% of cases (KAZNER and STEINHOFF 1978). Given the experience gathered in the past several years, one would expect that retrospective analysis of the earlier CT scan would result in even better overall results.

*Correct identification of an intracranial tumor depends on CT characteristics as well as on clinical data:*

1. Typical location
2. Characteristic age at first appearance of symptoms
3. Radiation absorption characteristics ("density") before and after contrast enhancement
4. Composition of the tumor
5. Configuration of the tumor

ZÜLCH, among others, emphasized the importance of the first two points in 1958, long before the introduction of computed tomography. The value of these characteristics in analysis of CT scans cannot be overemphasised. We have included these points in the discussion of the various tumor groups and selected the pictorial material accordingly. *Analysis of CT studies* themselves includes evaluation of the *analog picture,* the CT scan in the strictest sense

**Table 2.** Hounsfield numbers in tissue and fluid in the cranial cavity and the orbits (precontrast studies)

| Medium (tissue, fluid) | Mean Hounsfield numbers in the digital printout |
|---|---|
| Bone | to +1,000 |
| Calcification | from + 60 |
| Gray matter | + 32 to + 40 |
| White matter | + 28 to + 32 |
| CSF | + 3 to + 14[a] |
| Flowing blood | + 32 to + 44 |
| Clotted blood (recent) | + 64 to + 86 |
| Older blood clots | + 30 to + 60 |
| Glioma (uncalcified) | + 18 to + 40 |
| Glioblastoma (viable tissue) | + 29 to + 38 |
| Ependymoma | + 28 to + 50 |
| Medulloblastoma | + 36 to + 58 |
| Meningioma (uncalcified) | + 36 to + 56 |
| Neurinoma | + 28 to + 40 |
| Pituitary adenoma | + 35 to + 50 |
| Lipoma | −120 to − 40 |
| Malformative tumors (epidermoid, dermoid, teratoma) | −120 to + 10 |
| Metastases | + 22 to + 50 |
| Tumor cysts | + 6 to + 22 |
| Necrosis in brain tumors | + 19 to + 23 |
| Brain edema surrounding tumors | + 18 to + 26 |
| Recent brain infarction | + 22 to + 26 |
| Old brain infarction | + 10 to + 16 |
| Capsule of brain abscess | + 28 to + 34 |
| Contents of brain abscess | + 19 to + 23 |
| Fatty tissue in the orbits | − 90 to − 70 |

[a] High values due to partial volume effect in narrow ventricles

of the word, and the *numerical values,* which provide more precise information on the radiation absorption characteristics of the tumor than can be derived from observation of the gray shades of the analog picture. Exact analysis of digital values is most useful in the differential diagnosis of hypodense lesions – from brain edema to intracranial lipoma – and hyperdense zones – from recent hemorrhage to tumor calcification (see Table 2). The extent of an increase in density after contrast enhancement is also a significant factor in differential diagnosis, since a very strong increase in X-ray absorption suggests a vascular malformation or a highly vascularized lesion.

Our experience in the past 6 years has shown that a *large number of tumors exhibits a characteristic appearance in the CT scan,* which allows the prediction of the histological diagnosis in many cases. We have included a large number of these CT scans among the illustrations, because *certain characteristic patterns* recur in *many tumors.* The *most frequent locations* are also demonstrated. However, we have also included *atypical findings* in order to demonstrate the *limits of histological diagnosis derived from CT.*

We have placed considerable emphasis on *differential diagnosis in the CT scan* and have included a discussion of alternative diagnoses in the sections on individual tumors and tumor locations. The differential diagnosis of brain tumors necessarily includes nonneoplastic space-occupying lesions, and the latter are extensively discussed and illustrated in Chap. F.

The book is organized in such a manner that extensive tables with percentage data on the individual tumors and their locations are superfluous. ZÜLCH provided this data in his exemplary neuropathological analysis of intracranial tumors in 1958. The appearance of a tumor in the CT scan is often so characteristic that differential diagnosis is limited to a relatively small number of possibilities, so that extensive statistical data on histological type and location are of secondary importance in the analysis of CT scans in the majority of cases. With one exception, schematic illustrations were not included because nothing demonstrates the significant elements of a CT scan better than the CT picture itself.

In most cases the discussion of individual tumors includes information on the *biological* behavior and prognostic *significance* of the tumor. The classification used in this book resembles that proposed by ZÜLCH, which was included in the new WHO classification system (1980).

Grade I – benign: cure after "total extirpation" or at least 5-year survival
Grade II – semibenign: 3- to 5-year survival after surgery
Grade III – semimalignant: 2- to 3-year survival after surgery
Grade IV – malignant: 6- to 15-month survival after surgery

# 1. Autochthonous Brain Tumors

## a) Astrocytomas

| | |
|---|---|
| Incidence | Approximately 5% of all brain tumors |
| Characteristic age at diagnosis | 25–45 years |
| Sex distribution | Slight preponderance of males |
| Typical locations | Frontal, frontotemporal, frontoparietal, and pontine region |
| Characteristic clinical findings | Focal and generalized seizures, often over a period of years |
| Skull film | Displacement of pineal body in some cases |
| EEG | Focal seizure potentials in many cases |
| Echoencephalography | Often normal initially, with displacement of midline structures in later stages |
| Serial brain scintigraphy | Perfusion defects without radionuclide uptake in large tumors |
| Cerebral angiography | Often normal in early stages, with signs of a space-occupying lesion in later stages; no pathological tumor stain |

**Computed Tomography**

| | |
|---|---|
| Precontrast study | Circumscribed, homogeneous, relatively well-delineated hypodense zone near the cortex or diffuse spread in the frontotemporal white matter |
| Contrast medium uptake | No significant increase in density |
| Appearance after contrast enhancement | No significant change in comparison to the precontrast study |

**Differential diagnosis**

Anaplastic astrocytoma
Oligodendroglioma without calcification
Solitary metastasis without contrast uptake
Recent brain infarction
Circumscribed brain edema in a tumor at the base of the skull or high in the parietal region
Intracerebral hematoma in the stage of resorption
Superficial venous thrombosis
Circumscribed posttraumatic brain edema ("Type I" contusion)
Phlegmonous encephalitis
Multiple sclerosis
Hypodense artifacts, especially in the temporopolar region and the frontal area behind an air-filled frontal sinus

Slow-growing astrocytomas – fibrillary, protoplasmatic, and gemistocytic astrocytomas – are defined as grade II tumors in the WHO classification, although the lesions demonstrate all the microscopic characteristics of a benign tumor. We designated these tumors as grade I astrocytomas in earlier publications (cf. KAZNER et al. 1975; WENDE et al. 1978). Astrocytomas made up for 4.1% of all tumors in our collective and were most commonly found between the ages of 25 and 45 years, though they may also occur in children and adolescents. There is a slight preponderance in males.

### Typical Locations

The most common cerebral locations are the frontal, frontotemporal, temporal, and temporoparietal regions. Some tumors demonstrate diffuse growth in the white matter of the frontotemporal area. Astrocytomas are also found in the thalamus, the midbrain, and the pontine region (Fig. D1.2–11, 134–136).

### Characteristic Clinical Findings

Focal and generalized seizures are the most important clinical signs of astrocytomas and may be present for years before diagnosis is made. Neurological deficits and signs of increased intracranial pressure usually appear much later.

### Additional Diagnostic Procedures

Skull films and echoencephalograms do not provide specific diagnostic clues, while the EEG often reveals focal activity. Dynamic brain scans demonstrate perfusion defects in large tumors, though smaller lesions may go undetected. Increased nuclide uptake is not found in grade II astrocytomas. Cerebral angiography does not demonstrate pathological findings in the early stage, but signs of an intracranial space-occupying lesion appear as the tumor grows, though pathological tumor vessels are never demonstrated.

## Computed Tomography (Figs. D1.1–11)

### Precontrast Study

Slow-growing astrocytomas appear in the CT scan as rather sharply delineated, homogeneous hypodense zones that very often lie close to the convexity (Figs. D1.2, 5–7, 9). Tumors with dif-

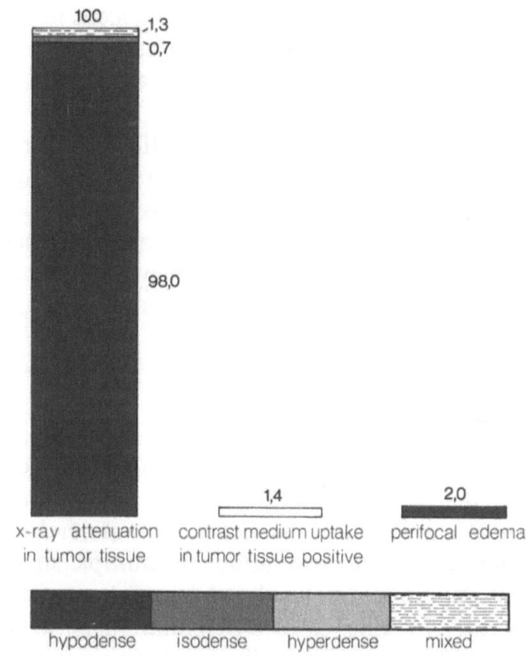


**Fig. D1.1.** X-ray attenuation, contrast medium uptake, and frequency of edema in astrocytomas (percent)

fuse growth patterns are usually found in the frontotemporal white matter and have indistinct borders (Figs. D1.3, 4, 8). Astrocytomas of the midbrain and the caudal brainstem cause distension of the pons (Figs. D1.134–136).

Absorption values in low-grade astrocytomas are considerably lower than those of adjacent normal brain tissue and are similar to those found in brain edema (18–24 HU). Our studies suggest that high water content is responsible for the low density of grade II astrocytomas. Water content is 81–82%, the same as that found in brain edema (LANKSCH et al. 1976).

*These findings apply to fibrillary and protoplasmatic astrocytomas but are not characteristic of gemistocytic astrocytomas,* which may contain areas of widely differing density, including extensive isodense zones (Figs. D1.10, 11).

### Postcontrast Study

Slow growing (fibrillary and protoplasmatic) astrocytomas *do not demonstrate visible contrast uptake.* However, statistical analysis reveals an increase in absorption values in the tumor of 2–3 HU, about the same as the general increase in density found in normal brain tissue after contrast enhancement. One may find contrast uptake in normal cortical tissue adjacent to tumors near the convexity. This phenomenon is sometimes misinterpreted as contrast uptake in the tumor itself (Figs. D1.5, 6).

Gemistocytic astrocytomas differ in this regard as well. We observed definite contrast uptake in two astrocytomas of this type (Figs. D1.10, 11); these are the only astrocytomas with positive contrast enhancement in Table 1. In addition, both tumors demonstrated slight perifocal edema.

### Differential Diagnosis

**Circumscribed brain edema** is the most common differential diagnosis. *Edema in recent brain infarction* is found in the distribution of cerebral arteries in most cases, although multiple small embolic infarctions result in a less characteristic picture. In some cases differentiation between a hypodense tumor and brain infarction is possible only with the help of serial studies, unless the clinical course provides conclusive evidence for the diagnosis.

Confusion with *circumscribed posttraumatic edema* (type I contusion, LANKSCH et al. 1977) is possible only when initial diagnostic studies are performed immediately after craniocerebral injury in a patient with a hitherto unknown tumor. This is not inconceivable, since injury may occur during a seizure. The correct diagnosis usually becomes evident in follow-up studies.

*Intracerebral hematomas in the resorption phase* may appear as zones of low density during the process of resorption and may therefore present a CT picture similar to that found in astrocytoma (Figs. F49, 50, p. 434). Perifocal edema in the white matter does not favor the diagnosis of astrocytoma. One sometimes finds *metastases that do not take up contrast medium* and therefore appear as circumscribed low density zones, which may be misinterpreted as astrocytoma if clinical data do not suggest a diagnosis of metastatic tumor.

It is not possible to differentiate between astrocytoma and *uncalcified oligodendroglioma* in the CT scan (Figs. D1.39–41).

One-third of *anaplastic astrocytomas* demonstrated CT findings similar to those in fibrillary and protoplasmatic astrocytomas. Even contrast enhancement may fail to differentiate among these tumors, since 17% of anaplastic astrocytomas do not take up contrast medium.

*Differential diagnosis is particularly difficult in tumors of the basal and high parietal regions.* In the latter, *perifocal edema* may be demonstrated, but not the tumor itself. The low density region of perifocal edema is then mistakenly interpreted as an astrocytoma (Fig. D9.13). Misinterpretations of this sort can be avoided if scans are performed up to the vertex or if coronary sections are used.

*Small basal meningiomas* with extensive perifocal edema may also lead to *misinterpretation* (Fig. D2.23). Additional scans with a different head position usually clarify the situation (Fig. D2.25).

*Artifacts* may simulate hypodense lesions, especially in the frontopolar and temporobasal regions (LANGE et al. 1976).

*Phlegmonous encephalitis* may have the same appearance as astrocytoma in the precontrast scan, and diagnosis requires special attention to the history and clinical data. Meningoencephalitis is sometimes encountered and may demonstrate contrast uptake in the cortex during late stages (Fig. F18). Abscess may also develop in cases of encephalitis, and produce extensive glial scars which appear as hypodense zones (status spongiosus, Fig. F19, p. 416).

Both recent and old lesions in *multiple sclerosis* may appear as hypodense areas that can be confused with astrocytoma if the history is not characteristic (Fig. F24, p. 421).

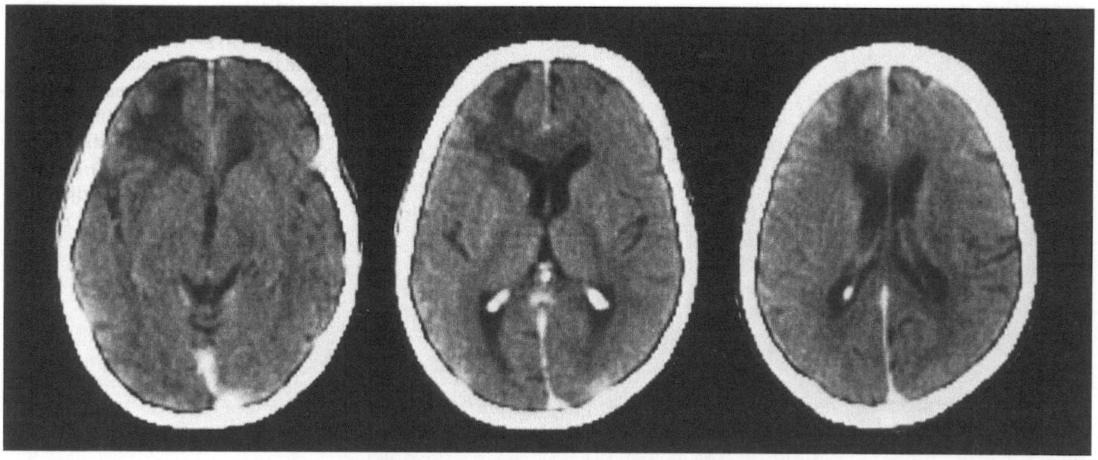

**Fig. D1.2.** Astrocytoma in the left frontal lobe with extension through the anterior corpus callosum to the right side in a 65-year-old man. The diffuse growth pattern resembles that found in perifocal edema. The tumor does not take up contrast media (postcontrast study)

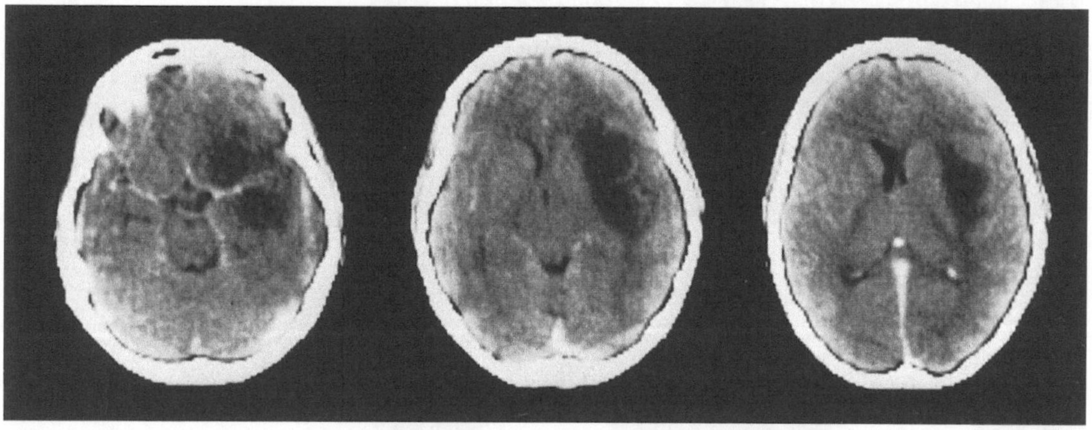

**Fig. D1.3.** Astrocytoma with a diffuse growth pattern in the right frontotemporal region. The right middle cerebral artery is surrounded by the tumor (as can clearly be seen in the picture on the left). Slight herniation of the uncus with slight brain stem compression. No contrast uptake, moderate displacement of normal structures (34-year-old female with seizures)

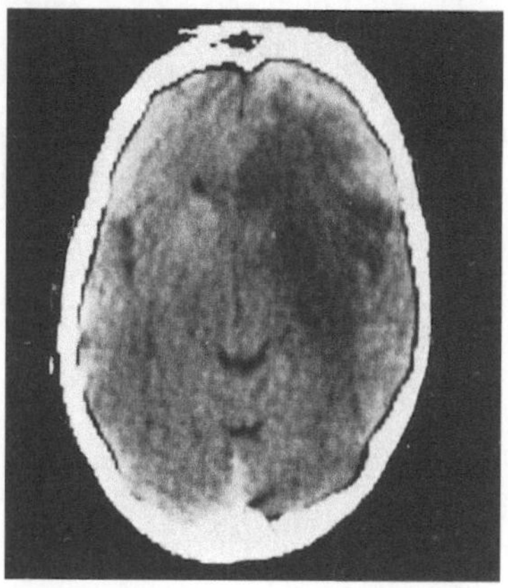

**Fig. D1.4.** Extensive astrocytoma of the white matter of the right hemisphere with diffuse growth pattern in a 40-year-old female with a history of seizures for 10 years. No significant contrast uptake in the tumor

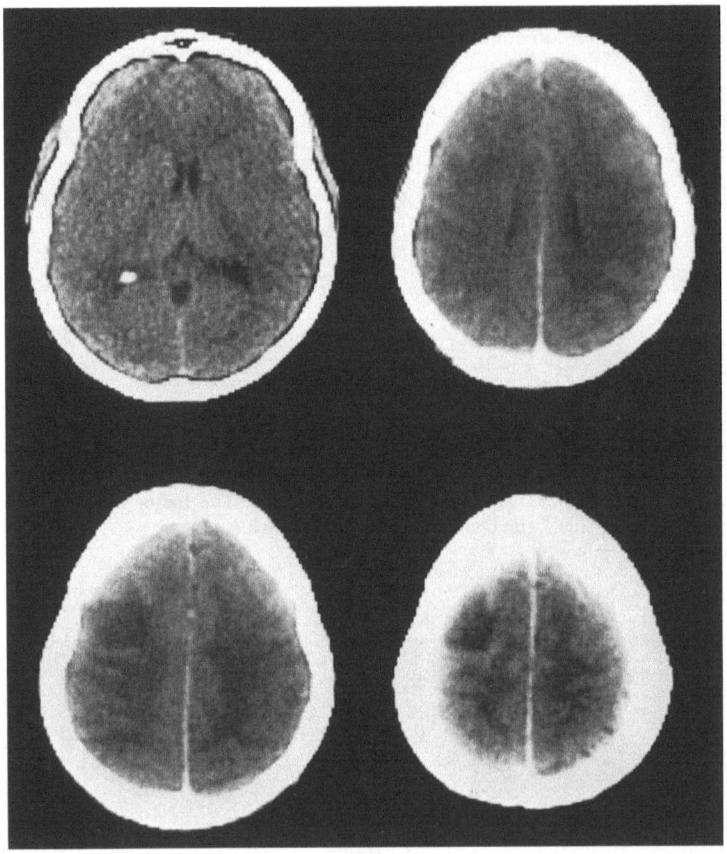

**Fig. D1.5.** Astrocytoma in the left precentral region in a 37-year-old woman with focal seizures and a speech disorder. The ventricular planes are entirely normal (upper pair). The tumor appears only as a hypodense zone high in the parietal region. Contrast uptake in adjacent cortical tissue simulates rim enhancement of the tumor

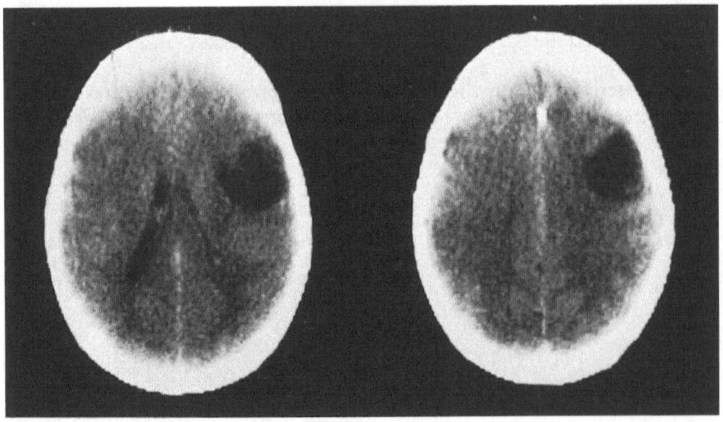

**Fig. D1.6.** Astrocytoma of the right precentral region in a 40-year-old male with focal seizures. Hypodense tumor (22 HU) without contrast uptake

**Fig. D1.7.** Astrocytoma in the right parietal region adjacent to the interhemispheric fissure in a 36-year-old male. Clear demonstration of the surrounding sulci indicates that the tumor has only limited space-occupying effects. No contrast uptake in the tumor itself. The small high-density zone at the medial margin of the tumor represents calcification in the falx ►

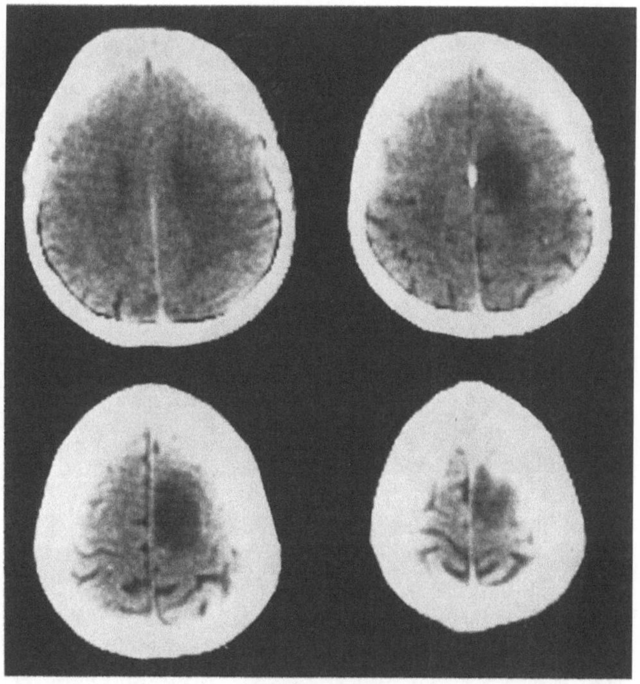

**Fig. D1.8.** Large astrocytoma in the white matter on the right with extension along the lateral ventricle. Bulging of the vault on the right (5-year-old child). Perifocal edema is evident around the hypodense tumor, unusual since edema in low-grade astrocytomas is usually indistinguishable from the tumor itself. Tumor growth around the anterior horn on the left may have occurred ▼

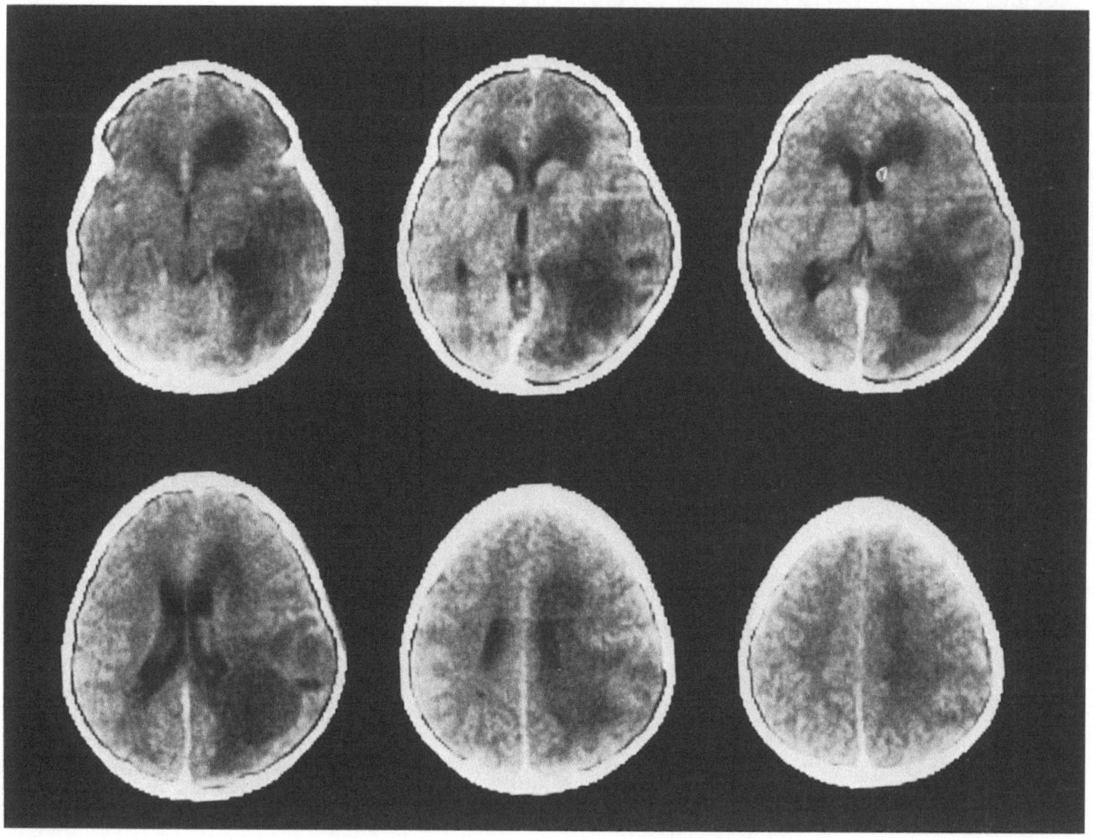

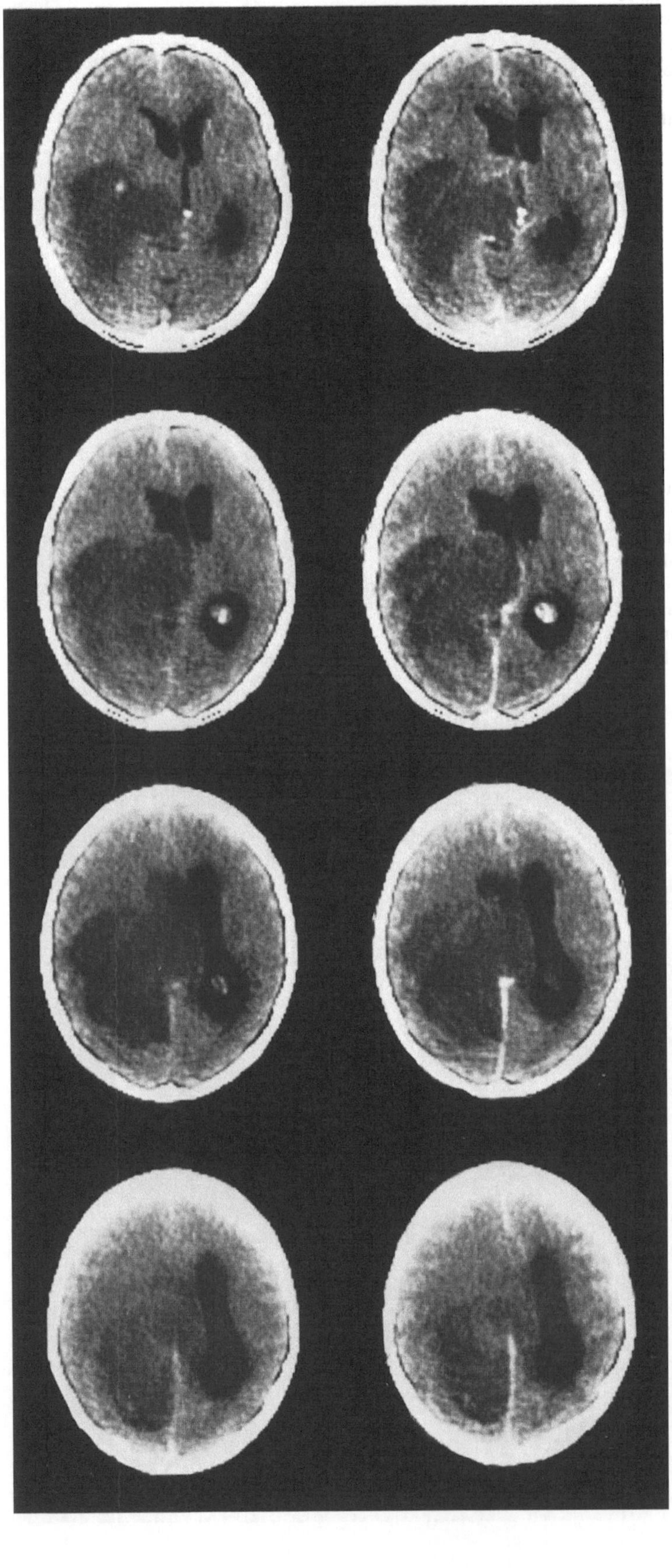

**Fig. D 1.9.** Very large astrocytoma in the left hemisphere with involvement of the basal ganglia in a 37-year-old man presenting with headache and papilledema. Ventricular dilatation on the right due to blockage of CSF pathways. No visible change in the hypodense tumor after contrast administration (postcontrast CT on the right). Analysis of the numerical values reveals an increase of 2–3 HU

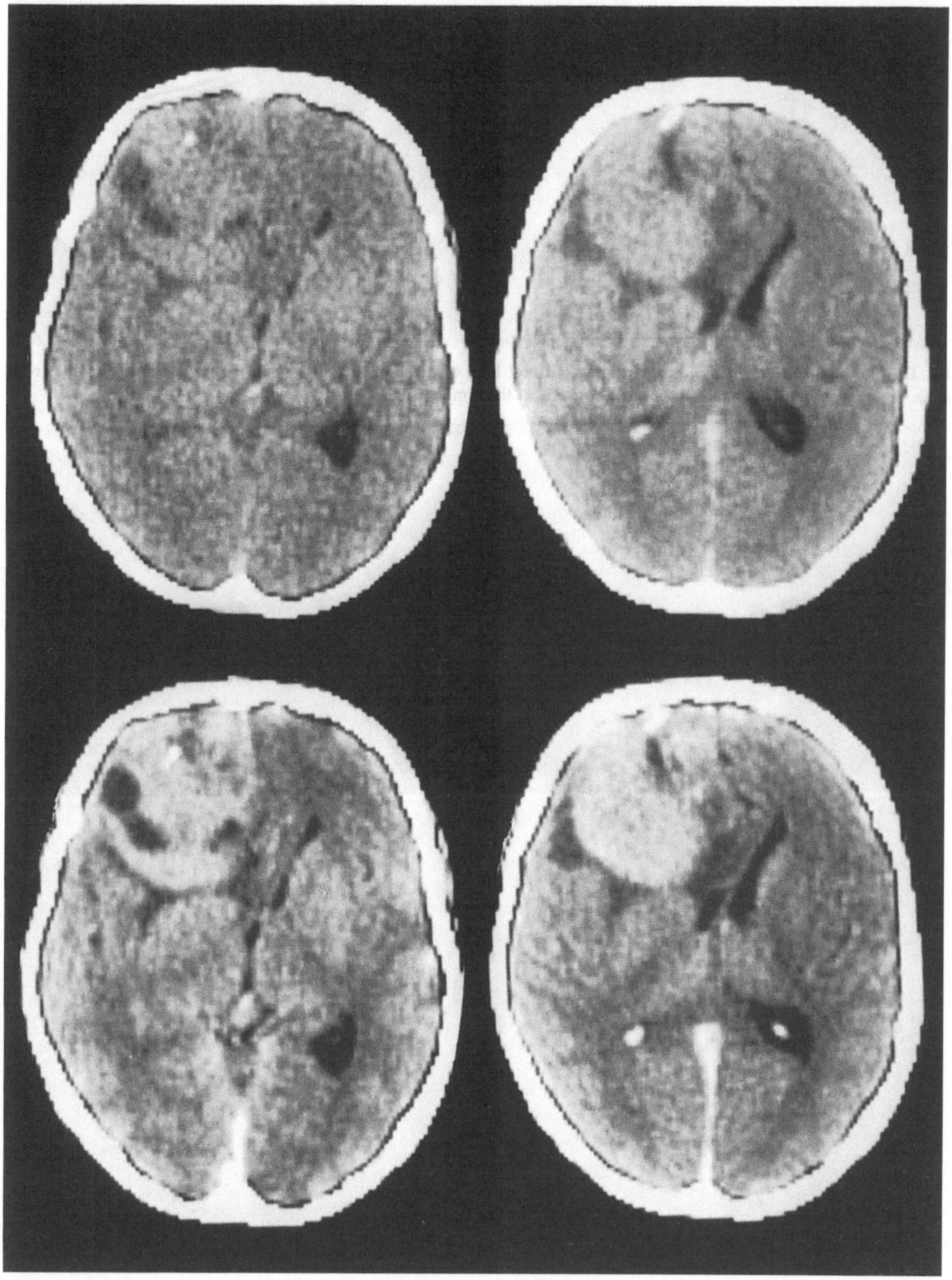

**Fig. D 1.10.** Gemistocytic astrocytoma in the left frontal lobe of a 35-year-old patient. The tumor is primarily isodense with small calcifications and low-density zones due to cysts. Limited perifocal edema. Increased density values after contrast administration (below). This differs considerably from CT studies of other low-grade (fibrillary and protoplasmatic) astrocytomas

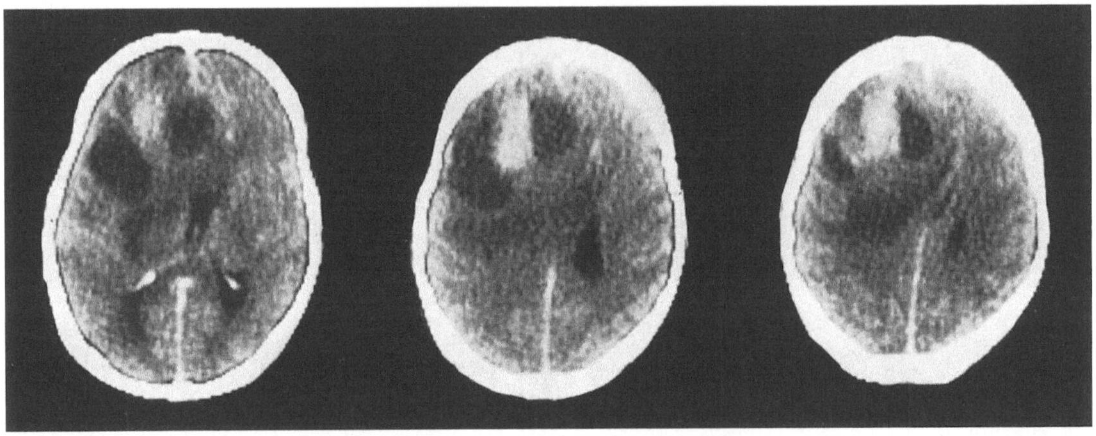

**Fig. D1.11.** Gemistocytic astrocytoma in the left frontal lobe with marginal cysts and perifocal edema in a 34-year-old male. Significant contrast uptake in the solid portions of the tumor (postcontrast CT)

## b) Anaplastic Astrocytomas

| | |
|---|---|
| Incidence | Approximately 4% |
| Characteristic age at diagnosis | 35–55 years |
| Sex distribution | Slight preponderance of males |
| Typical locations | Frontal, frontoparietal, temporal, and temporoparietal regions |
| Characteristic clinical findings | Seizures; neurological deficits depending on location of the tumor; headache |
| Skull film | Frequent displacement of the pineal body |
| EEG | Frequent focal seizure potentials |
| Echoencephalography | Displacement of midline structures in most cases |
| Serial brain scintigraphy | Perfusion defects common; slight to moderate nuclide uptake in the tumor in delayed scans |
| Cerebral angiography | Signs of a space-occupying lesion; capillary blush rare |

**Computed Tomography**

| | |
|---|---|
| Precontrast study | Quite inhomogeneous; hypodense or isodense zones are common, sometimes in combination |
| Contrast medium uptake | Positive in the great majority of cases |
| Appearance after contrast enhancement | Varied; ring figures or solid tumors, some with large cysts; may sometimes resemble grade II astrocytoma; slight to moderate perifocal edema common |

**Differential Diagnosis**

Glioblastoma
Anaplastic oligodendroglioma without calcification
Solitary metastasis
Ependymoma
Malignant lymphoma
Pilocytic astrocytoma
Astrocytoma in the absence of contrast uptake

**In Rare Cases**

Brain abscess, acute disseminating encephalomyelitis, leukemic infiltrate, old intracerebral hematoma

This group made up 4.2% of all intracranial tumors in our series. It may occur at any age but is most commonly found between the ages of 35 and 45 years with a slight preponderance of males. Prognosis is that of a grade III tumor.

### Typical Locations

The tumors are most commonly found in the frontal, frontoparietal, temporal, and temporoparietal regions. The lesions have also been demonstrated in the parietal lobe, in the thalamus, and in the pontine region, but they are rarely found in the cerebellum (Fig. D1.13–27).

### Characteristic Clinical Findings

Clinical features include seizures, localizing neurological deficits, and headache.

### Additional Diagnostic Procedures

Skull films do not reveal specific changes in patients with anaplastic astrocytomas, though displacement of the calcified pineal body may be found in large tumors. The EEG often demonstrates focal activity, and the echoencephalogram usually shows displacement of midline structures. Dynamic brain scans produce a variety of results. Large cysts cause perfusion defects, while solid portions of the tumor show slight nuclide uptake. Large solid astrocytomas may demonstrate homogeneous radionuclide uptake. Transitional forms related to glioblastoma may be observed as well.

Cerebral angiography demonstrates signs of a mass lesion, while tumor vascularization is rarely found except in highly malignant astrocytomas with pathological vessels at their centers. A capillary blush sometimes appears. Large cysts result in an avascular space.

## Computed Tomography (Figs. D1.12–27)

### Precontrast Study

All astrocytomas with portions demonstrating higher-grade malignancy were included among the anaplastic astrocytomas, even when most of the tumor was composed of slow-growing tissue. As a result the findings in this group are *very inhomogeneous* (Fig. D1.12).

Solid tumors may appear hypodense, isodense, or hyperdense, and combinations of two or even all three types are possible (Figs. D1.24, 25). Sharply delineated cysts may be found in the CT scan in some cases, with density of the cyst ranging from 15–22 HU, depending on the protein content of the cyst fluid (Figs. D1.16, 18).

*A few isodense anaplastic astrocytomas may produce very discrete tumor signs in the CT scan and may be overlooked as a result* (Fig. D1.20; see Table 1).

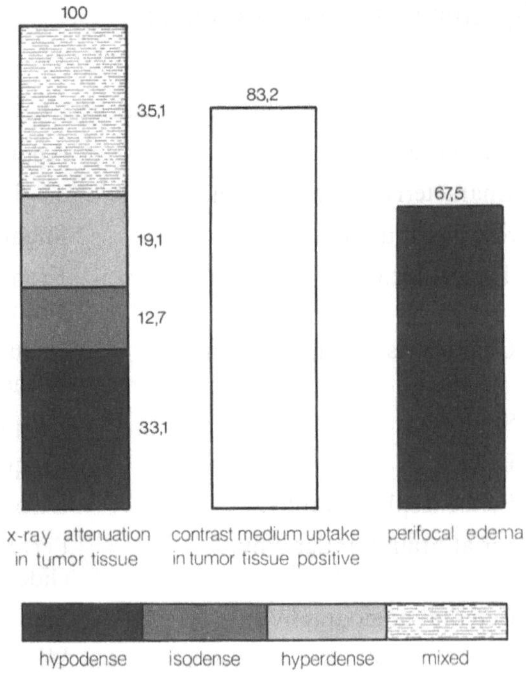


**Fig. D1.12.** X-ray attenuation, contrast medium uptake, and frequency of edema in anaplastic astrocytomas (in percent)

Slight to moderate *perifocal brain edema* was present in 67.5% of the anaplastic astrocytomas in our collective. Tumor and accompanying edema often cause pronounced displacement of midline structures. Grade III edema is rare in these tumors (5.1%). The tumor itself usually appears as a distinct isodense structure within the hypodense zone of edema (Fig. D1.24). In some cases the actual neoplasm may be hypodense, and as a result it is not possible to differentiate between tumor and edema in the precontrast study.

### Postcontrast Study

Contrast enhancement was positive in 83% of the 157 patients in our series, but 17% of anaplastic astrocytomas did not take up contrast medium. The latter were hypodense astrocytomas which contained small areas of anaplasia. This inconsistent response to contrast media suggests that hypodense tumors which do not take up contrast media may represent a transitional stage between astrocytoma and anaplastic astrocytoma.

The *appearance of anaplastic astrocytomas after contrast enhancement varies considerably,* but our experience indicates that the following findings are rather typical.

a) A narrow ring, sometimes interrupted, which encompasses a sharply delineated zone of low density, usually a cyst; one sometimes finds a solid tumor nodule which takes up contrast at the lateral margin of the cyst (Figs. D1.16–18)
b) A hypodense, sharply delineated area with slight inhomogeneous contrast medium uptake resulting in a blurred figure (Fig. D1.14).

Large solid isodense tumors with density measuring 32–40 HU in the procontrast scan showed an average increase in density of 11 HU after contrast enhancement (range 8–16 HU).

**Differential Diagnosis**

The protean manifestations of anaplastic astrocytomas in CT scans necessarily entail a wide range of possibilities in differential diagnosis.

The **hypodense tumors** suggest less malignant *astrocytomas* or oligodendrogliomas without calcification. In our series the hypodense zone in anaplastic tumors was usually larger than that found in other astrocytomas (Figs. D1.14, 15, 17).

**Ring structures** in the tumor are also found with *glioblastoma, brain abscess,* and *metastases. Pilocytic astrocytomas* may also produce similar findings (see p. 107 ff.).

*Malignant lymphoma, solitary brain metastasis, ependymoma, and rare leukemic infiltrates* as well as *acute disseminating encephalomyelitis* with contrast enhancement should be considered in the differential diagnosis of **solid tumors with homogeneous contrast medium uptake.**

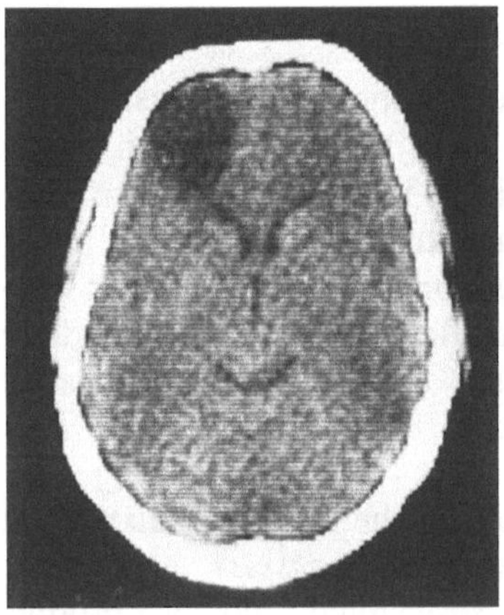

**Fig. D1.13.** Astrocytoma in the left frontal lobe of a 33-year-old patient with seizures. No contrast uptake in the hypodense portions of the tumor. Histological examination revealed areas of anaplasia, therefore classification of the tumor as anaplastic astrocytoma

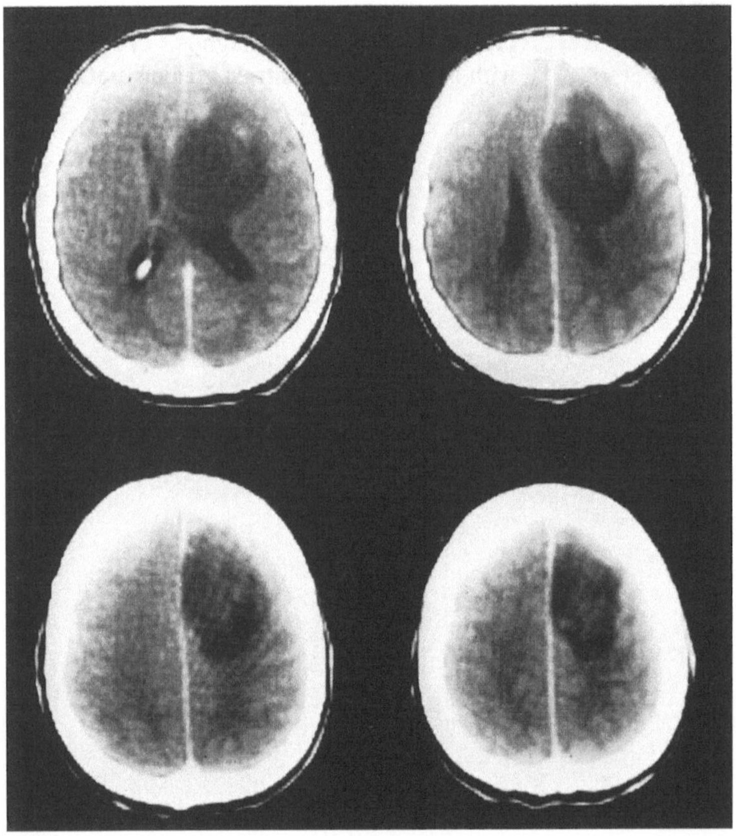

**Fig. D1.14.** Large anaplastic astrocytoma in the right precentral region with extension into the right lateral ventricle in a 40-year-old patient with a history of seizures for several years and progredient left hemiparesis. Sharply delineated, primarily hypodense tumor with indistinct areas of contrast uptake indicating anaplasia

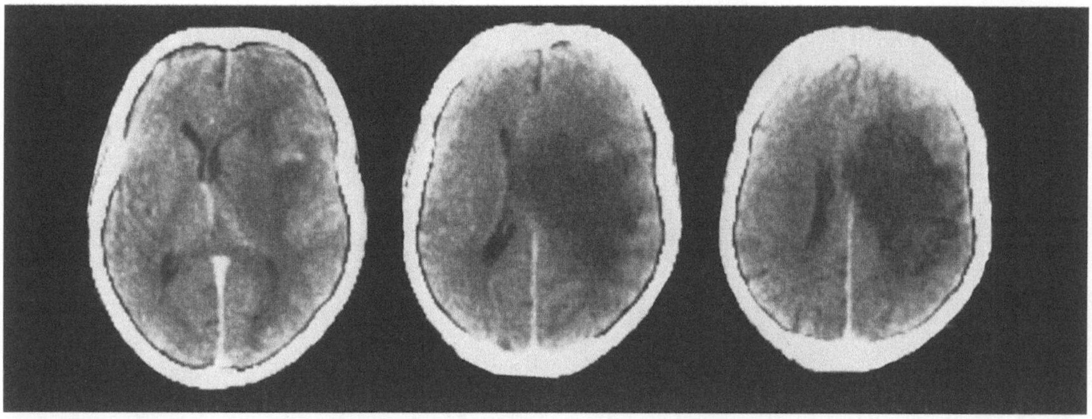

**Fig. D 1.15.** Anaplastic astrocytoma in the central portions of the right hemisphere in a 43-year-old male. Discrete zone of contrast enhancement within the large hypodense tumor (pictures on the left and in the middle)

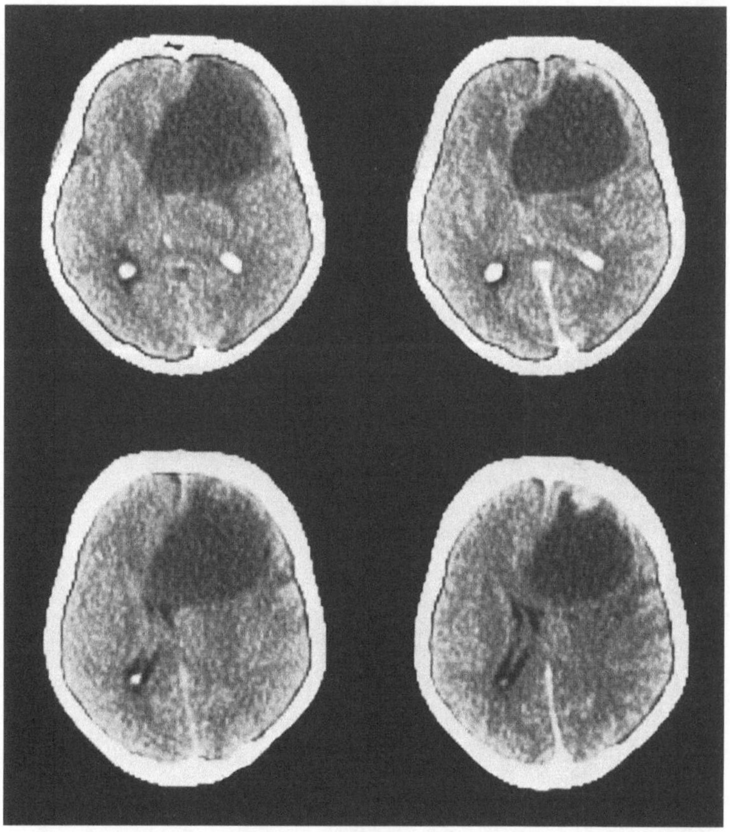

**Fig. D 1.16.** Right frontal anaplastic astrocytoma in a 60-year-old female. The large hypodense zone proved to be a cyst at operation. Contrast administration shows a slight increase in density at the margin of the cyst and a small solid tumor nodule in the cortex (postcontrast studies on the right). Similar findings are observed in pilocytic astrocytoma

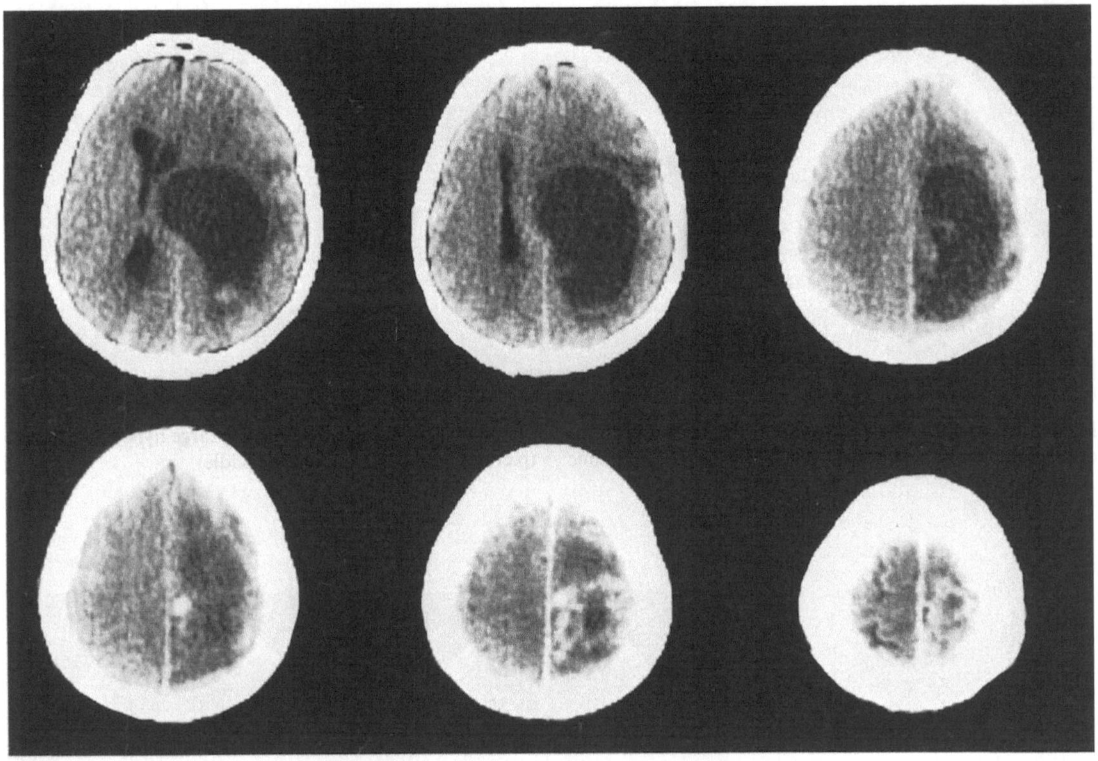

**Fig. D 1.17.** Anaplastic astrocytoma in the central and parietal portions of the right hemisphere with demonstration of a large centrally located cyst and solid tumor tissue with inhomogeneous contrast uptake in the right parietal region (54-year-old patient). Postcontrast CT

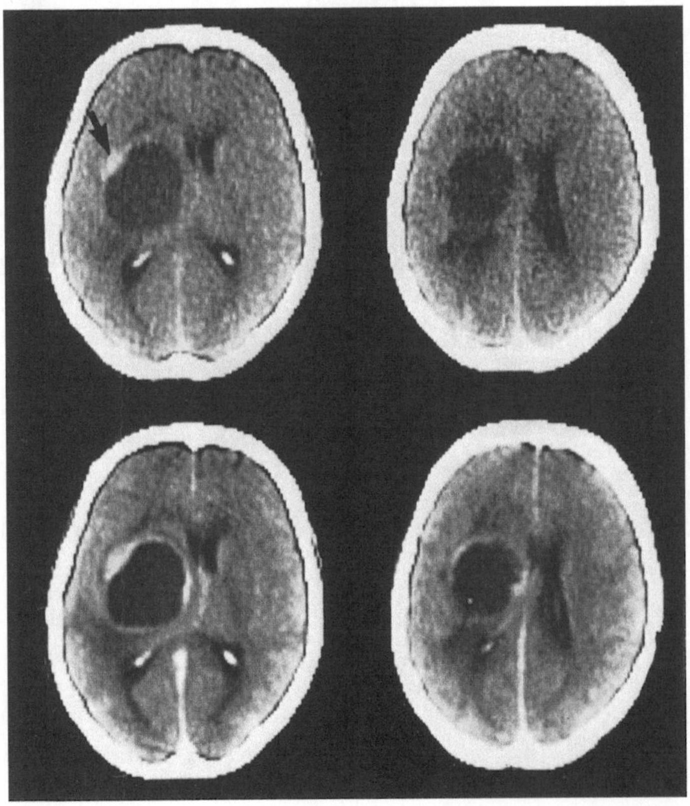

**Fig. D 1.18.** Anaplastic astrocytoma in the basal ganglia on the left. Large cyst and slight marginal contrast uptake in the solid portions of the tumor. Small hematoma in the anterior wall of the cyst (arrow). This tumor could be mistaken for pilocytic astrocytoma (58-year-old female). Precontrast CT above, postcontrast CT below

**Fig. D1.19.** Anaplastic astrocytoma in the right posterior temporal region with mixed density and inhomogeneous contrast uptake in a 51-year-old female

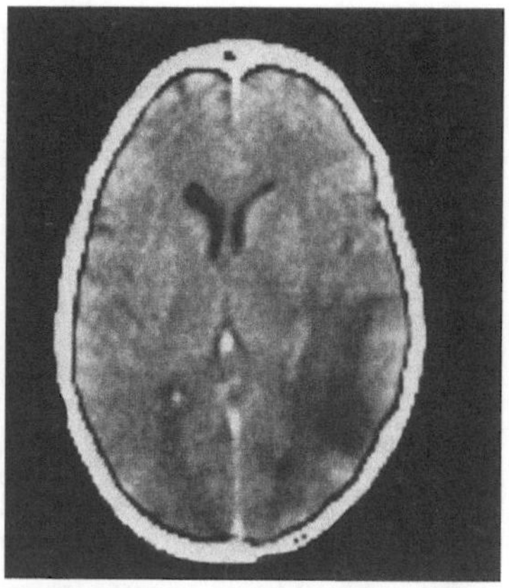

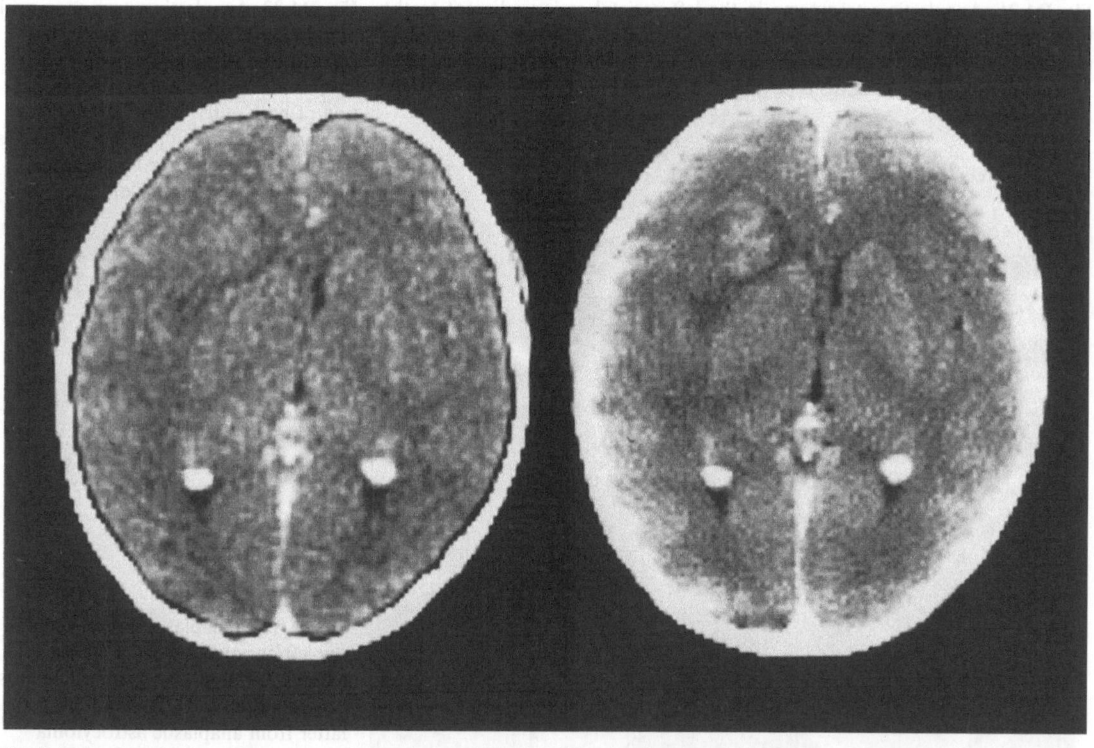

**Fig. D1.20.** Anaplastic astrocytoma deep in the frontal white matter of a 36-year-old male with psychomotor seizures. Precontrast studies reveal only a small semicircular hypodense zone at the medial border of the isodense tumor. Postcontrast studies (right) demonstrate a slight inhomogeneous increase in density within the tumor

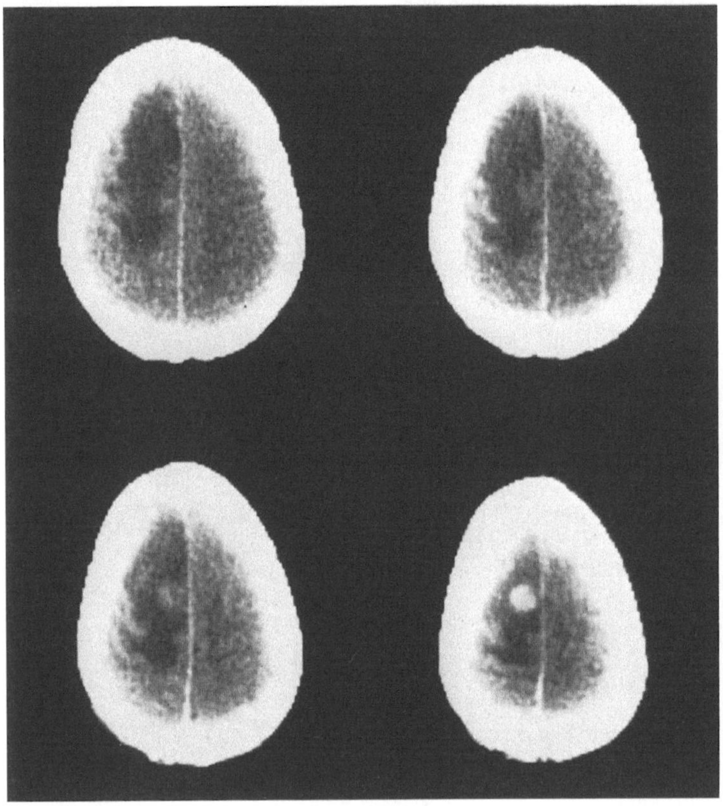

▲

**Fig. D 1.21.** Anaplastic astrocytoma in the left parietal region adjacent to the interhemispheric fissure, surrounded by grade II edema. The actual tumor nodule measures only 15 mm in diameter and is limited to the highest parietal slice. Misinterpretation as metastasis is possible (38-year-old man). Postcontrast study

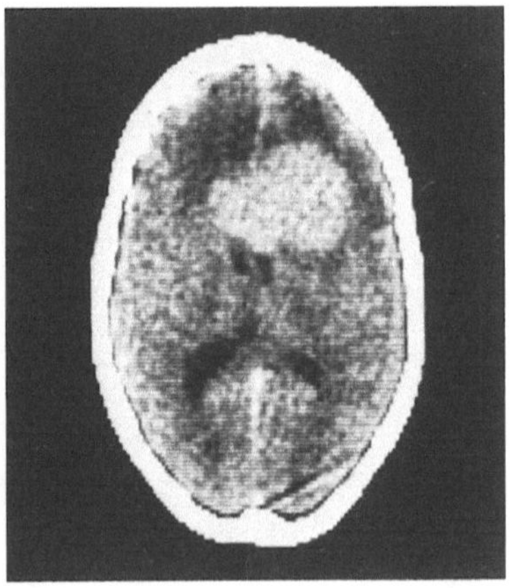

▲

**Fig. D 1.22.** Anaplastic astrocytoma with homogeneous contrast uptake in the right frontal white matter with extension to the left hemisphere and amputation of both anterior horns. The tumor appeared isodense in precontrast studies but was well delineated by perifocal edema (39-year-old female)

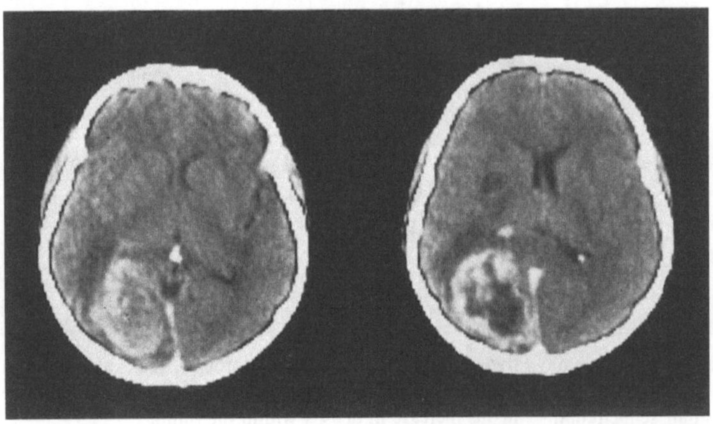

**Fig. D 1.23.** Anaplastic astrocytoma in the left occipital lobe of a 50-year-old patient. CT studies suggest a diagnosis of glioblastoma. Differentiation of the latter from anaplastic astrocytoma may prove difficult or impossible even at histological examination. Postcontrast study

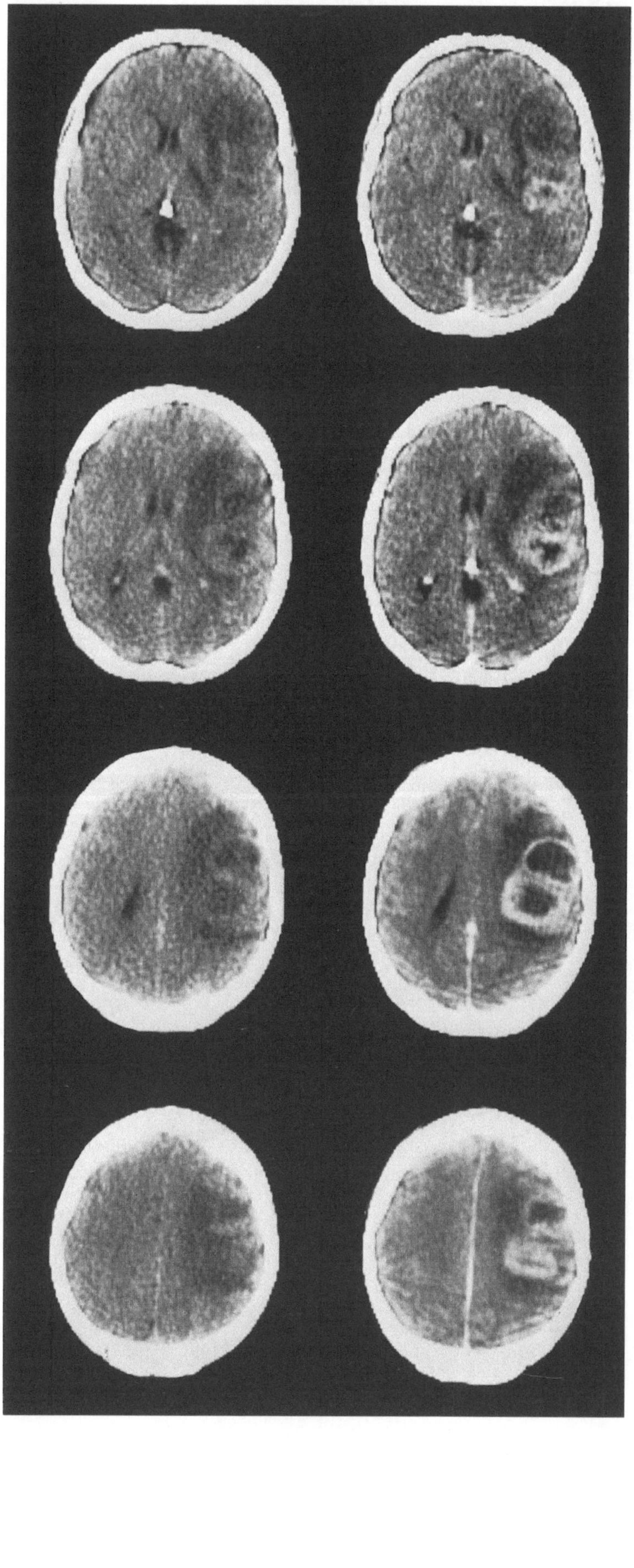

**Fig. D1.24.** Anaplastic astrocytoma with transition to glioblastoma in a 60-year-old patient. Precontrast studies (series on the left) demonstrate a tumor composed of several ring structures in the right temporoparietal region. Significantly increased density after contrast administration with improved delineation of the actual tumor from perifocal edema (series on the right)

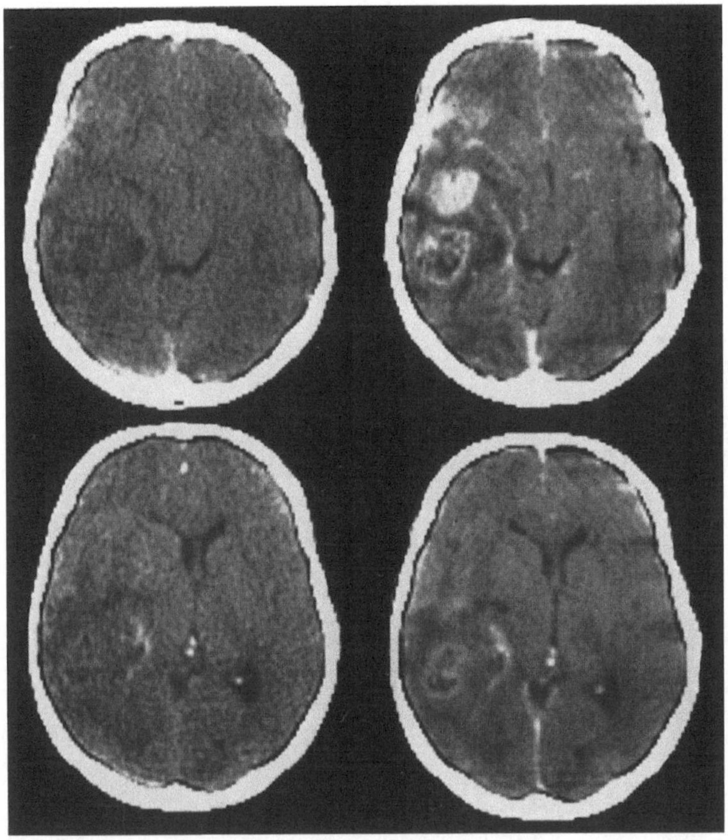

**Fig. D 1.25.** Anaplastic astrocytoma in the left temporal lobe with demonstration of two distinct tumor nodules with different CT patterns. Conspicuously little perifocal edema. (36-year-old man). Precontrast CT on the left, postcontrast CT on the right

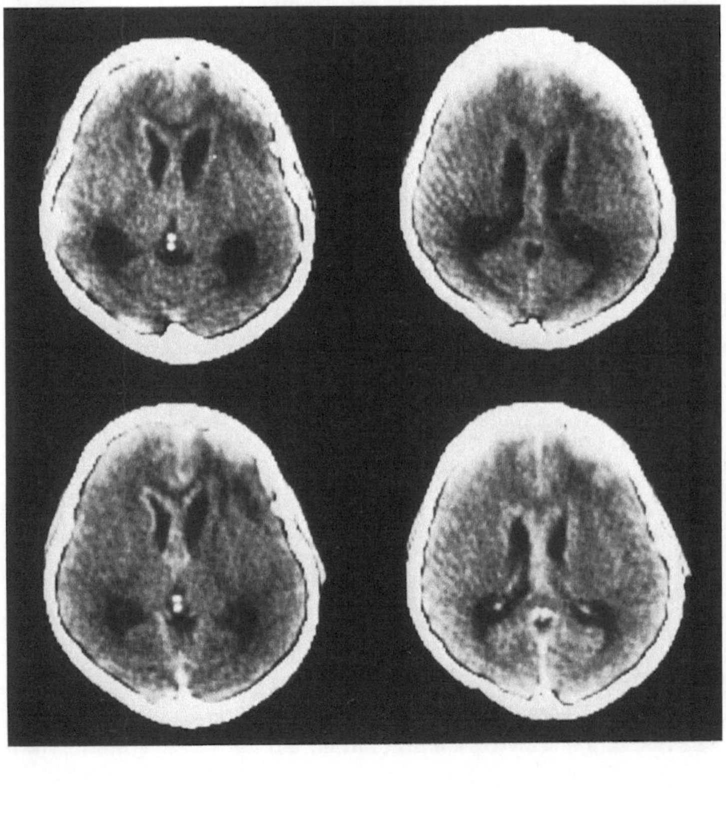

**Fig. D 1.26.** Recurrence of a right frontal anaplastic astrocytoma in a 30-year-old patient. The tumor spreads along the walls of the ventricles and in the septum pellucidum. (Precontrast CT above, postcontrast CT below)

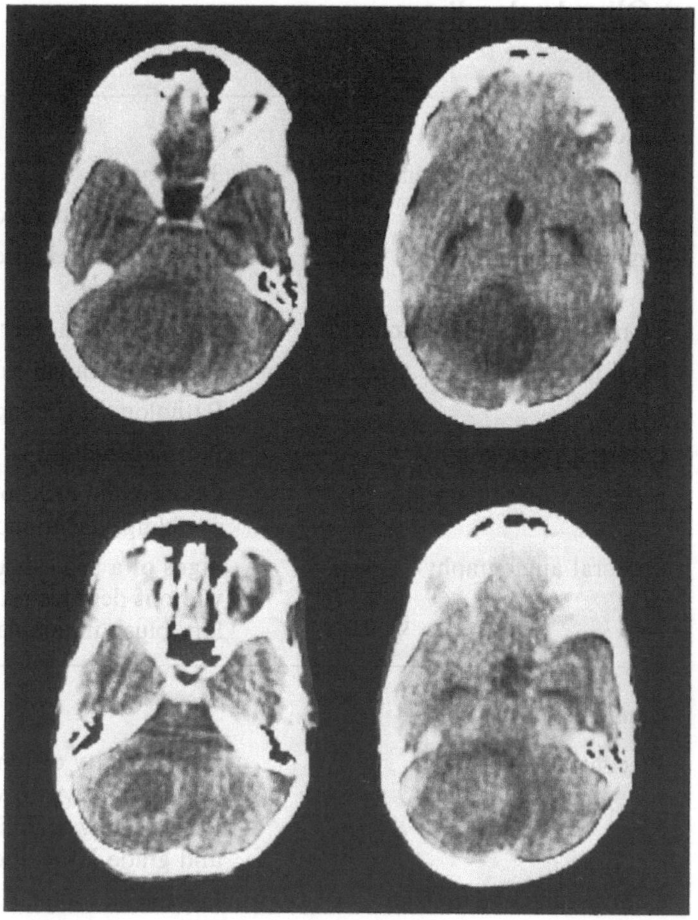

**Fig. D1.27.** Anaplastic astrocytoma in the left cerebellar hemisphere of the type usually found in the cerebral hemispheres. Isodense to hypodense values in the precontrast CT (above) with ring enhancement in the postcontrast CT (below). (11-year-old boy with signs of cerebellar dysfunction). The lesion may be mistaken for a pilocytic astrocytoma, since appearance in CT studies is identical

## c) Oligodendrogliomas

| | |
|---|---|
| Incidence | 2–10% |
| Characteristic age at diagnosis | 30–55 years |
| Sex distribution | Slight preponderance of males |
| Typical locations | Frontal, frontoparietal, frontotemporal, and temporal region |
| Characteristic clinical findings | Seizures, often over a period of several years |
| Skull film | Fine intracranial calcifications in many cases |
| EEG | Pathological findings in most cases |
| Echoencephalography | Normal findings or slight midline displacement |
| Serial brain scintigraphy | Occasional perfusion defect; radionuclide uptake resembling that found in other anaplastic gliomas |
| Cerebral angiography | Signs of a space-occupying lesion in all large tumors without demonstration of pathological vessels; capillary blush in anaplastic oligodendrogliomas only |

**Computed Tomography**

| | |
|---|---|
| Precontrast study | The majority of tumors demonstrates irregularly shaped zones with very high density due to calcification; otherwise findings similar to those in grade II and grade III astrocytomas |
| Contrast medium uptake | Positive in anaplastic oligodendrogliomas only (grade III) |
| Appearance after contrast enhancement | Areas with different density values corresponding to the inhomogeneous composition of the tumor; only slight perifocal edema in most cases |

**Differential Diagnosis**

Astrocytoma (and the diagnostic alternatives to this lesion) in the absence of calcification
Pilocytic astrocytoma of the cerebral hemispheres
Gangliocytoma
Calcified meningioma
Ependymoma
Calcified arteriovenous malformation
Cavernous hemangioma
Sturge-Weber syndrome (encephalotrigeminal syndrome)
Tuberculoma
Cysticercosis

Reports on the incidence of oligodendrogliomas in the literature vary considerably (CUSHING, 1.3%; KERNOHAN and SAYRE, 5%; ZÜLCH, 9.6%); in our series oligodendroglioma comprised 4.5% of all tumors. Greatest incidence is found between the ages of 30 and 55 years, with males afflicted somewhat more frequently than females.

The tumors are classified from grade I – with well-delineated calcified tumors – to grade III with anaplastic oligodendrogliomas.

### Typical Locations

These tumors are found almost exclusively in the cerebral hemispheres in the frontal, frontoparietal, frontotemporal, temporoparietal and temporo-occipital regions, in the thalamus, and the corpus callosum.

### Characteristic Clinical Findings

The overwhelming majority of patients with oligodendroglioma present with focal or generalized seizures. Paresis may develop in later stages.

### Additional Diagnostic Procedures

Plain skull films reveal fine intracranial calcifications in some cases. These may take the form of irregularly distributed specks or may demonstrate a garland-like pattern resembling cortical gyri. Other preliminary studies do not provide characteristic findings that suggest the diagnosis of oligodendroglioma.

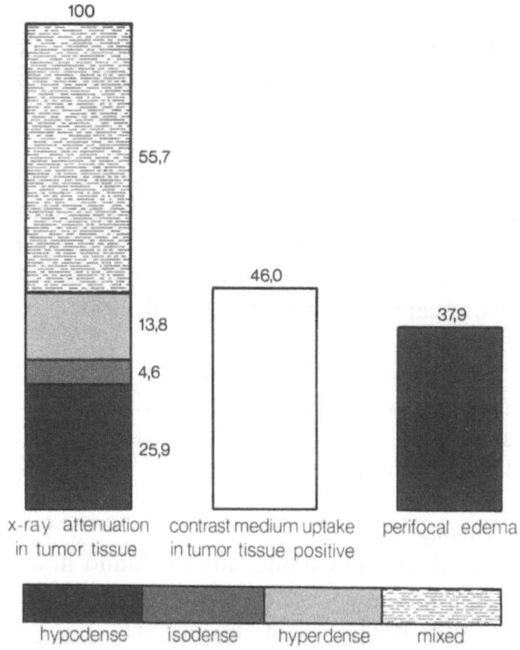


**Fig. D 1.28.** X-ray attenuation, contrast medium uptake, and frequency of edema in oligodendrogliomas (percent)

## Computed Tomography (Figs. D1.28–48)

### Precontrast Study

*Calcification is characteristic of oligodendroglioma and appears in approximately 70% of cases* (Figs. D1.29–37). Calcification may be limited to a few specks but more often appears as a large irregular area of very high density, which may follow the contours of cortical gyri (Figs. D1.30, 35). The calcified focus is sometimes surrounded by hypodense tumor (Fig. D1.33). However, surrounding tissue may also appear isodense, and the true extent of the tumor is not recognizable (Fig. D1.30). In a number of cases we found a much larger tumor at operation than we had expected on the basis of visible calcification in the CT scan.

Oligodendrogliomas are sometimes homogeneously isodense and therefore not detectable in a few of these cases. CT studies rarely demonstrate cysts in oligodendrogliomas (Fig. D1.45).

Approximately one-fourth of all oligodendrogliomas in our series appeared as a hypodense zone of the sort found in fibrillary or protoplasmatic astrocytoma without evidence of calcification (Figs. D1.39–41).

*Calcification is less frequently seen in anaplastic oligodendroglioma,* which most often demonstrates a combination of isodense and hypodense zones (Figs. D1.43, 44). Entirely isodense and slightly hypodense anaplastic oligodendrogliomas are also found (Figs. D1.46, 47). The appearance of edema in anaplastic oligodendroglioma will be discussed below.

Hemorrhage is a rare finding in anaplastic oligodendroglioma (Fig. D1.48).

### Postcontrast Study

Low-grade oligodendrogliomas do not take up contrast media, while anaplastic and polymorphic oligodendrogliomas (grade III) usually demonstrate a significant increase in density in the solid uncalcified portions of the tumor (Figs. D1.37, 42–46). Contrast application results in homogeneous enhancement or a ring structure in rare cases. Both figures may be surrounded by perifocal edema, in some cases involving the entire hemisphere. This type of edema can be found in 70%–80% of all anaplastic oligodendrogliomas. Computed tomography usually fails to differentiate between perifocal edema and hypodense tumor in low-grade oligodendrogliomas.

**Differential Diagnosis**

Aside from oligodendroglioma the following intracranial lesions may demonstrate *pathological supratentorial calcification* in the CT scan.

1. *Pilocytic Astrocytoma.* This tumor is usually located in the temporal lobe and often contains cysts, but it may also be found in the parietal or occipital lobes and may demonstrate homogeneous calcification (Figs. D1.128, 129).

2. *Gangliocytoma.* This is a very rare tumor usually located in the temporobasal region, occasionally in the frontal or parietal lobe. Both calcification and cysts are common.

3. *Meningioma.* Meningiomas rarely demonstrate calcification similar to that found in oligodendroglioma. Differentiation is usually fairly easy after contrast enhancement.

4. *Ependymoma.* The tumor is most often found in the triangle formed by the parietal, temporal, and occipital lobes. One finds both calcification and large cysts in typical cases. Incidence is highest in younger patients.

5. *Arteriovenous Malformation.* Arteriovenous malformations may resemble oligodendrogliomas in the plain CT scan, but the diagnosis is almost always evident after contrast enhancement. Definitive diagnosis is the province of cerebral angiography.

6. *Sturge-Weber Syndrome (Encephalotrigeminal Syndrome).* The conspicuous cavernous hemangioma in the cutaneous distribution of the second and third branches of the trigeminal nerve makes this diagnosis obvious. Intracranial findings include very extensive garland-like calcification, usually in the temporo-parieto-occipital region. Diagnostic problems may arise when the facial hemangioma is absent and intracranial calcification is limited (Fig. F59).

7. *Tuberculoma.* Circumscribed solitary calcification may be found in tuberculoma. These lesions are currently quite rare in Central Europe, but frequent in Central and South America.

8. *Cysticercosis.* One most often finds multiple circular calcifications, and this facilitates diagnosis. The disease is quite rare in Europe.

9. *Other Types of Calcification.* Old intracerebral hematomas may also demonstrate calcification in rare cases. The same is true of brain abscess treated conservatively.

The differential diagnosis of hypodense oligodendroglioma is discussed in detail in the section on grade II astrocytoma (see p. 24).

## d) Mixed Gliomas

In addition to astrocytomas and oligodendrogliomas there is a group of mixed tumors composed of portions of both types of tumor and designated mixed glioma or oligoastrocytoma. Five percent of gliomas with low-grade malignancy belong to this group. In Table 1 the mixed gliomas are grouped with oligodendrogliomas, because both of these tumors are quite variable in their appearance in CT scans. One finds solid isodense and hypodense regions, calcification, and – occasionally – cysts, a picture also found in oligodendroglioma. Figures D1.49–52 provide representative CT findings in these tumors.

In a few cases mixed gliomas may have anaplastic characteristics and may take up contrast media (Fig. D1.52).

## e) Diffuse Gliomatosis

Diffuse gliomatosis of the brain is an extremely rare condition with diffuse growth of astrocytic or oligodendrocytic tumor cells throughout one or both cerebral hemispheres. The brain stem may also be involved. The condition may also be termed "astrocytomatosis cerebri" or "oligodendrogliomatosis cerebri," depending on the predominant tumor cell type. Local anaplasia resembling glioblastoma has also been observed.

Unilateral diffuse gliomatosis appears as a generalized increase in volume of one cerebral hemisphere. In the two such cases we observed, brain tissue density was normal, and contrast studies were negative (Figs. D1.53, 54). The CT picture closely resembles an isodense chronic subdural hematoma, though the latter can always be delineated with administration of large doses of contrast medium (Fig. F52, p. 436).

In a third patient with a diffusely growing astrocytoma we found involvement of both cerebral hemispheres, with calcification in the tumor and focal anaplasia which demonstrated contrast enhancement (Fig. D1.55).

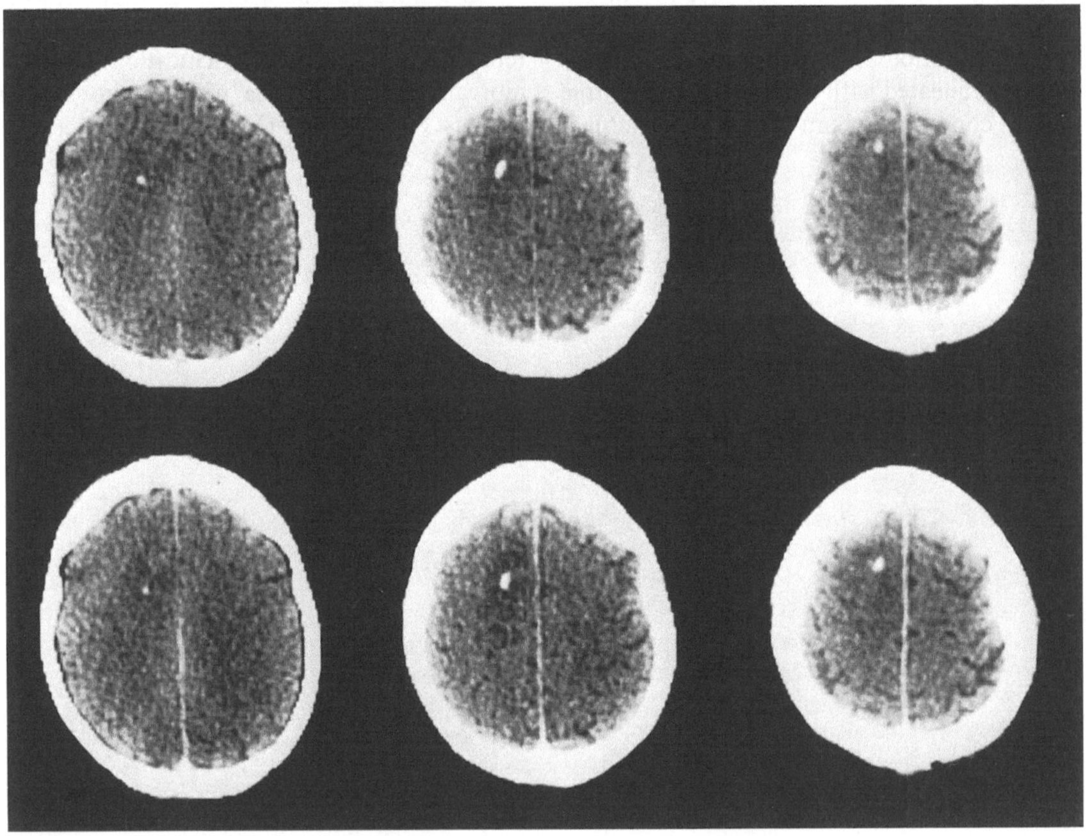

**Fig. D1.29.** Oligodendroglioma in the left precentral region in a 30-year-old male with seizures. The tumor is slightly hypodense and ill-defined against the surrounding brain tissue. Fine nodular calcification at the center of the tumor. Absence of contrast uptake (below)

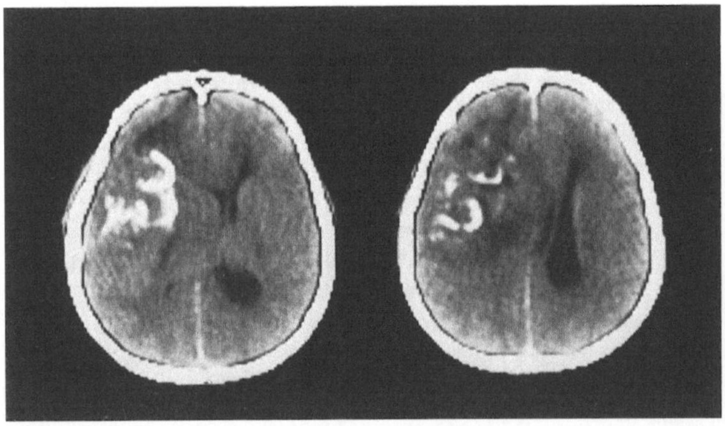

▲

**Fig. D1.30.** Oligodendroglioma of the left frontotemporal region in a 51-year-old female. Garland-like calcification within a tumor area of isodense and hypodense attenuation values. Significant mass effect. Absence of contrast uptake. Typical CT appearance of oligodendroglioma

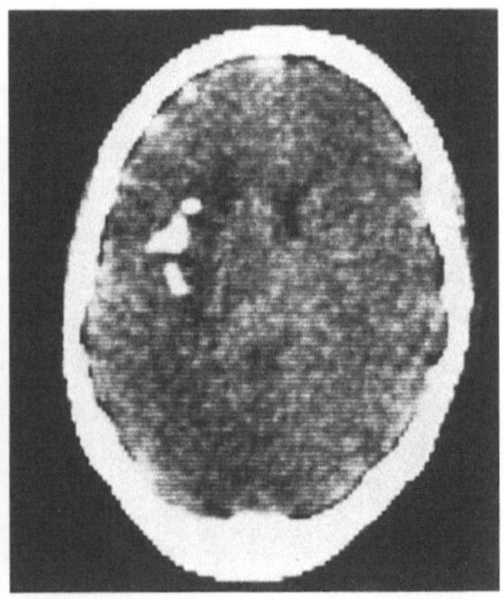

▲

**Fig. D1.31.** Oligodendroglioma in the left frontotemporal white matter in a 32-year-old female. Several zones of calcification and a hypodense tumor region. Typical CT appearance (precontrast CT)

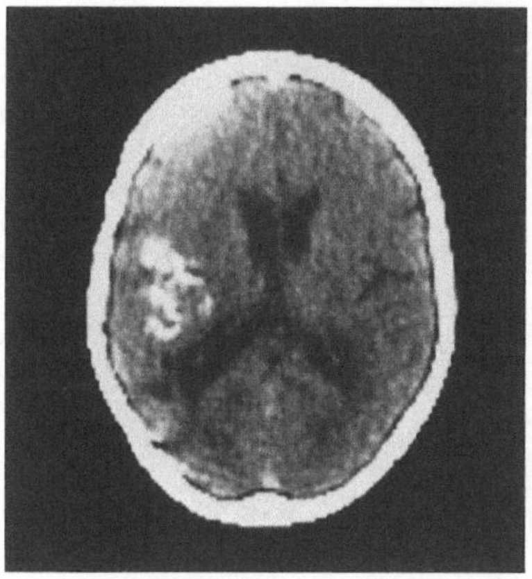

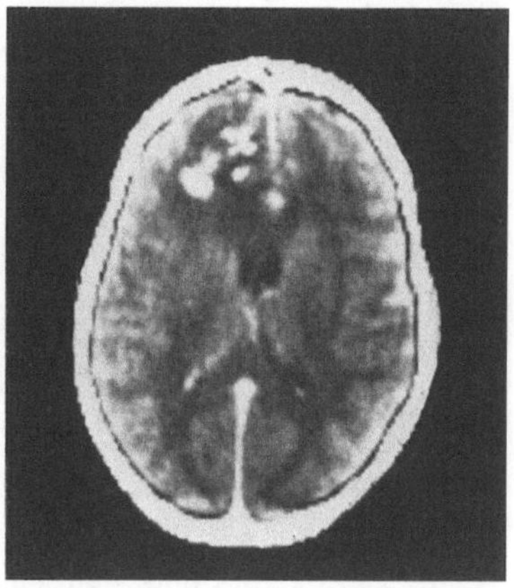

**Fig. D1.32.** Oligodendroglioma in the left temporal region of a 66-year-old male. Extensive calcification following the cortical gyri in the insular cistern. At operation the tumor proved to be larger than expected from the CT scan, since isodense portions of the tumor were discovered (precontrast study)

**Fig. D1.33.** Oligodendroglioma in the left frontal lobe of a 29-year-old male. Typical calcification within the hypodense tumor which extends into the anterior part of the corpus callosum and the right cerebral hemisphere. Absence of significant contrast uptake in the tumor

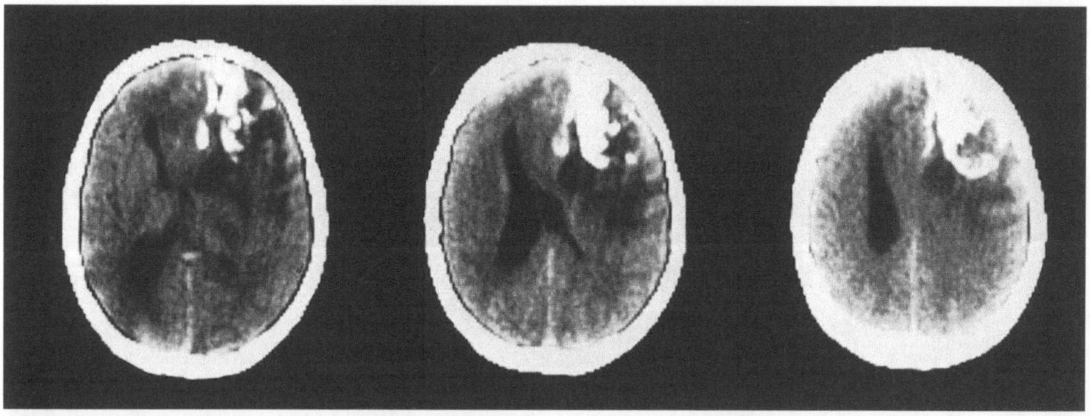

**Fig. D1.34.** Large anaplastic oligodendroglioma in the right precentral region with widely varying density values within the tumor. Irregular calcifications, cysts, and isodense zones. The tumor involves the anterior corpus callosum and the septum pellucidum. Significant perifocal edema. Slight contrast uptake in the frontomedial portions of the tumor (middle)

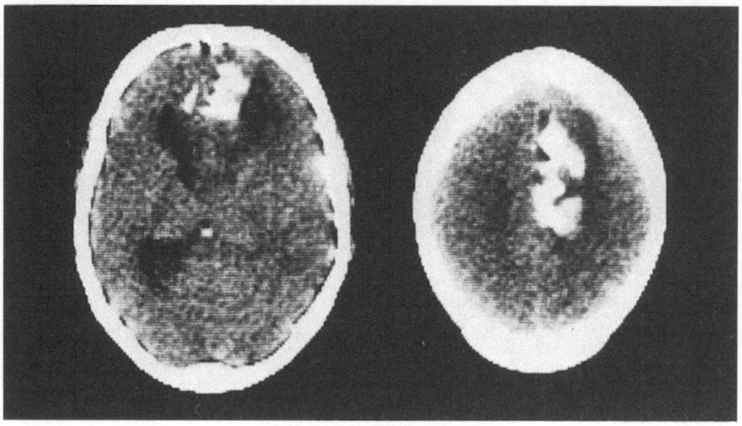

**Fig. D1.35.** Oligodendroglioma in the right fronto precentral region of a 36-year-old man with seizures. Calcifications following the gyri are the characteristic pattern of this tumor. Isodense and hypodense zones are found in the anterior portions of the tumor and extend to the corpus callosum and the septum pellucidum. Exact demarcation of the tumor is not possible in the CT (precontrast study)

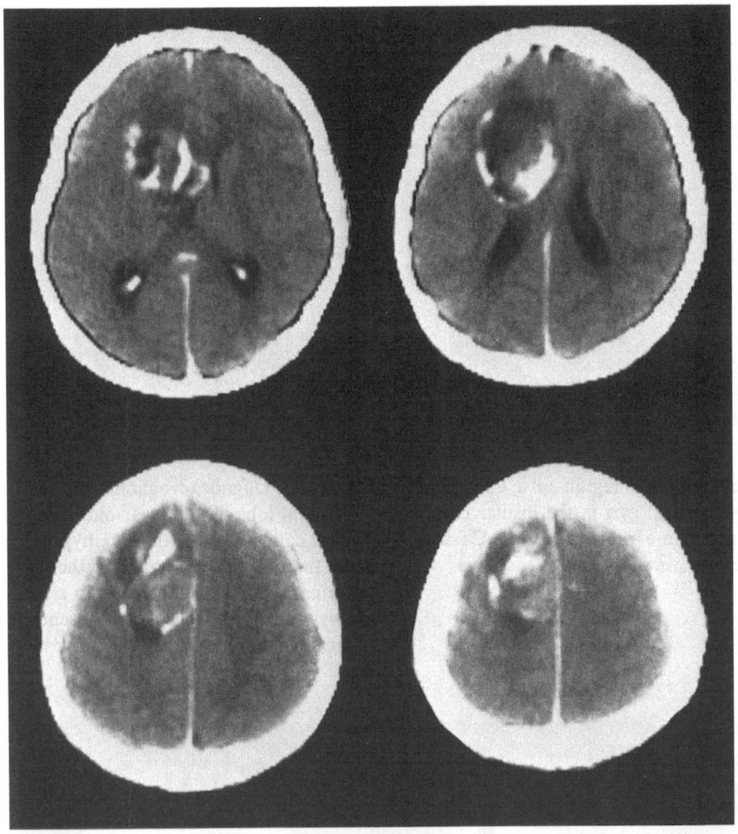

**Fig. D1.36.** Oligodendroglioma in the left precentral region with anaplastic portions in a 25-year-old patient. Typical CT pattern in the tumor: shell-like calcifications with isodense and hypodense zones. The tumor has penetrated the corpus callosum near the septum pellucidum and is relatively well delineated. Absence of significant contrast enhancement (postcontrast CT)
◄

**Fig. D1.37.** Anaplastic oligodendroglioma in the left temporal lobe. Typical calcifications within an isodense and hypodense area (upper series, precontrast CT). Postcontrast CT reveals enhancement in the solid uncalcified portions of the tumor which demonstrates the true extent of the lesion. Improved demarcation of perifocal edema (lower series)
▼

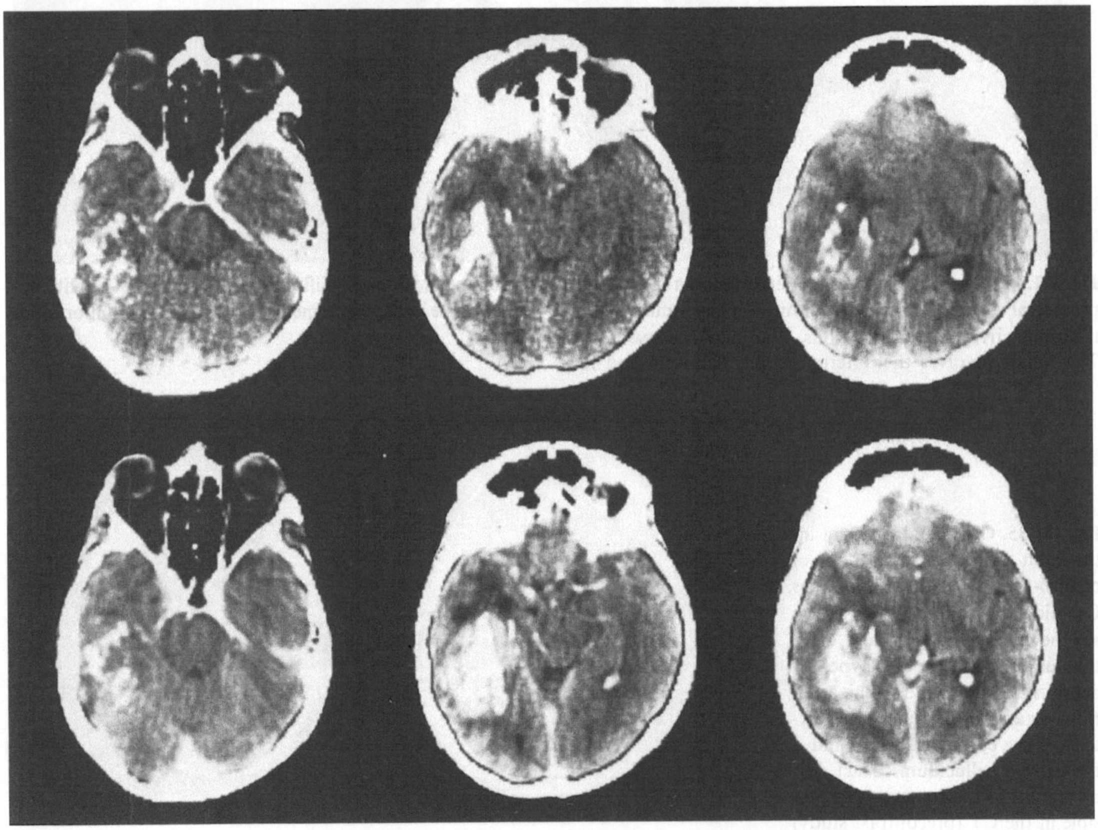

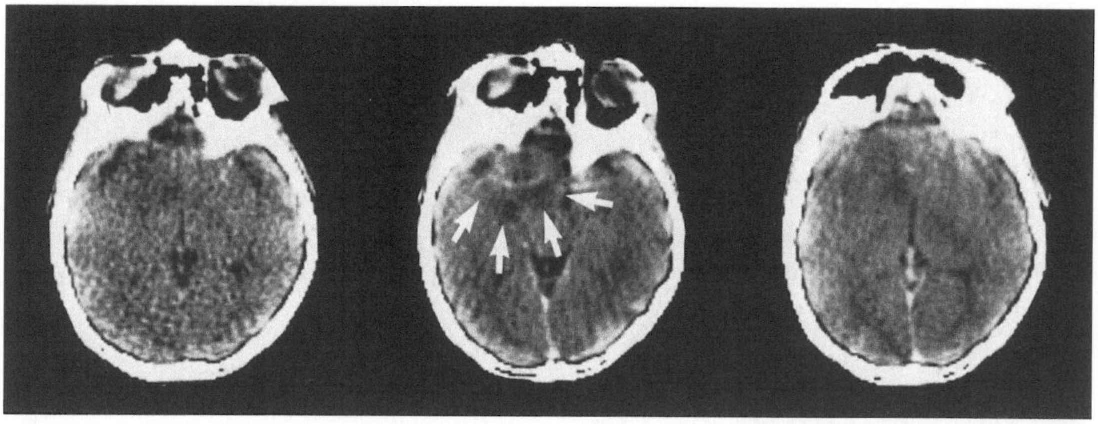

**Fig. D1.38.** Oligodendroglioma in the pole of the left temporal lobe with isodense and hypodense portions in a 22-year-old patient with psychomotor seizures (arrows). Demonstration of the tumor was possible only in special sections parallel to the orbit (left: precontrast CT; right and middle: postcontrast CT)

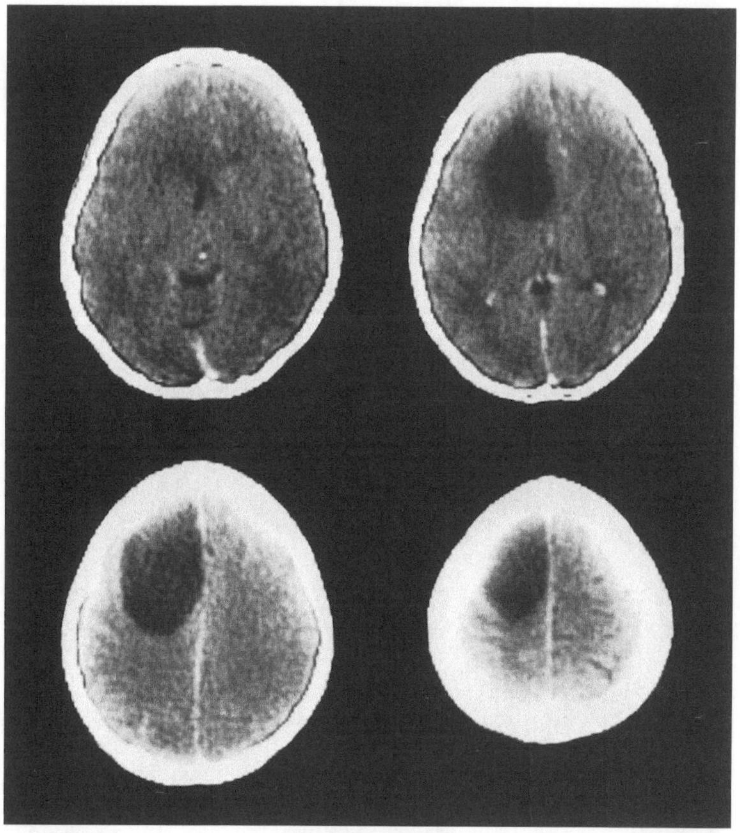

**Fig. D1.39.** Oligodendroglioma in the left precentral region of a 31-year-old patient. Absence of calcification and homogeneous hypodense values within the tumor do not allow differentiation from astrocytoma. No significant increase in attenuation values in postcontrast CT

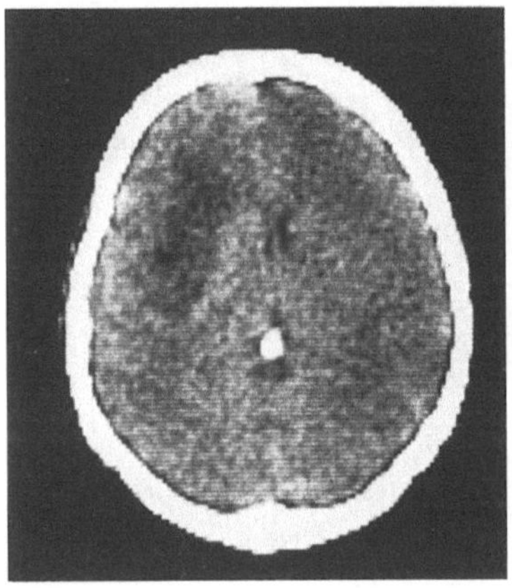

▲
**Fig. D1.40.** Oligodendroglioma in the left frontotemporal white matter in a 33-year-old man. Absence of calcification does not allow differentiation from astrocytoma at the same location

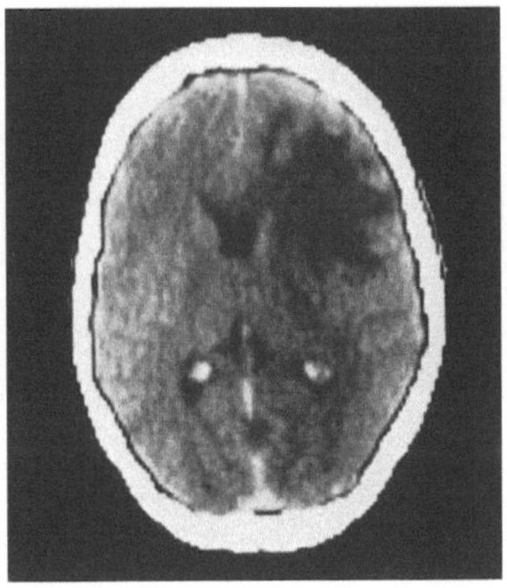

▲
**Fig. D1.41.** Oligodendroglioma in the right frontotemporal white matter with indistinct borders. Extension of the tumor follows the distribution of the white matter. Density values within the tumor identical to those of low-grade astrocytoma (22 HU). Differentiation of these tumor types is not possible with CT studies

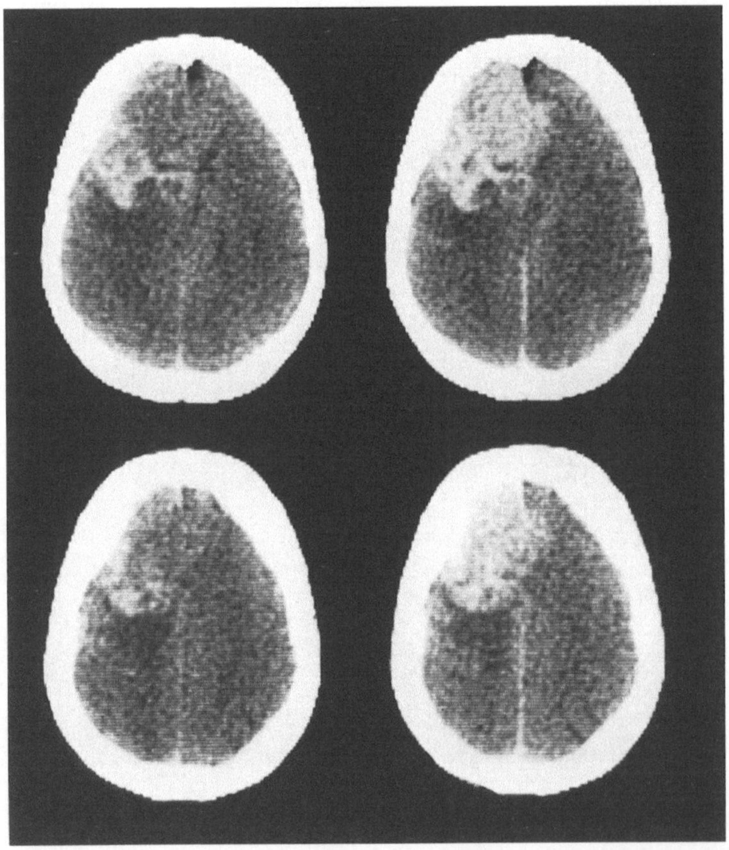

**Fig. D1.42.** Anaplastic oligodendroglioma in the left precentral region of a 55-year-old male. Precontrast studies (left) reveal hyperdense and isodense values in the tumor tissue. Hypodense values due to perifocal edema at the parietal margin of the tumor. Postcontrast studies demonstrate the true extent of the tumor, which has extended over the midline and infiltrated the corpus callosum. Falx meningioma was considered as a possible alternative in the differential diagnosis of this tumor

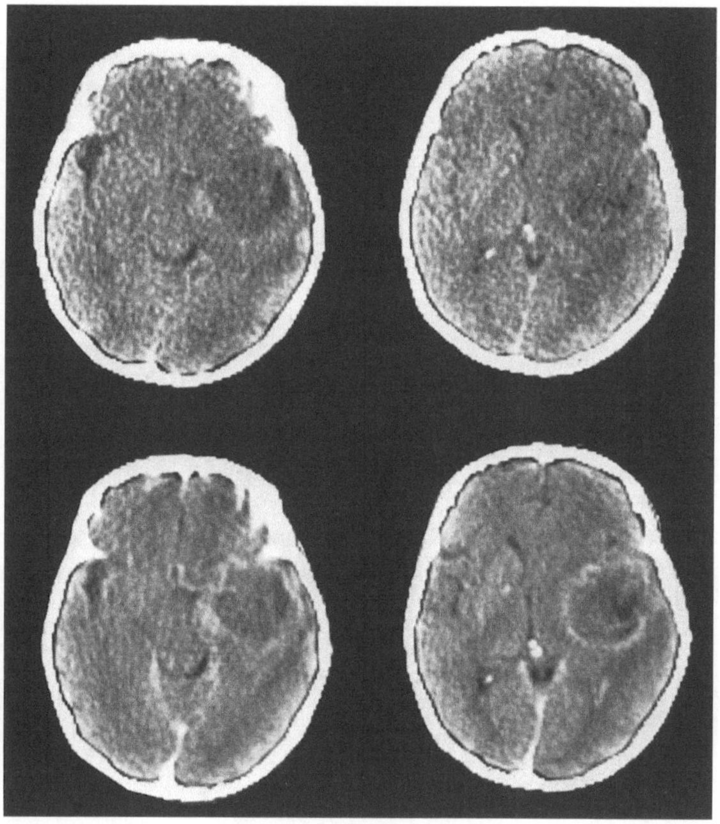

**Fig. D1.43.** Anaplastic oligodendroglioma in the right temporal lobe of a 51-year-old patient. Precontrast studies (above) demonstrate ring structures with a central hypodense area. Postcontrast studies (below) reveal slight contrast enhancement at the margins of the tumor. CT findings are similar to those in glioblastoma

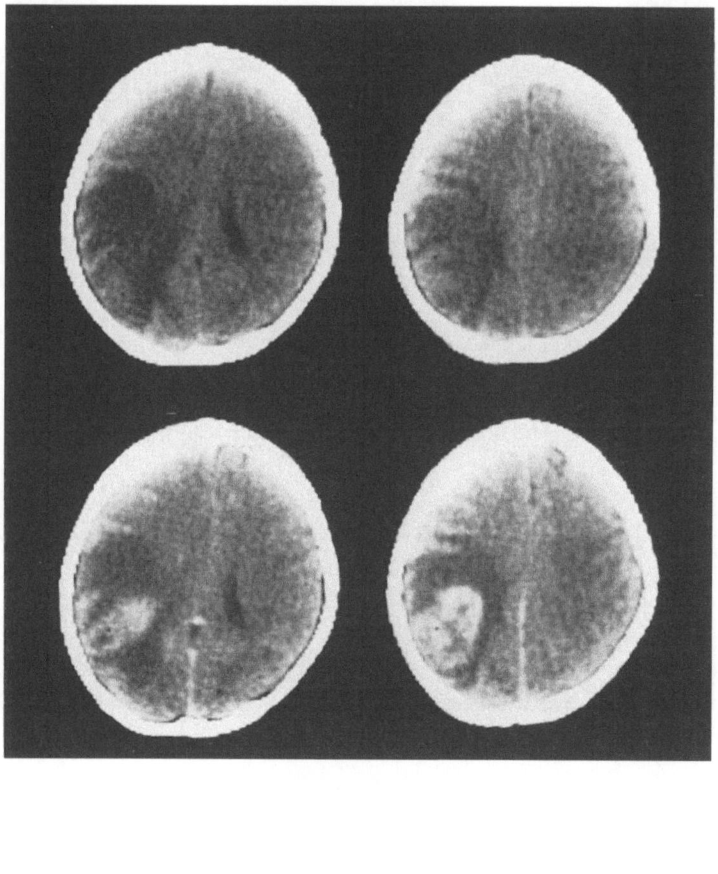

**Fig. D1.44.** Anaplastic oligodendroglioma in the left parietal region of a 42-year-old patient. Precontrast studies (above) show a circumscribed isodense area within an extensive hypodense zone. Postcontrast studies (below) demonstrate a large almost homogeneous tumor nodule with grade II perifocal edema. CT findings alone do not allow differentiation between this tumor and anaplastic astrocytoma, glioblastoma, or metastasis

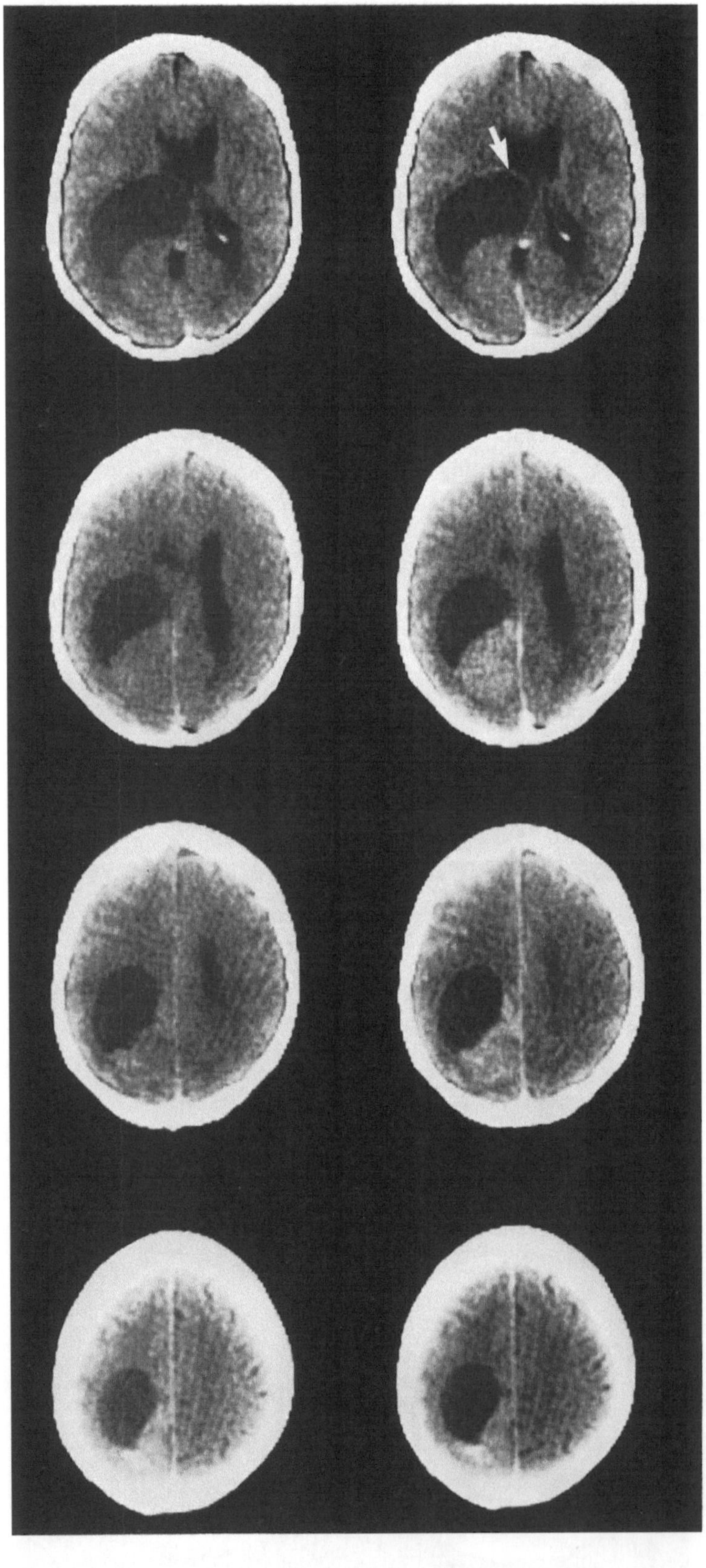

**Fig. D 1.45.** Very extensive anaplastic oligodendroglioma in the central and posterior segments of the left cerebral hemisphere with isodense, hypodense, and hyperdense portions (corresponding to solid tumor, cysts, and calcification). Postcontrast studies demonstrate contrast enhancement in the solid portions of the tumor and slight enhancement at the margin of the cyst with clear demarcation of the latter from the left lateral ventricle (arrow). Precontrast studies on the left, postcontrast studies on the right (36-year-old male)

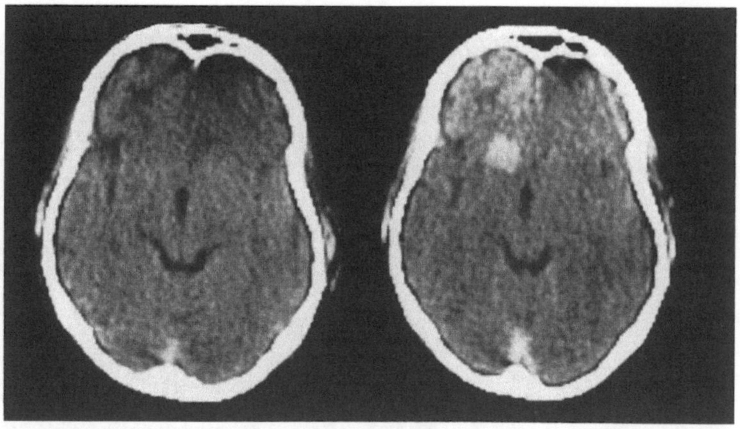

**Fig. D 1.46.** Primarily isodense anaplastic oligodendroglioma near the left basal ganglia of a 32-year-old male. Precontrast CT is completely normal and fails to demonstrate the tumor, perifocal edema, or signs of displacement. Postcontrast CT (right) reveals homogeneous contrast enhancement of the tumor located below the head of the caudate nucleus

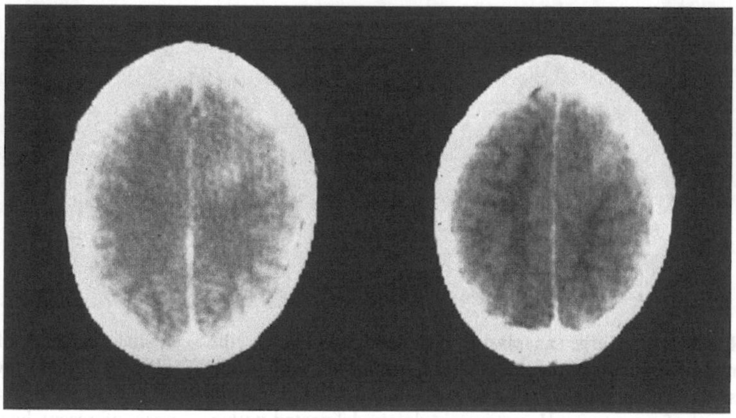

**Fig. D 1.47.** Anaplastic oligodendroglioma in the white matter of the right cerebral hemisphere of a 15-year-old boy with seizures. The primarily isodense tumor demonstrates slight homogeneous contrast enhancement. (Postcontrast CT)

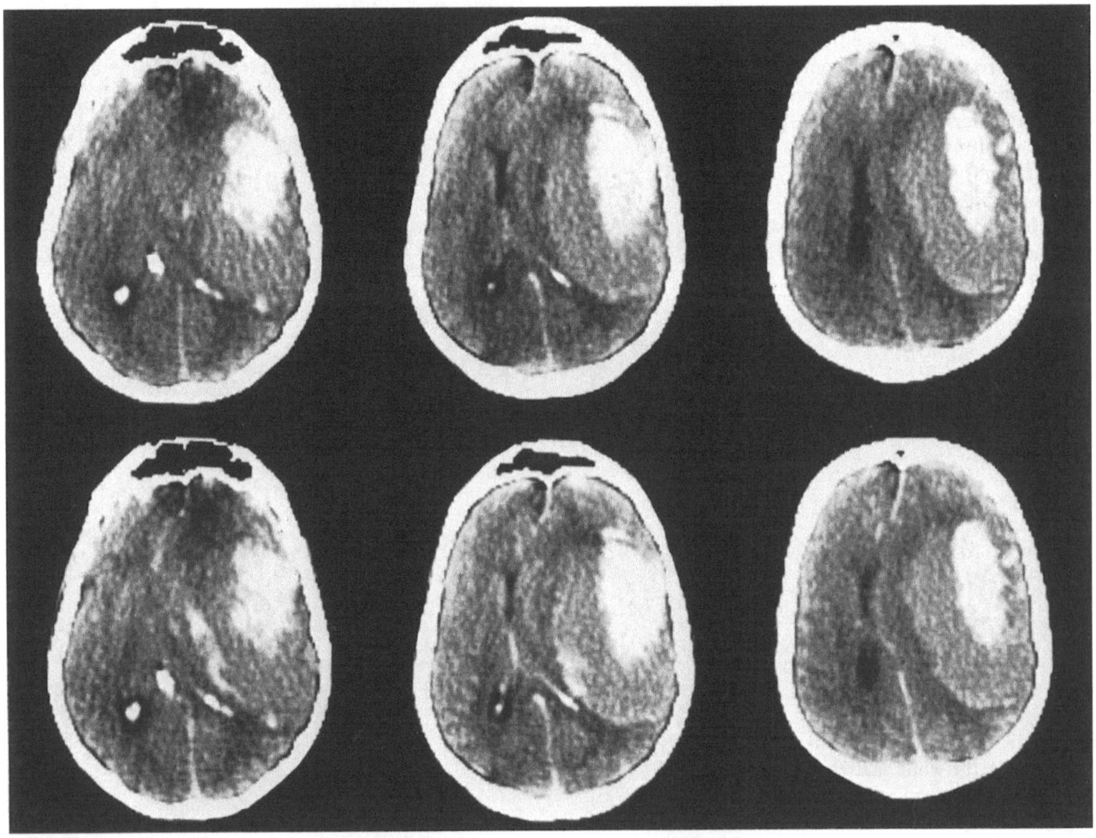

**Fig. D 1.48.** Large anaplastic oligodendroglioma in the middle segments of the right cerebral hemisphere with extensive recent hemorrhage in a 60-year-old patient with abrupt onset of symptoms. Hematoma is clearly delineated within the slightly hyperdense portion of the tumor. Postcontrast studies (below) reveal marginal contrast enhancement in the medial segments of the tumor near the lateral ventricle, which suggested the diagnosis of hemorrhage within a tumor. Extreme displacement of midline structures. CT diagnosis of recent hemorrhage is based on very high density values (+80 to +84 HU)

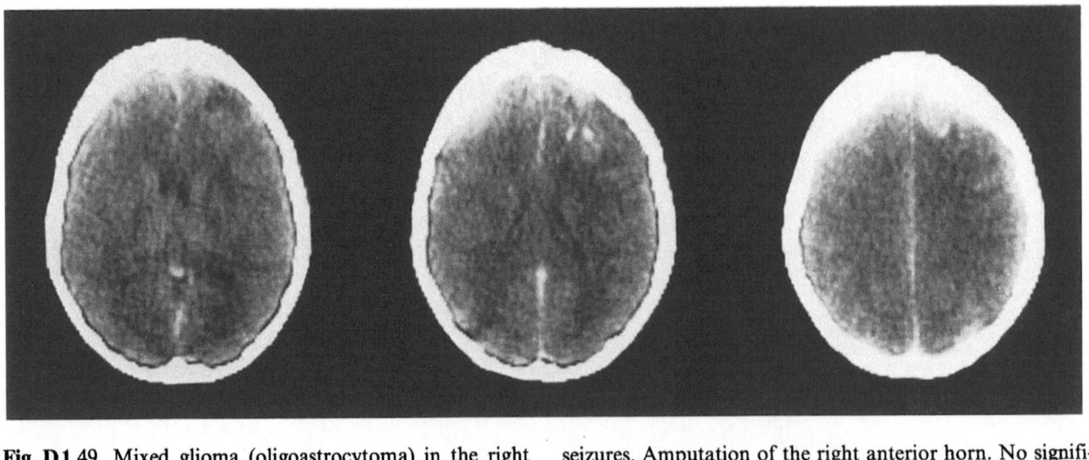

**Fig. D 1.49.** Mixed glioma (oligoastrocytoma) in the right frontal region with isodense, hyperdense, and hypodense zones in the right frontal lobe of a 26-year-old female with seizures. Amputation of the right anterior horn. No significant contrast enhancement of the tumor (postcontrast CT)

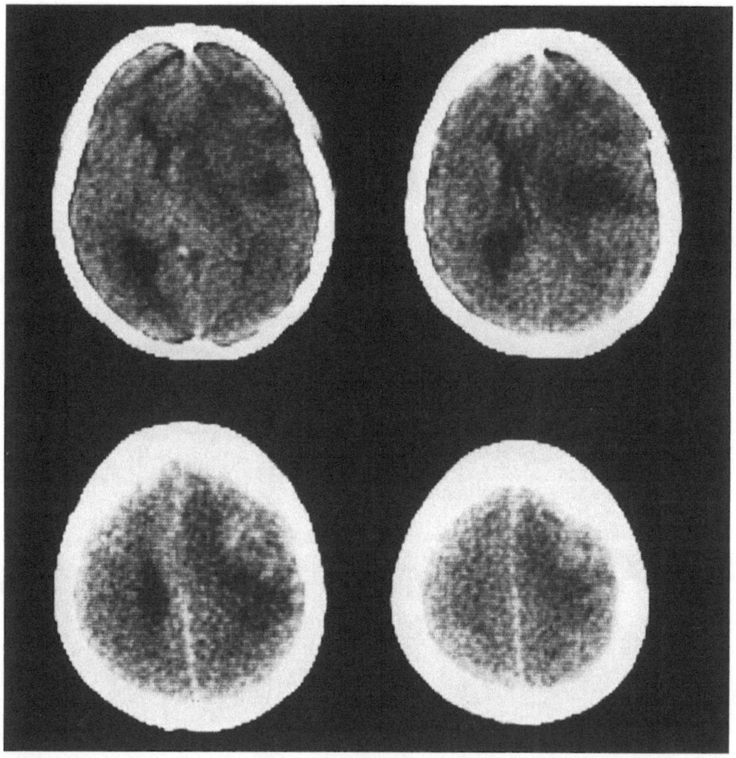

**Fig. D1.50.** Mixed glioma (oligoastrocytoma) in the right frontal lobe of a 42-year-old female with seizures. The tumor contains areas of varying density. Spotty contrast enhancement suggests anaplasia within the tumor

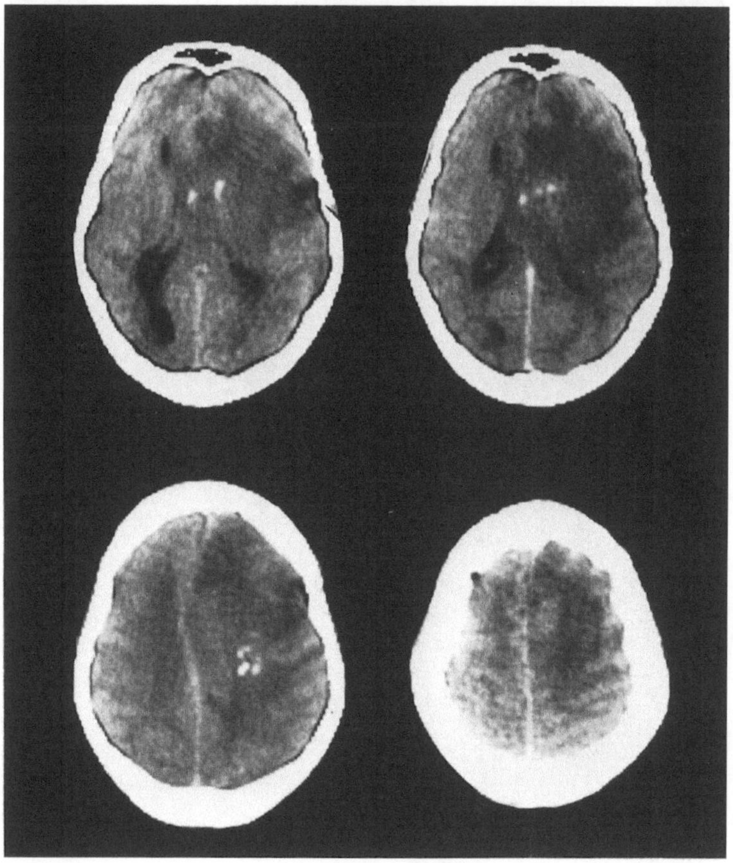

**Fig. D1.51.** Mixed glioma (oligoastrocytoma) in the right cerebral hemisphere with infiltration of the corpus callosum in a 30-year-old man with seizures. The tumor is predominantly hypodense. Central hyperdense spots due to circumscribed calcifications. CT appearance identical to that of oligodendroglioma. Absence of significant contrast enhancement

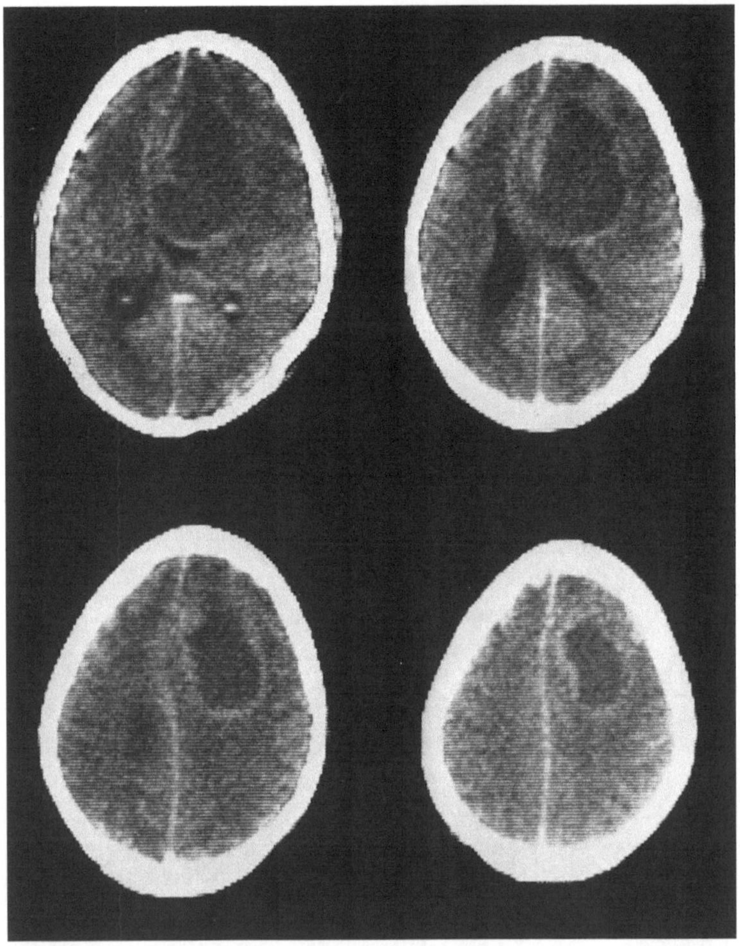

**Fig. D1.52.** Mixed glioma in the right precentral region with extension to the corpus callosum in a 23-year-old male with an organic brain syndrome and seizures. CT shows a large cystic tumor with marginal contrast enhancement as in glioblastoma. Histological examination resulted in the diagnosis of anaplastic oligoastrocytoma. Postcontrast study

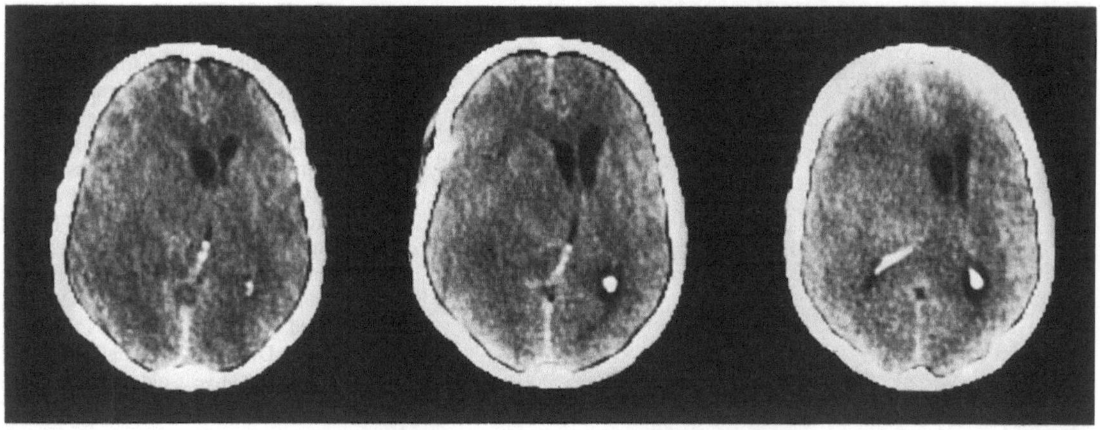

a

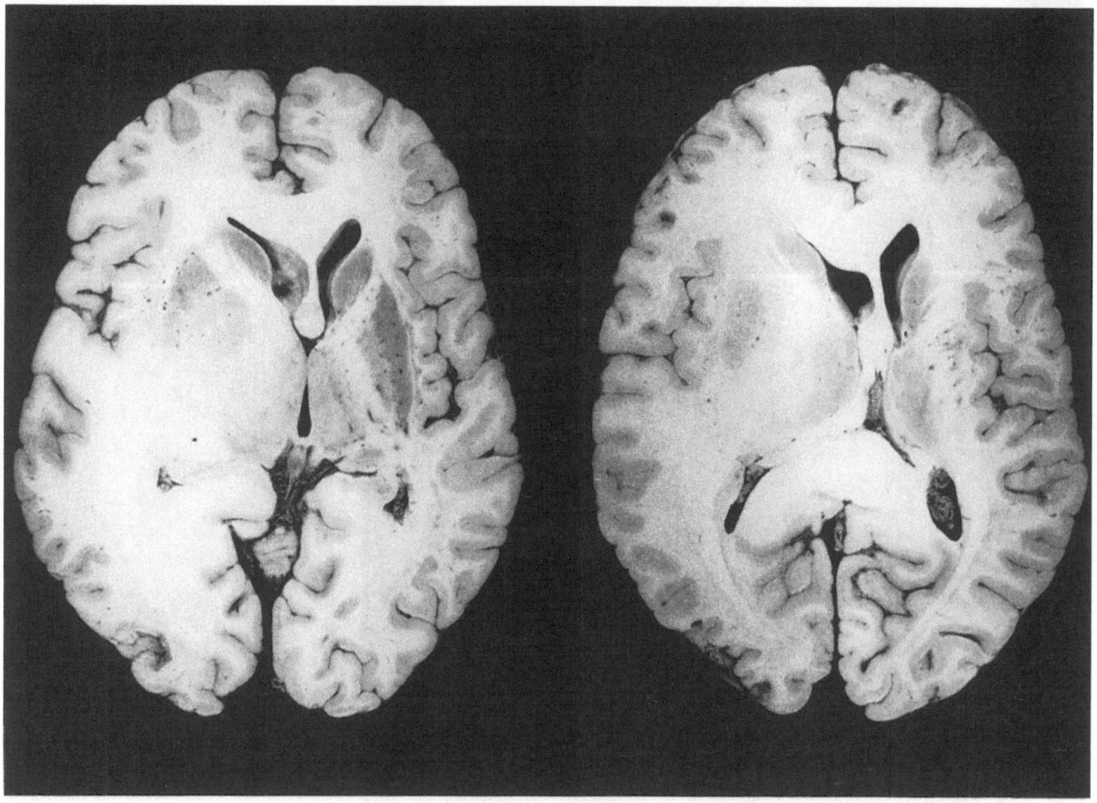

b

**Fig. D1.53** a, b. Diffuse gliomatosis of the left cerebral hemisphere in a 72-year-old male. (**a**) Diffuse enlargement of the entire left hemisphere in the CT scan without changes in X-ray absorption. Initial diagnosis was isodense chronic subdural hematoma. (**b**) The postmortem examination showed diffuse distension of the left cerebral hemisphere with partial extinction of the structures of the basal ganglia. Marked thickening of the corpus callosum. Histological examination provided the diagnosis of diffuse astrocytic gliomatosis. (Courtesy of Priv.-Doz. Dr. Gisela EBHARDT, Neuropathological Institute, Free University of Berlin)

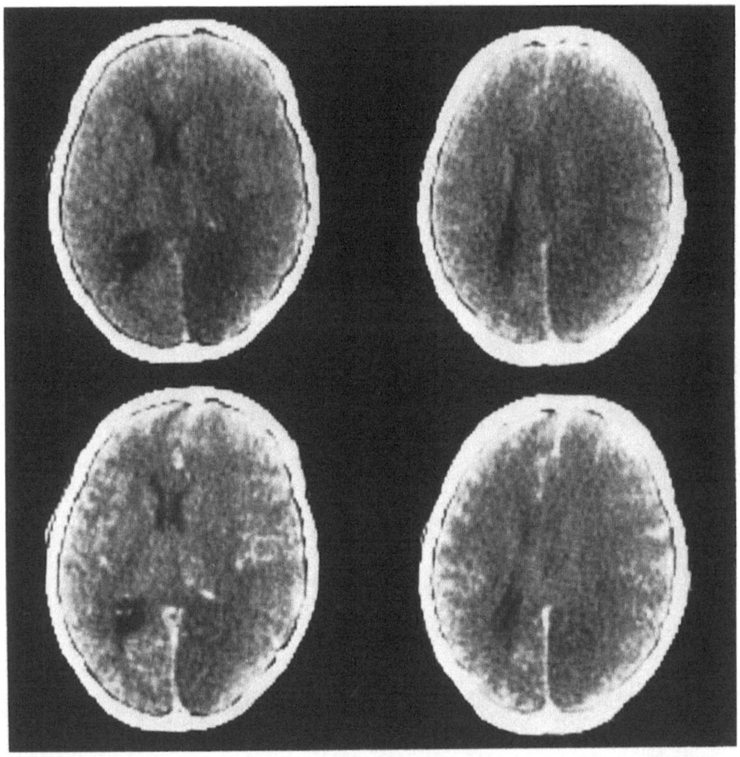

**Fig. D1.54.** Diffuse gliomatosis of the entire right hemisphere without evident alteration of attenuation values. The large hypodense zone in the left occipital lobe is the result of infarction due to thrombosis of the transversal and rectus sinuses. Density values in the rectus sinus are increased in precontrast studies (above right). Postcontrast studies (below) reveal diffuse spotty contrast enhancement in the congested and dilated veins, typical of sinus thrombosis. Diagnosis was confirmed at autopsy. (34-year-old female)

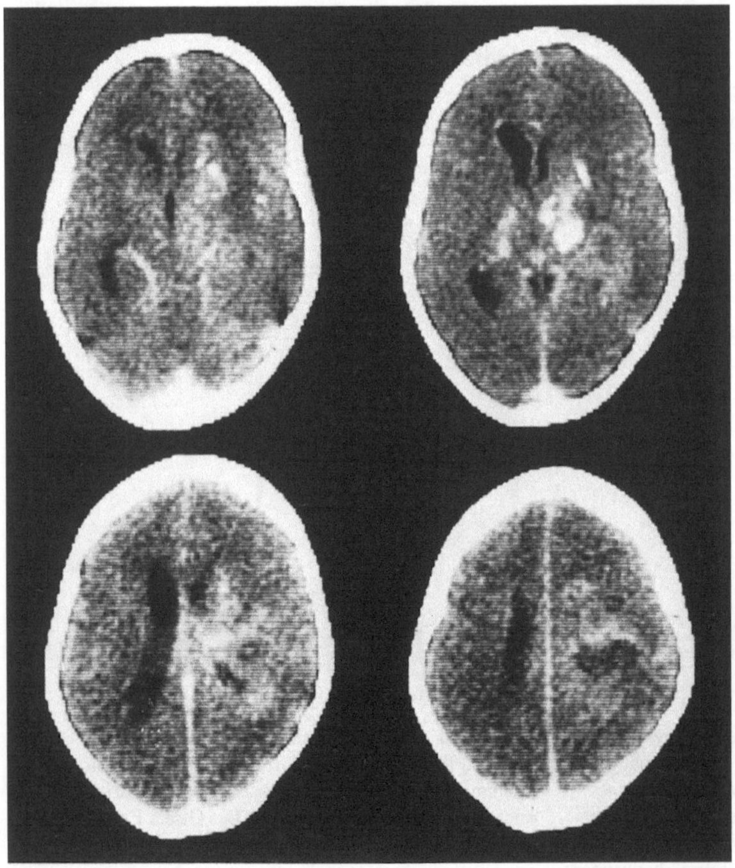

**Fig. D1.55a**

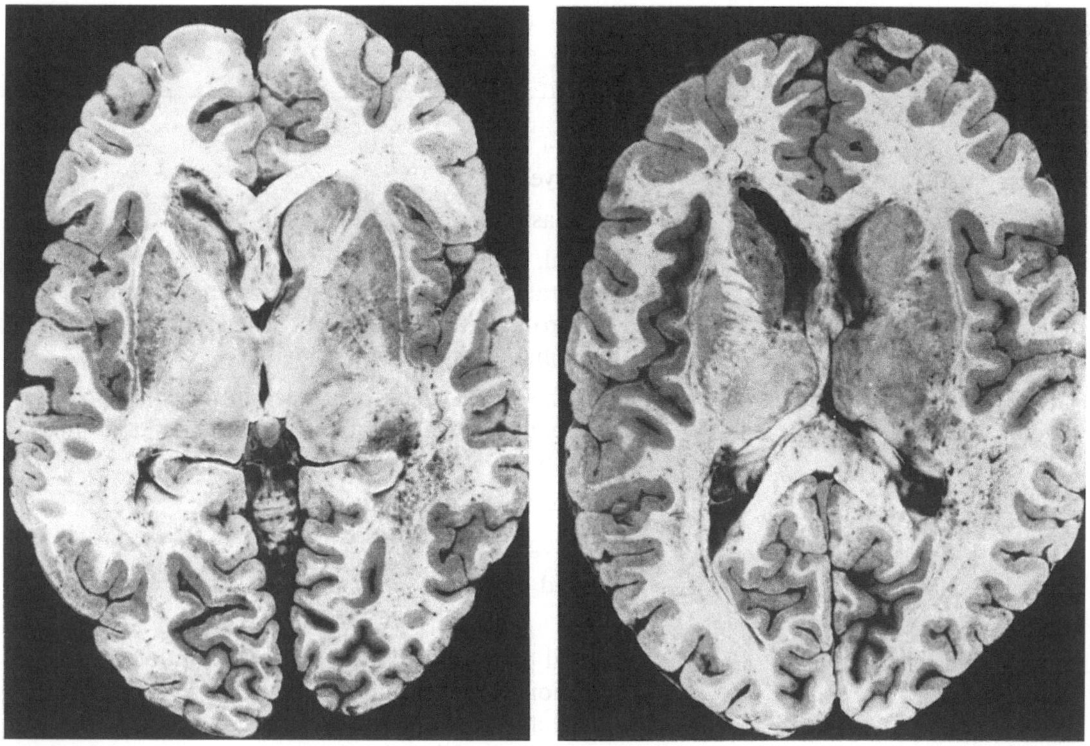

**Fig. D1.55b**

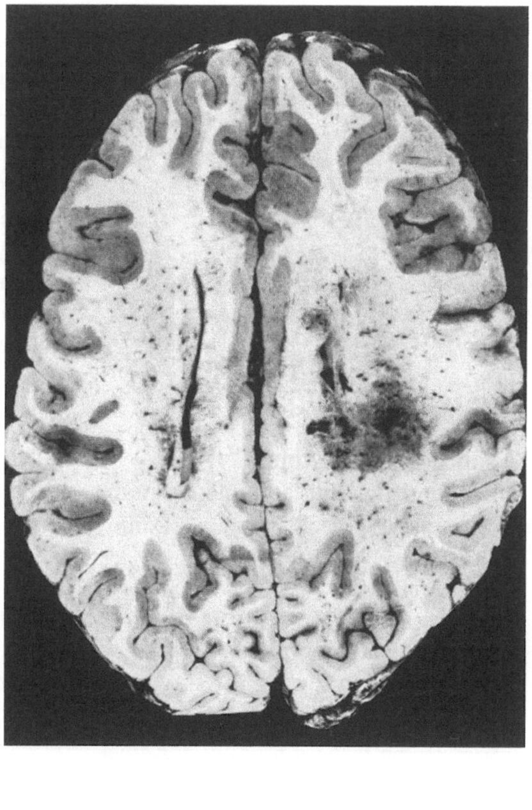

**Fig. D1.55.** (**a**) Diffuse growth of astrocytoma in both cerebral hemispheres with multifocal anaplasia and calcification. Significant contrast enhancement in postcontrast CT studies. (**b**) Brain specimen from the same patient shows diffuse tumor growth in both cerebral hemispheres (12-year-old child with seizures)

## f) Glioblastomas

| | |
|---|---|
| Incidence | 12–20% |
| Characteristic age at diagnosis | 40–65 years |
| Sex distribution | Twice as common in males as in females |
| Typical locations | Frontal, frontomedial, frontolateral, frontodorsal, temporal, temporomedial including basal ganglia, temporo-parieto-occipital, corpus callosum ("butterfly glioma"), and occipital region |
| Characteristic clinical findings | Short history; signs of increased intracranial pressure; major neurological deficits; organic brain syndrome |
| Skull film | Displacement of the pineal body |
| EEG | Pathological findings in almost all cases |
| Echoencephalography | Marked displacement of midline structures in most cases |
| Serial brain scintigraphy | Typical pattern of radionuclide distribution in the perfusion phase; progressive increase in radionuclide uptake and characteristic changes in distribution from early to delayed scans |
| Cerebral angiography | Signs of a space-occupying lesion with demonstration of typical tumor vessels: arteriovenous fistulas with early filling veins, sinusoid vessels; failure to demonstrate vessels in 10% of tumors due to necrosis |

**Computed Tomography**

| | |
|---|---|
| Precontrast study | Combination of isodense and hypodense zones; marked displacement of normal structures; hemorrhage in some cases |
| Contrast medium uptake | Positive in almost all cases |
| Appearance after contrast enhancement | Ring structures and garland figures with increased density in many cases, sometimes combined with solid tumor nodules; centrally located hypodense zones due to necrosis or cysts; extensive perifocal edema in most cases |

**Differential Diagnosis**

Anaplastic astrocytoma
Oligodendroglioma and ependymoma
Brain abscess
Metastasis
Gliosarcoma
Pilocytic astrocytoma of the cerebral hemispheres
Atypical meningioma
Brain infarction during the stage of disruption of the blood-brain barrier
Old intracerebral hematoma with rim enhancement

*Glioblastomas are the most common autochthonous brain tumors.* CUSHING reported finding glioblastoma in 10.3% of all brain tumors, while ZÜLCH found 12.2% in a series of 9,000 tumor patients. In our collective, glioblastoma comprised 19% of 3,750 tumors. The lesion is most common in the middle aged and the elderly, with peak incidence between 40 and 65 years of age. Glioblastoma is rarely found in children. Males are affected almost twice as often as females.

Glioblastomas demonstrate infiltrative and destructive growth. Extensive necrosis and hemorrhages at different stages are typical of this tumor. As a result the macroscopic appearance is extremely variegated. It is classified as a grade IV tumor.

### Typical Locations

Glioblastomas may be found in all regions of the cerebral hemispheres, the basal ganglia, and the brain stem. ZÜLCH has observed the following typical locations: frontolateral, frontodorsal, frontobasal, parietolateral, parietodorsal, occipitolateral, occipitobasal, temporolateral, and temporomedial regions with extension into the basal ganglia. The tumor may also be found in the region of the corpus callosum – the so-called "butterfly glioblastoma," in the thalamus, the quadrigeminal region, and the pons. Cerebellar glioblastomas are rare.

### Characteristic Clinical Findings

The period from first appearance of symptoms to diagnosis is very short in the majority of patients, with a maximum of 3–4 months. Signs of increased intracranial pressure develop very quickly, and severe neurological deficits appear as a function of tumor location. An organic brain syndrome is sometimes observed. Epileptic seizures may be the presenting sign.

### Additional Diagnostic Procedures

Plain skull films provide indirect evidence of a space-occupying lesion when there is displacement of the calcified pineal gland. Displacement of midline structures is frequent and can be documented with echoencephalography. The EEG almost always reveals focal activity and severe generalized changes. Dynamic brain scans show characteristic radionuclide uptake in the tumor, which increases in the late phase and demonstrates changes in shape which are characteristic of this tumor. The perfusion pattern is rather typical in glioblastomas (Fig. D1.57).

Glioblastomas are highly vascular tumors containing arteriovenous fistulas as well as small pathological vessels, which may be considered pathognomonic of glioblastoma in the angiogram. In our series 70% of histologically verified glioblastomas were correctly identified on the basis of angiographic studies alone. KRAYENBÜHL and YASARGIL (1965) reported similar results.

## Computed Tomography (Figs. D1.56–98)

### Precontrast Study

As one might expect from the morphology of the tumor, the CT scan reveals a *very inhomogeneous density pattern* (Figs. D1.56, 58–65). Isodense and hypodense areas predominate as a result of the juxtaposition of vital tumor tissue, necrosis, and perifocal edema. Seventy-one percent of patients with glioblastoma in our collective demonstrated mixed absorption patterns in precontrast CT scans (Fig. D1.56). The remaining 29.0% were distributed fairly evenly

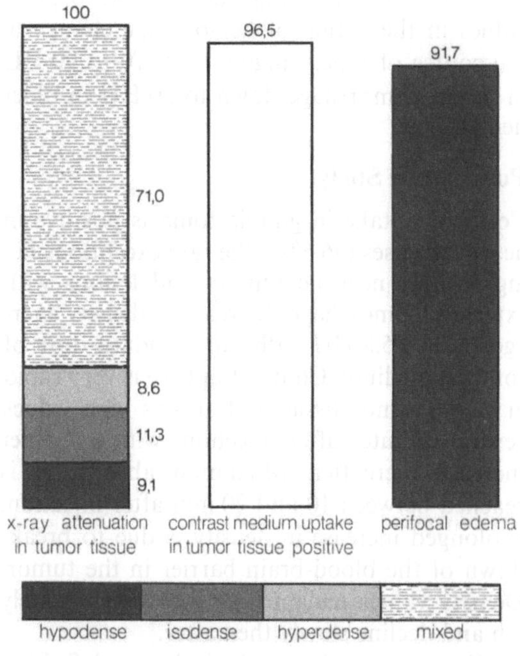


**Fig. D 1.56.** X-ray attenuation, contrast medium uptake, and frequency of edema in glioblastoma (percent)

among homogeneously hypodense, isodense, and hyperdense absorption values.

Density values in solid nonnecrotic tumor tissue differ only slightly from that of normal brain tissue. This may be explained by the nonuniform structure of the tumor, especially insofar as pathological vessels are concerned. The computer analysis reveals absorption values averaging 33–34 HU in solid tumor tissue, with a range of $\pm 4$ HU.

Glioblastomas very often contain *necrotic areas,* and *cysts* are also found. Both of the latter are low-density structures, with absorption values between 16 and 23 HU. Mean density values range from 16 to 20 HU in cysts and from 19 to 23 HU in areas of necrosis, so that overlap may occur. Cysts are usually more sharply delineated than necrotic areas. Calcification is extremely rare in glioblastoma.

Precontrast CT scans failed to demonstrate glioblastoma in only 2.3% of tumors in our series; contrast studies demonstrated the tumor in some of these cases (see Table 1), while only follow-up CT studies provided the diagnosis in a small number of cases.

*Intensely hyperdense zones in glioblastoma are very suggestive of recent or past hemorrhage into the tumor* (glioma apoplecticum) (Figs. D1.65–67). However, the tumor is not always evident when a hematoma is demonstrated in the first CT scan (Fig. D1.68). Absorption values in the region of hemorrhage change in the course of time, ranging from 70 to 90 HU in recent hemorrhage down to 30 HU in older hematomas.

**Postcontrast Study**

Contrast uptake in glioblastoma is positive in nearly all cases (96.5%), the rare exceptions being entirely necrotic tumors and lesions with extensive hemorrhage. Increase in density averaged $12.6 \pm 5.8$ HU with our standard dose of contrast medium. Contrast uptake is very rapid in viable tumor tissue and attains high values several minutes after injection, with a further increase thereafter. Maximum absorption is reached between 10 and 20 min after injection. Prolonged increase in density is due to breakdown of the blood-brain barrier in the tumor. Density values remain high for approximately 1 h and decline slowly thereafter.

Contrast uptake results in better definition of the tumor and often provides the first delineation of the actual glioblastoma within the characteristically extensive perifocal brain edema (Figs. D1.58, 60, 61). Contrast administration results in better differentiation between solid and necrotic or cystic portions of the tumor (Fig. D1.59).

Glioblastomas often appear as *ring lesions or garland-like structures* after contrast enhancement (Figs. D1.58–61, 71–79, 81–85, 87–98). This is a function of the projection in the particular scan. Ring structures of all types were found in 83.9% of glioblastomas in our series. Glioblastomas may also contain large solid nodular structures.

Glioblastomas which appear *exclusively as homogeneous nodules of solid tumor tissue* in the CT scan have been demonstrated *much less frequently* since the introduction of thinner slices and higher density resolution (Fig. D1.62).

Approximately 5% of glioblastomas contain *large cysts* and show a relatively narrow border of solid tissue or a marginal knot of tumor tissue (Figs. D1.59, 73). *Demonstration of contrast medium uptake in cyst fluid* is rare. Sedimentation of contrast material within the cyst may be observed (see Fig. D1.74). This phenomenon is a reliable criterion for differentiation of cystic and necrotic tumor portions (AFRA et al. 1980).

*Glioblastoma in the earliest stages* presents, with an area of low density which does not readily take up contrast media. Follow-up studies are absolutely necessary in these cases. A circumscribed area of tumor which increases in density after contrast enhancement usually appears within days or weeks (Fig. D1.70).

Glioblastoma very often is associated with *brain edema,* in 91.7% of cases in our series. Edema varies greatly in extent; grade I edema was found in 24.5%, grade II in 57.7%, and grade III in 17.8%. Size of the glioblastoma has no influence on the extent of edema, and a relatively small glioblastoma may produce edema extending throughout an entire hemisphere, while large glioblastomas may show a very small margin of edema (Figs. D1.69, 94).

Clinical findings and CT analysis allowed a correct diagnosis of glioblastoma in 70% of cases, and the diagnosis glioblastoma was included among the probable differential diagnoses in an additional 12% (STEINHOFF et al. 1977). Accuracy has increased to over 80% in the last 100 patients with glioblastoma examined with CT systems offering improved density resolution.

*The following criteria are characteristic of glioblastoma:*

1. Demonstration of an irregular ring which sometimes has a garland-like appearance. Contrast enhancement of the ring usually diminishes in the course of steroid therapy
2. Single or multiple irregular centrally located low-density zones which represent necrotic areas
3. Typical locations, such as the corpus callosum, basal ganglia, and frontal and temporal lobe.

## Differential Diagnosis

Differential diagnosis includes all lesions which demonstrate a ring structure after contrast enhancement, unless located in the posterior fossa, where glioblastoma is extremely rare (one case in our series). Table 3 shows the frequency of ring structures in the postcontrast CT with the most common intracranial tumors and in brain abscess (KAZNER et al. 1978).

**Table 3.** Incidence of ring enhancement in CT studies of brain tumors and abscess (KAZNER et al. 1978)

| Diagnosis | Number of patients | Ring enhancement (not including combination of ring and solid tumor nodule) | |
|---|---|---|---|
| | | *n* | % |
| Pilocytic astrocytoma | 76 | 25 | 33 |
| Anaplastic astrocytoma | 109 | 25 | 22.9 |
| Oligodendroglioma | 117 | 12 | 10.3 |
| Glioblastoma | 523 | 282 | 53.9 |
| Ependymoma | 37 | 5 | 14 |
| Meningioma | 410 | 8 | 2.0 |
| Neurinoma | 138 | 13 | 9.4 |
| Pituitary adenoma | 243 | 12 | 4.9 |
| Hemangioblastoma | 30 | 4 | 13 |
| Craniopharyngioma | 67 | 4 | 6 |
| Other brain tumors | 468 | 24 | 5.1 |
| Metastases | 363 | 102 | 28.1 |
| Total | 2,581 | 516 | 20.0 |
| Brain abscess | 44 | 38 | 86 |

### *1. Brain Abscess*

The history and clinical findings offer the greatest help in establishing the diagnosis of brain abscess. Differentiation in the CT scan may be extremely difficult or impossible if the history is not characteristic. The ring found in brain abscess represents the highly vascularized capsule and almost always appears as a sharply delineated round or oval shape with uniform thickness. This is rare in glioblastoma, while the garland-like formations and the nodules extending from the ring to the center of the lesion, typical of glioblastoma, are not found in brain abscess. This is also true of chambered abscesses, though the latter may simulate a knot of tumor in certain projections and lead to confusion in differential diagnosis. Very thin rings suggest a diagnosis of tumor rather than brain abscess.

In our experience *quantitative analysis of absorption values in the capsule and the contents of the abscess does not contribute significantly to differentiation,* since absorption values in individual cases may be similar to those found in glioblastoma. MAUERSBERGER (1981) reported consistently low density values in abscess contents. However, we have found that density may vary greatly and is an unreliable criterion for differential diagnosis. Mean absorption values in 20 brain abscesses ranged from 19 to 23 HU, with lower values in only one case, but we have measured similar absorption values in necrotic and cystic portions of glioblastomas.

Cerebral angiography contributes to differential diagnosis of glioblastoma and brain abscess only when vessels typical of glioblastoma are demonstrated or when a characteristic abscess capsule appears at angiography. *In some cases biopsy is the only means of establishing the diagnosis and excluding an operable brain abscess.*

### *2. Intracranial Metastases*

Differential diagnosis is relatively easy in cases of known primary tumor, though one is well advised to consider the possibility of an autochthonous brain tumor in a patient with a primary tumor of another organ, as our own experience has shown. Multiple intracerebral lesions suggest metastases even when there is no evidence of a primary tumor, but *multifocal glioblastomas* also occur, however, rarely (Figs. D1.94–97), and comprise 1% of glioblastomas in our collective. An irregular ring with garland-like structures is an extremely rare CT finding in metastasis. Therefore, multifocal glioblastoma is a likely differential diagnosis when two intracranial tumors with garland-like structures appear after contrast enhancement.

### *3. Anaplastic Astrocytoma*

Ring structures in anaplastic astrocytoma are usually narrow and surround a cyst (Figs. D1.16–18), while such a finding is extremely rare in glioblastoma (Fig. D1.59). A homogeneous tumor nodule without zones of decreased density due to necrosis is found in anaplastic astrocytoma but rare in glioblastoma. However, a number of anaplastic astrocytomas are virtually identical to glioblastoma in the CT scan (Figs. D1.23–25).

### *4. Brain Infarction*

The stage of brain infarction accompanied by a serious disorder in the blood-brain barrier, which occurs in the 2nd and 3th week, may have the same appearance as a glioblastoma after contrast enhancement (Figs. F86, 88). In these cases, the history, clinical findings, and little or no displacement of intracerebral structures 3 weeks after the acute event suggest a vascular process. Follow-up CT studies and other techniques such as serial isotope scanning aid in diagnosis.

### *5. Other Space-Occupying Lesions*

*It may be almost impossible to differentiate between CT findings in atypical meningioma, usually malignant forms with ring structures, and glioblastoma.* Plain skull films, dynamic scintigraphy, and angiography may provide important diagnostic clues. Glioblastomas located near the interhemispheric fissure may be confused with atypical meningioma of the falx cerebri, and vice versa (Figs. D1.83, D2.26).

*Intracerebral hematomas undergoing resorption* may also demonstrate ring structures after contrast enhancement (ZIMMERMAN et al. 1977). WEISBERG (1980) has shown that this phenomenon is a very common finding with intracerebral hematomas at certain stages (see also p. 432).

Neither CT nor angiography allows certain discrimination between gliosarcoma and glioblastoma (Figs. D1.99). Cerebral pilocytic astrocytoma may occasionally mimic atypical glioblastoma. The same is true of highly malignant ependymoma (Figs. D1.161, 162).

**Fig. D 1.**57 a–d. Glioblastoma in the left precentral region of a 66-year-old male. Ring structures after contrast enhancement representing the solid portion of the tumor. Slight perifocal edema (grade I) and minimal displacement of midline structures (**a**). Dynamic brain scintigraphy confirmed the diagnosis. Radionuclide angiography: Radionuclide uptake in the tumor during the late arterial phase, with elimination of radionuclide in the venous phase (**b**). Slight radionuclide uptake with central defect in the left precentral region during the early phase of the static brain scan (**c**). Significant increase in radionuclide uptake in the late phase (**d**). These findings are typical of glioblastoma ▶

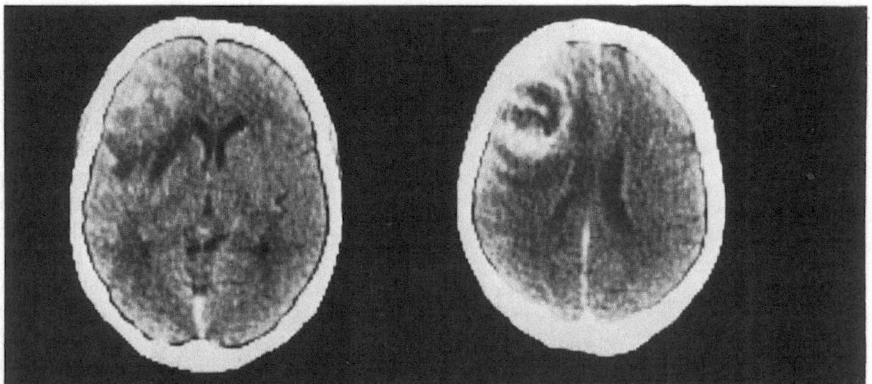
a

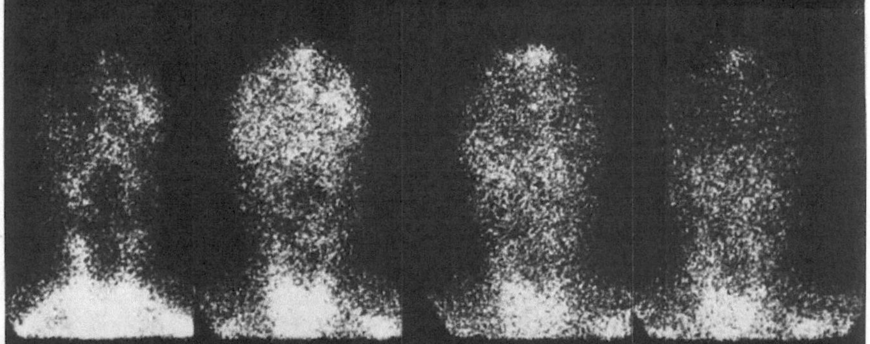
b

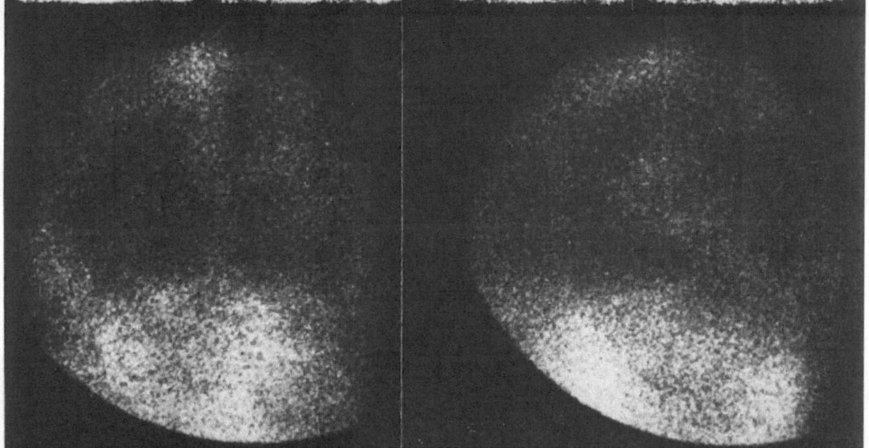
c

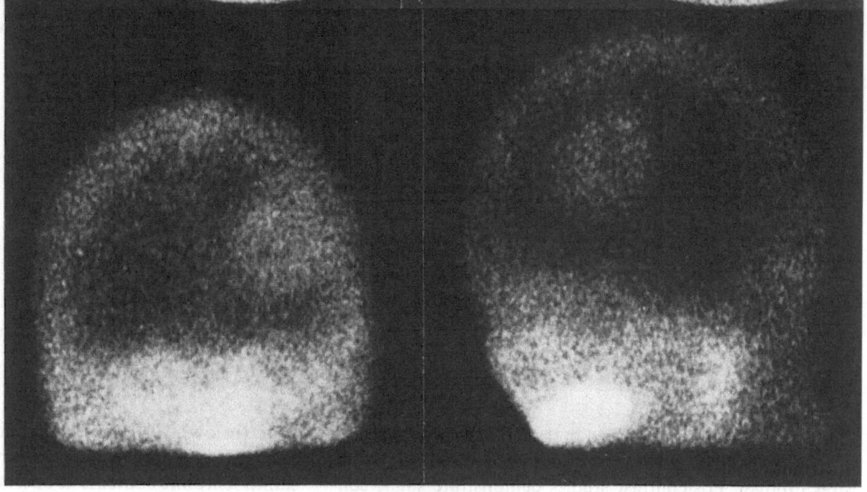
d

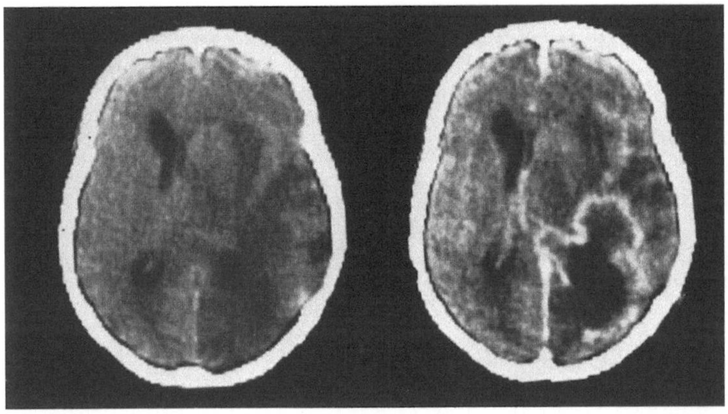

**Fig. D 1.58.** Extensive glioblastoma in the right occipitotemporal region of a 54-year-old female. Precontrast CT (left) demonstrates predominantly hypodense values with some isodense zones within the tumor. Differentiation between the actual tumor and perifocal edema is not possible. Postcontrast CT reveals garland-like contrast enhancement in the solid marginal regions of the tumor, typical of glioblastoma (right). Clear demarcation of central necrosis and perifocal edema. Extreme displacement of midline structures

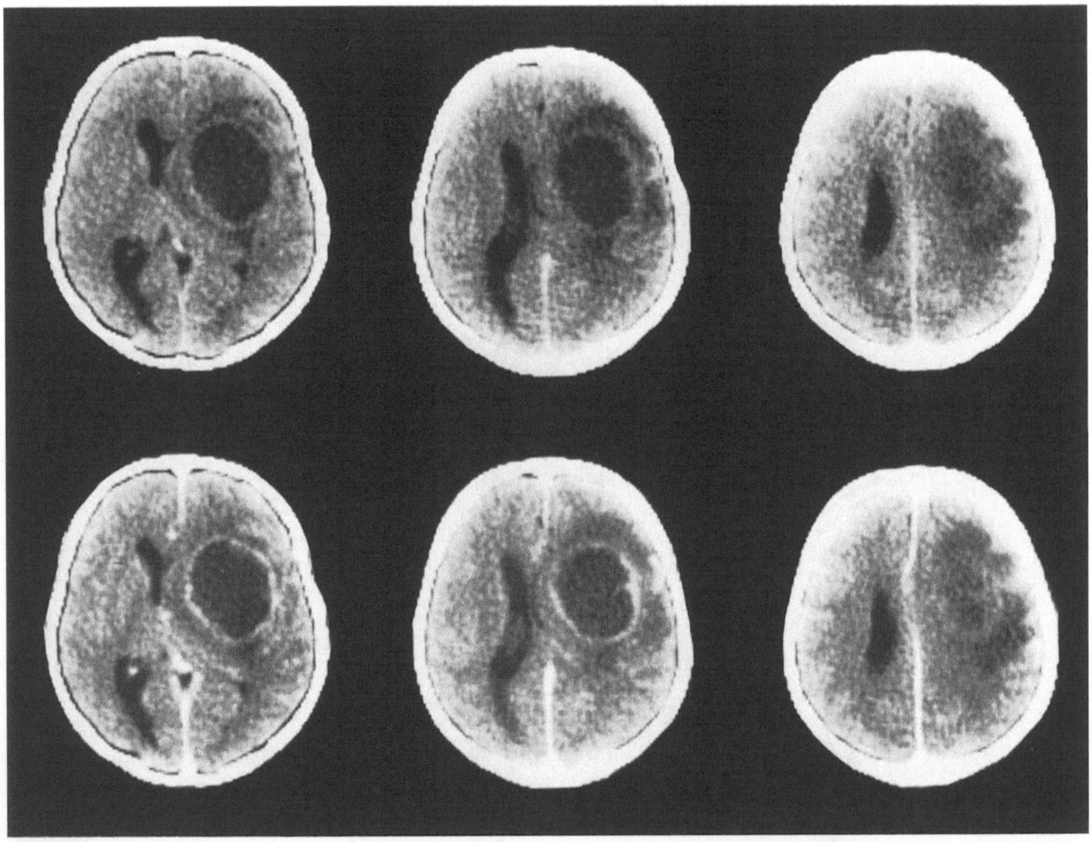

**Fig. D 1.59.** Glioblastoma deep in the frontotemporal region in a 43-year-old male. Precontrast studies reveal ring structures (above). Postcontrast studies demonstrate slight contrast enhancement in the solid marginal portions of the tumor (below). The central hypodense zone was originally thought to represent necrosis but proved to be a cyst with xanthochromic contents at operation (density 18 HU). Confusion with brain abscess is possible

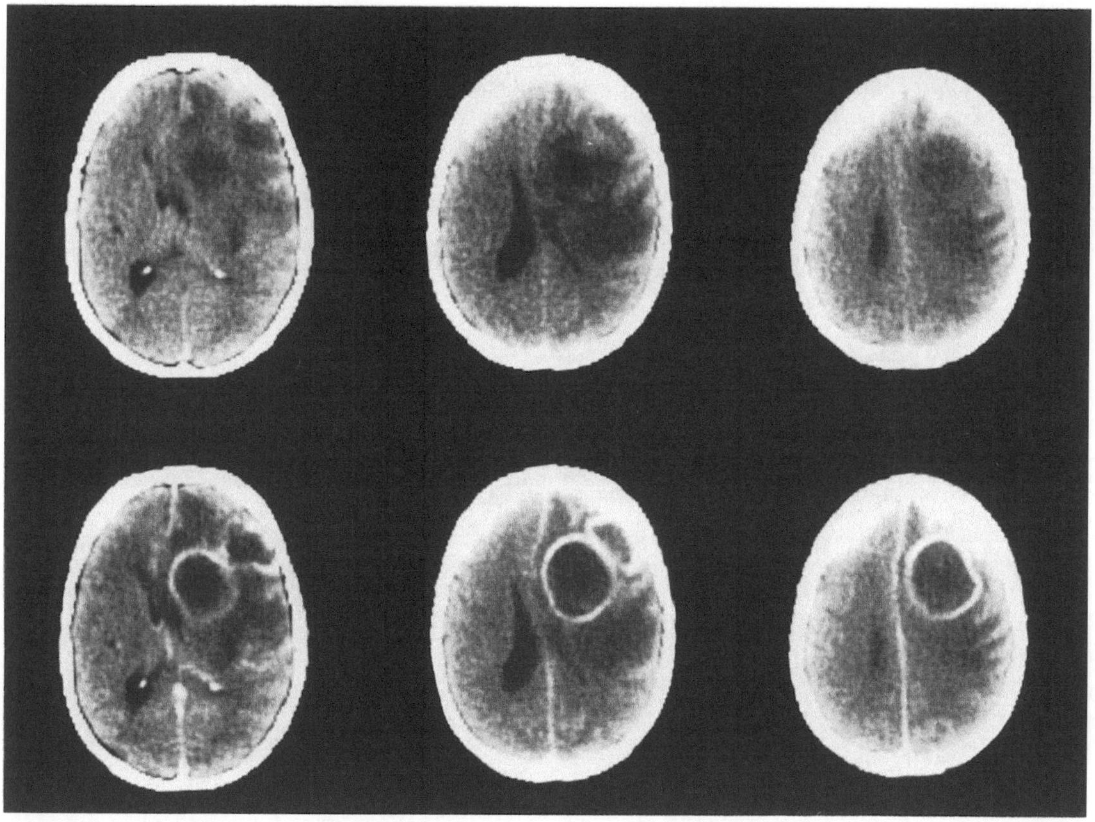

**Fig. D 1.60.** Glioblastoma in the right precentral region with extension to the basal ganglia in a 65-year-old female. Precontrast CT (above) shows a space-occupying lesion in the right frontoprecentral region but fails to demonstrate the actual tumor. Postcontrast CT (below) reveals two sharply delineated contiguous ring structures. CT diagnosis: multichambered brain abscess or glioblastoma. The central hypodense zone was caused by necrosis (density values 20 HU)

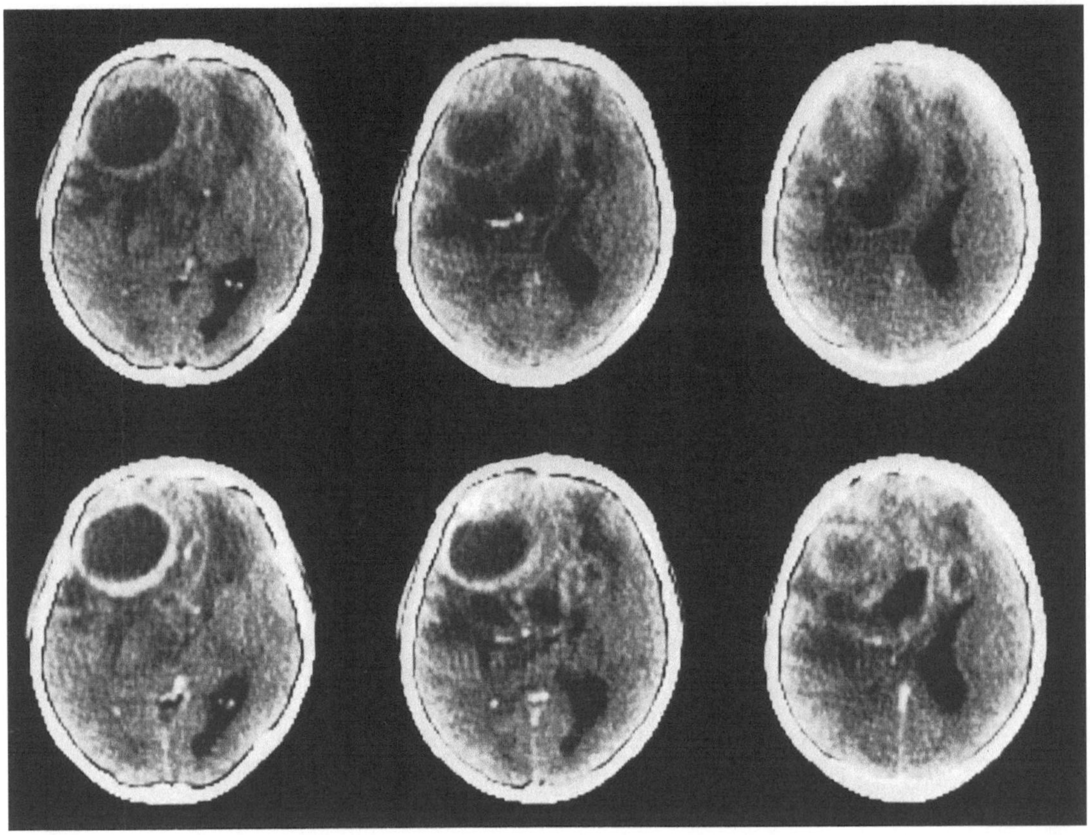

**Fig. D1.61.** Very large glioblastoma in the left frontal lobe with extension to the basal ganglia and through the corpus callosum to the contralateral hemisphere. Wide range of density values in the precontrast study, including calcification at the posterior margin of the tumor (*above*). Clear demonstration of rings and garland structures in viable tissue after contrast administration (*below*). Dilatation of the posterior segment of the right lateral horn secondary to blockage of the foramen of Monro. (46 year old female)

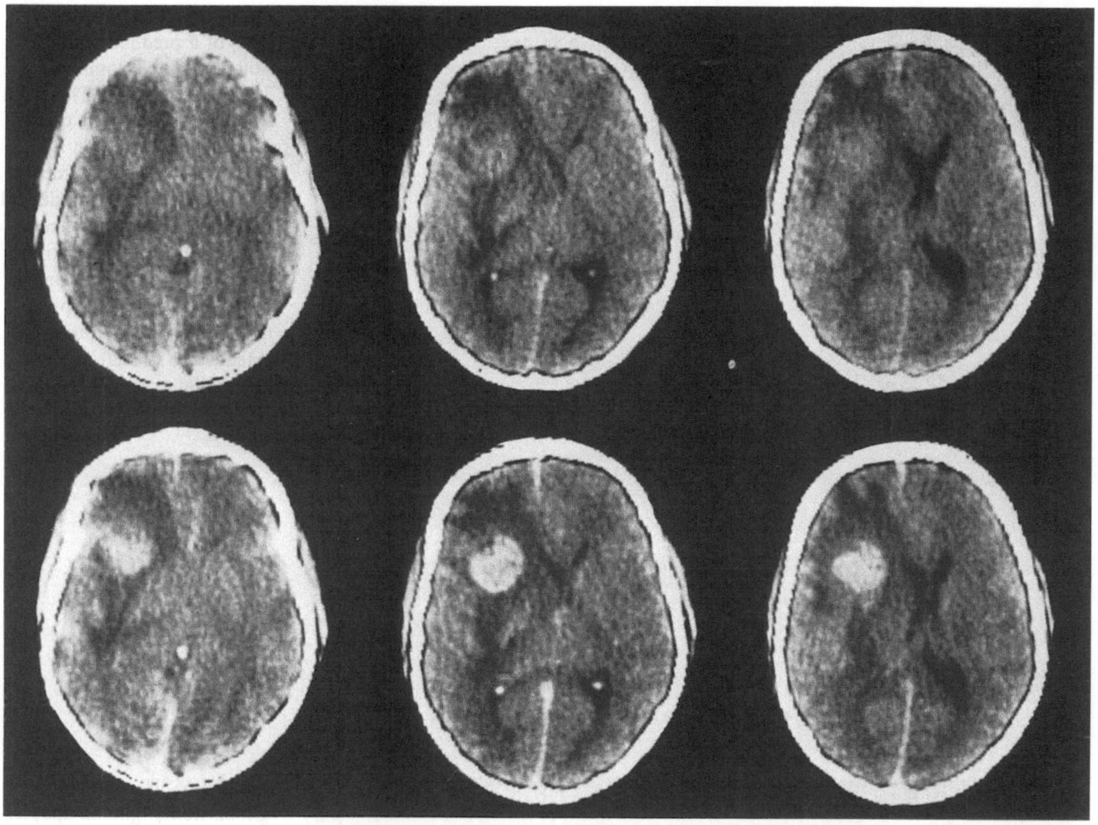

▲

**Fig. D 1.62.** Glioblastoma deep in the frontal white matter at the border of the basal ganglia in a 42-year-old patient with signs of increased intracranial pressure. Precontrast studies (above) reveal a spherical slightly hyperdense region (mean density 44 HU) surrounded by perifocal edema. Postcontrast studies (below) demonstrate a homogeneous increase in density within the tumor (so-called nodular type). Density increase 18 HU with standard dose of contrast medium (1 ml per kilogram body weight)

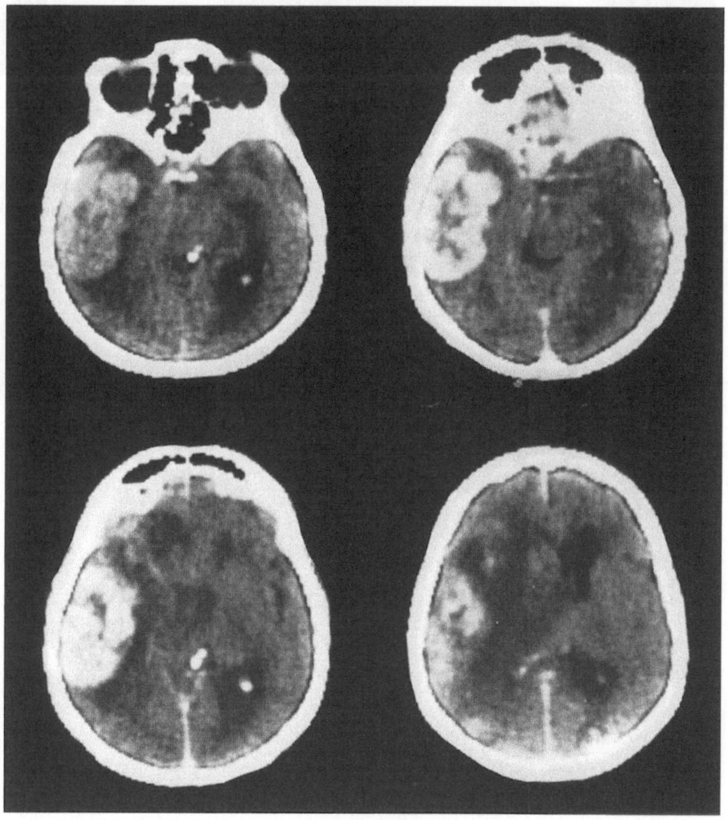

►

**Fig. D 1.63.** Glioblastoma in the left temporal lobe of a 72-year-old patient. The neoplasm consists primarily of solid tumor tissue with hyperdense values in the precontrast CT (above left). Very strong contrast enhancement. A meningioma with regressive changes is compatible with these CT findings. Grade III perifocal edema

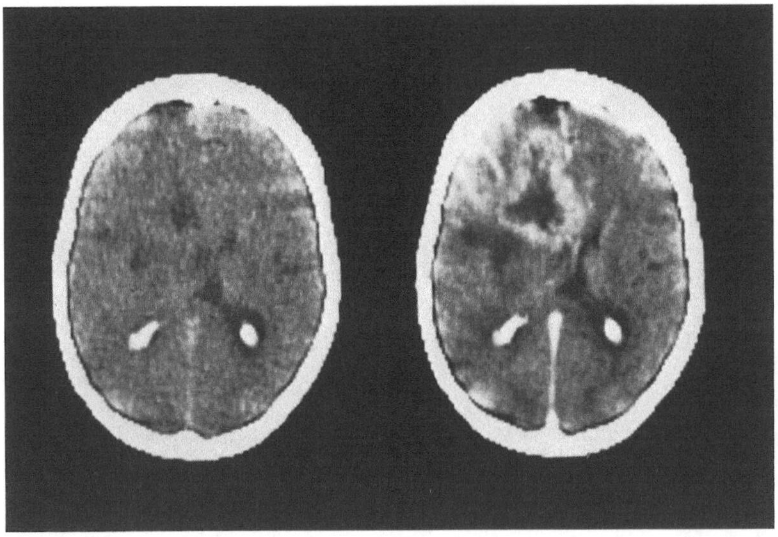

**Fig. D 1.64.** Precontrast CT (left) of a predominantly isodense glioblastoma in a 70-year-old patient. There is a small hypodense zone due to central necrosis within the isodense tumor. Obliteration of the left lateral ventricle and the anterior horns. Postcontrast CT (right) demonstrates typical garland enhancement of the tumor; the necrosis is more evident. The tumor has extended to the left anterior horn. Slight perifocal edema

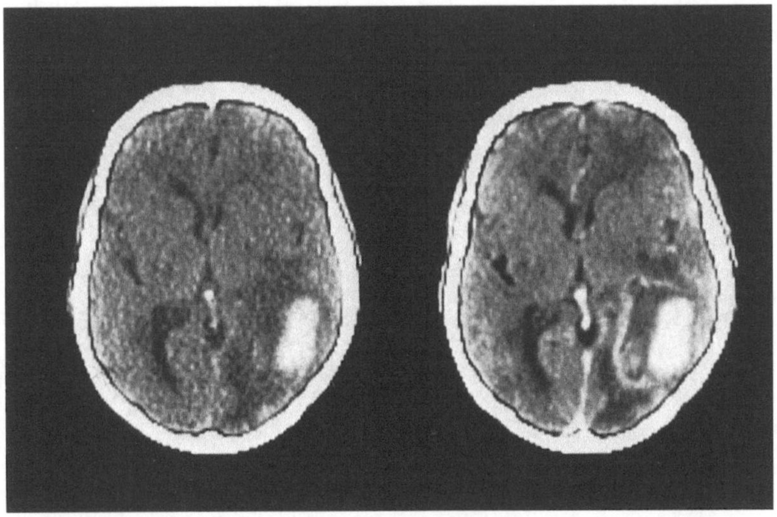

**Fig. D 1.65.** Hemorrhage in a glioblastoma (glioma apoplecticum) in a 65-year-old patient with abrupt onset of symptoms. Precontrast CT (left) reveals a hyperdense zone with density values around 80 HU suggesting freshly clotted blood. There is an extensive hypodense zone near the hemorrhage. These findings are not typical of a recent spontaneous intracerebral hematoma. Postcontrast CT (right) demonstrates the source of hemorrhage. Ring structures appear after contrast enhancement and surround the hematoma. This confirms the diagnosis of hemorrhage within a tumor

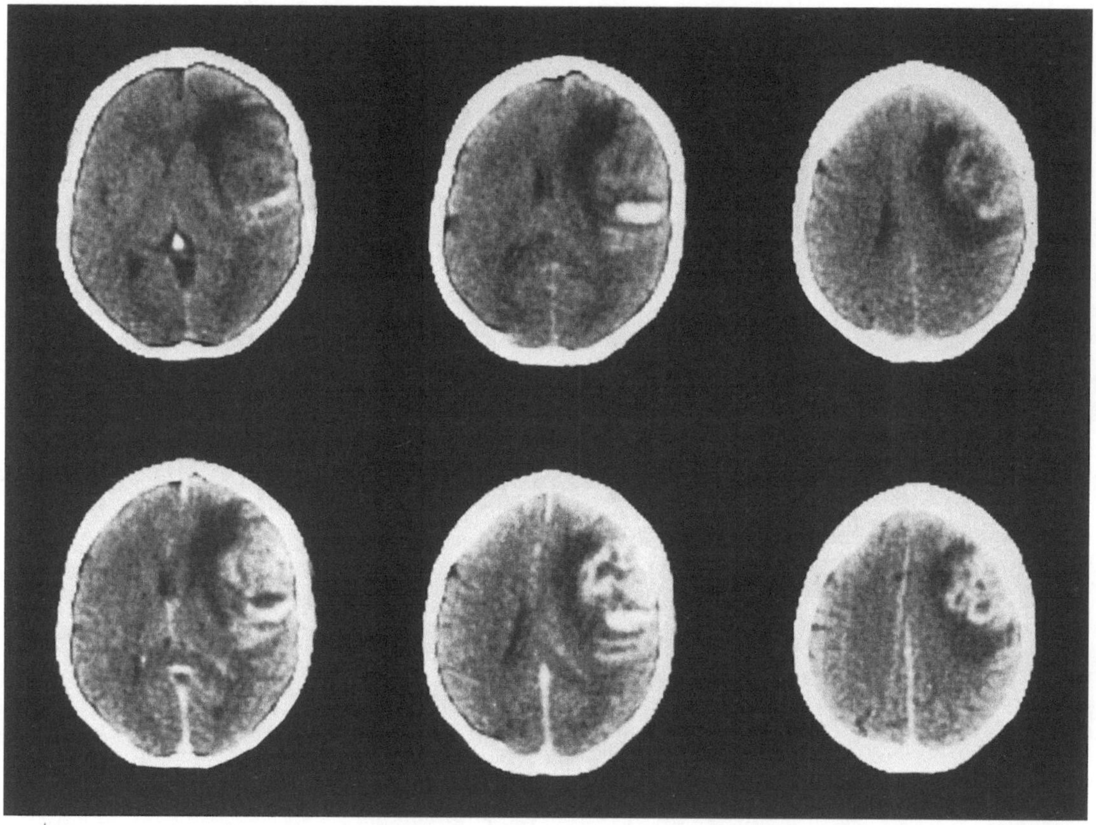

**Fig. D1.66.** CT findings several days after hemorrhage within a glioblastoma in the right precentral region in a 69-year-old patient. Precontrast studies (above) demonstrate a hyperdense zone with a fluid level within the tumor. Postcontrast studies (below) reveal very strong contrast enhancement in viable tumor tissue. Several necrotic zones are visible. Grade II perifocal edema

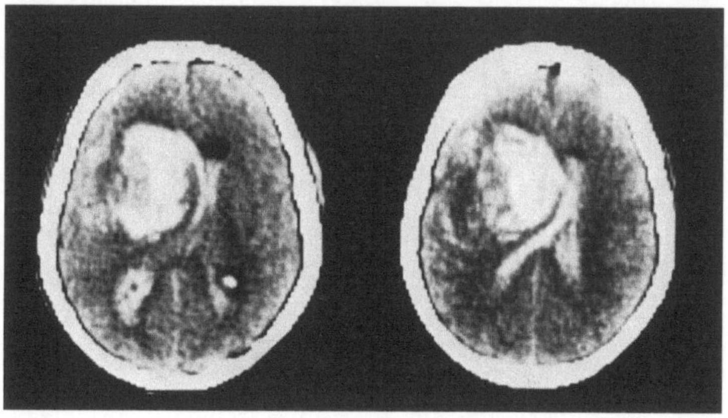

**Fig. D1.67.** Massive hemorrhage penetrating the ventricular system in a case of glioblastoma in a 72-year-old patient. Angiographic studies had provided a diagnosis of glioblastoma deep in the left temporal lobe a short time before acute deterioration

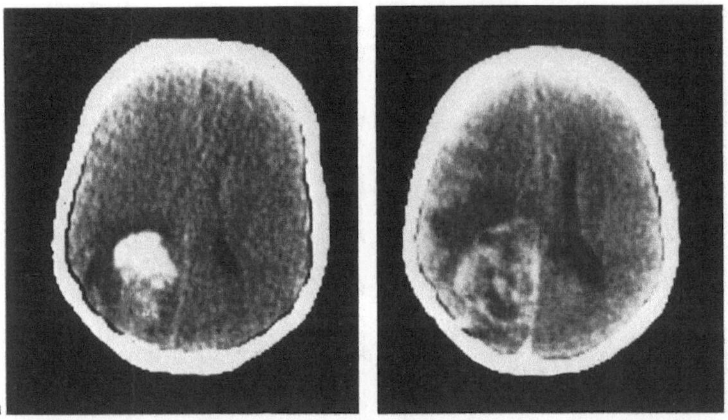

a b

**Fig. D1.68** a, b. Hemorrhage within a glioblastoma in the left parietooccipital region in a 54-year-old man. Follow-up study. (**a**) July 13, 1978: Large hematoma in the left parietooccipital region. No evidence of tumor during surgical evacuation of the hemorrhage. Histological studies of the material were also negative. (**b**) Oct 10, 1979: Slow and progredient deterioration with development of dysphasia and hemiparesis on the right. CT studies reveal an inhomogeneous tumor diagnosed as glioblastoma and confirmed at operation

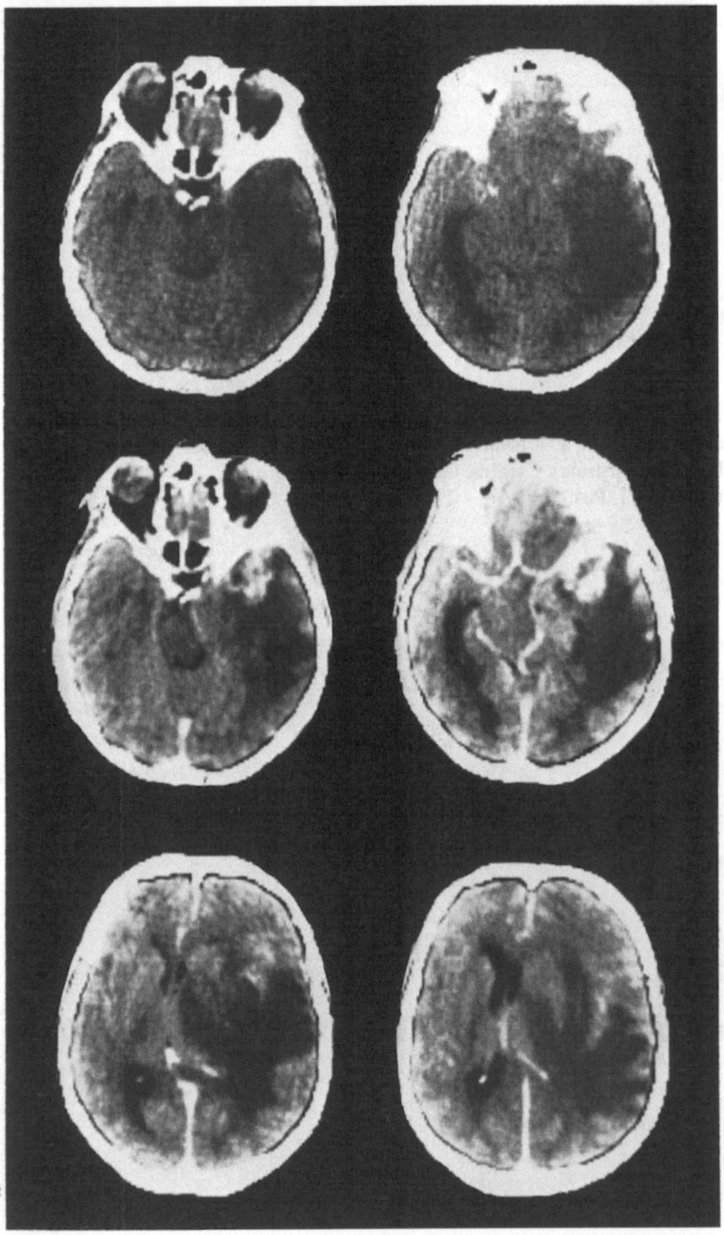

a b c

**Fig. D1.69** a–c. Glioblastoma in the right temporal lobe of a 44-year-old patient. (**a**) Precontrast studies demonstrate a large hypodense zone in the right temporal lobe without demarcation of the tumor itself. (**b**) Demonstration of a relatively small tumor with central necrosis at the pole of the right temporal lobe. Extreme displacement of midline structures with herniation of the medial segments of the right temporal lobe and its vessels at the tentorium. (**c**) Grade III perifocal edema extending throughout the entire right hemisphere. (**b**) and (**c**) postcontrast CT

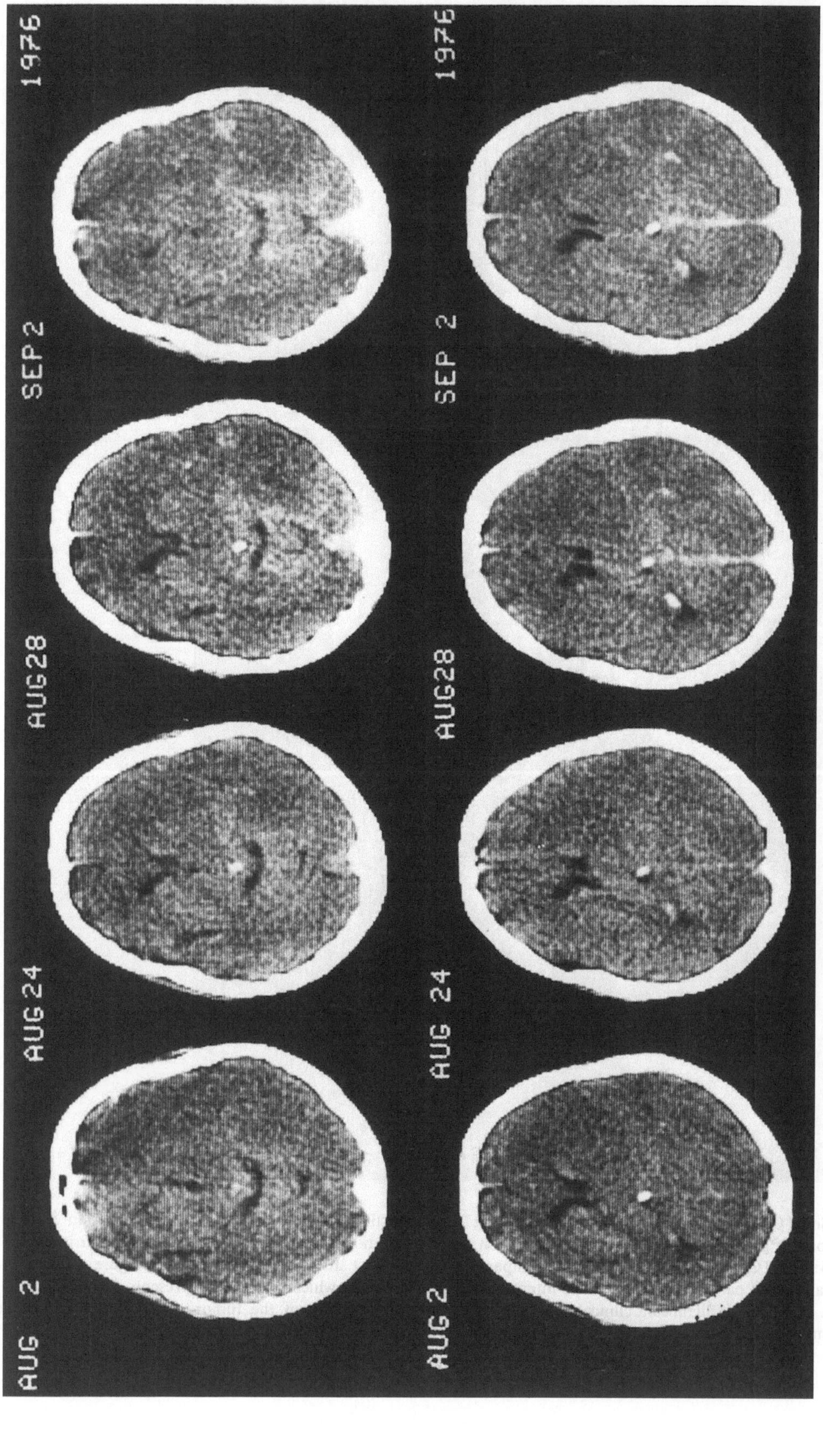


**Fig. D1.70.** Glioblastoma in the right temporal lobe of a 50-year-old patient. Serial study, Aug 2, 1976: Signs of a space-occupying lesion in the right hemisphere with compression of the right trigonum. Tentative diagnosis of isodense chronic subdural hematoma excluded by angiography. Progredient displacement of normal structures and slight decrease in density over a large area of the right hemisphere. Postcontrast studies on Aug 28, 1976 demonstrated circumscribed contrast enhancement in a small zone near the cortex of the right temporal lobe. Identical findings on Sept 2, 1976. Examination of the surgical specimen after resection of the right temporal lobe revealed a glial tumor extending throughout the temporal lobe with characteristic features of glioblastoma in a circumscribed region

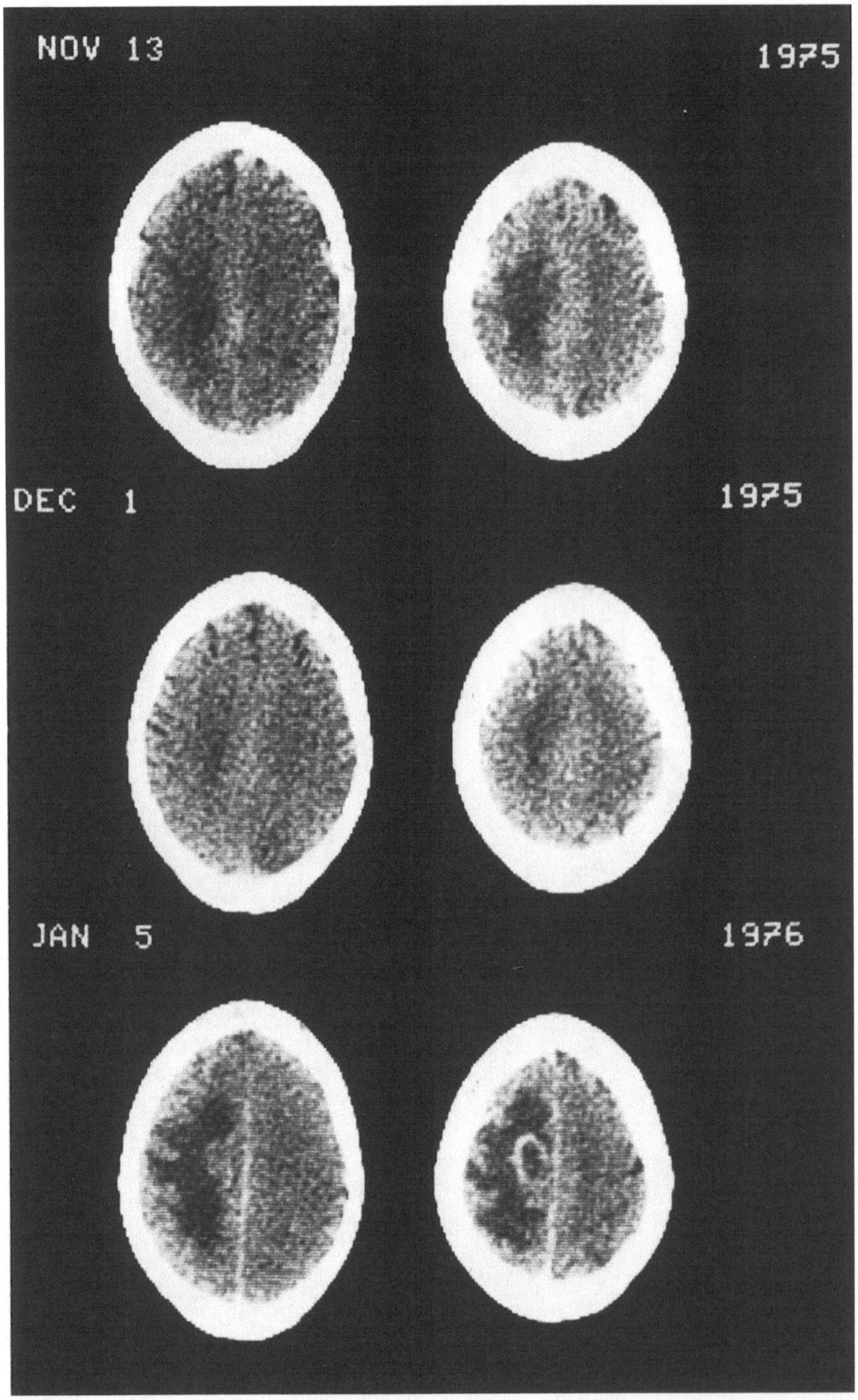


**Fig. D1.71.** Serial CT studies in a 59-year-old patient leading to the diagnosis of glioblastoma in the left parietal region. Nov 13, 1975: Initial CT made after onset of right hemiparesis demonstrates a left parietal hypodense zone interpreted as infarction. Dec 1, 1975: Significant clinical improvement after treatment with dexamethasone with CT demonstration of reduction in size of the hypodense zone. Jan 5, 1976: Deterioration in the clinical state 2 months after initial CT. Postcontrast studies demonstrate a ring figure within a hypodense zone which obviously represents perifocal edema. Surgical resection of the tumor, which was classified as glioblastoma at histological examination

**Fig. D1.72.** Large glioblastoma in the right frontal region. Ring structures after contrast administration; typical frontal edema with a funnel-shaped distribution ending at the basal ganglia. A sharply delineated hypodense zone at the center of the tumor proved to be necrotic tissue at operation. CT findings suggest both glioblastoma and abscess as possible diagnoses. Postcontrast study

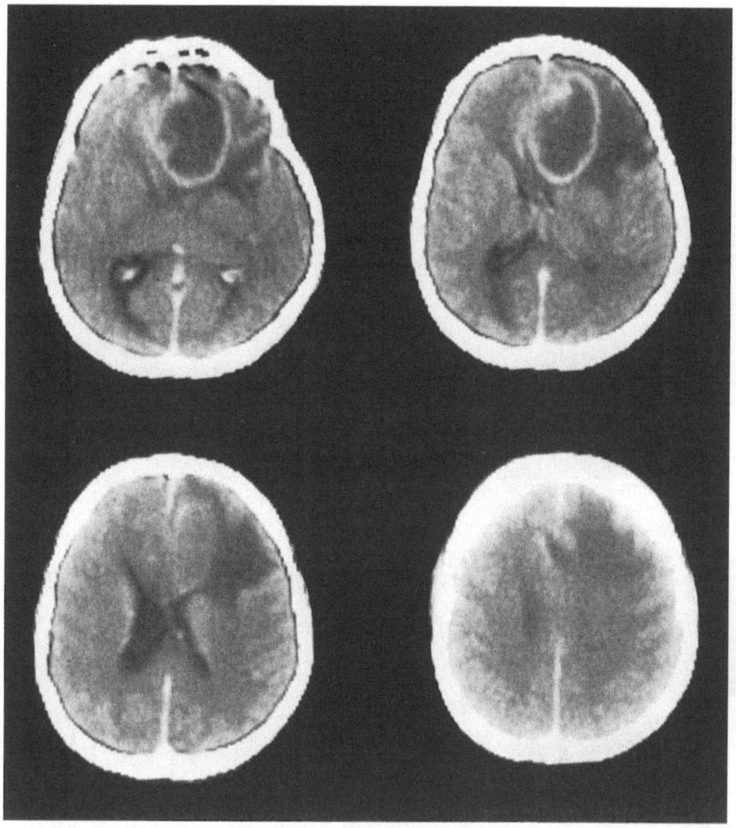

**Fig. D1.73.** Large cystic glioblastoma in the right temporal lobe of a 67-year-old patient. Discrete ring-like contrast enhancement of the neoplasm with several intramural tumor nodules. Significant displacement of the midbrain with compression of the ambient cistern (left). Typical finger-shaped edema in the ventricular plane with demonstration of the upper tumor pole (right). Postcontrast study

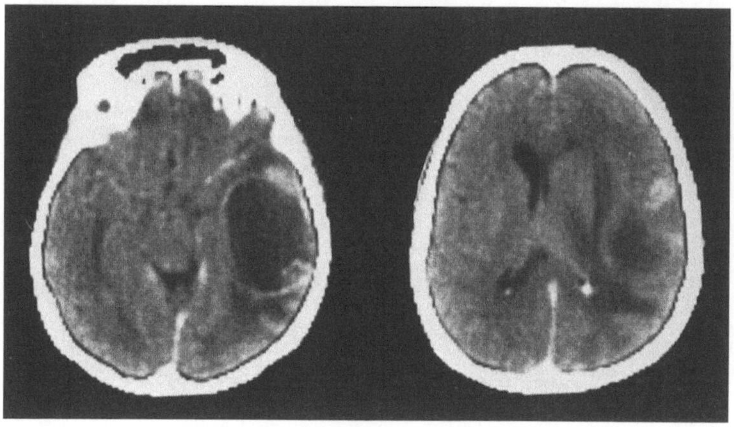

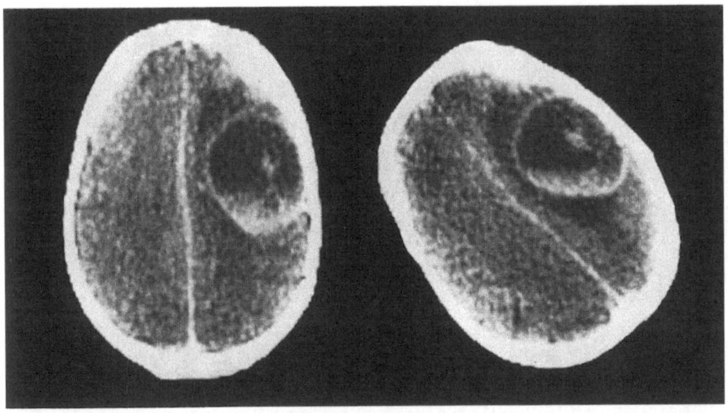

**Fig. D 1.74.** Glioblastoma with a large cyst in the right precentral region. Postcontrast CT demonstrates a ring structure in the marginal solid portions of the tumor as well as a small tumor nodule within the cyst. There is some contrast medium located posteriorly in the cyst. Repeated CT in oblique position demonstrates gravity-dependent sedimentation of the contrast material

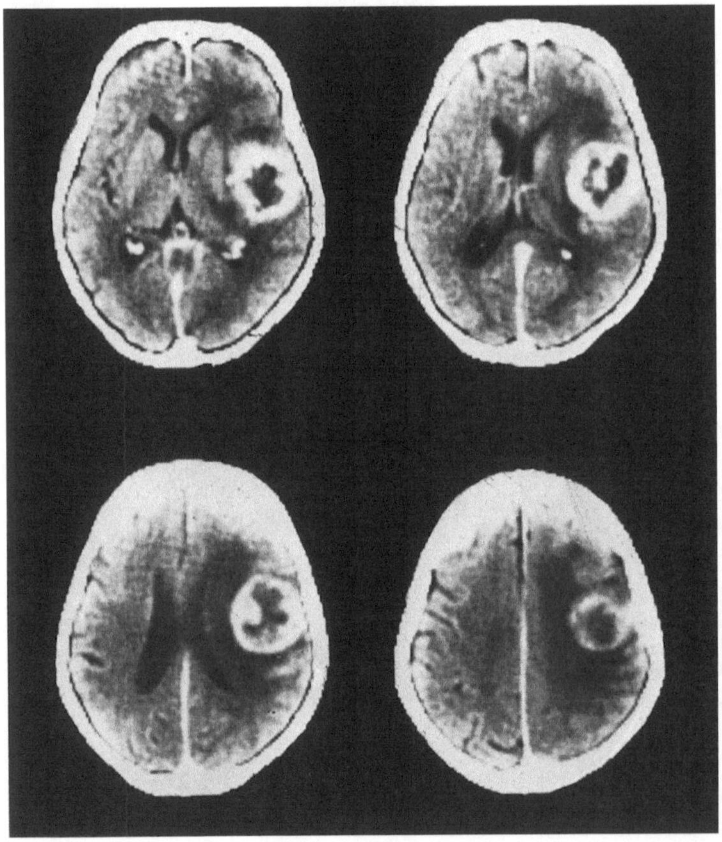

**Fig. D 1.75.** Typical glioblastoma with extensive perifocal edema in the right temporoparietal region. Only slight displacement of midline structures. Intense contrast enhancement in the solid tumor is due to a large dose of contrast medium (100 ml of 60% contrast medium; 63-year-old patient)

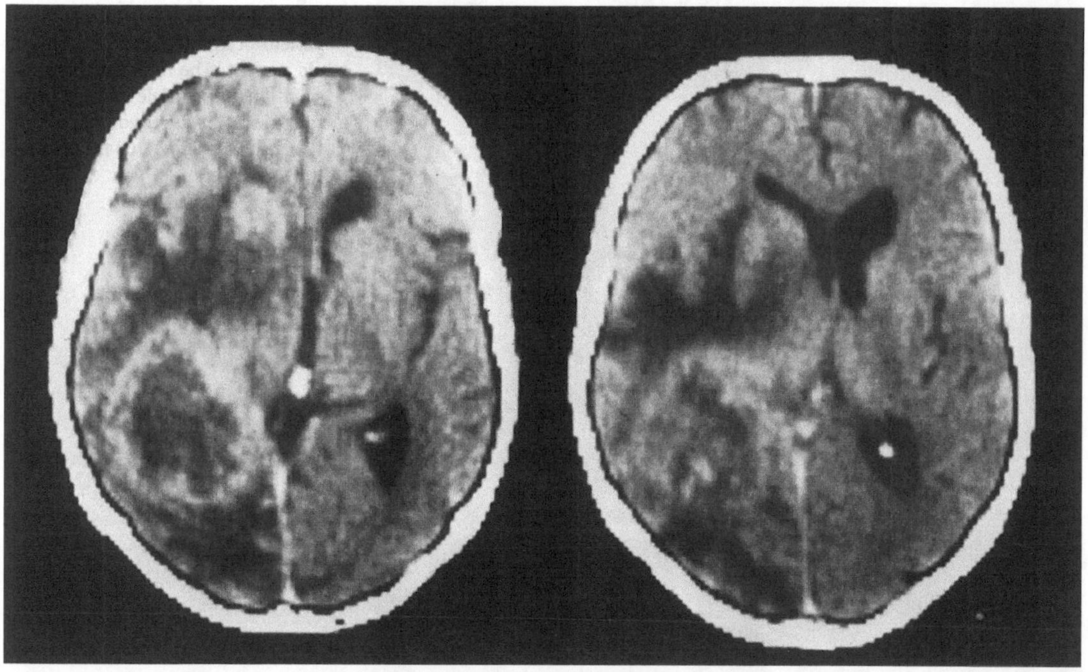

**Fig. D1.76.** Glioblastoma in the left temporo-occipital region with extension to the trigonum. Slight contrast enhancement with garland figures and typical finger-shaped edema

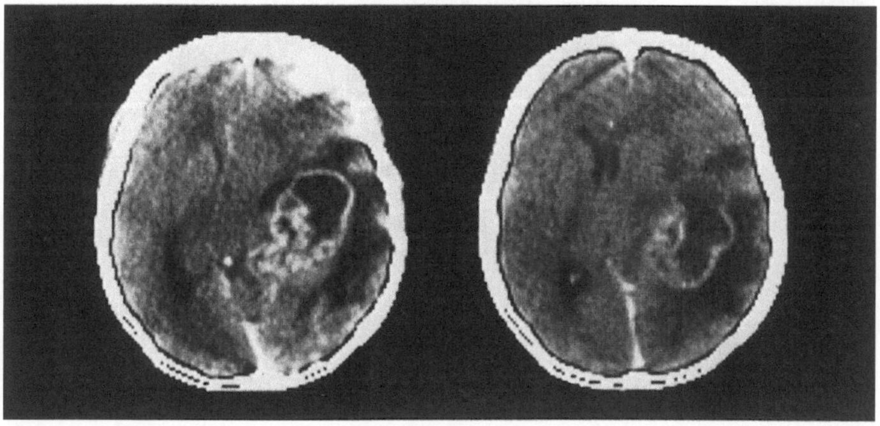

**Fig. D1.77.** Glioblastoma deep in the right temporal lobe with penetration of the ventricles near the trigonum in a 46-year-old patient. One large zone of necrosis as well as many smaller necrotic areas in the medial portions of the tumor. Postcontrast study

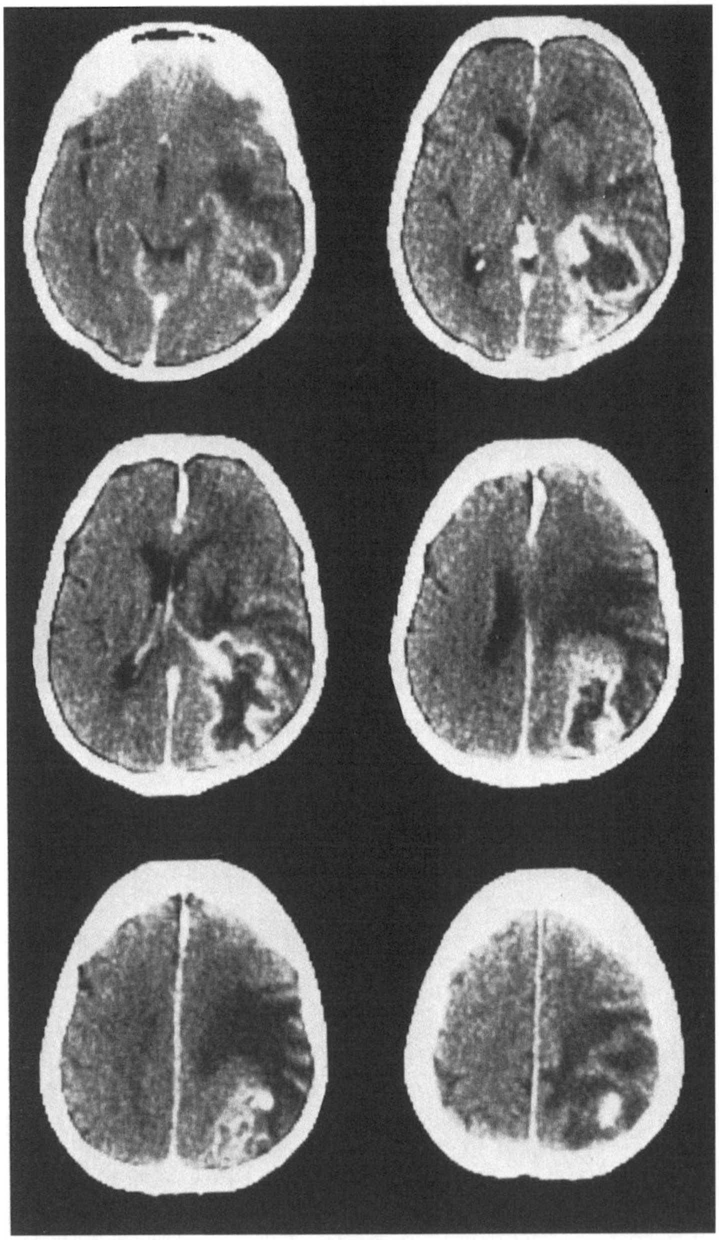

**Fig. D 1.78.** Typical appearance of a glioblastoma in the right temporo-parieto-occipital region of a 56-year-old patient. The tumor involves the right lateral ventricle and the choroid plexus in the trigonum. Grade II perifocal edema (100 ml of contrast medium)

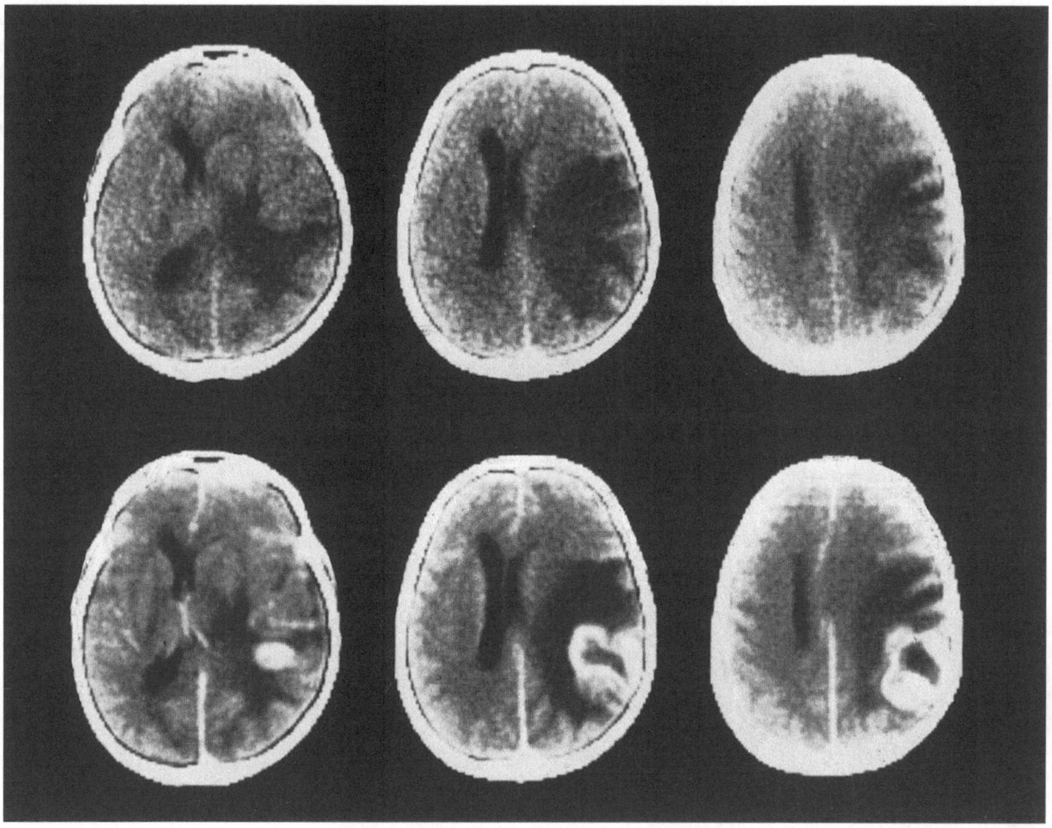

**Fig. D 1.79.** Glioblastoma near the cortex in the right temporo-parieto-occipital region of a 47-year-old patient. Delineation of the actual tumor from extensive perifocal edema is impossible in the precontrast study (above). Postcontrast studies demonstrate a tumor composed of ring structures and larger solid nodules (below). Metastases may produce similar findings in CT studies, as may meningiomas at the convexity in very rare cases

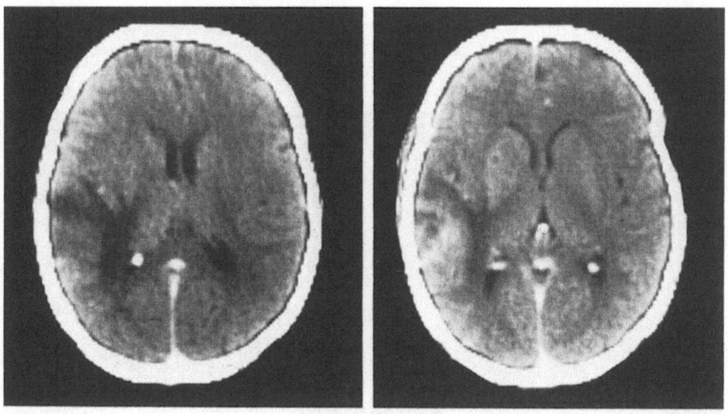

a b

**Fig. D 1.80** a, b. Glioblastoma in the posterior left temporal lobe of a 56-year-old patient; serial study. **(a)** Jan 26, 1979: isodense zone with finger-shaped edema at its medial border. No evidence of midline displacement, though the left choroid plexus is displaced medially. Acute onset of right hemiparesis led to the diagnosis of past hemorrhage. **(b)** June 16, 1979: reduction in perifocal edema and displacement of the choroid plexus during dexamethasone therapy. Demonstration of slight contrast uptake near the cortex in the posterior portion of the left temporal lobe. Diagnosis of a tumor which proved to be glioblastoma at operation

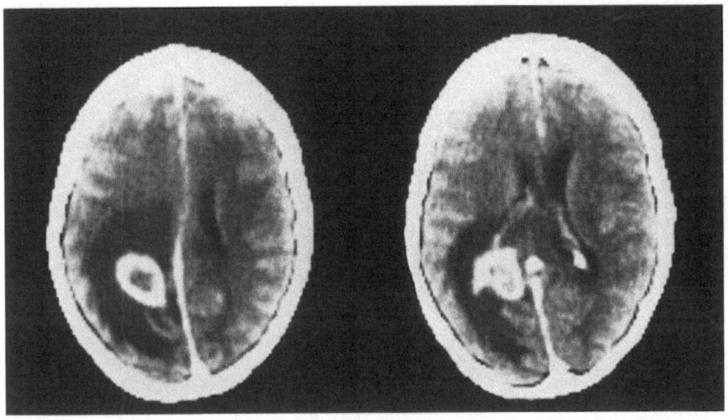

**Fig. D1.81.** Small glioblastoma between the trigonum and the pineal body on the left. Grade III perifocal edema. Strong contrast enhancement due to administration of 100 ml of contrast medium

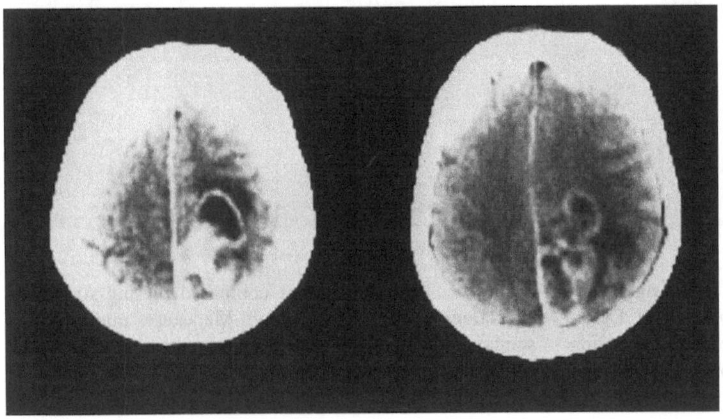

**Fig. D1.82.** Very irregularly shaped glioblastoma in the right postcentral region with slight perifocal edema in a 79-year-old patient (100 ml of contrast medium)

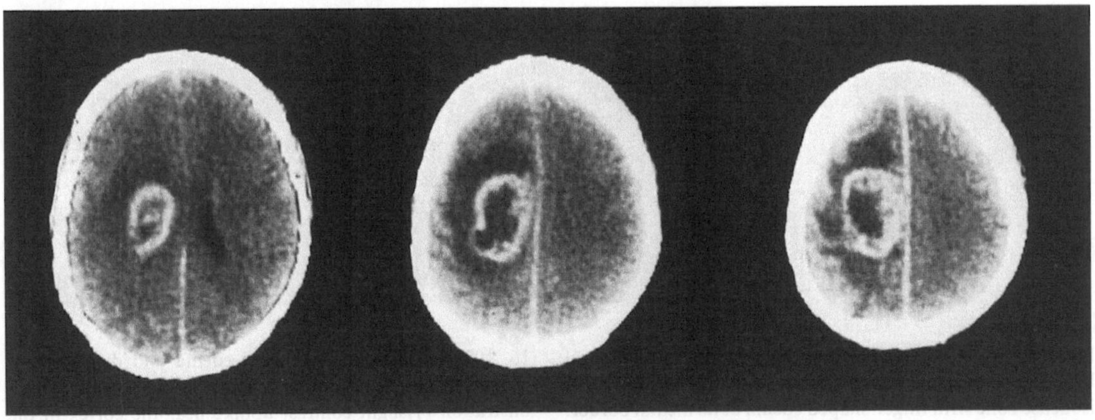

**Fig. D1.83.** Glioblastoma in the left central region of a 46-year-old-man with right hemiparesis. CT findings typical of glioblastoma. Compression of the left lateral ventricle from above (left). Postcontrast study

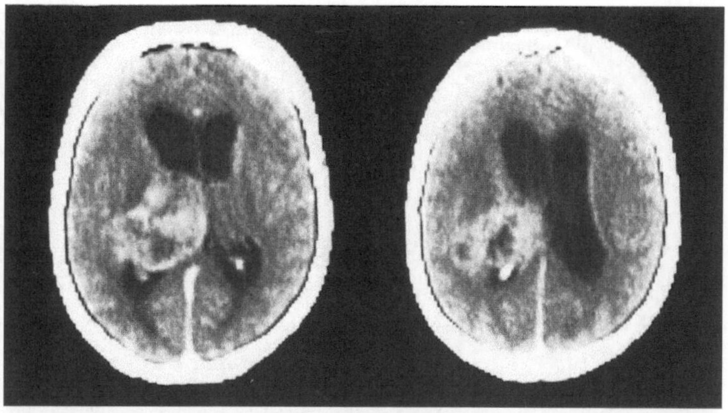

**Fig. D1.84.** Glioblastoma in the left basal ganglia with blockage of the foramen of Monro and obliteration of the third ventricle in a 59-year-old patient. CT findings typical of glioblastoma. Postcontrast study

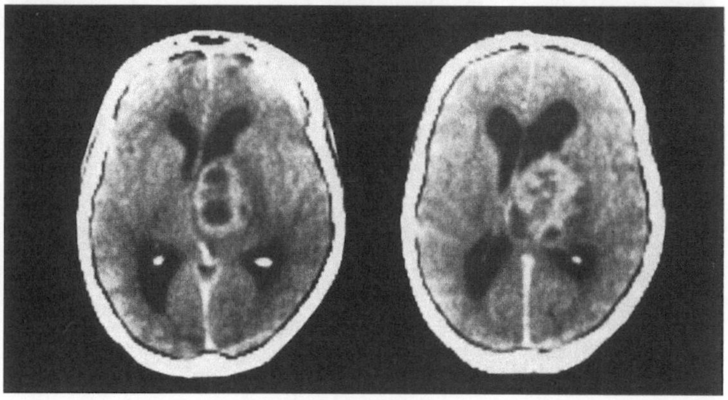

**Fig. D1.85.** Glioblastoma in the basal ganglia on the right with blockage of the CSF passages in a 56-year-old patient. Perifocal edema is very limited since there is no contact with the white matter. Postcontrast study

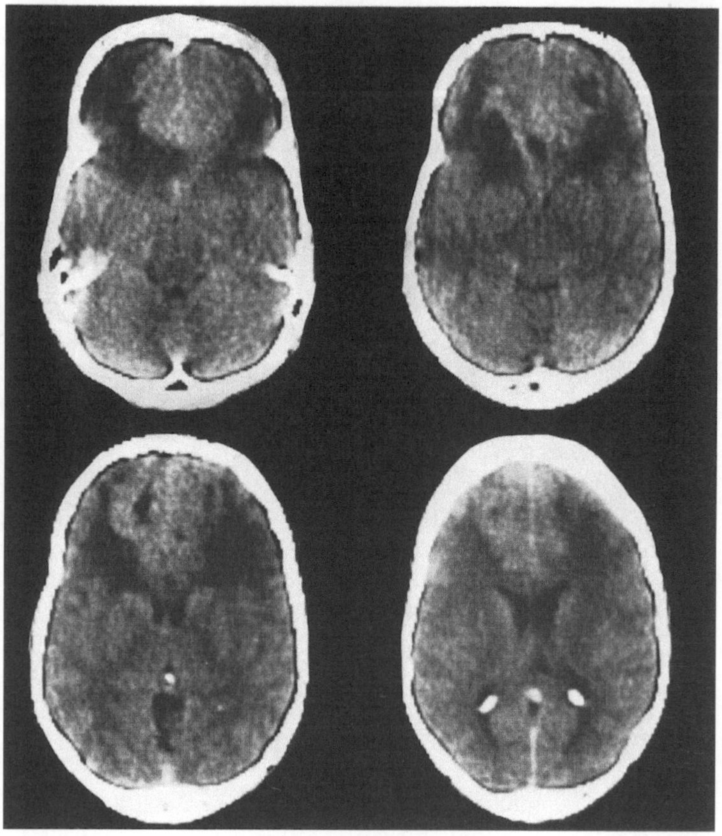

**Fig. D1.86.** Bifrontal glioblastoma with only slight contrast enhancement. Several small cysts and zones of necrosis are visible within the tumor, which has displaced the anterior horns posteriorly. Bilateral frontal edema similar to that found in meningioma of the olfactory groove (36-year-old patient with headache, visual disorders, and papilledema). Postcontrast study

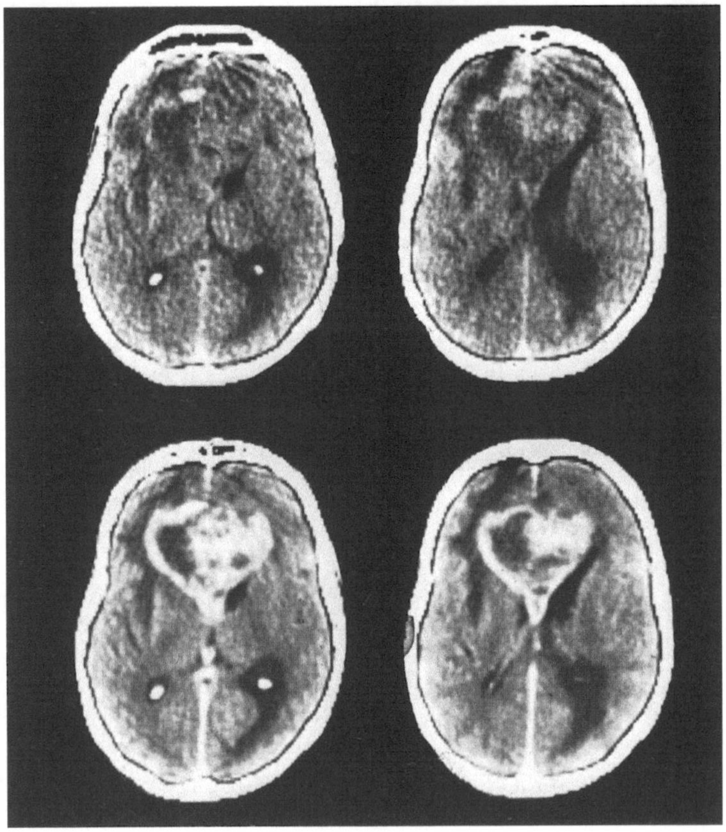

**Fig. D1.87.** Butterfly glioblastoma near the anterior corpus callosum with involvement of the septum pellucidum. The tumor demonstrates inhomogeneous density values as well as a small marginal calcification in the precontrast CT (above). Postcontrast CT studies demonstrate the true extent of the tumor, which contains a number of necrotic areas (below)

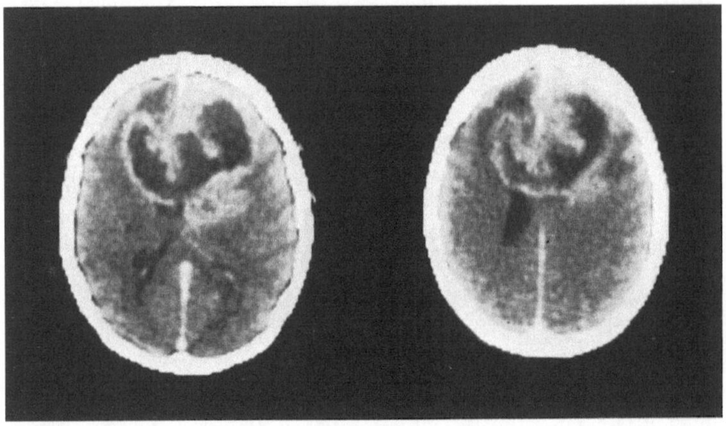

**Fig. D1.88.** Butterfly glioblastoma in the anterior corpus callosum with strong contrast enhancement in the solid portions of the tumor. Large central zone of necrosis. Sixty-four year-old patient with severe organic brain syndrome (postcontrast study)

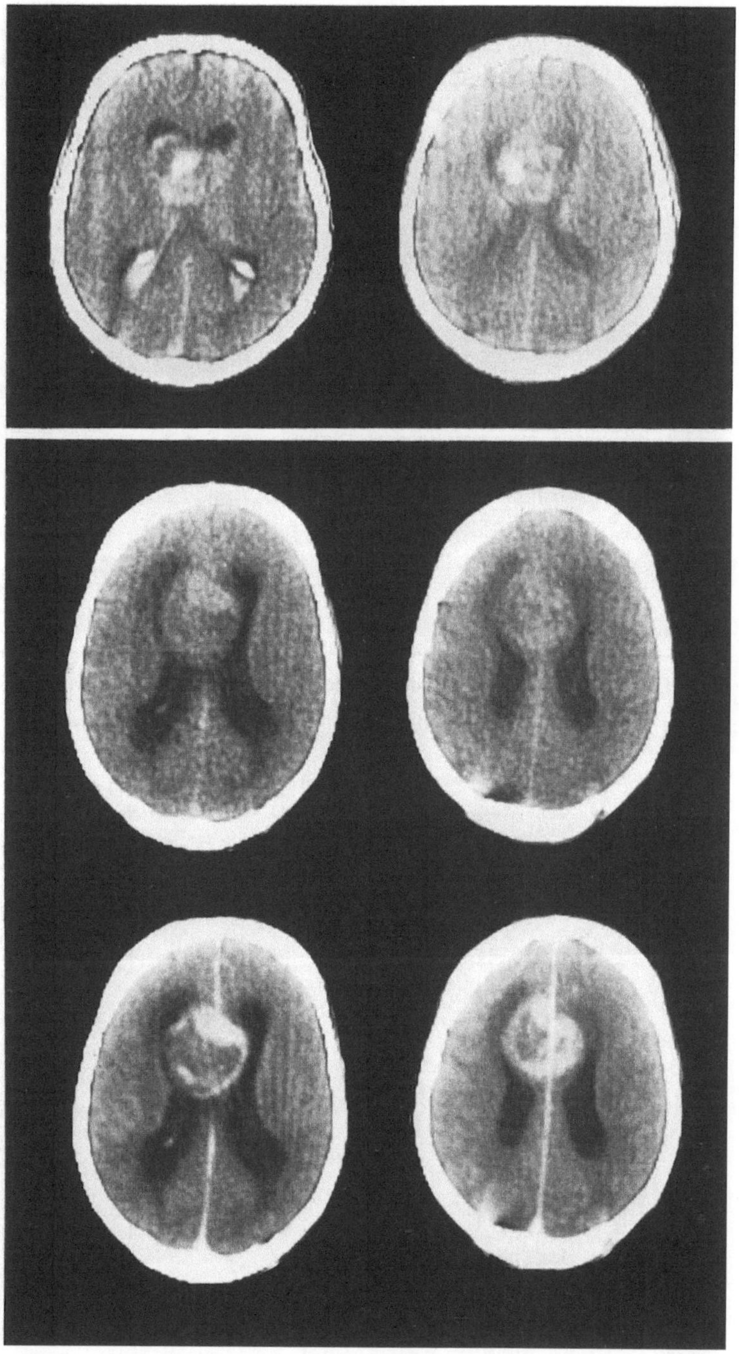


**Fig. D1.89** a–c. Glioblastoma of the corpus callosum in a 50-year-old man. Follow-up study. (**a**) Initial CT studies after an acute disorder of consciousness. Demonstration of a strongly hyperdense zone in the corpus callosum. Diagnosis of hemorrhage. (**b, c**) Follow-up study 2 weeks later. Precontrast (**b**) and postcontrast CT (**c**). Increase in size of the space-occupying lesion with dilatation of the lateral ventricles. Ring-like contrast enhancement within the tumor. Hemorrhage is no longer evident in the CT pictures

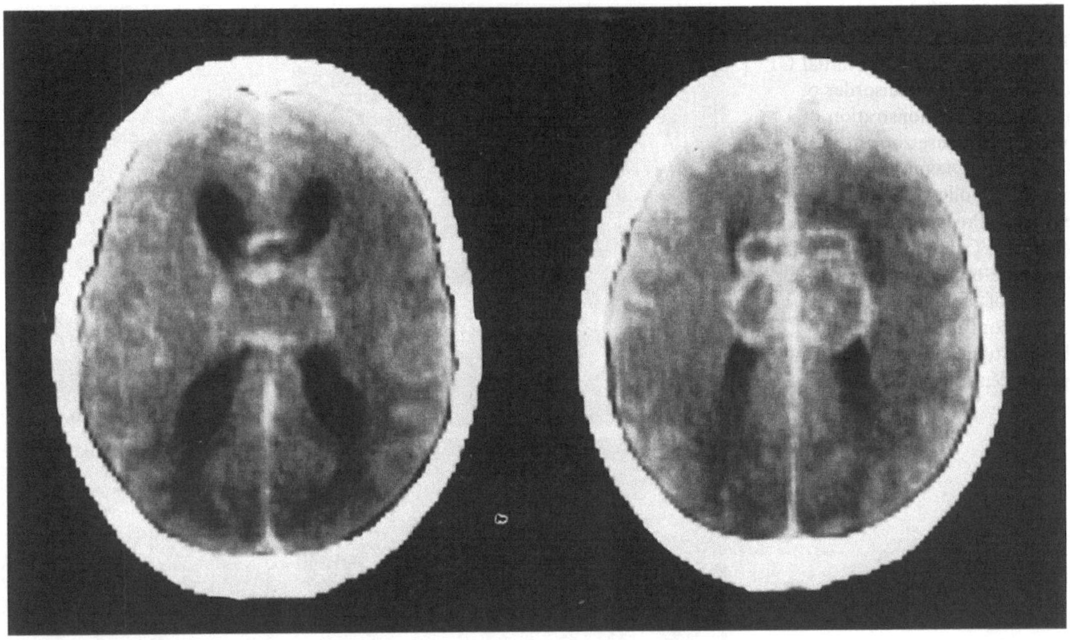

Fig. D1.90. Glioblastoma in the middle portions of the corpus callosum with typical garland figures after contrast enhancement

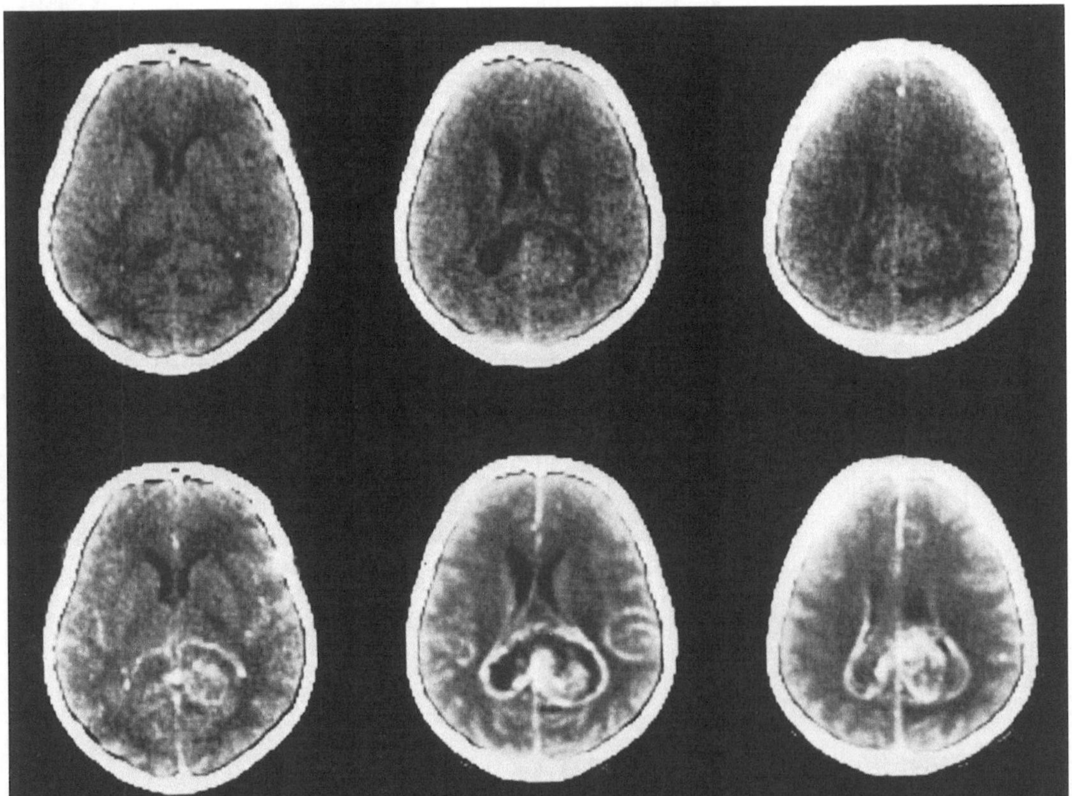

Fig. D1.91. Glioblastoma in the posterior corpus callosum and the lamina tecti in a 50-year-old patient. Findings typical of glioblastoma after contrast enhancement (below) (100 ml of contrast medium)

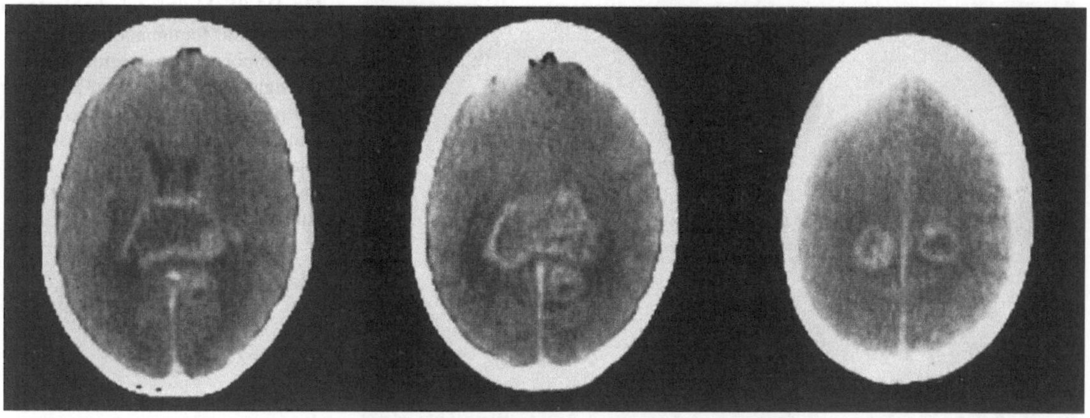

**Fig. D1.92.** Glioblastoma of the corpus callosum. Two apparently separate tumors are demonstrated in the high parietal cross section (right). These are in fact the upper portions of the tumor's butterfly figure

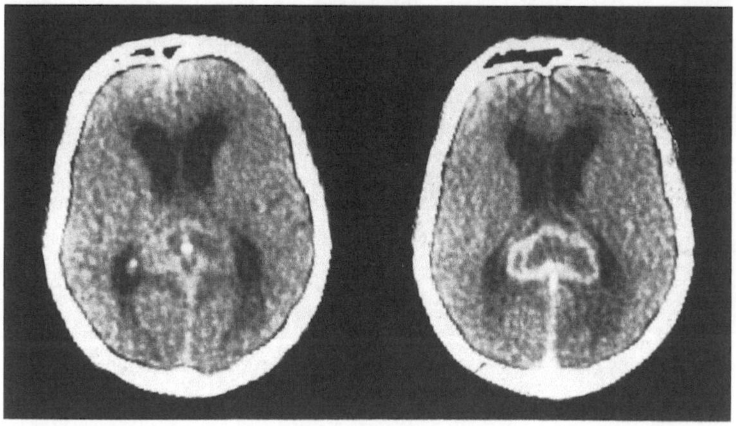

**Fig. D1.93.** Glioblastoma of the lamina tecti with extension toward the trigonum of both lateral ventricles. Extreme hydrocephalus due to compression of the aqueduct (50-year-old patient). Postcontrast study

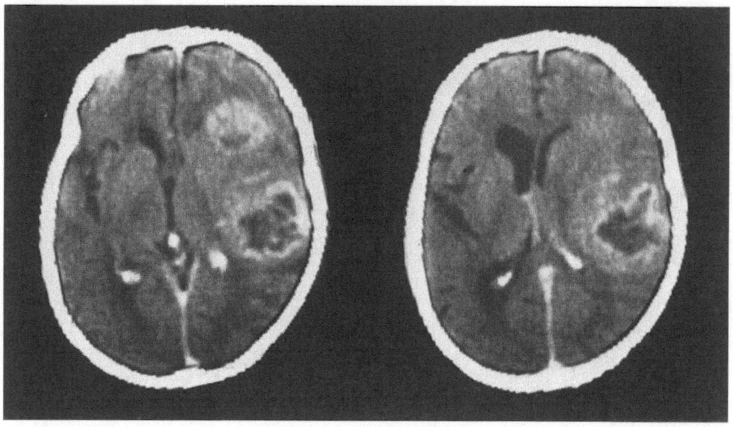

**Fig. D1.94.** Multifocal glioblastoma with clearly separated tumor nodules in the right frontal white matter and the right temporal lobe. Histological studies confirmed the diagnosis. Postcontrast study

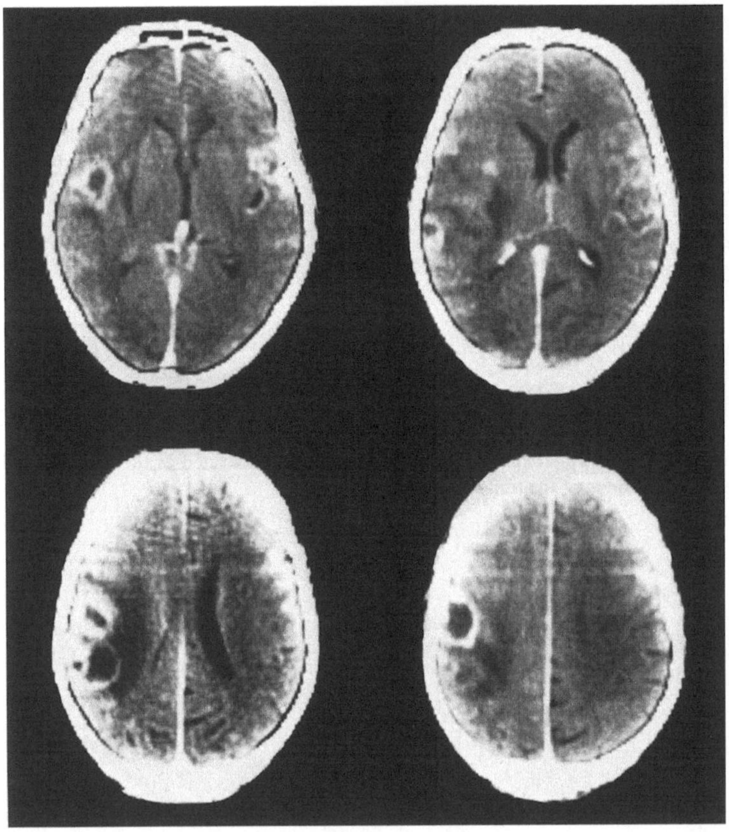

**Fig. D 1.95.** Multifocal glioblastoma with several tumor nodules in the left temporoparietal region and in the right temporal lobe in a 60-year-old patient. The CT findings suggest a diagnosis of multiple metastases. Diagnosis was established by histological examination. Postcontrast study

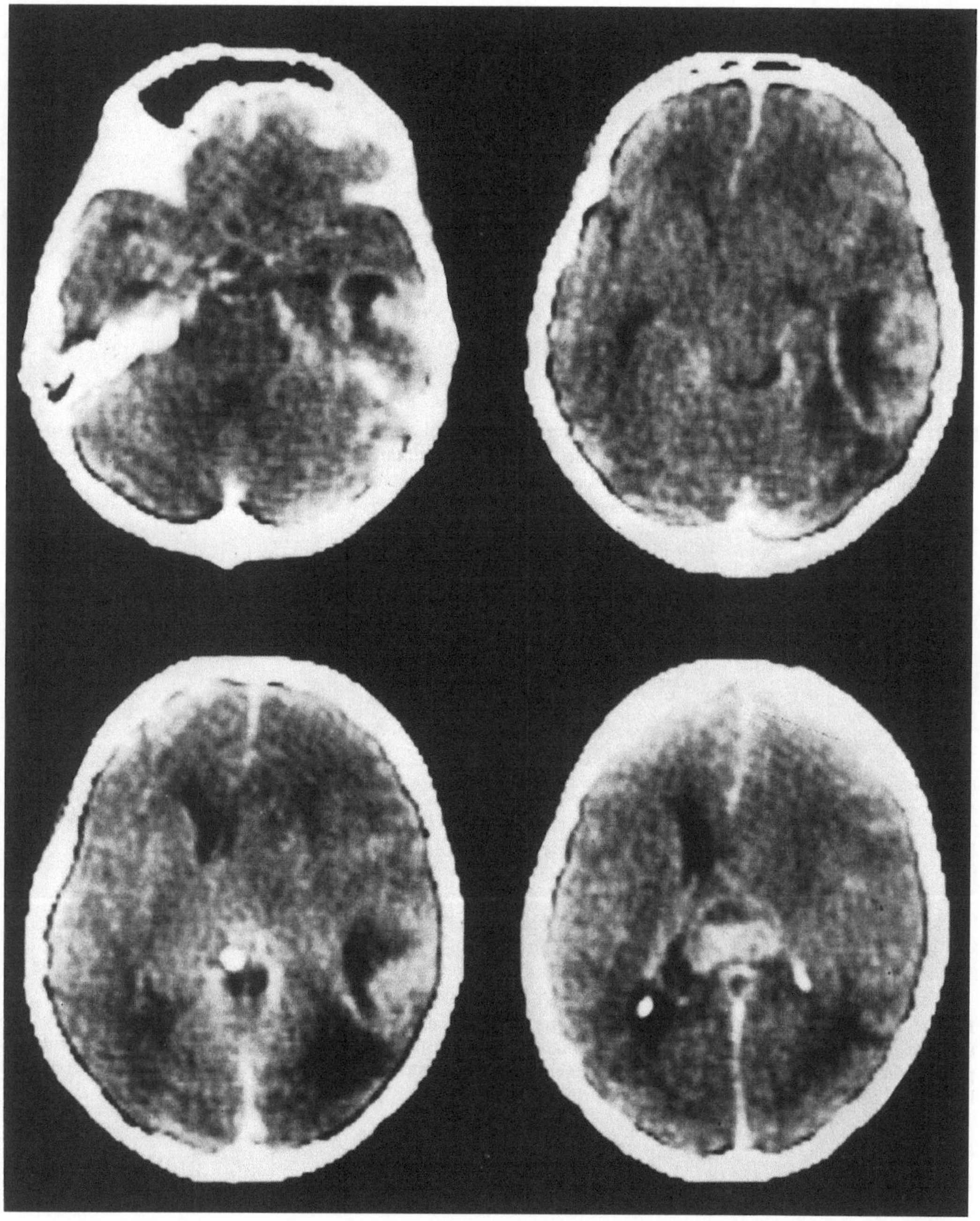

**Fig. D1.96.** Multifocal glioblastoma with tumor nodules in the posterior portion of the right temporal lobe and in the corpus callosum in a 65-year-old patient. Diagnosis was confirmed by histological examination. Postcontrast study

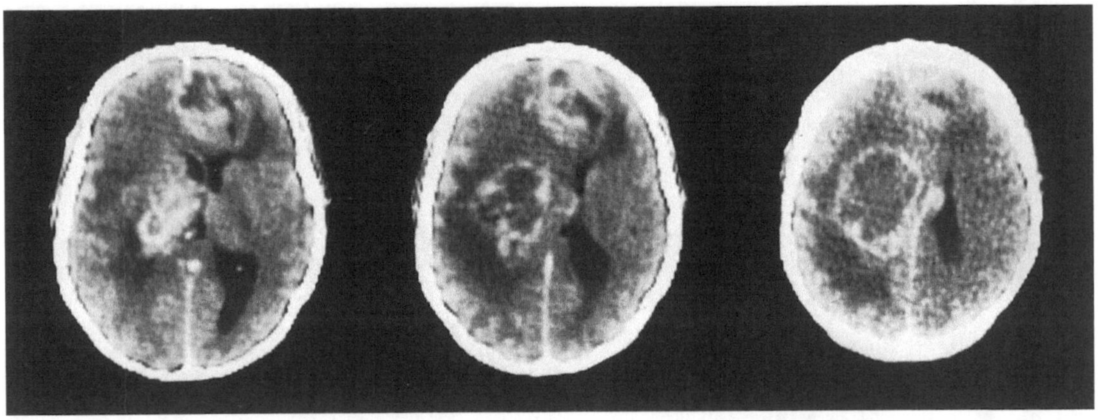

**Fig. D1.97.** Multifocal glioblastoma with nodules in the right frontal lobe and the basal ganglia on the left in a 47-year-old patient with right hemiparesis and a severe organic brain syndrome. Both tumor nodules demonstrate typical characteristics of glioblastoma: garland figures in viable tumor after contrast administration as well as extensive central necrosis. Postcontrast study

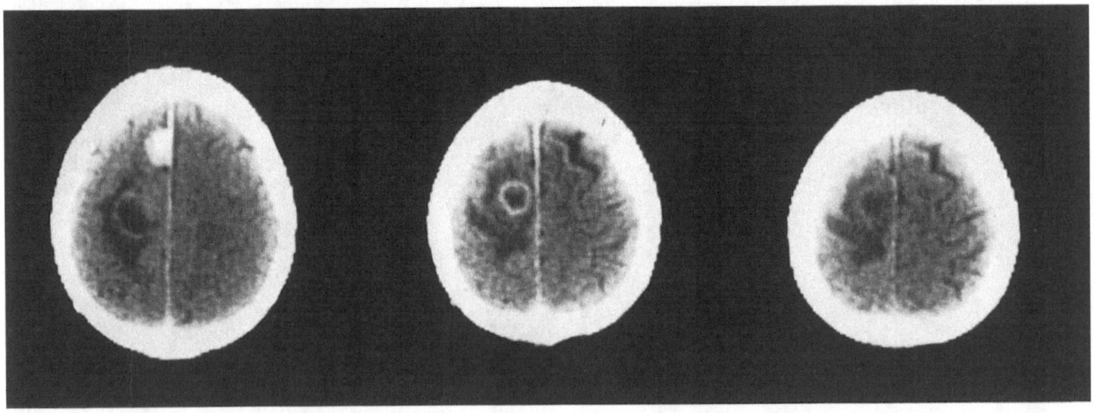

**Fig. D1.98.** Multiple tumors in the left parietal region in an 85-year-old patient with slowly progredient right hemiparesis. Small glioblastoma with ring enhancement in the left central region with grade I–II perifocal edema. A small falx meningioma, which had not produced symptoms, is visible anterior to the glioblastoma. Both diagnoses confirmed by histological examination. Postcontrast study

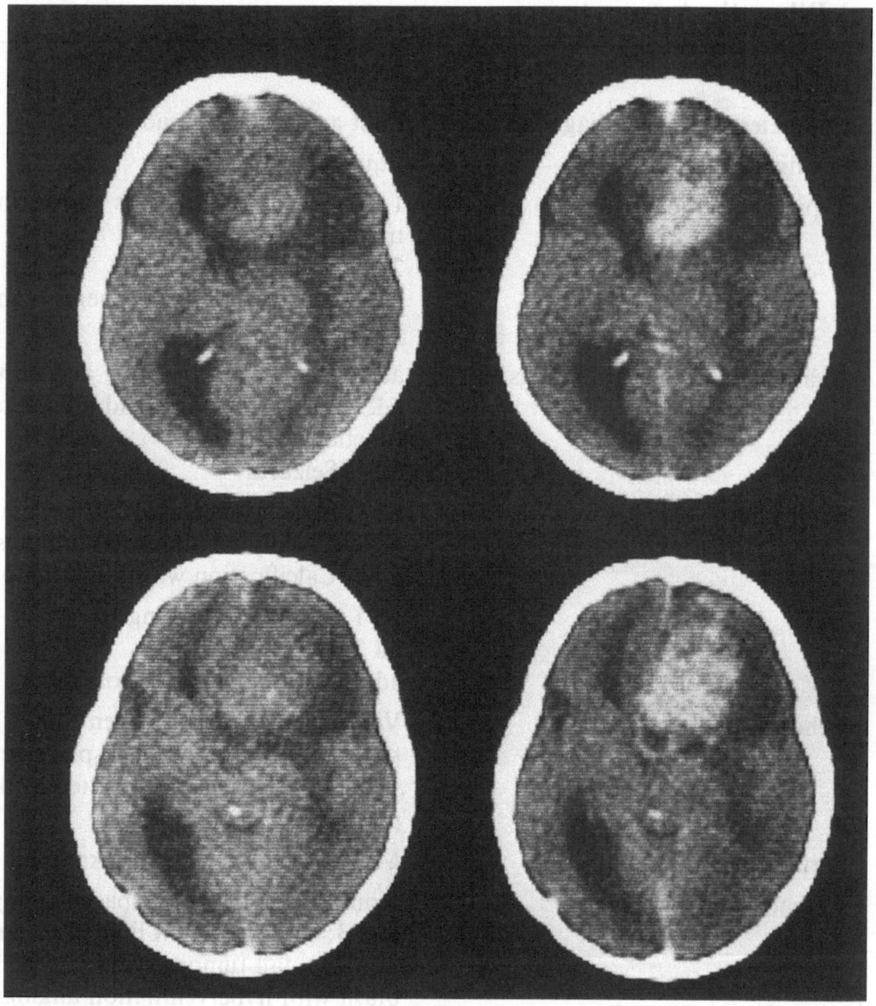

**Fig. D1.99.** Gliosarcoma of the right frontal region with penetration to the right anterior horn in a 57-year-old patient. The tumor appears isodense in precontrast studies (left) and demonstrates inhomogeneous contrast enhancement in postcontrast studies (right). The large solid tumor is not typical of most glioblastomas but may be found in anaplastic ependymoma or astrocytoma

## g) Pilocytic Astrocytomas

| | |
|---|---|
| Incidence | 3–6% |
| Characteristic age at diagnosis | First and second decades |
| Sex distribution | Equal distribution |
| Typical locations | 1. Cerebellar hemispheres and vermis, fourth ventricle and pons<br>2. Chiasmal region<br>3. Rarely cerebral hemispheres with predilection for the temporal lobe |
| Characteristic clinical findings | ad 1. Headache, vomiting, and ataxia<br>ad 2. Visual disorders and disorders of hypothalamic function<br>ad 3. Seizures |
| Skull film | ad 1. Signs of increased intracranial pressure<br>ad 2. Usually no abnormal findings<br>ad 3. Calcification within the tumor in some cases |
| EEG | ad 1. Nonspecific changes<br>ad 2. No findings<br>ad 3. Focal activity in most cases |
| Echoencephalography | Ventricular dilatation when tumor located in the posterior fossa; little or no displacement of midline structures when tumor located in the cerebral hemispheres |
| Serial brain scintigraphy | Marked radionuclide uptake in all large tumors |
| Cerebral angiography | Nonspecific signs of a space-occupying lesion in 1 and 3; demonstration limited to large tumors at location 2; small tumor vessels and delicate capillary blush with hyperventilation angiography |
| Additional contrast studies | ad 1. Central ventriculography demonstrates displacement of the fourth ventricle or delineates the contour of the tumor<br>ad 2. Demonstration of the chiasmal region with pneumoencephalography |

| | |
|---|---|
| **Computed Tomography** | |
| Precontrast study | ad 1. Hypodense or, more rarely, isodense zone; combination of both types, sometimes calcification<br>ad 2. Isodense or hyperdense zone in most cases<br>ad 3. Inhomogeneous absorption pattern with calcification and cysts in some cases |
| Contrast medium uptake | Strongly positive in solid uncalcified portions of the tumor |
| Appearance after contrast enhancement | ad 1. and 3.: Solid tumor nodules, partly combined with cysts or ring stuctures<br>ad 2. Solid tumors in most cases |

Continuation see p. 91

Continuation

**Differential Diagnosis**

ad 1. Atypical medulloblastoma or ependymoma
Hemangioblastoma
Cerebellar abscess

ad 2. Craniopharyngioma
Pituitary adenoma
Histiocytosis X

ad 3. Anaplastic astrocytoma
Glioblastoma
Oligodendroglioma
Gangliocytoma
Cavernous hemangioma
Metastasis

The following histological diagnoses are currently grouped under the term "pilocytic astrocytoma" because the histological features are virtually identical: *cystic and solid cerebellar astrocytoma, cerebellar spongioblastoma, polar spongioblastoma, optic nerve glioma, hypothalamic glioma, juvenile astrocytoma, and infundibuloma.*

Total resection of the tumor in either the cerebral hemispheres or the cerebellum results in cure, and the pilocytic astrocytoma is therefore classified as a grade I tumor. Reports in the literature suggest that pilocytic astrocytoma comprises 6%–7% of brain tumors (ZÜLCH 1975; CUSHING series), though they made up only 3% of tumors in our collective. Pilocytic astrocytoma may occur in all age groups but demonstrates a predilection for children and adolescents with an equal distribution between the two sexes.

## Typical Locations

Pilocytic astrocytoma is most often located in the *cerebellar region* – in the vermis cerebelli, the cerebellar hemisphere, the 4th ventricle, or the caudal brain stem. Pilocytic astrocytoma is the third most common tumor in the *chiasma region*. It may also be found in the *cerebral hemispheres*, most often in the medial portion of the temporal lobe, in the *basal ganglia*, and the *quadrigeminal region*.

## Characteristic Clinical Findings

Symptoms and signs are related to location of the tumor. Headache, vomiting, and ataxia are found in cerebellar tumors, disorders of vision when the optic nerve or the chiasma is involved, diencephalic signs with cachexia, especially in young children, when the tumor is located in the hypothalamus, and epileptic seizures when the tumor is located in the cerebral hemispheres.

## Additional Diagnostic Procedures

Plain skull films demonstrate indirect signs of increased intracranial pressure only when the tumor is located in the posterior fossa, though calcification may be observed on occasion. EEG shows pathological findings in tumors of the cerebral hemispheres. Echoencephalography demonstrates hydrocephalus when the pilocytic astrocytoma is located in the posterior fossa but does not usually show displacement of midline structures in cerebral tumors of this histological type. Cerebral serial scintigraphy reveals intense nuclide uptake in all large tumors but there are no pathognomonic scintigraphic features in pilocytic astrocytoma. Cerebral angiography demonstrates displacement of major vessels without characteristic findings. Pneumoencephalography and ventriculography are capable of demonstrating the tumor but do not suggest the histological diagnosis.

## Computed Tomography (Figs. D1.100–133)

### Precontrast Study

Absorption values may show a wide range in pilocytic astrocytoma since cysts and calcification may occur in the same tumor (Fig. D1.100).

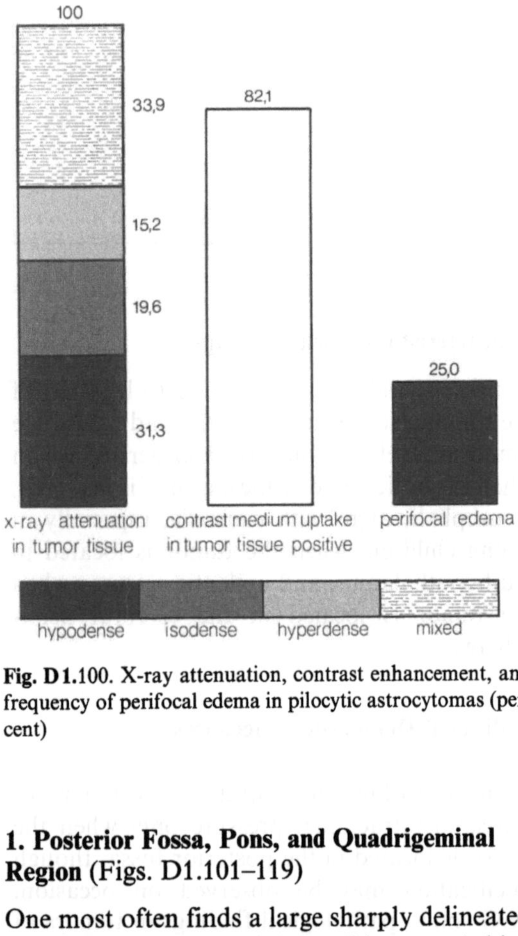


**Fig. D1.100.** X-ray attenuation, contrast enhancement, and frequency of perifocal edema in pilocytic astrocytomas (percent)

### 1. Posterior Fossa, Pons, and Quadrigeminal Region (Figs. D1.101–119)

One most often finds a large sharply delineated hypodense zone containing solid tumor (which demonstrates somewhat higher density than the cystic or edematous areas before contrast enhancement). Solid tumor usually appears slightly hypodense, rarely isodense in comparison with adjacent, normal cerebellar tissue (Figs. D1.101–104). The more hypodense areas usually represent either cysts (density 18–20 HU) or perifocal edema (18–26 HU). Extremely high density values indicate either hemorrhage or calcification in the tumor itself (Figs. D1.111, 112).

The 4th ventricle is usually compressed and sometimes displaced laterally by the tumor. Cranial displacement and enlargement of the 4th ventricle may be found when a tumor is located in the lower segments of the cerebellum, but the 4th ventricle may be completely compressed when tumor extends throughout the cerebellum. Tumors are occasionally found within the 4th ventricle entirely surrounded by CSF (Fig. D1.115). In these cases the origin of the tumor is not visible; the ventricles are dilated and may demonstrate periventricular lucency especially around the anterior horns (Fig. D1.103).

### 2. Chiasmal Region (Figs. D1.120, G12)

Partial or total obliteration of the opticochiasmatic cistern or the third ventricle is a typical finding in the plain CT scan in pilocytic astrocytomas, which are often isodense (Fig. D1.120). Calcification may be present and small cysts are sometimes found. Rostral extension may result in blockage of the foramen of Monro which causes unilateral or bilateral ventricular dilatation. If the tumor reaches the optic nerve, there are corresponding changes in the nerve which are clearly visibly in the precontrast CT (Fig. G12, p. 471).

### 3. Cerebral Hemispheres and Basal Ganglia (Figs. D1.121–133)

One finds a wide variety of density values – hypodense in cystic tumors, isodense in solid lesions, and hyperdense in calcified tumors. Solid isodense tumors are recognizable in the plain CT scan only when perifocal edema or calcification is present. However, *perifocal edema is found in only 25% of pilocytic astrocytomas, less frequently than in any other cerebral tumor* with contrast medium uptake.

### Postcontrast Study

With few exceptions pilocytic astrocytomas demonstrate a pronounced increase in density after contrast enhancement in the solid uncalcified portions of the tumor. Increase in density averages 12–14 HU with application of a standard contrast dose, and the enhancement is often visible for a long period of time.

Cysts and perifocal edema are more clearly delineated as a result of increased density in the solid uncalcified portions of the tumor. Ring structures may appear (Figs. D1.107, 108, 127).

In our experience cerebellar pilocytic astrocytoma may take *three different forms:*

1. Large cyst with a small marginal tumor
2. Large solid tumor with a cyst and ring enhancement of varying size
3. Relatively small solid tumor without cyst

## Differential Diagnosis

### 1. Posterior Fossa

Rare atypical *medulloblastomas* with isodense or hypodense structures may resemble pilocytic astrocytoma, and contrast enhancement is of little help in differentiation, since both tumors demonstrate a pronounced increase in density after contrast enhancement. However, contrast with time studies show clearly different curves (see p. 150).

It may be difficult to differentiate pilocytic astrocytoma from uncalcified *ependymoma* of the fourth ventricle. There was not a single case of calcified pilocytic astrocytoma at this location in our collective.

*Angioblastomas* may produce similar CT findings, but these tumors are most common in the middle aged and are extremely rare in children (only 2 of 41 angioblastomas in our study). The increase in absorption in the solid portions of angioblastoma is considerably greater than in pilocytic astrocytoma as a result of the vascularity of the former.

*Cerebellar abscess* may resemble pilocytic astrocytoma with a ring structure in the CT scan (Fig. F11, p. 411), but the history and clinical course usually suggest the diagnosis.

### 2. Chiasmal Region

Differentiation between *craniopharyngioma* and calcified pilocytic astrocytoma is not possible with the CT scan alone. Additional clinical and radiological parameters including skull films and endocrinological studies may not provide evidence for definitive diagnosis in individual cases. *Pituitary adenoma* of the suprasellar region demonstrates typical radiological and endocrinological findings which allow differentiation from pilocytic astrocytoma of the chiasma or the hypothalamus in nearly every case.

### 3. Cerebral Hemispheres

Pilocytic astrocytomas in the cerebral hemispheres present such a variety of findings in the CT scan that it is not possible to define pathognomonic CT criteria which allow certain differentiation from other tumors (Figs. D1.121–133). The range of diagnostic alternatives is reduced to *gangliocytoma, meningioma and cavernous hemangioma* when the tumor is located in the median portion of the temporal lobe.

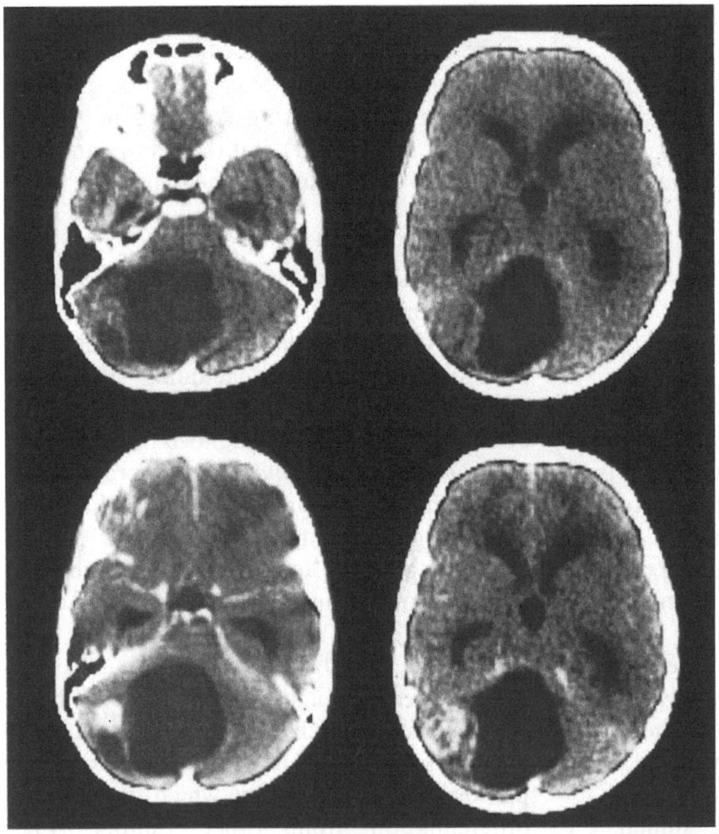

**Fig. D1.101.** Pilocytic astrocytoma in a 10-year-old boy with signs of left cerebellar dysfunction. Precontrast CT studies (above) show a large cystic lesion in the posterior fossa, extending to the left. Postcontrast studies (below) reveal a solid tumor at the edge of the cyst in the left lateral portions. The tumor itself has slightly hypodense values in the precontrast CT. Dilatation of the ventricular system with slight periventricular lucency

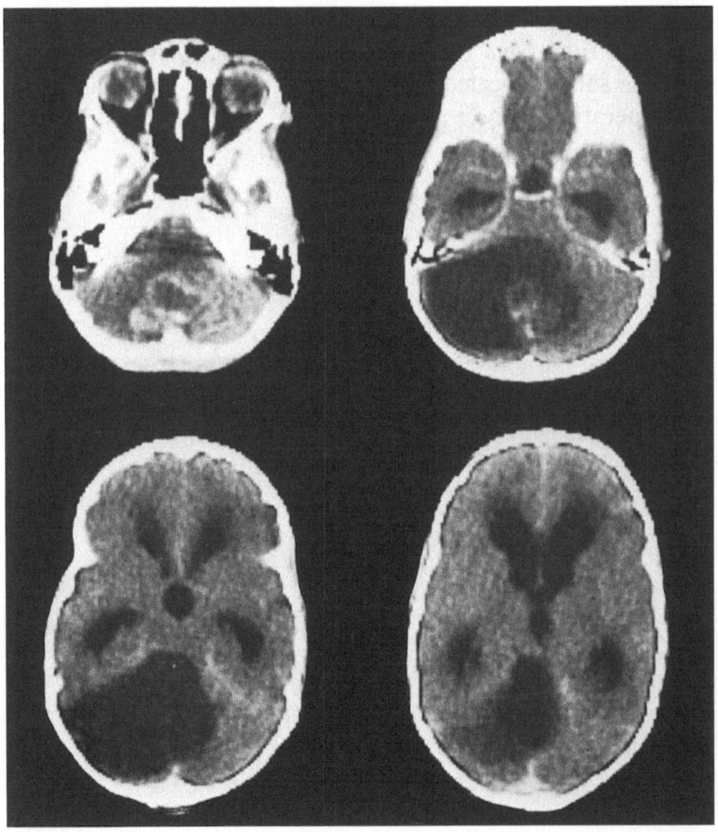

**Fig. D1.102.** Pilocytic astrocytoma of the cerebellum. Large cystic lesion which almost completely fills the posterior fossa on the left and extends to the right side. A small tumor nodule with a hypodense zone at its center is demonstrated at the margin of the cyst in the lower segments of the cerebellum. The tumor appeared slightly hypodense in precontrast CT studies. Pronounced hydrocephalus with slight periventricular lucency in a 12-year-old girl with signs of cerebellar dysfunction. Postcontrast study

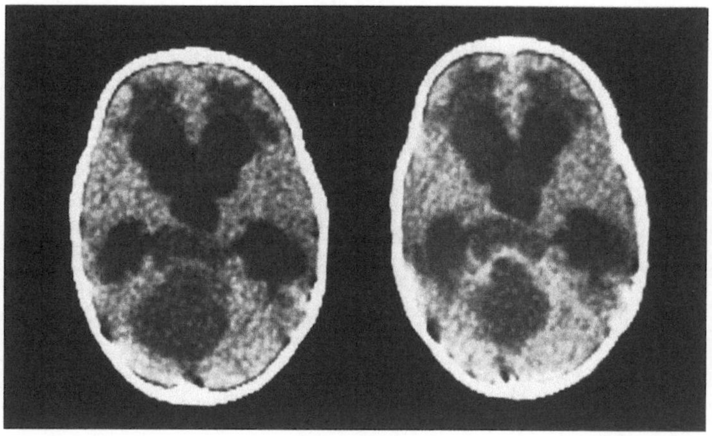

**Fig. D1.103.** Pilocytic astrocytoma of the vermis cerebelli and the midbrain in a 9-year-old girl. The tumor contains hypodense zones (cysts) and has caused obliteration of the third ventricle with consequent hydrocephalus accompanied by extensive periventricular lucency. The few solid portions of the tumor take up contrast media (right)

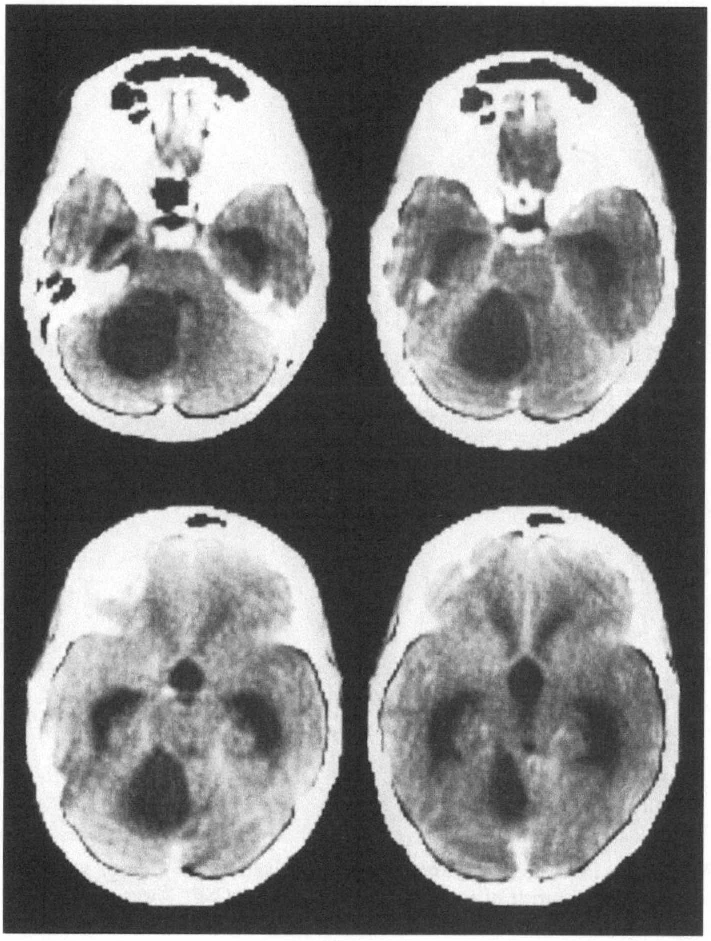

**Fig. D1.104.** Pilocytic astrocytoma in the left cerebellar hemisphere and the caudal brain stem in a 30-year-old woman. CT studies reveal only a sharply delineated hypodense zone (cyst) but not the solid tumor nodule in the caudal brain stem. Misinterpretation as angioblastoma is obvious. Postcontrast study

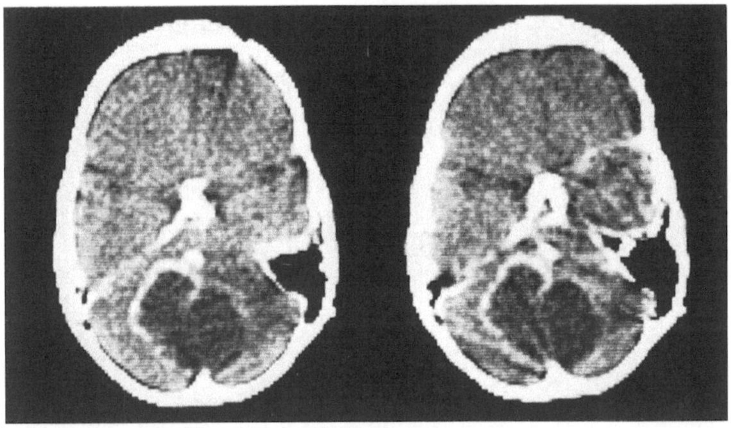

**Fig. D1.105.** Pilocytic astrocytoma with a large cyst and marginal contrast enhancement in a 9-year-old girl. A calcified craniopharyngioma is also demonstrated. Both diagnoses confirmed at histological examination. Postcontrast study

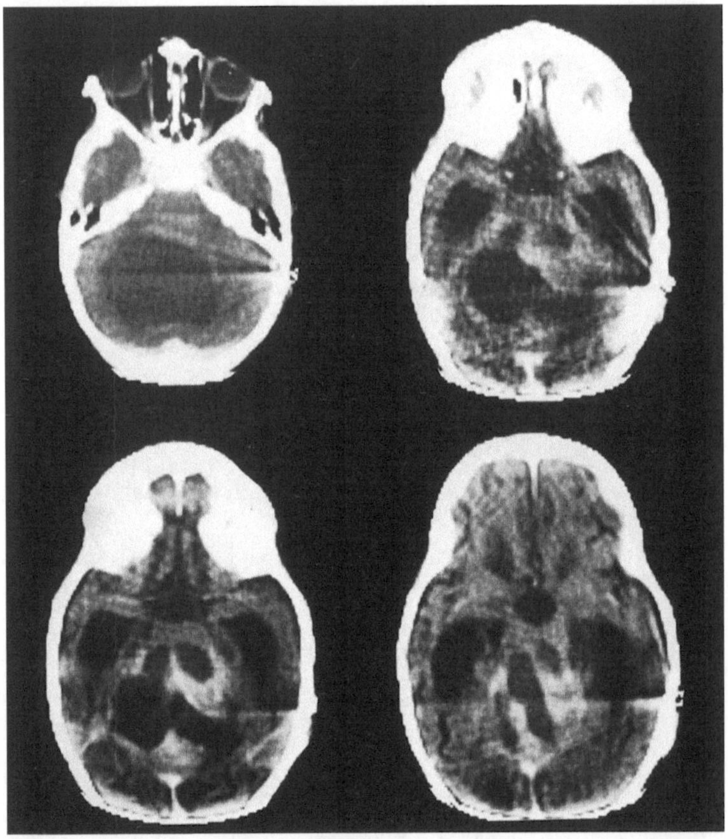

**Fig. D1.106.** Pilocytic astrocytoma in the cerebellar vermis and the fourth ventricle of a child who had received a CSF shunt 6 months earlier (artifacts). Multiple large and small cysts, strong contrast enhancement in solid tumor tissue. Demarcation against the brain stem is not possible in the CT study. The tumor, which originated in the roof of the fourth ventricle, was resected in toto at operation. There was extreme dilatation of the fourth ventricle, but the floor of the ventricle had not been infiltrated by tumor. Precontrast studies revealed an extensive hypodense zone in the posterior fossa. Postcontrast study

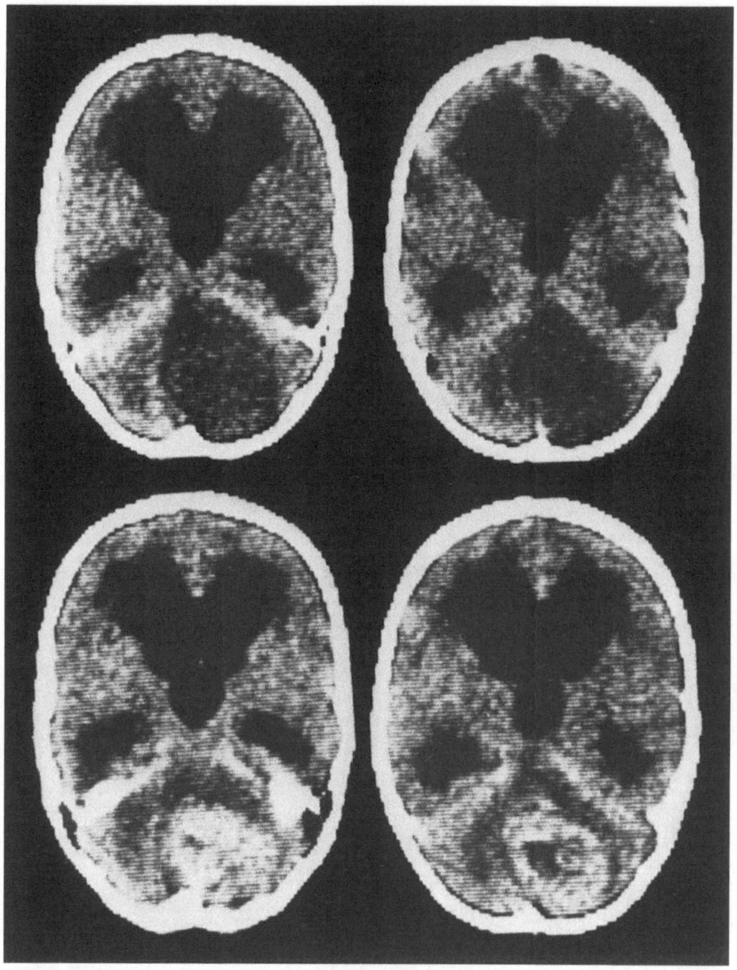

**Fig. D 1.107.** Large pilocytic astrocytoma in the vermis cerebelli and the right cerebellar hemisphere in a 2-year-old girl with signs of cerebellar dysfunction and increased intracranial pressure. Precontrast studies (above) demonstrate a large hypodense zone in the posterior fossa as well as pronounced hydrocephalus with periventricular lucency. Postcontrast studies (below) demonstrate a large solid tumor with strong contrast enhancement and a small central hypodense zone which proved to be a cyst at operation. Slight perifocal edema

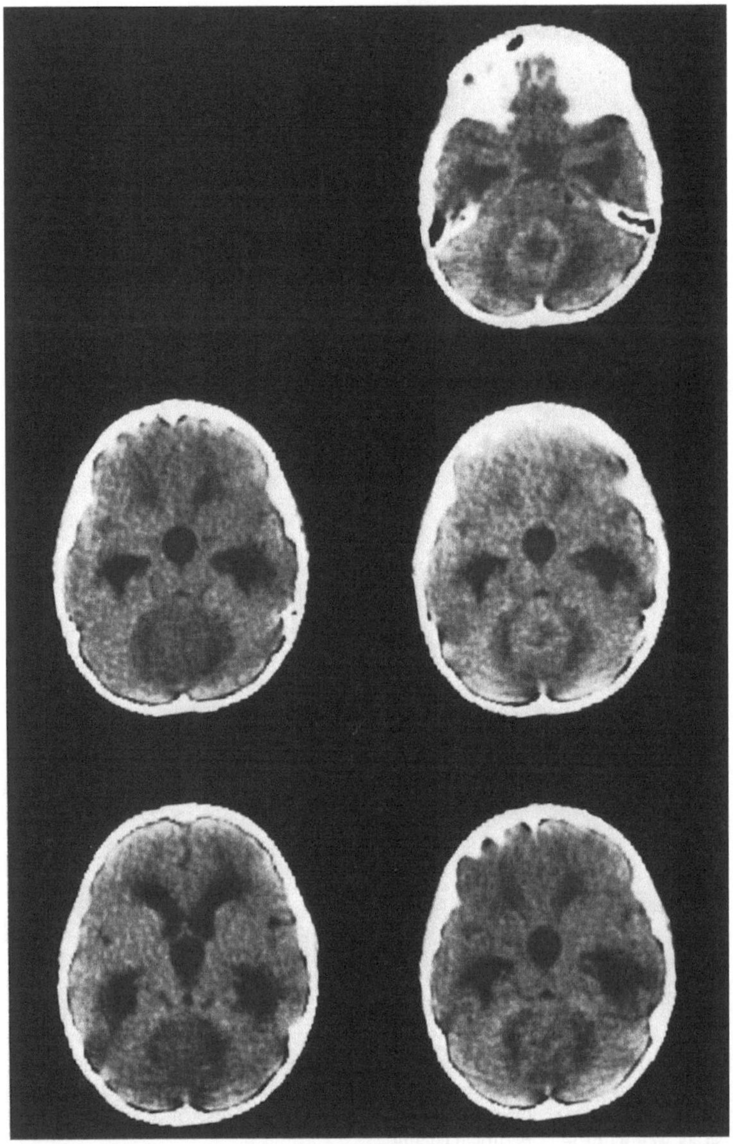

**Fig. D 1.108.** Pilocytic astrocytoma of the vermis cerebelli in a $6^1/_2$-year-old boy with signs of cerebellar dysfunction. Precontrast studies (left) demonstrate a solid hypodense tumor which strongly suggests a diagnosis of pilocytic astrocytoma. Postcontrast studies show slight contrast enhancement in the solid portions of the tumor with a small central hypodense zone (cyst). Differentiation between medulloblastoma and pilocytic astrocytoma on the basis of contrast studies alone is not possible; analysis of the precontrast study provides the diagnosis

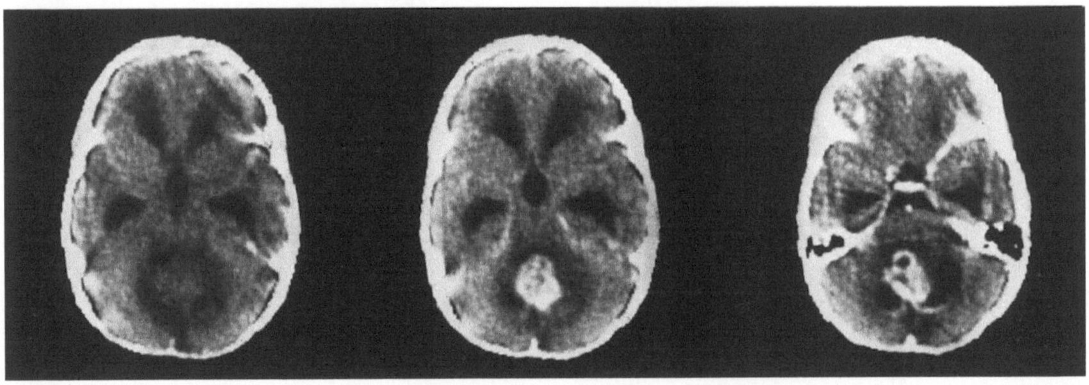

**Fig. D 1.109.** Pilocytic astrocytoma at the roof of the fourth ventricle and in the vermis cerebelli in a 9-year-old girl. Precontrast studies reveal a slightly hypodense tumor with perifocal edema. Significant contrast enhancement of solid tumor nodule (middle and right) as well as demonstration of adjacent cystic portions. Moderate hydrocephalus with slight periventricular lucency. The precontrast study provides the key to the histological diagnosis

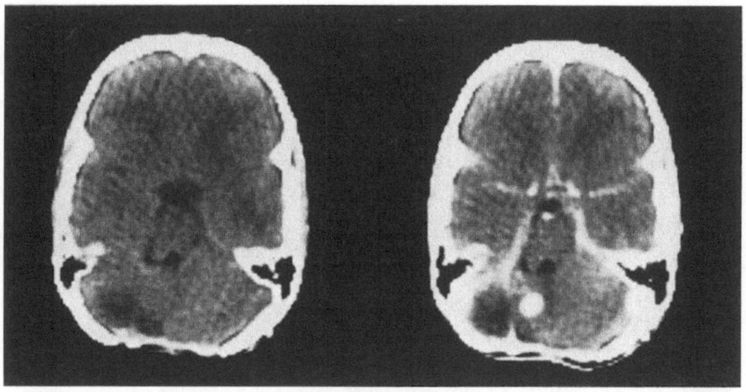

**Fig. D1.110.** Recurrence of pilocytic astrocytoma in the left cerebellar hemisphere. The actual tumor nodule is demonstrated only after contrast enhancement (right). Precontrast studies show hypodense zones in the region of the previous surgical intervention (left) which could be interpreted as sequelae of operation (13-year-old girl)

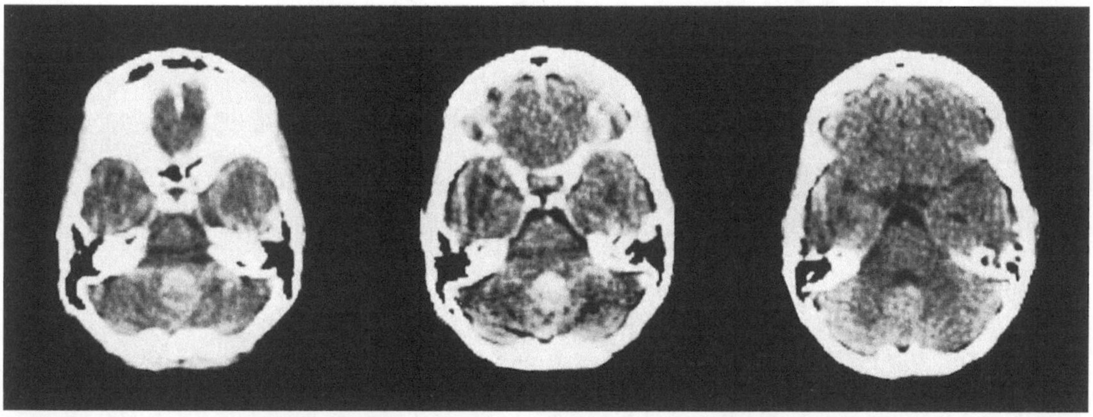

**Fig. D1.111.** Pilocytic astrocytoma with hemorrhage in a 15-year-old girl who presented with signs of acute subarachnoid hemorrhage. Demonstration of a spherical hyperdense zone 2 cm in diameter at the outlet of the fourth ventricle. Administration of a contrast medium did not result in significantly increased values. At operation solid tumor was found only at the margins, while the rest of the lesion was composed of clotted blood

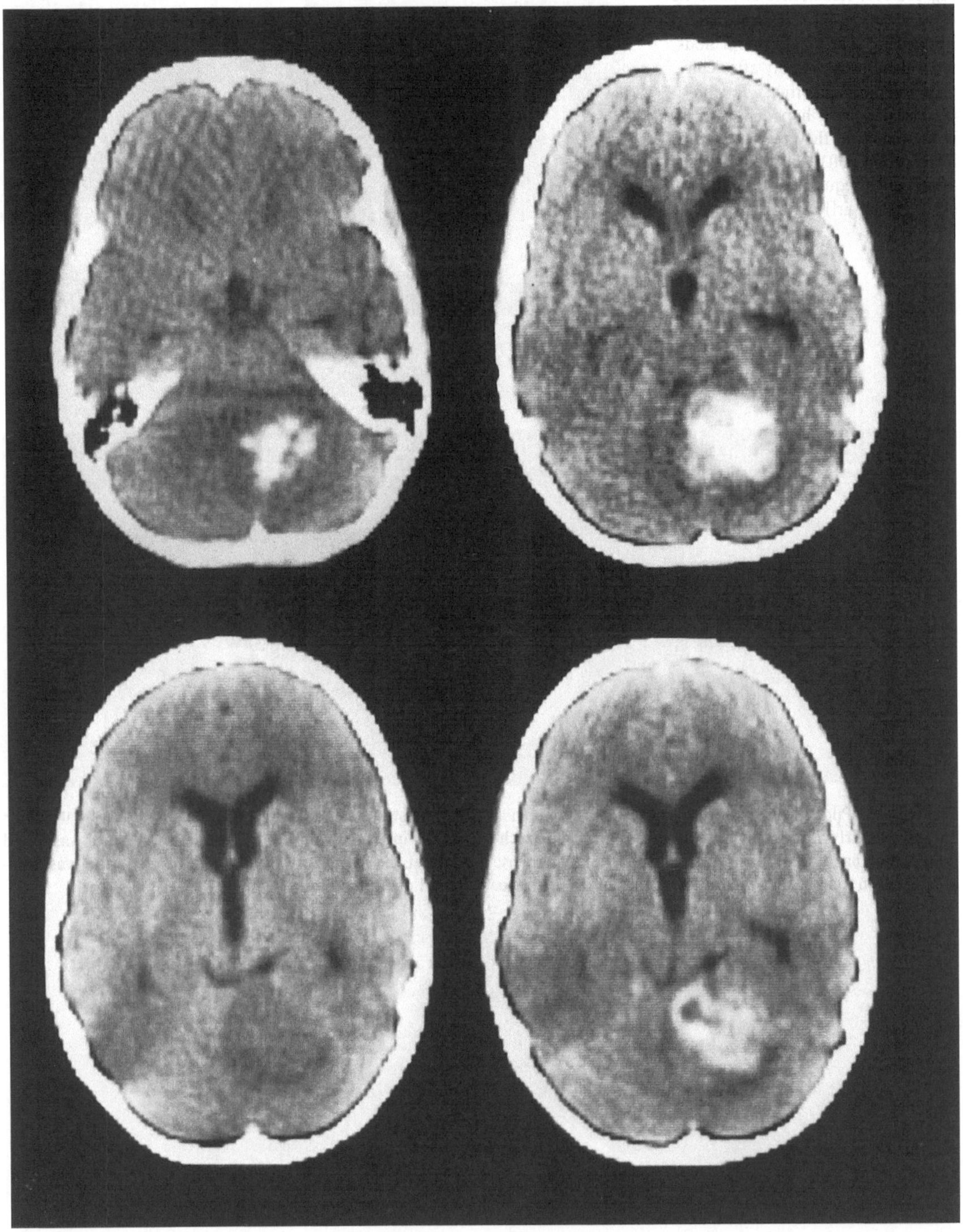

**Fig. D1.**112. Pilocytic astrocytoma in the right cerebellar hemisphere in a 13-year-old girl with signs of cerebellar dysfunction. Precontrast studies reveal a tumor with hypodense areas and calcification (left). The solid uncalcified portions of the tumor demonstrate strong contrast enhancement (right)

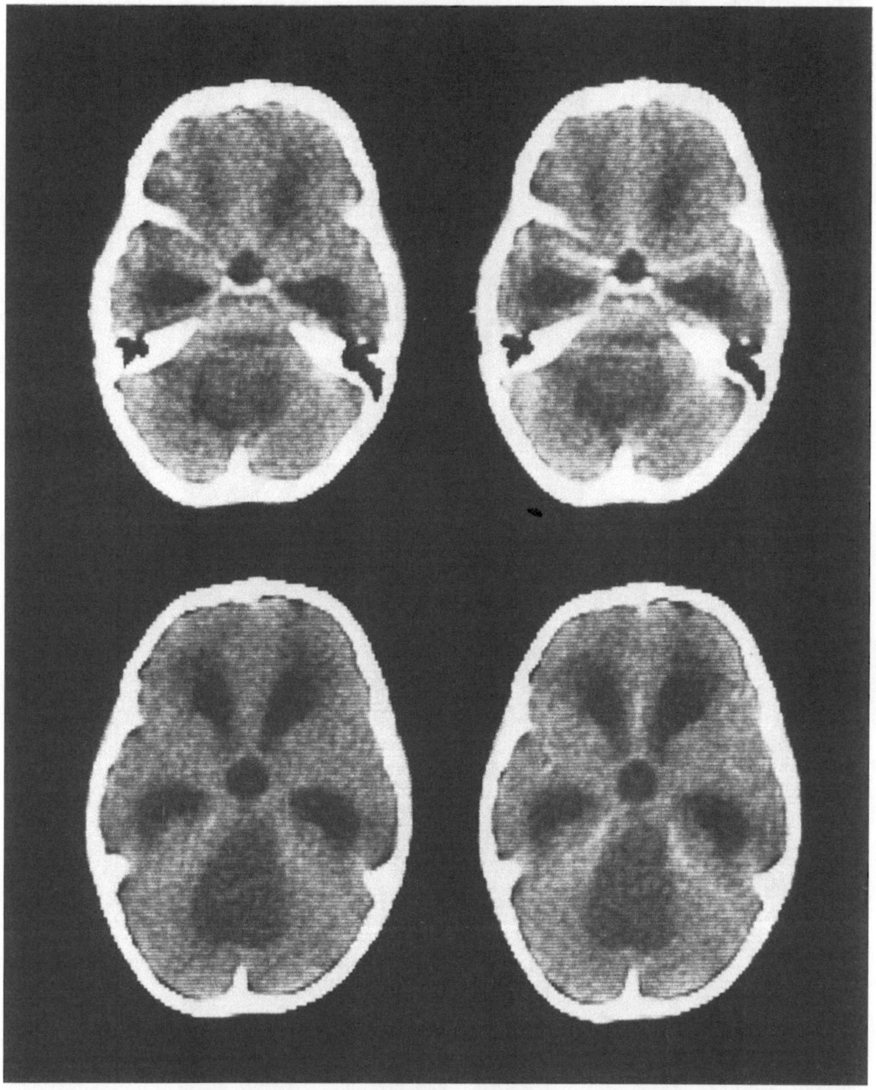

**Fig. D1.113.** Variant of pilocytic astrocytoma in a 7-year-old boy. The tumor is located in the vermis cerebelli with extension to the midbrain. It demonstrates hypodense values both before and after administration of contrast medium. At operation a solid glassy tumor was removed; histological examination revealed a variant form of pilocytic astrocytoma

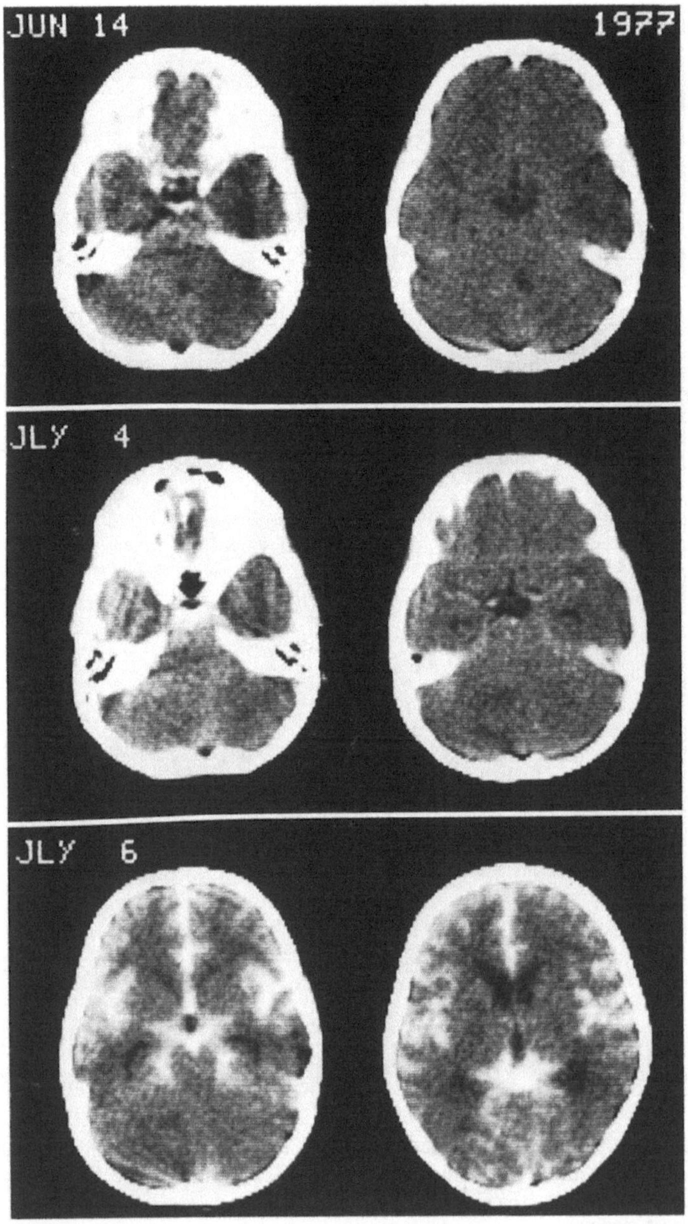


a

b

c

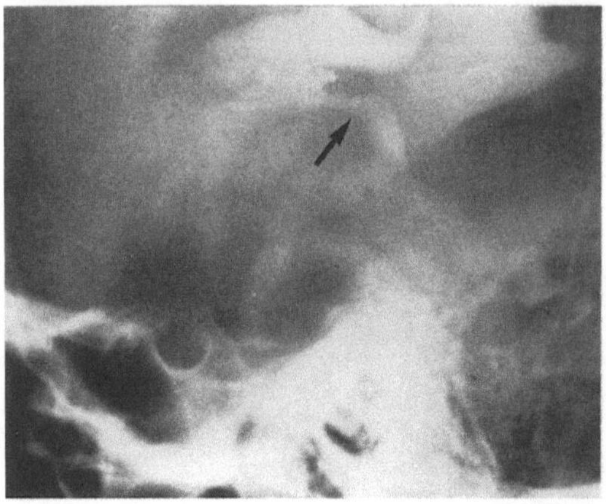

d

**Fig. D1.**114 a–e. Follow-up study in a 7-year-old boy with an anaplastic pilocytic astrocytoma of the brain stem and the cerebellum. The CT studies were performed as progredient cerebellar dysfunction appeared. (**a**) Initial CT studies demonstrate slight displacement of the fourth ventricle to the right (with no other pathological findings). (**b**) In follow-up studies 18 days later the fourth ventricle was obliterated and there was some dilatation of the temporal horns of the lateral ventricles (right). (**c**) CT studies with intrathecal instillation of metrizamide demonstrate slight torsion of the brain stem and further increase in the width of the ventricles. (**d**) Deformation of the aqueduct demonstrated by central ventriculography which confirms the diagnosis of a tumor in the posterior fossa. (**e**) A tumor with a small cyst originating in the brain stem and projecting from the left into the fourth ventricle was found at operation (view through the microscope)

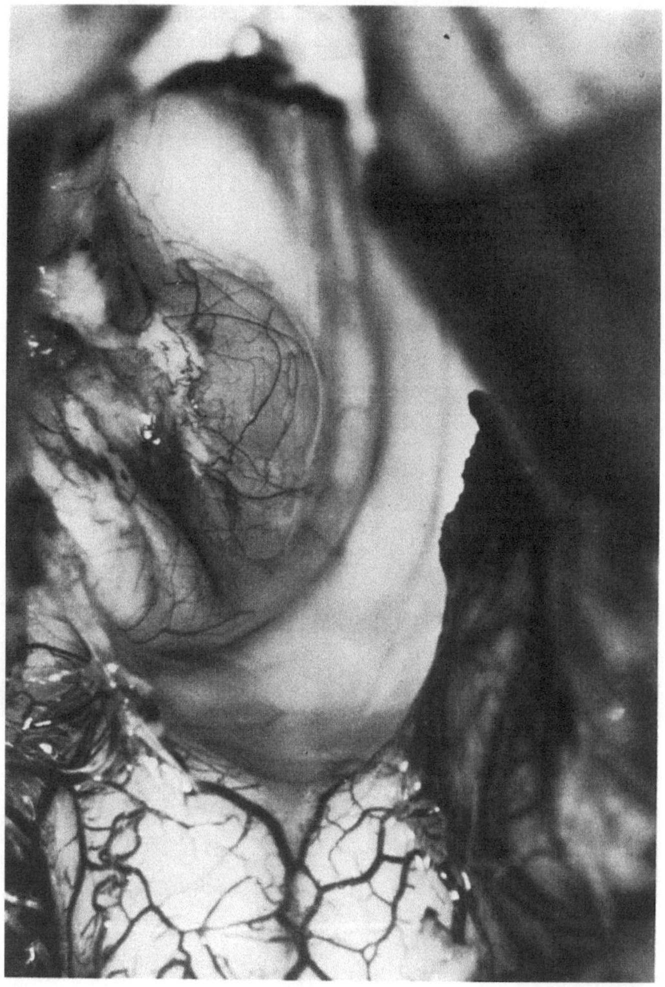

**Fig. D1.114e**

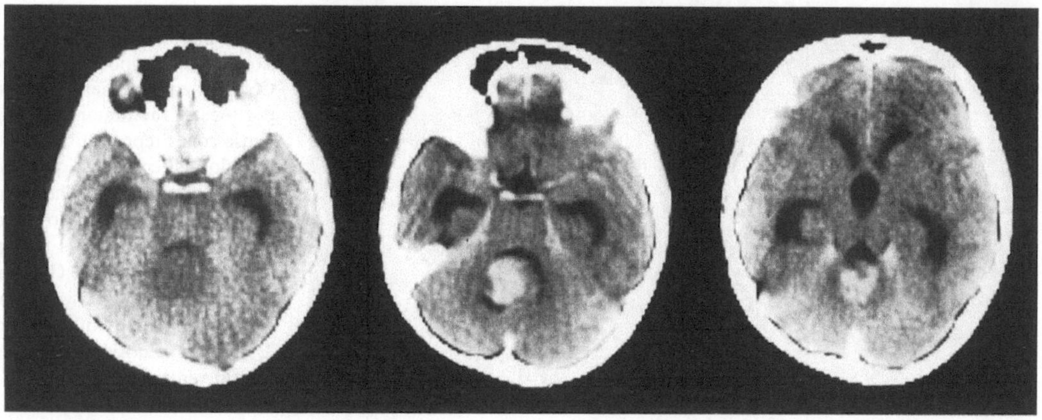

**Fig. D1.115.** Pilocytic astrocytoma in an 8-year-old boy. The tumor is primarily hypodense (left) and demonstrates homogeneous contrast enhancement. The lesion seems to be surrounded by CSF (middle), but the origin of the tumor is not demonstrable in the CT scan. The absorption values permit a histological diagnosis. At operation the origin of the tumor was found in the brain stem in the lower segments of the rhomboid fossa

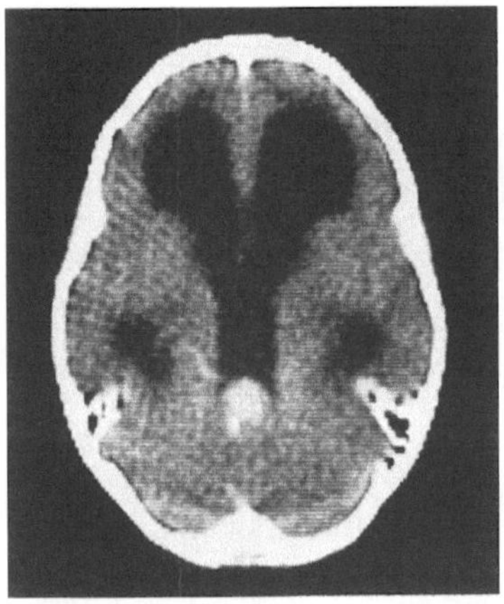

**Fig. D1.116.** Pilocytic astrocytoma in the aqueduct with extreme hydrocephalus in a 15-year-old boy. Strong contrast enhancement in the solid tumor nodule. CT studies were performed after ataxic gait was noted following slight craniocerebral injury

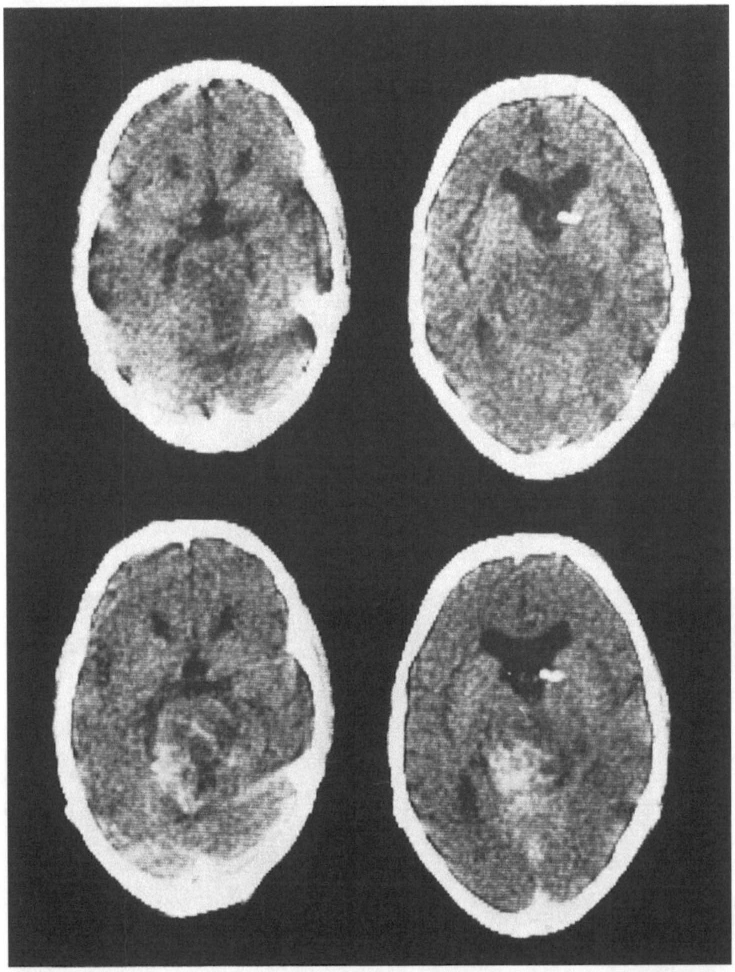

**Fig. D1.117.** Pilocytic astrocytoma of the midbrain. Tumor tissue is isodense and hypodense (above). Contrast enhancement in the solid portions of the tumor with hypodense zones representing small cysts. Histological confirmation of the diagnosis at operation. The high density figure projecting into the right anterior horn represents the tip of a ventricular catheter. A CSF shunt had been implanted 3 years previously for therapy of a presumed "aqueduct stenosis" (diagnosis by central ventriculography)

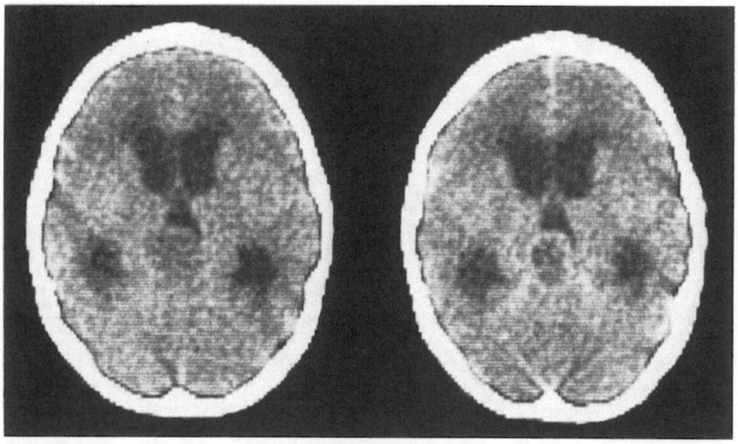

**Fig. D1.118.** Pilocytic astrocytoma in the pineal region with obliteration of the third ventricle in a 13-year-old girl, with signs of a lesion in the lamina tecti as well as the cerebellar vermis. The solid portions of the tumor are hypodense (left), as is the case in most pilocytic astrocytomas. This permits differentiation from a genuine pinealoma. A marginal ring structure is observed after contrast enhancement (right). Histological confirmation of the diagnosis

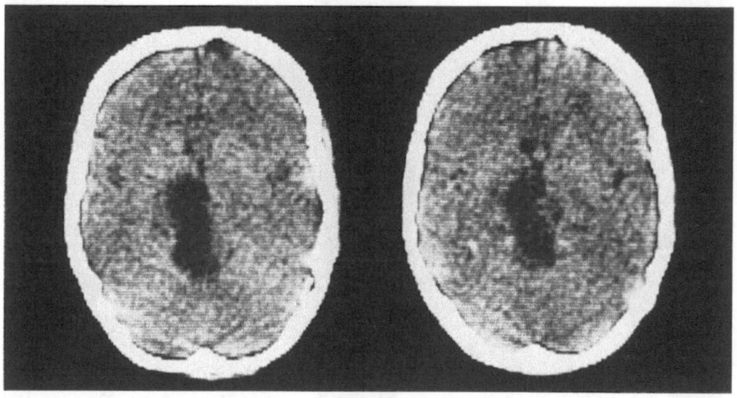

**Fig. D1.119.** Pilocytic astrocytoma of the brain stem and the left cerebral peduncle in a 21-year-old patient. An initial diagnosis of epidermoid was made on the basis of CT studies, since there was sharp demarcation of the hypodense zone (CSF density) and absence of contrast enhancement in this area. Histological studies of the surgical specimen resulted in the diagnosis of pilocytic astrocytoma

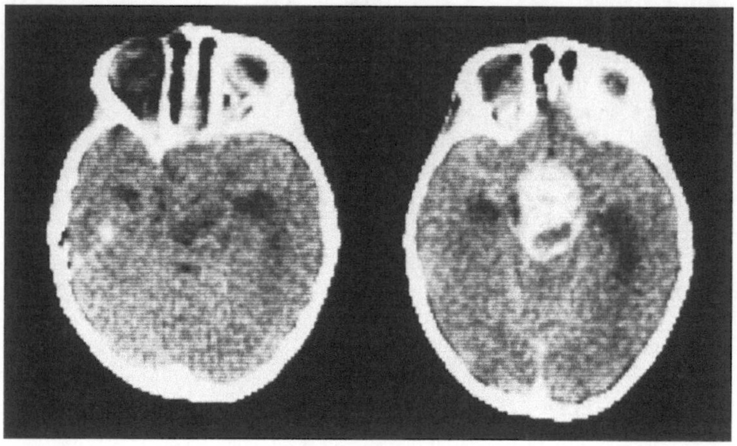

**Fig. D1.120.** Pilocytic astrocytoma of the hypothalamic region in a 6-year-old girl with signs of a diencephalic disorder. The tumor is isodense to hypodense in precontrast CT scan (left). Strong contrast enhancement in the solid portions of the tumor (right). Histological confirmation of the diagnosis

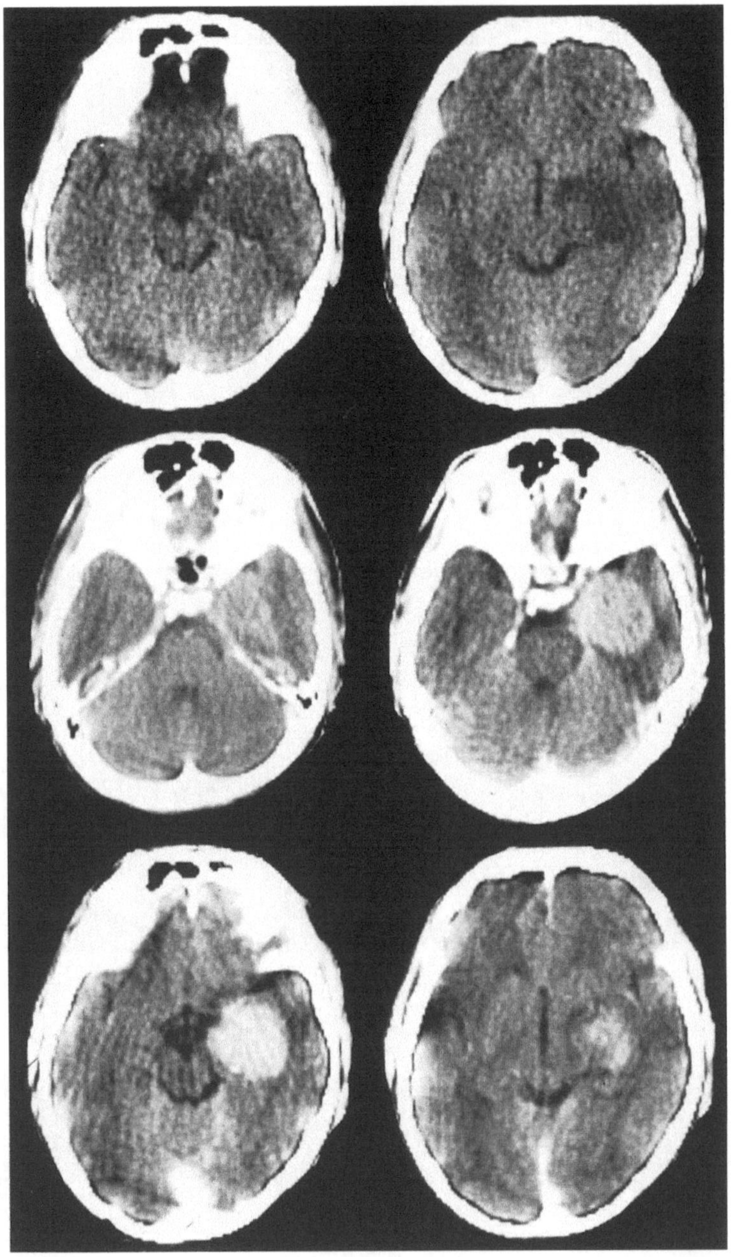

**Fig. D 1.121.** Pilocytic astrocytoma in a 17-year-old patient with seizures. The tumor appears hypodense in precontrast studies (above); post-contrast studies reveal homogeneous contrast enhancement in a tumor located in the medial portions of the right temporal lobe (lower group of four pictures). The tumor extends into the chiasmatic and ambient cisterns

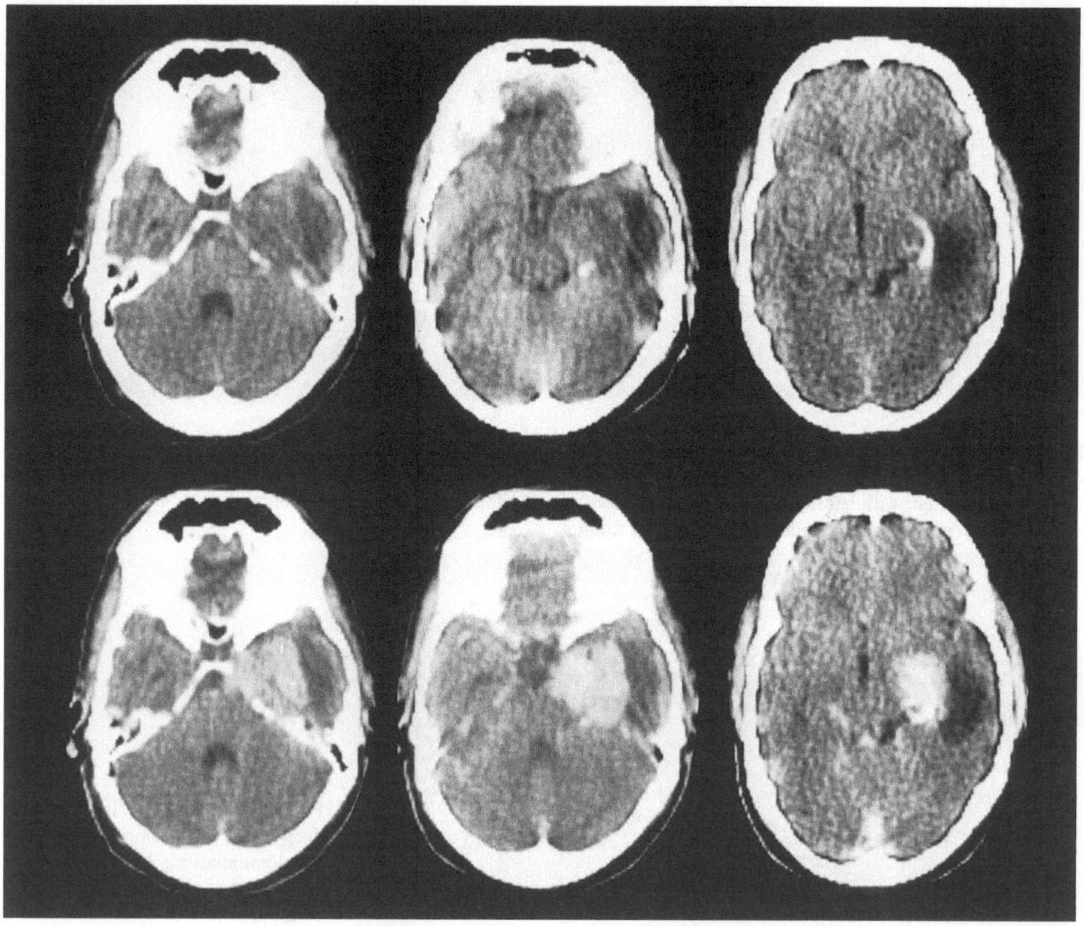

**Fig. D1.122.** Pilocytic astrocytoma in the right temporal lobe of a 17-year-old patient with seizures. The tumor demonstrates a wide variety of absorption values in precontrast CT studies (above): slightly hypodense values in the solid portions of the tumor, calcification, and crescent-shaped zones of very low density representing a cyst. Strong contrast enhancement in the solid tumor portions (below)

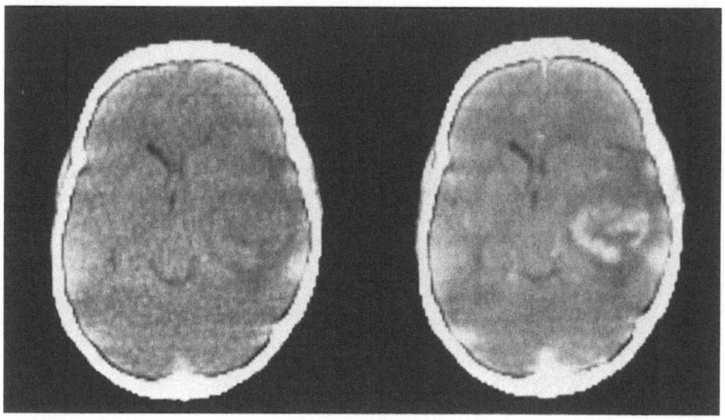

**Fig. D1.123.** Pilocytic astrocytoma in the right temporal lobe of an 11-year-old girl. Precontrast studies demonstrate isodense absorption values in the solid portions of the tumor (left). Ring structures and slight perifocal edema after contrast enhancement (right)

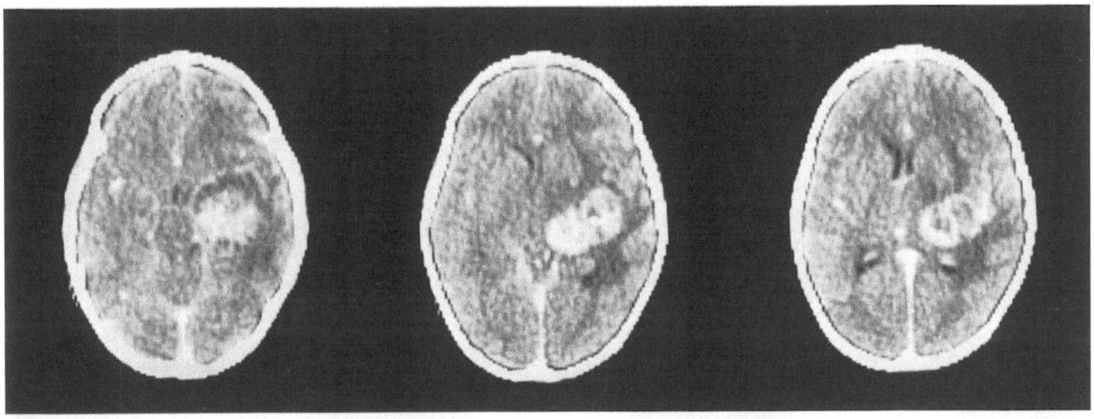

**Fig. D 1.124.** Pilocytic astrocytoma deep in the right temporal lobe with penetration of the thalamus on the right in a $3^1/_2$-year-old girl with left hemiparesis. Inhomogeneous density values after contrast enhancement in the tumor caused by cystic structures. Grade I–II perifocal edema. Postcontrast study. Diagnosis confirmed at histological examination of surgical specimen

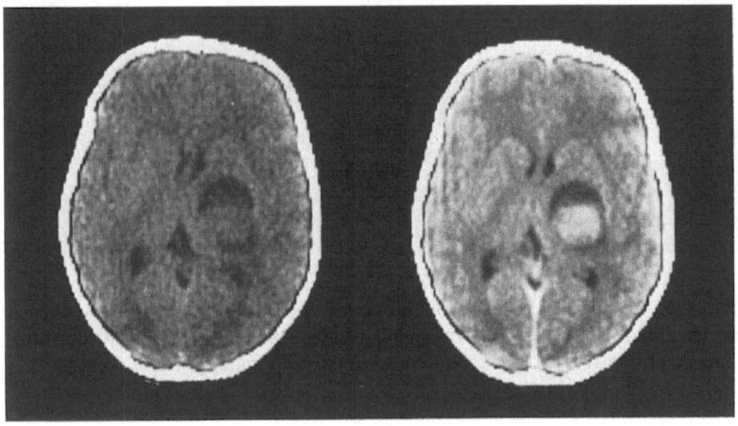

**Fig. D 1.125.** Pilocytic astrocytoma deep in the right temporal lobe and basal ganglia in a 7-year-old boy with progredient left hemiparesis. Demonstration of solid tumor within a cyst. The tumor is slightly hypodense in precontrast studies (left) with strong contrast enhancement (right). Diagnosis confirmed at histological examination of surgical specimen

**Fig. D1.126.** Large tumor in the basal ganglia on the left with extension to the left cerebral peduncle and hypothalamus in a 17-month-old child. The lesion appears hypodense with varying density values in precontrast CT studies and fulfills the CT criteria of a pilocytic astrocytoma. No histological confirmation of the diagnosis to date. Pronounced ventricular dilatation with periventricular lucency (precontrast CT on the left, postcontrast CT on the right)

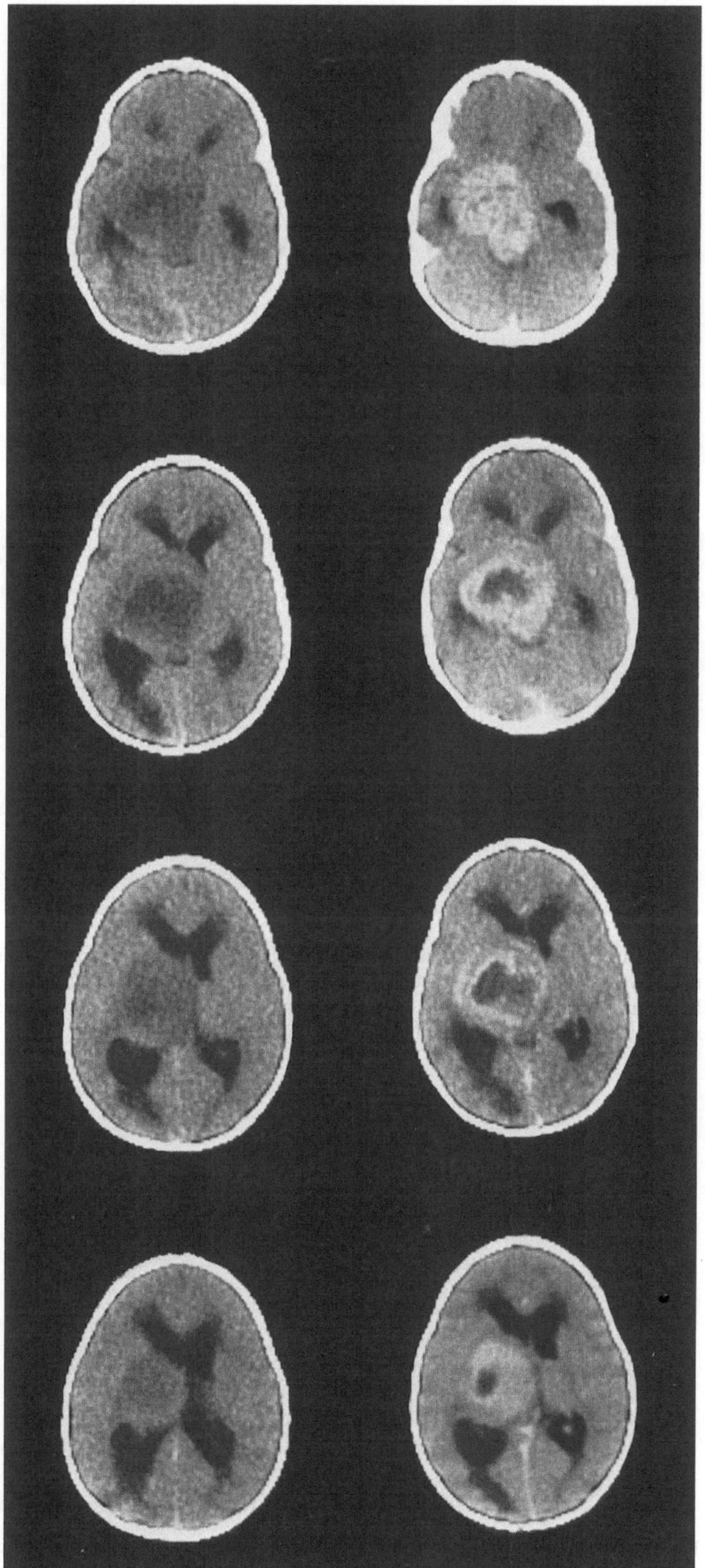

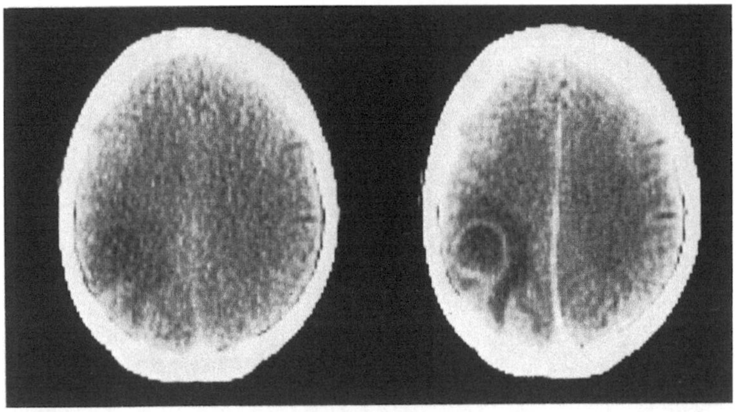

**Fig. D 1.127.** Pilocytic astrocytoma in the left parietal region of a 38-year-old patient. Precontrast studies demonstrate a hypodense lesion (left), while postcontrast studies show a ring structure (right). Grade I perifocal edema. CT findings suggested the diagnosis of anaplastic astrocytoma

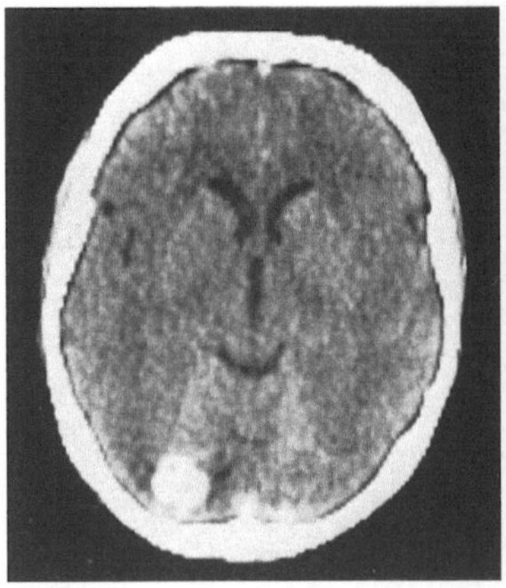

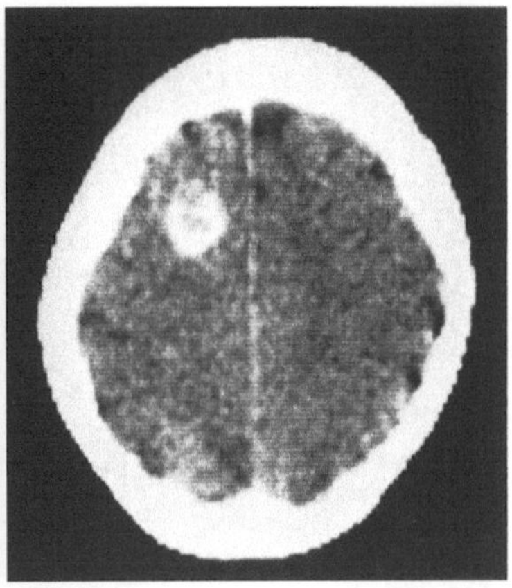

**Fig. D 1.129.** Pilocytic astrocytoma in the left precentral region in a 66-year-old patient. The tumor is almost entirely calcified. Nevertheless, oligodendroglioma hardly has to be considered in differential diagnosis ◄

▲

**Fig. D 1.128.** Pilocytic astrocytoma in the left occipital lobe in a 31-year-old man. Demonstration of a spherical calcified lesion in the left occipital lobe. There is a small zone of normal tissue between the tumor and the vault. Intracerebral tumors rarely cause such findings. Calcified meningioma originating in the tentorium may produce similar appearance in horizontal slice (see Fig. D 2.67 b)

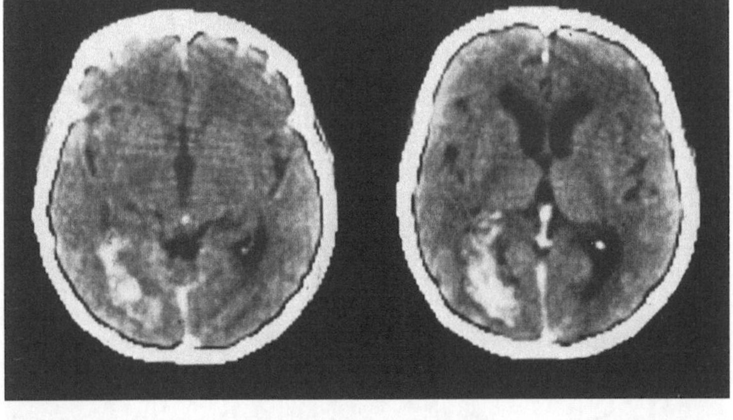

**Fig. D 1.130.** Pilocytic astrocytoma in the left occipital lobe with penetration of the lateral ventricle in a 55-year-old patient with intermittent right homonymous hemianopsia. Irregularly shaped tumor with strong contrast enhancement, initially diagnosed as arteriovenous malformation. No space-occupying effect, no perifocal edema. Postcontrast study

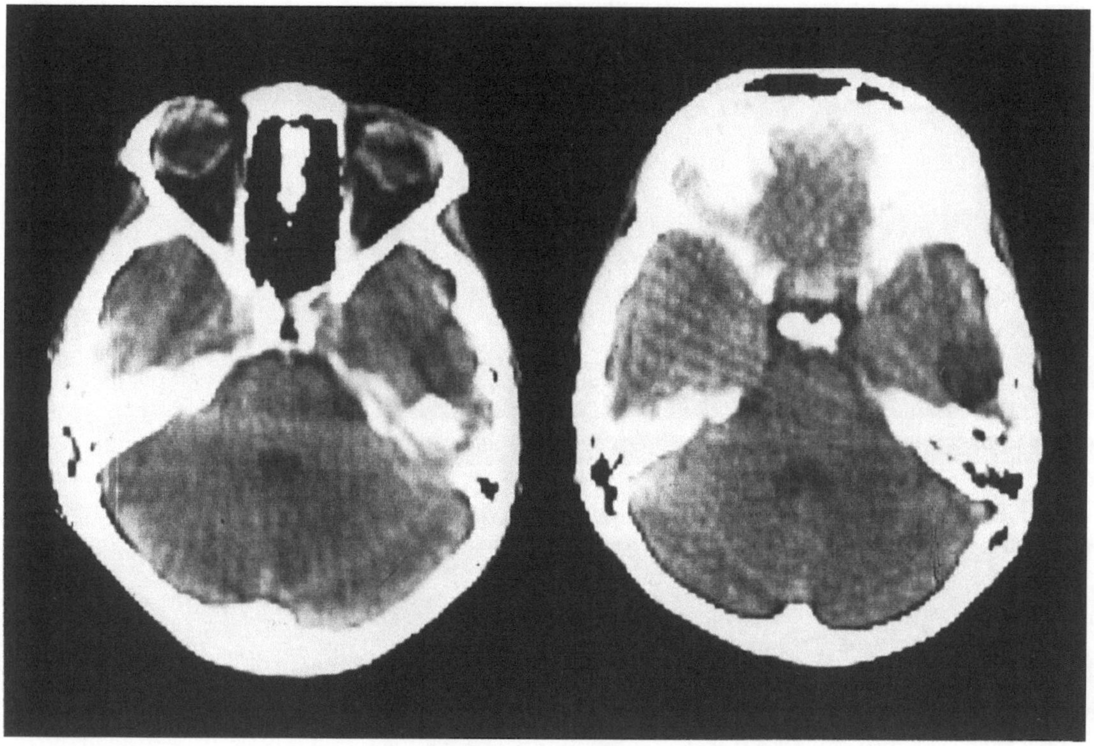

**Fig. D1.131.** Pilocytic astrocytoma in the basal sections of the right temporal lobe in a 23-year-old patient with psychomotor epilepsy. There is a small spherical hypodense zone which does not take up contrast. The lesion was overlooked at first analysis of the CT pictures

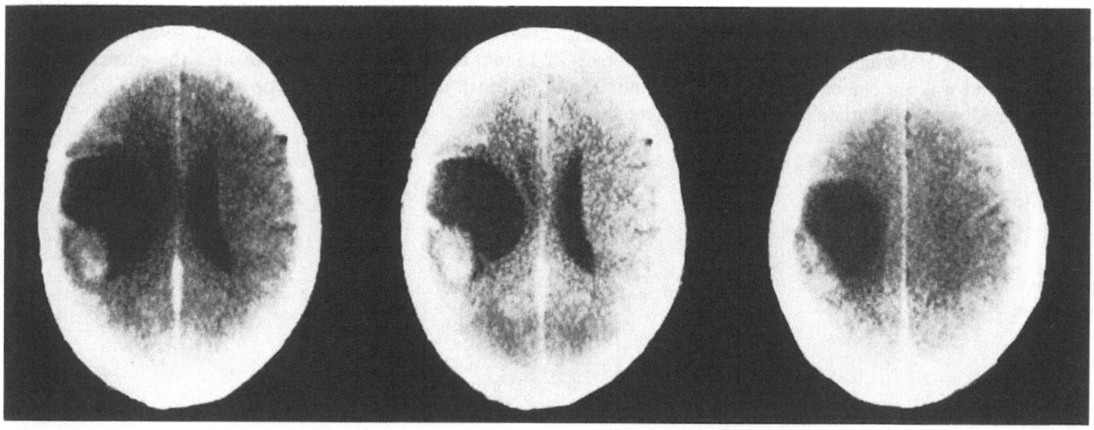

**Fig. D1.132.** Pilocytic astrocytoma with a large cyst and small marginal solid tumor nodule in the right parietal lobe in a 41-year-old patient. Significant contrast enhancement within the solid tumor. (Studies courtesy of Doz. Dr. Hammer, Department of Radiology, Wagner-Jauregg-Hospital, Linz, Austria)

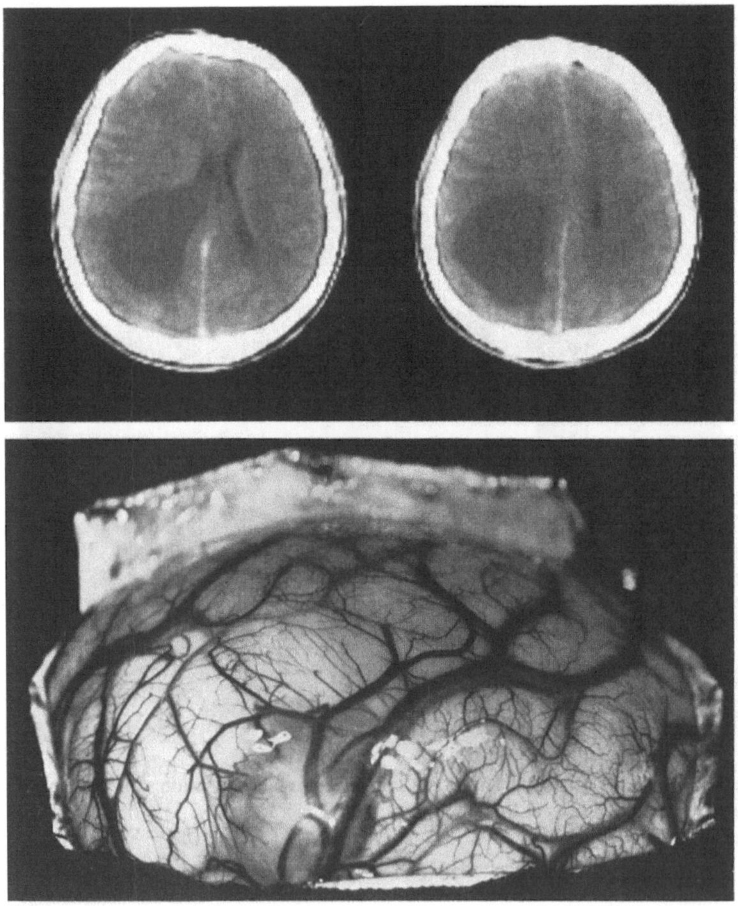

a

b

**Fig. D1.133.** (**a**) Pilocytic astrocytoma with a large cyst in a 19-year-old patient with progredient right hemiparesis. The solid portion of the tumor was located high in the parietal region and was not demonstrated in the CT scan. The cyst contained strongly xanthochromic fluid, with the result that density values are much higher than those of CSF (24–26 HU). (**b**) Demonstration of a solid tumor nodule 15 mm in diameter in the cortex near the interhemispheric fissure in the same patient at operation

## h) Pontine Gliomas

These tumors are usually slow-growing fibrillary or pilocytic astrocytomas and rarely anaplastic astrocytomas or glioblastomas. Medulloblastomas are found exceptionally in the pontine region. The tumor most often occurs in children younger than 10 years of age. Pontine neoplasms in adults are usually cerebral metastases, rarely glioblastomas. Gliomas of the pons comprise approximately 1% of all brain tumors.

Pontine tumors most often cause cranial nerve deficits in combination with lesions of the motor and sensory tracts. The slow-growing pontine gliomas cause increased intracranial pressure only in later stages after hydrocephalus has developed. CSF circulation may remain intact for a long period. Early occlusive hydrocephalus with signs of increased intracranial pressure is found in rare cases of rapidly growing tumors.

Before the introduction of CT, diagnosis of pontine tumors was established by pneumoencephalography, which demonstrates the enlarged pons and dorsal displacement of the aqueduct and the fourth ventricle. Angiography reveals stretching of the posterior cerebral arteries and displacement of veins in large pontine tumors. Other diagnostic procedures are uncharacteristic with the exception of special echoencephalographic techniques.

### Computed Tomography (Figs. D1.134–143)

#### Precontrast Study

The plain CT scan is diagnostic in the majority of pontine tumors. Enlargement of the pons results in some degree of dorsal displacement of the fourth ventricle, which appears as a narrow irregularly shaped, sharply delineated, hypodense zone adjacent to the dorsal border of the tumor (Figs. D1.134–137, 139, 140, 143). In some cases pontine tumors may result in narrowing of the interpeduncular cistern and dorsal indentation of the pentagon (Figs. D1.141–143).

Slightly more than half of all pontine gliomas demonstrate hypodense absorption values (averaging 19–26 HU). The remainder of these tumors comprises isodense, slightly hyperdense, or mixed density lesions. Cysts appear as rather sharply delineated low density structures within the pons (Fig. D1.141). Pontine tumors are often associated with slight to moderate ventricular dilatation, but the ventricle system may be entirely normal in some cases (Fig. D1.139). Large pontine gliomas may cause a significant disorder of CSF circulation which results in pronounced hydrocephalus.

#### Postcontrast Study

Our studies show that approximately 60% of pontine gliomas demonstrate contrast medium uptake in the solid portions of the tumor, which allows better delineation of the tumor in relation to normal brain structures. Approximately half of hypodense pontine gliomas take up contrast media and demonstrate ring enhancement or nodular structures, sometimes a combination of the two (Figs. D1.137, 138). Contrast enhancement also shows whether the tumor has extended to the cerebral peduncles or the thalamus.

*Diagnosis of a pontine glioma is sometimes not possible with CT in the early stage of the disease,* as 3 of our 44 cases showed. Pontine tumors are best demonstrated in the projection used for examination of the posterior fossa. In some cases the orbital scanning plane may be useful, with the brain stem perpendicular to the axis of the system. This reduces artifacts resulting from the petrous bones (Fig. D1.137).

#### Differential Diagnosis

Hypodense pontine tumors which do not take up contrast media are usually *fibrillary astrocytomas*. Tumors with a ring or nodular structures after contrast enhancement are *pilocytic astrocytomas* or *anaplastic astrocytomas,* but CT studies do not allow certain differentiation between the two. In one case of a very large cyst with slightly higher density than CSF a preliminary diagnosis of epidermoid was made. At operation the tumor proved to be a pilocytic astrocytoma with a large cyst and a small solid portion, which had escaped detection in the CT scan (Fig. D1.119).

*Medulloblastoma of the pons* shows intense homogeneous contrast enhancement of the entire midbrain (Fig. D1.190). *Ependymoma* may resemble pontine glioma in some cases (cf. Fig. D1.145).

As in other regions of the brain, *metastases in the pons* may vary considerably in appearance.

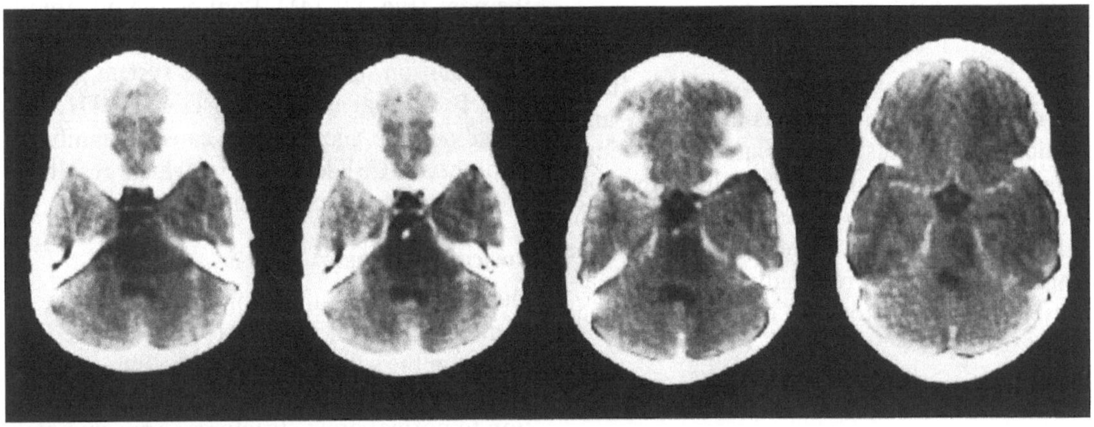

**Fig. D1.134.** Bulbopontine astrocytoma in a $4^1/_2$-year-old girl with cranial nerves palsy and disorder of the pyramidal tracts. The tumor itself is extremely hypodense (18 HU, left). Contrast administration was not followed by a significant increase in density (19.5 HU). At the level of the pons the tumor is located more on the right and extends to the right cerebral peduncle

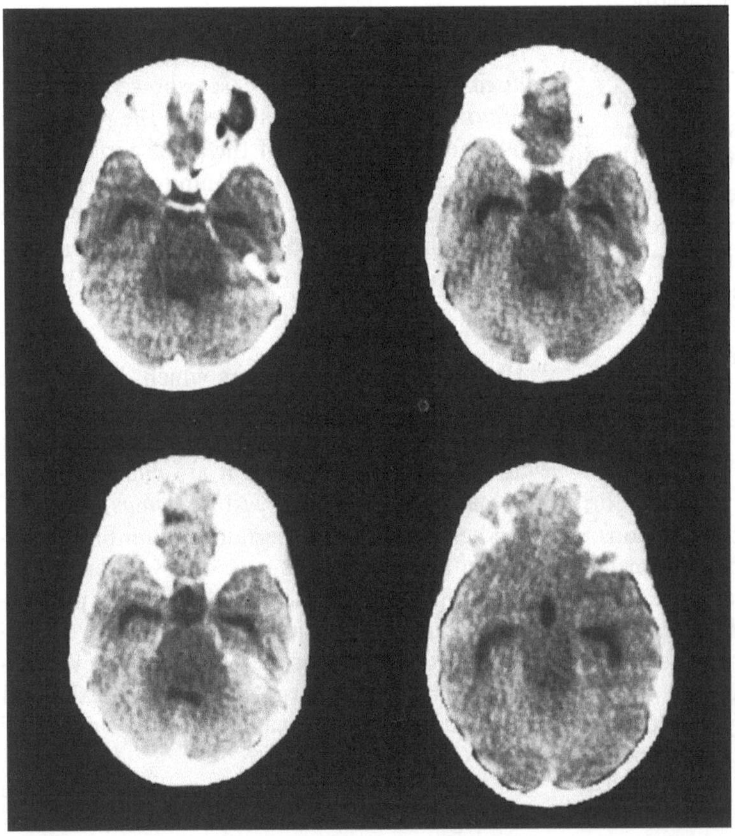

**Fig. D1.135.** Pontine astrocytoma in a 9-year-old girl with involvement of the cranial nerves, the pyramidal tracts, and ataxia. The pons itself is distended and appears hypodense, while the fourth ventricle is displaced posteriorly. Dilatation of the inferior horns as sign of moderate hydrocephalus. Postcontrast studies (below left) do not reveal a significant increase in density within the tumor as compared to precontrast CT scans (above right). Histological confirmation of the diagnosis

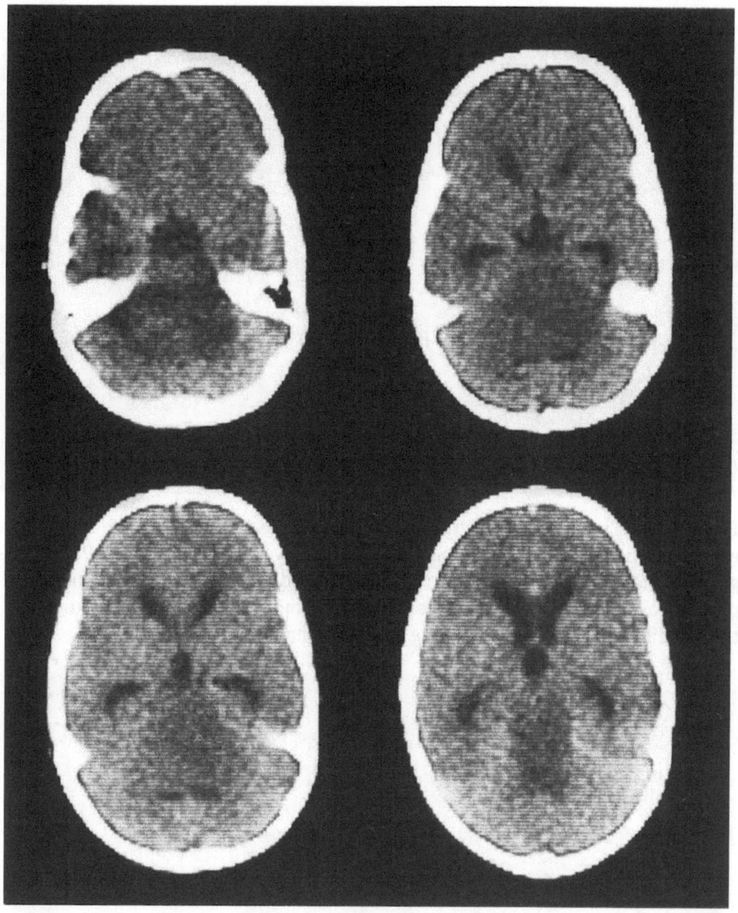

**Fig. D1.136.** Very large pontine glioma (probably astrocytoma) in a 4-year-old boy with involvement of the cranial nerves and the pyramidal tracts. The pons is grossly distended, and there is extreme posterior displacement of the fourth ventricle. The tumor itself appears as a hypodense zone with indistinct borders measuring more than 5 cm in diameter (13-mm slices)

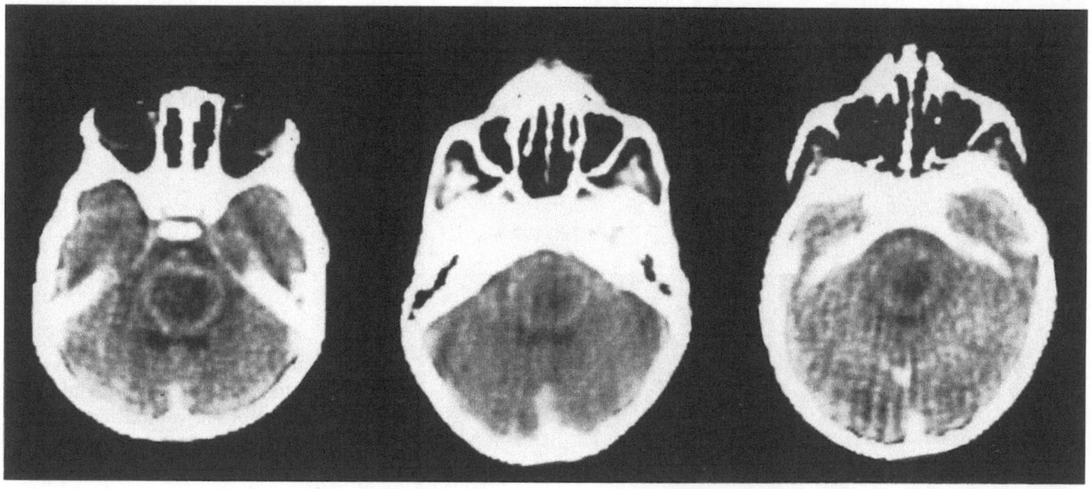

**Fig. D1.137.** Pontine glioma with ring structures after contrast enhancement in a 2-year old child. Anaplastic or pilocytic astrocytoma. Standard position (left) and special studies with extreme dorsal flexion of the head (middle and right)

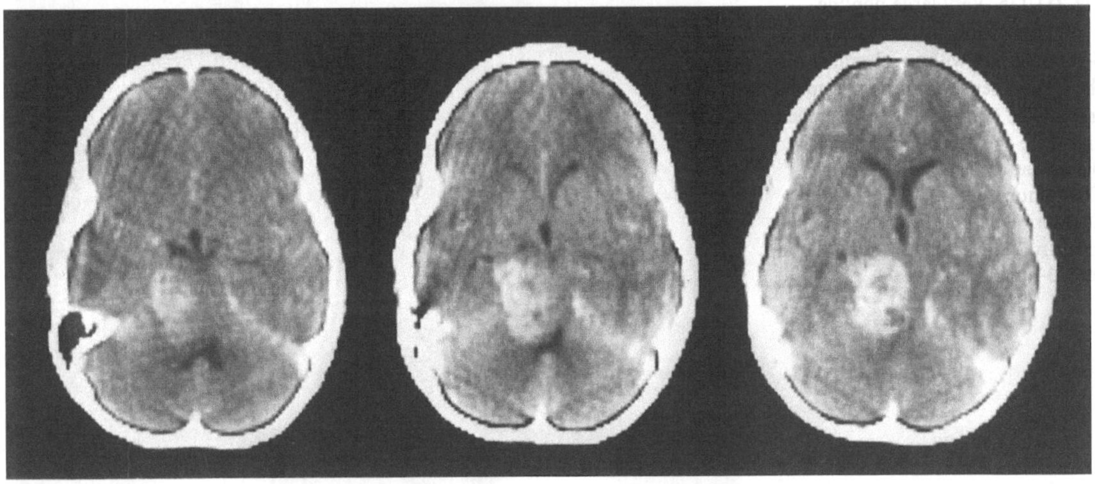

**Fig. D1.138.** Tumor in the upper section of the pons extending to the left cerebral peduncle and thalamus in a 7-year-old girl with rapidly progredient right hemiparesis and cranial nerve involvement. The tumor appeared isodense in precontrast studies and demonstrated strong contrast enhancement with the exception of two small zones which may represent necrosis. Postcontrast study. Rapid deterioration in the clinical state suggested a diagnosis of anaplastic astrocytoma or glioblastoma

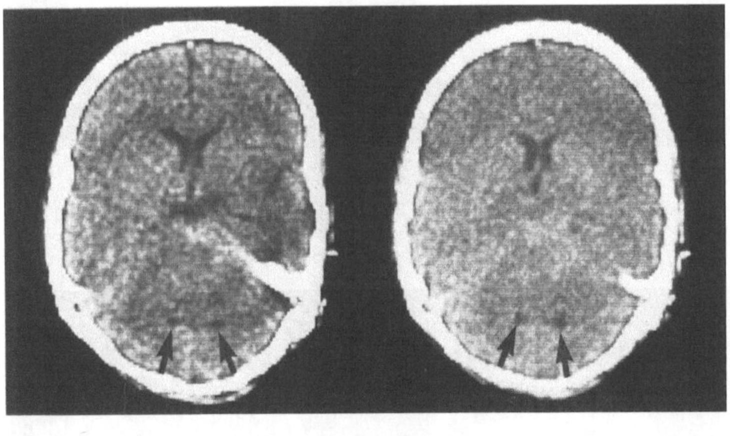

**Fig. D1.139.** Very large isodense pontine glioma with extreme dorsal displacement of the fourth ventricle, which is visible only in the form of two small zones of CSF density (arrows). No evidence of hydrocephalus (13-year-old girl). Precontrast study

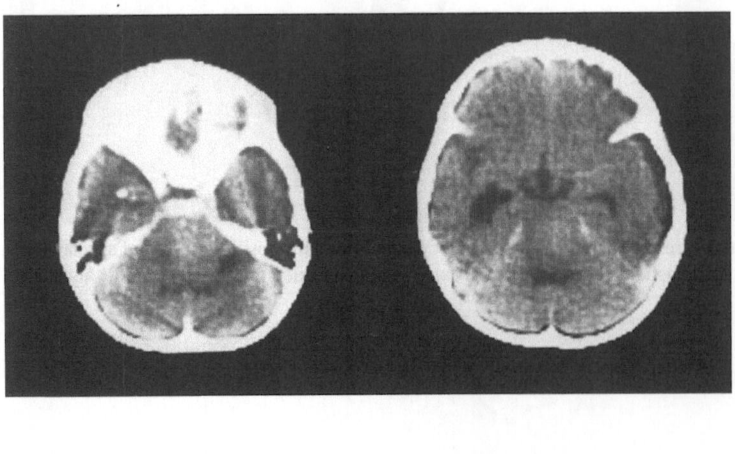

**Fig. D1.140.** Slightly hyperdense pontine glioma in a 5-year-old boy. The tumor has caused significant distension of the pons and the medulla oblongata as well as typical dorsal displacement of the fourth ventricle. A subdural effusion is visible on the right, probably secondary to combined chemotherapy and dexamethasone. No evidence of contrast uptake within the tumor. Postcontrast study

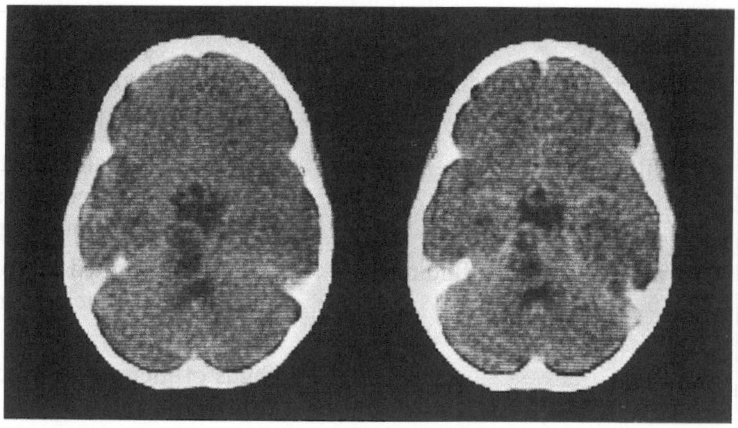

**Fig. D 1.141.** Tumor with isodense and hypodense zones, probably representing cysts, at the border between the left cerebral peduncle and the pons. Indentation in the left posterior section of the pentagon caused by the tumor. Postcontrast studies reveal slightly increased density values within the tumor (right). Eight-year-old girl with cranial nerve deficits and right hemiparesis. No histological diagnosis

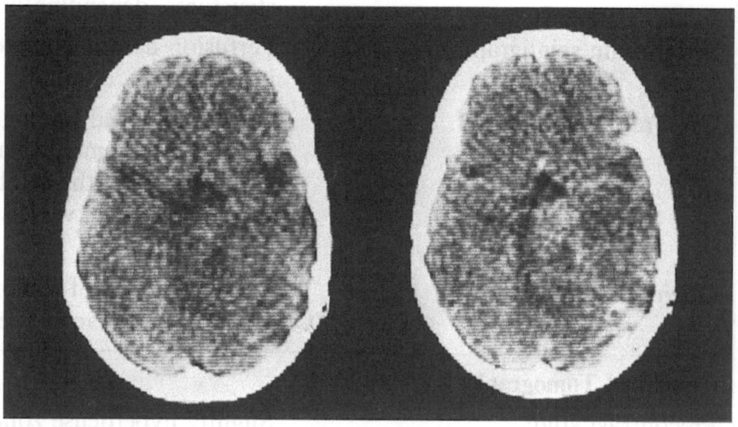

**Fig. D 1.142.** Pontine tumor with isodense and hypodense regions and indistinct borders (left) in a $7^1/_2$-year-old girl with disorders of the left pyramidal tracts. The tumor extends from the pons to the right cerebral peduncle. Postcontrast studies reveal a significant increase in density within the tumor (right), which fills the right posterior section of the pentagon

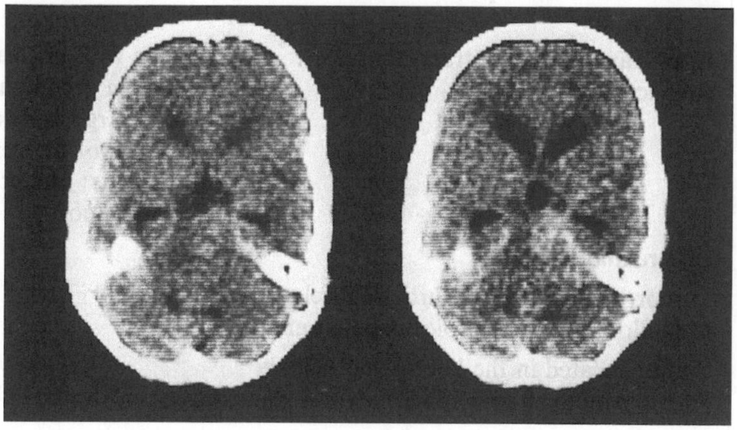

**Fig. D 1.143.** Large pontine tumor with isodense and hyperdense zones. Significant contrast enhancement within portions of the tumor between the pons and the right cerebral peduncle (right). Note the pronounced dorsal displacement of the fourth ventricle with typical accumulation of CSF in both lateral recesses. Eight-year-old child with cranial nerve deficits and disorders of the left pyramidal tract. No histological diagnosis, but a presumption of anaplastic astrocytoma

## i) Ependymomas

| | |
|---|---|
| Incidence | 1–4% |
| Characteristic age at diagnosis | First and second decades |
| Sex distribution | Strong preponderance of males |
| Typical locations | Lateral, third, and fourth ventricles; cerebral hemispheres in children and adolescents; temporo-parieto-occipital and frontal regions |
| Characteristic clinical findings | Symptoms limited to vomiting when tumor located in the fourth ventricle; signs of increased intracranial pressure |
| Skull film | Signs of increased intracranial pressure; occasional calcification |
| EEG | Severe pathological changes are common with tumors in the cerebral hemispheres |
| Echoencephalography | Ventricular dilatation or displacement of midline structures, depending on tumor location |
| Serial brain scintigraphy | Perfusion defects common; slight radionuclide uptake in the tumor, especially in delayed scans |
| Cerebral angiography | No pathological findings with tumors in the fourth ventricle; extreme displacement of normal vessels with tumors of the cerebral hemispheres in many cases; pathological vessels in some cases of malignant ependymomas |
| Other contrast studies | Demonstration of tumors on the floor of the fourth ventricle by means of central ventriculography |

**Computed Tomography**

| | |
|---|---|
| Precontrast study | Slightly hyperdense zone fairly common, with calcification in some cases; large hypodense zones (cysts) in cerebral tumors |
| Contrast medium uptake | Slight increase in density in solid portions of the tumor |
| Appearance after contrast enhancement | Solid tumor with unclear demarcation from the caudal brain stem accompanied by fine calcifications in some cases; large cysts and occasional calcification in ependymomas of the cerebral hemispheres in children and adolescents; moderate perifocal edema surrounding cerebral tumors |

**Differential Diagnosis**

Tumor located in the fourth ventricle:
Medulloblastoma and plexus papilloma

Tumor located in the lateral ventricle:
Plexus papilloma and subependymal giant cell astrocytoma, subependymoma

Location in the third ventricle:
Tumors of the pineal body, pilocytic astrocytoma, plexus papilloma, and colloid cyst

Location in the cerebral hemispheres:
Pilocytic astrocytoma, anaplastic astrocytoma, glioblastoma, monstrocellular sarcoma, gangliocytoma, and metastasis

Incidence of ependymoma in the literature ranges from 1% to 4%; we encountered 54 such tumors in the 3,750 cases in our series (1.4%).

Incidence is highest in the 1st and 2nd decades, but ependymoma may occur in adults as well. ZÜLCH found a predominance in males, with a ratio of 3:2. Cerebral extraventricular ependymoma in children and anaplastic ependymoma in adults are both highly malignant tumors classified in grades III and IV. Ependymoma in the fourth ventricle may also prove malignant, especially in children ("ependymal medulloblastoma"). All other ependymomas are classified as grade I or grade II tumors.

Subependymomas (grade I) and papillary ependymomas (grade II) are subgroups with intraventricular sites.

### Typical Locations

Ependymomas are typically found within the ventricles, most often in the lateral ventricles, the third ventricle, and on the floor of the fourth ventricle.

Cerebral extraventricular ependymoma is the most common supratentorial tumor in children and is most often found in the white matter near the lateral ventricle, usually reaching the convexity. The junction of the parietal, temporal, and occipital lobes is a classic location for the tumor, but we have also found a large number in the frontal lobe. The tumors lie in close proximity to the lateral ventricles and often demonstrate large cysts as well as occasional calcification. Discrete calcification may also be found in intraventricular ependymomas.

### Characteristic Clinical Findings

Vomiting is the presenting sign in children with tumors of the fourth ventricle and direct involvement of the area postrema. Other intraventricular ependymomas cause disorders of CSF circulation which may result in occlusive hydrocephalus with typical clinical symptoms such as headache and vomiting.

Epileptic seizures may be observed in cerebral ependymoma in adolescents, though signs of increased intracranial pressure are present in most cases, since these tumors may become very large. In contrast, neurological deficits are rare.

### Additional Diagnostic Procedures

Plain skull films demonstrate secondary signs of increased intracranial pressure such as separation of the sutures in children or pronounced gyric impressions in older patients. Calcification is occasionally found in cerebral ependymoma. The EEG may be highly abnormal in supratentorial ependymomas but the changes are unspecific when the tumor is located in the ventricle.

Echoencephalography may demonstrate ventricular dilation or displacement of midline structures, depending on location of the tumor.

Dynamic brain scans are highly sensitive in demonstration of cerebral ependymomas, but the technique cannot provide evidence of a particular histological type.

Angiography demonstrates vascular displacement, but only in larger intraventricular tumors. Cerebral ependymomas are also associated with pronounced vascular displacement. Pathological vessels are rare, but some angiographic findings resemble those in glioblastoma, and a capillary blush has been recorded. Large cysts can also be demonstrated as avascular spaces.

Ventriculography is of interest only in diagnosis of ependymoma on the floor of the fourth ventricle. The tumor appears as a knobby irregular structure with projection into the ventricular lumen. The ventriculogram suggests that the tumor has close relations with the floor of the fourth ventricle.

## Computed Tomography (Figs. D1.144–163)

### Precontrast Study

Ependymomas often demonstrate slightly increased density in the plain scan, regardless of location. Fine calcification throughout the tumor is especially common in tumors of the fourth ventricle and the caudal brain stem (Figs. D1.145, 149). Cerebral ependymomas often demonstrate extensive zones of reduced density representing cysts (Fig. D1.156). Calcification is not unusual in cerebral ependymoma (Fig. D1.157). This often results in a mixed density tumor in the precontrast CT scan.

120

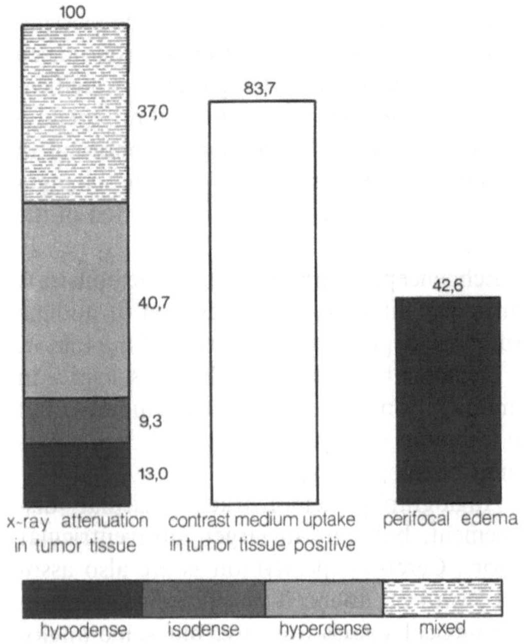


## Postcontrast Study

Contrast uptake is the rule in ependymoma (Figs. D1.145, 150, 156, 157, 161–163) and was found in 41 of 49 patients (83.7%). Contrast uptake would appear to be less pronounced in ependymomas of the fourth ventricle than in the cerebral hemispheres, where the increase in density averaged 14 HU with our standard dose of contrast medium.

*Ependymomas of the fourth ventricle* may be of different sizes, but their appearance after contrast enhancement is typical (Figs. D1.145–148). *A remnant of the fourth ventricle is often visible dorsal to the tumor itself* (Figs. D1.145, 148).

The CT scan occasionally shows the characteristic irregular surface of the tumor (Fig. D1.145). The origin of the tumor on the floor of the fourth ventricle is not demonstrable in the horizontal CT scan in a large number of cases.

One may suspect that the tumor has its origin on the floor of the fourth ventricle if the tumor obliterates the usual borders of the pons and the medulla oblongata and if CSF is only visible on the dorsal side of the tumor (Figs. D1.145, 148). If the origin of the tumor lies caudad in the brain stem and the CT section somewhat higher, one may gain the mistaken impression that the tumor is surrounded by CSF (Fig. D1.147). However, this is only a projection effect. Ventriculography may provide more reliable information in such cases.

*Ependymoma of the third ventricle* is most often found in the caudal portion of this chamber and may cause compression and displacement of the lamina tecti. Indistinct demarcation of the tumor against the thalamus is seen in many cases (Figs. D1.150, 151).

*Ependymomas in the lateral ventricles* are almost always located near the foramen of Monro and usually cause unilateral or bilateral hydrocephalus (Figs. D1.152, 153a and b). We have also found variants of ependymoma in the posterior horn and trigonum (Figs. D1.154, 155).

Typical CT findings in *anaplastic ependymoma of the cerebral hemisphere* are related to the age of the patient. In children and adolescents the tumor is most often located at the junction of the parietal, temporal, and occipital lobes as well as in the frontal lobe. Very large cysts and calcification are also found in addition to solid portions of the tumor (Figs. D1.156, 157). Hemorrhage within the tumor is occasionally demonstrated in this age group (Fig. D1.160). Cysts and calcification are less common in adults, while the typical location at the junction of the three cerebral lobes is the same as in children (Figs. D1.161, 162).

*Perifocal edema* is not demonstrable in ependymomas within the ventricles, but it is a common finding in cerebral extraventricular ependymomas, usually classified as grade I edema (61%).

## Differential Diagnosis

Tumors in the fourth ventricle suggest *medulloblastoma* and *plexus papilloma* as the most common alternatives in differential diagnosis. Medulloblastoma is generally more clearly demarcated from the brain stem in the CT scan, and calcification is rare. Contrast uptake is usually more intense in medulloblastoma than in ependymoma, and the surface of the medulloblastoma is smoother than that of ependymoma.

Plexus papilloma located in the fourth ventricle is usually a spherical sharply delineated tumor with surface irregularities. Contrast uptake is generally very intense, and calcification may be observed. *Angioblastomas* are rarely found in the fourth ventricle, and *pilocytic astrocytomas* are almost as rare (Figs. D1.111, 115). In two patients we observed *ectopic pinealomas* within the fourth ventricle (Fig. D1.251). *Subependymal giant cell astrocytoma* is a possible diagnostic alternative to *ependymoma of the lateral ventricle,* since both tumors have the same origin near the foramen of Monro at the head of the caudate nucleus (Figs. D1.164–169). Additional calcified flecks in the wall of the ventricle favor a diagnosis of subependymal giant cell astrocytoma. *Subependymomas* of the lateral ventricles are usually hypodense and show only slight contrast enhancement (Figs. D1.153a, b).

*Tumors of the middle and posterior segments of the lateral ventricle* may be either plexus papillomas, papillary ependymomas, or intraventricular meningiomas. Differentiation between plexus papilloma and papillary ependymoma may be impossible (Figs. D1.155, 237).

The differential diagnosis of *tumors in the anterior portion of the third ventricle* includes colloid cysts near the foramen of Monro (Fig. D6.17) and meningiomas in rare cases. Differential diagnosis of tumors in the posterior segment of the ventricle has to include tumors of the lamina tecti such as pinealoma, germinoma, teratoma, and pilocytic astrocytoma.

*Pinealoma and germinoma* cannot be differentiated from ependymoma in the CT scan. Most of these tumors are isodense or slightly hyperdense and demonstrate intense contrast uptake. Identification of a *pineal teratoma* is relatively easy, since this malformation is very irregular and typically contains fatty elements with extremely low density. *Pilocytic astrocytoma* of the lamina tecti cannot be differentiated with certainty from ependymoma of the third ventricle, although cystic elements favor a diagnosis of pilocytic astrocytoma.

The differential diagnosis of *cerebral ependymoma in children* must include pilocytic astrocytoma with large cysts, monstrocellular sarcoma, and gangliocytoma. All of these tumors can demonstrate cysts as well as calcification, and certain differentiation in the CT scan may not be possible in individual cases. However, we found that ependymomas in our series tended to be much larger than pilocytic astrocytomas and gangliocytomas.

*Cerebral ependymoma in adults may present with the same CT characteristics as anaplastic astrocytoma and glioblastoma.* As a result differentiation is not possible with CT studies alone. It is of some interest that solid portions of ependymoma tended to be much larger than those of the other tumor groups in our series. Age at diagnosis is another important characteristic, since the majority of our patients with cerebral ependymomas was about 20 years old.

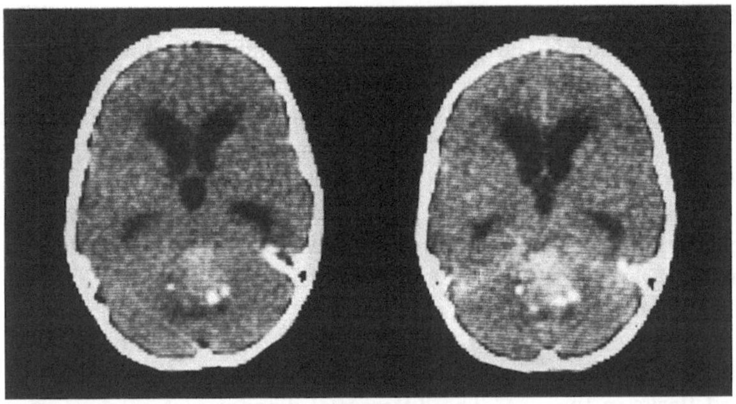

**Fig. D 1.145.** Typical ependymoma originating at the floor of the fourth ventricle in a 7-year-old girl. Most of the tumor appears hyperdense with a number of small calcifications in the precontrast study (left). Postcontrast studies reveal positive contrast enhancement (right). A small pool of CSF is evident on the dorsal side of the tumor. The border between the brain stem and the tumor is indistinct. Pronounced hydrocephalus secondary to blockage of the fourth ventricle

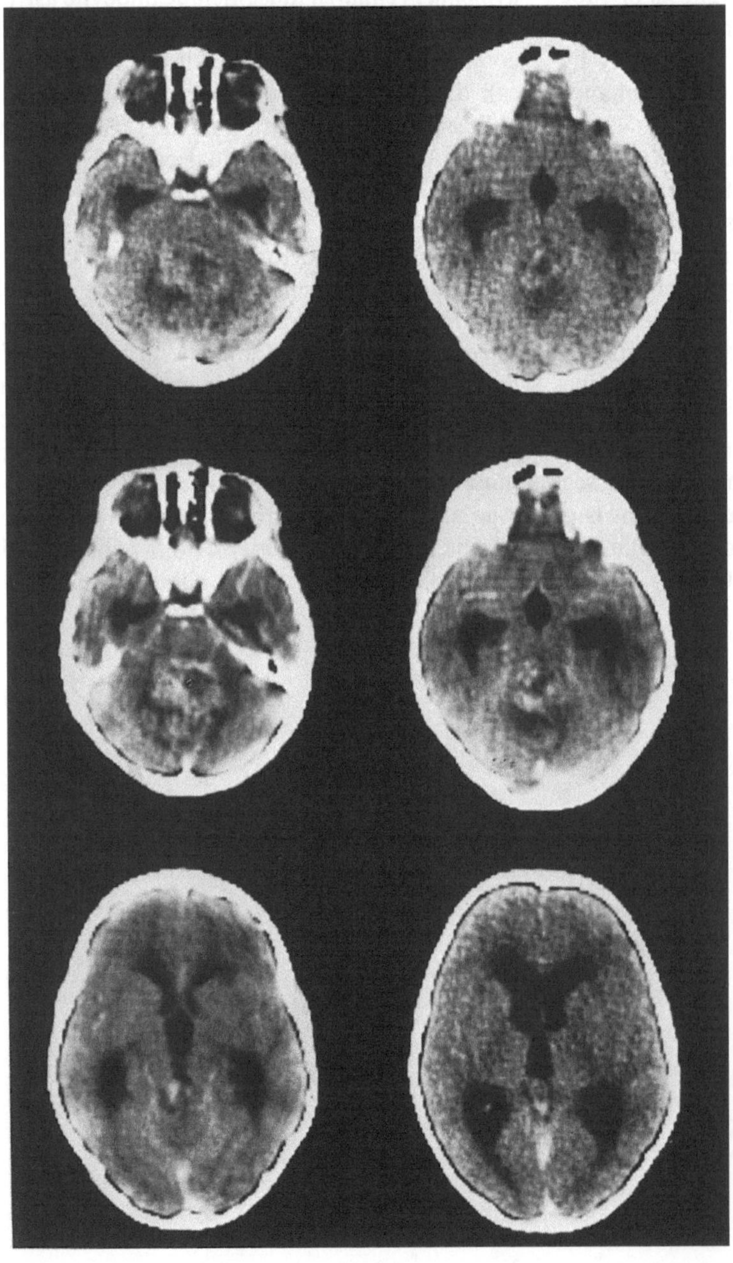

**Fig. D 1.146.** Ependymoma originating in the fourth ventricle with extension through the aqueduct to the third ventricle in a 10-year-old child. Most of the tumor is found within the fourth ventricle. The tumor itself is very inhomogeneous with necrosis at the center and slight perifocal edema. The solid portions of the tumor are hyperdense in the precontrast study (above). Distinct contrast enhancement and excellent delineation of the tumor portions extending to the third ventricle (below right). Pronounced hydrocephalus with periventricular lucency at the temporal horns

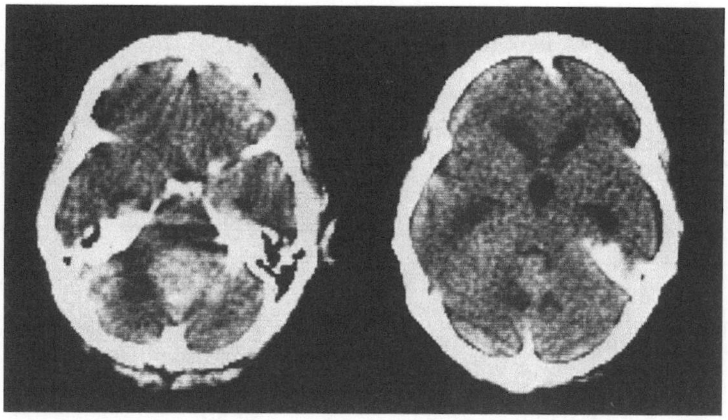

**Fig. D 1.147.** Ependymoma in the fourth ventricle of a 30-year-old male. The tumor appears as a slightly hyperdense lesion surrounded by CSF in the precontrast study (right). The postcontrast study (left) demonstrates a very large homogeneous tumor nodule that is not clearly delineated against the brain stem due to the presence of artifacts

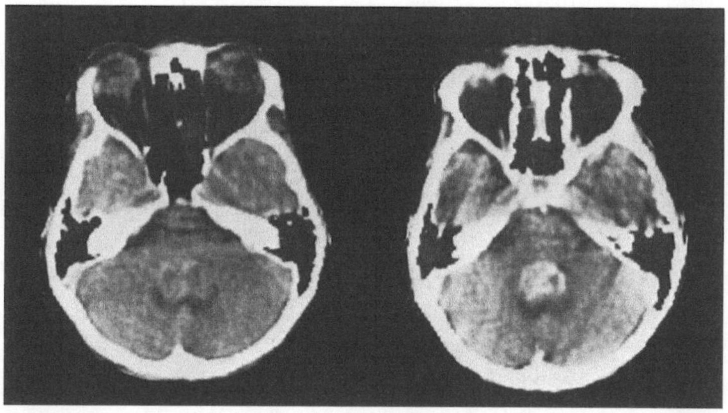

**Fig. D 1.148.** Ependymoma in the fourth ventricle of a 46-year-old male. The tumor demonstrates mixed density in the precontrast study (left). The fourth ventricle is displaced dorsally. Positive contrast enhancement (right). Small pool of CSF at the right anterior edge of the tumor

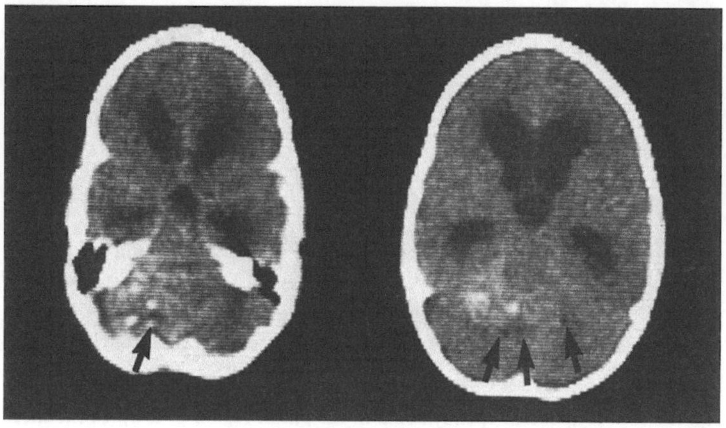

**Fig. D 1.149.** Ependymoma of the pons and the left cerebellar hemisphere with numerous small calcifications in a 2-year-old girl. Delineation of the tumor against the brain stem is not possible. The small CSF pools dorsal to the tumor (arrows) suggest a diagnosis of pontine tumor

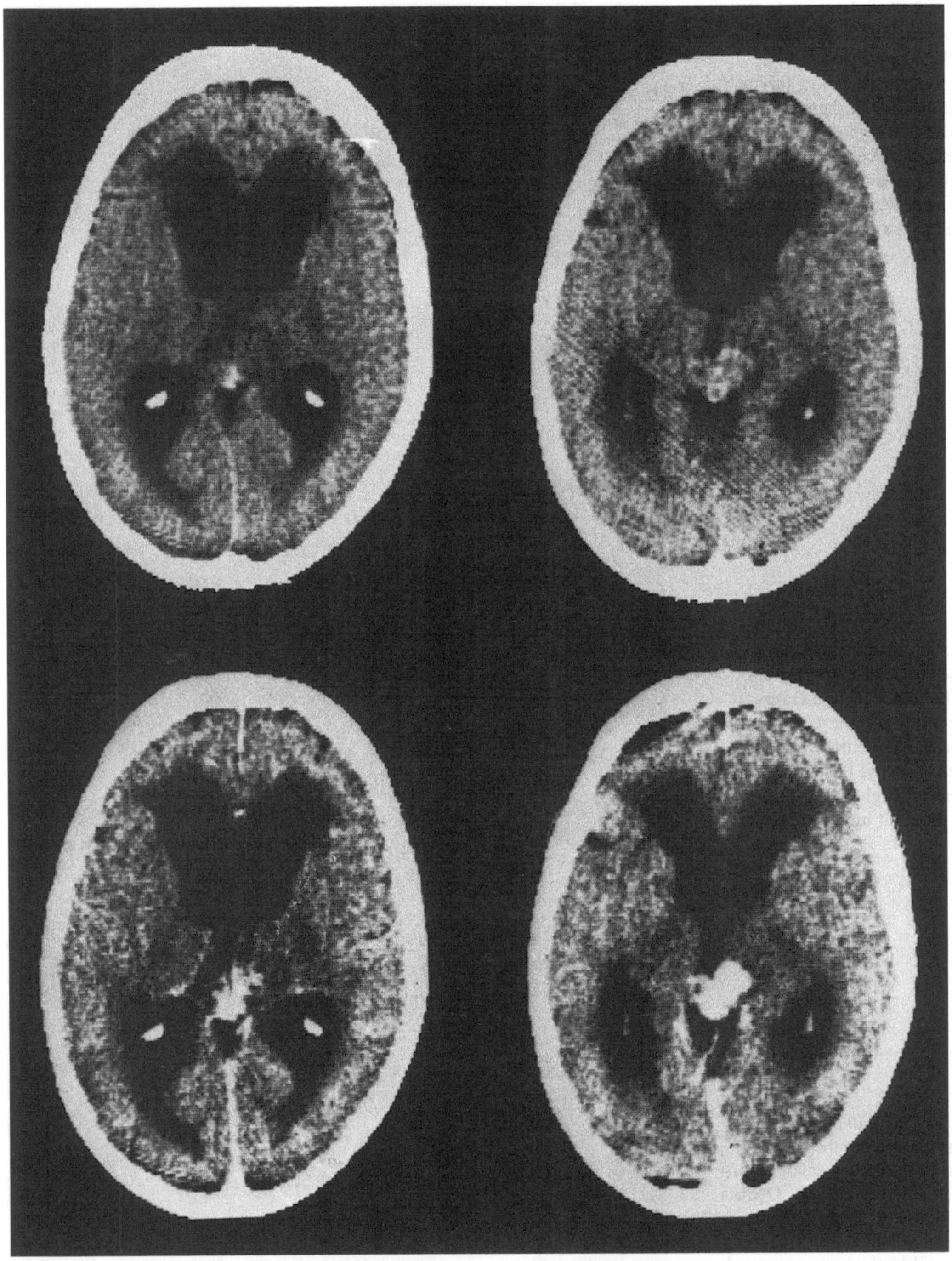

**Fig. D1.150.** Hyperdense ependymoma in the pineal region and the posterior portion of the third ventricle with extension to the right thalamus in a 44-year-old patient with vertical gaze paralysis and signs of increased intracranial pressure. Strong contrast enhancement within the tumor (below). Pronounced occlusive hydrocephalus with periventricular lucency (CT studies courtesy of Prof. Dr. Witt, Department of Radiology, Rudolf-Virchow-Krankenhaus, Berlin; studies made with Somatom 2)

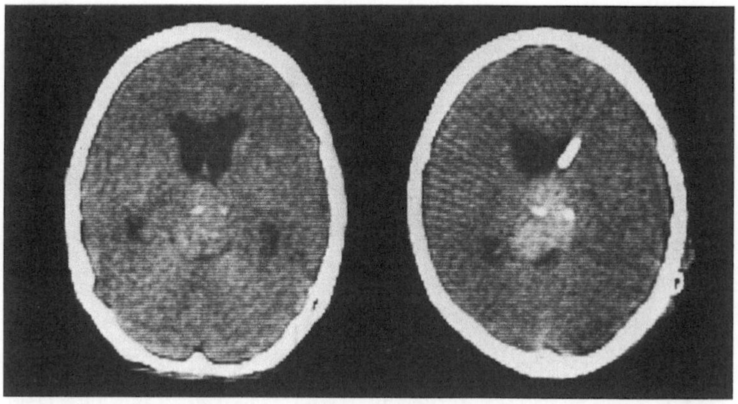

**Fig. D1.151.** Large tumor in the quadrigeminal region and the third ventricle in a 10-year-old boy with Parinaud syndrome. Precontrast CT shows isodense to slightly hyperdense tumor with spotty calcification (left). Postcontrast CT shows distinct contrast enhancement in the solid uncalcified portions of the tumor (right). The tumor fulfills CT criteria of intraventricular ependymoma. Histological diagnosis is not available since the tumor was judged inoperable due to its indistinct lateral borders

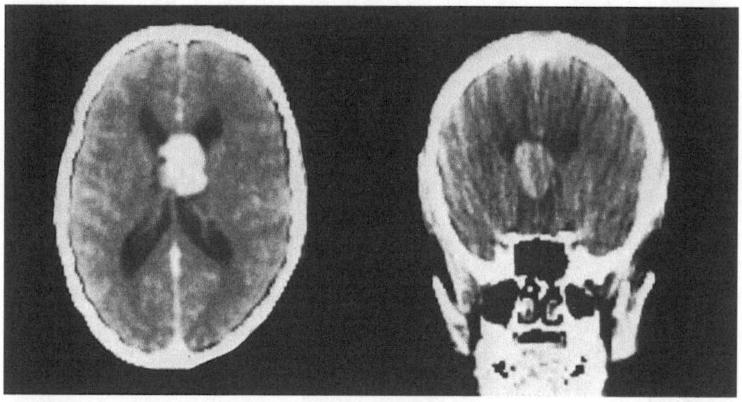

**Fig. D1.152.** Ependymoma in the right lateral ventricle at the foramen of Monro in horizontal and coronary projections. Strongly positive contrast enhancement within the tumor (14-year-old girl). Postcontrast study

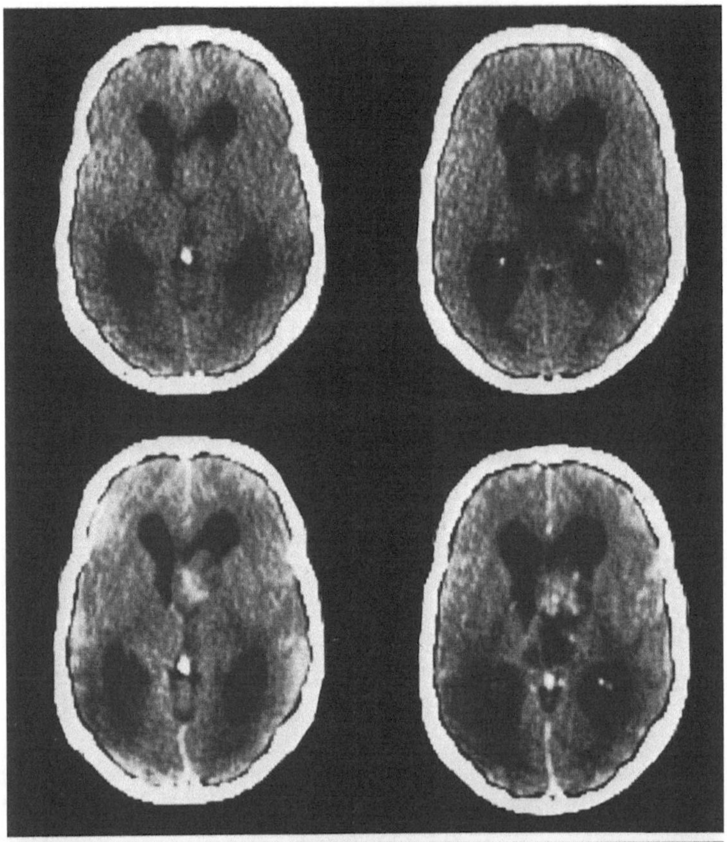

**Fig. D1.**153a. Subependymoma in the anterior portion of the right lateral ventricle between the foramen of Monro and the head of the caudate nucleus in a 49-year-old patient with signs of increased intracranial pressure. The isodense tumor lies within the ventricle and is easily recognized in the precontrast study (above). Inhomogeneous contrast enhancement (below). Pronounced hydrocephalus

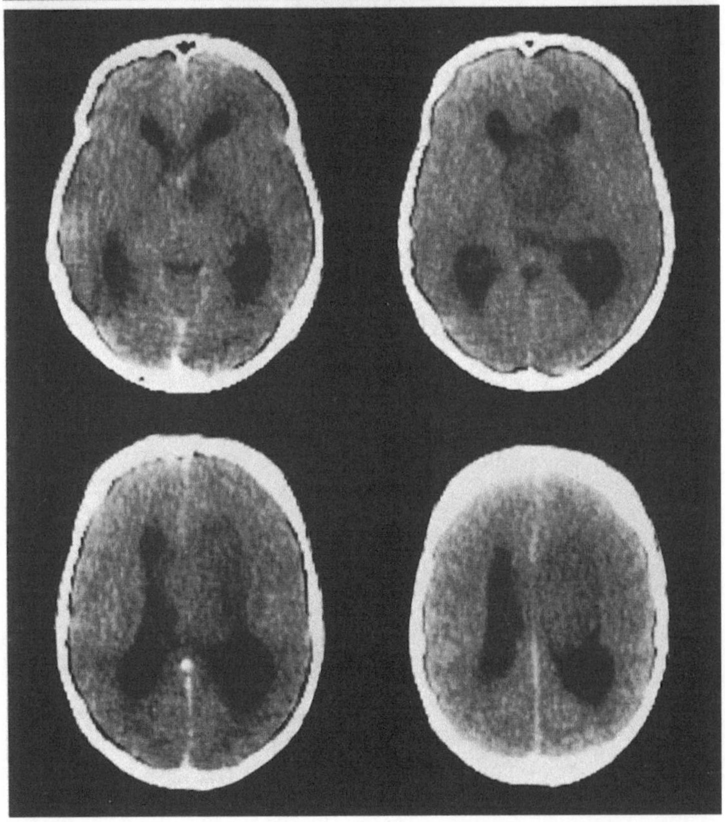

**Fig. D.1.**153b. Subependymoma in the anterior and middle sections of the right lateral ventricle with origin near the foramen of Monro on the right. Predominantly hypodense tumor with limited contrast enhancement at one location (above left)

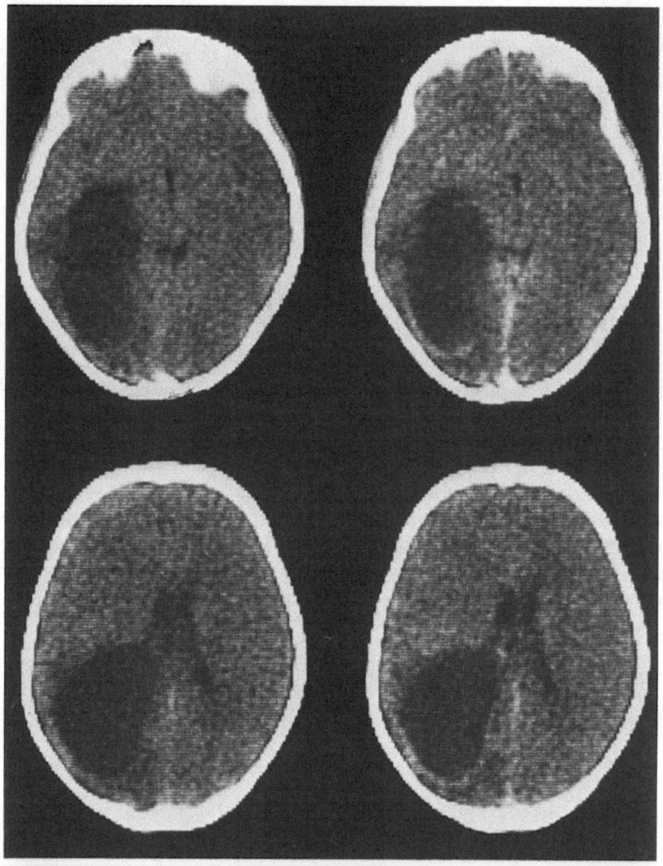

**Fig. D1.154.** Subependymoma in the left trigonum and posterior horn in a $6^1/_2$-year-old girl. Narrow solid portion of the tumor with contrast enhancement within the wall of the large cyst (right)

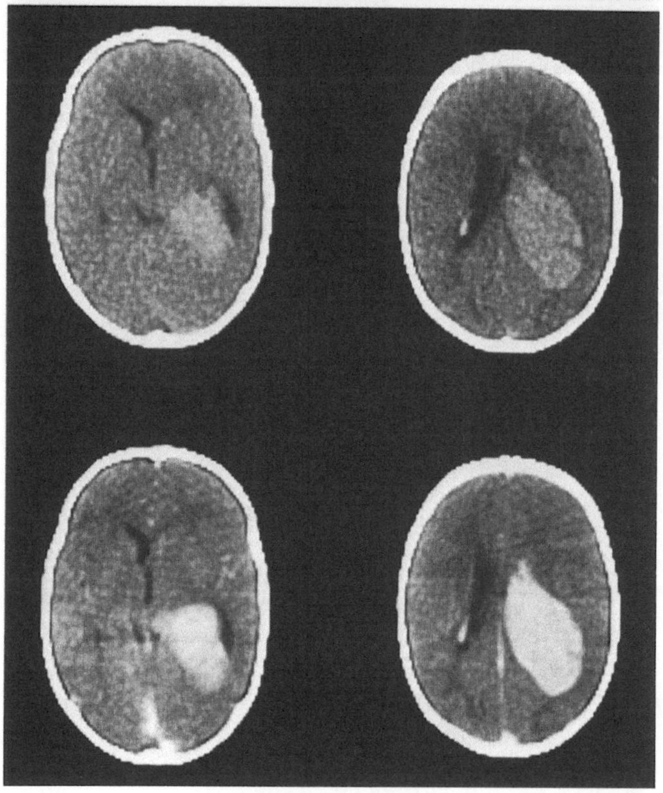

**Fig. D1.155.** Papillary ependymoma in the right lateral ventricle of an 11-month-old infant. Precontrast studies reveal a hyperdense tumor (above) with a further increase in density in the postcontrast study (below). Differentiation from plexus papilloma is hardly possible (cf. Fig. D1.237)

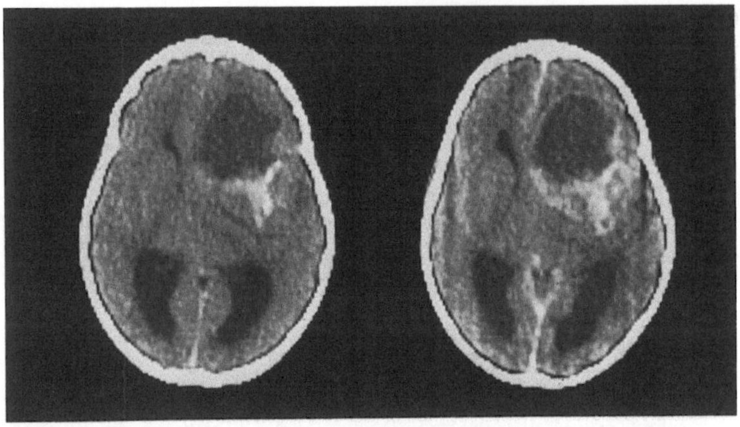

a

**Fig. D1.156** a, b. Ependymoma of the cerebral hemispheres in a 7-year-old girl. Serial studies. (**a**) Cystic calcified tumor with positive contrast enhancement (right) in the right frontotemporal region with obliteration of the right anterior horn and subsequent blockage of the foramen of Monro with resultant dilatation of both occipital horns. Characteristic CT findings in ependymoma of the cerebral hemispheres. (**b**) Follow-up study 3 months after partial removal of the tumor. Extensive recurrence of the tumor with slightly hyperdense values in precontrast CT studies (above) and positive contrast enhancement (below)

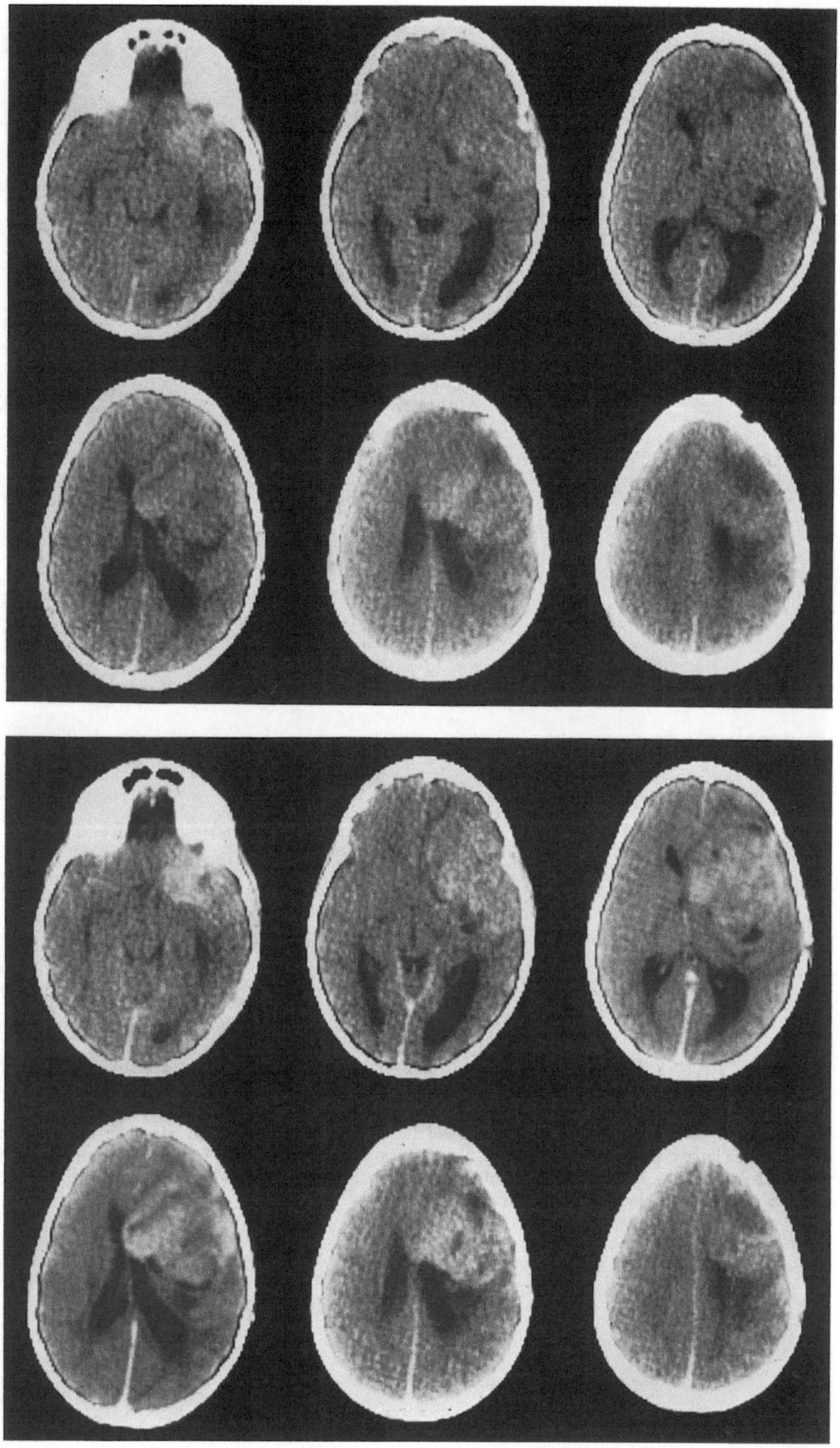

b

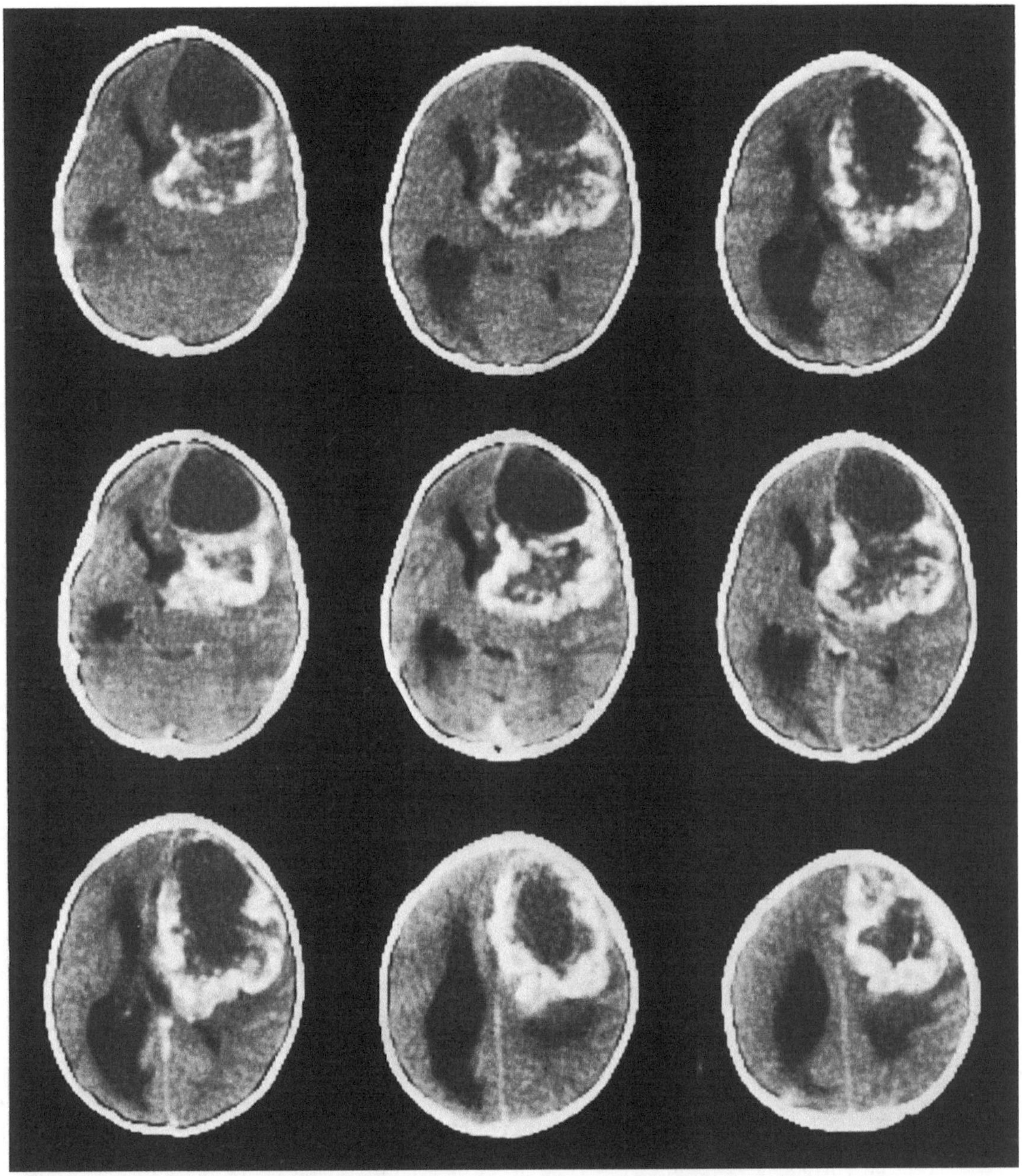

**Fig. D1.157.** Typical ependymoma of the cerebral hemispheres with a large cyst and extensive garland-like calcification in a 2-year-old boy. Extreme dilatation of the left lateral ventricle secondary to blockage of the foramen of Monro as well as perifocal edema in the white matter visible in the highest cross sections. (Precontrast studies above, postcontrast studies middle and below)

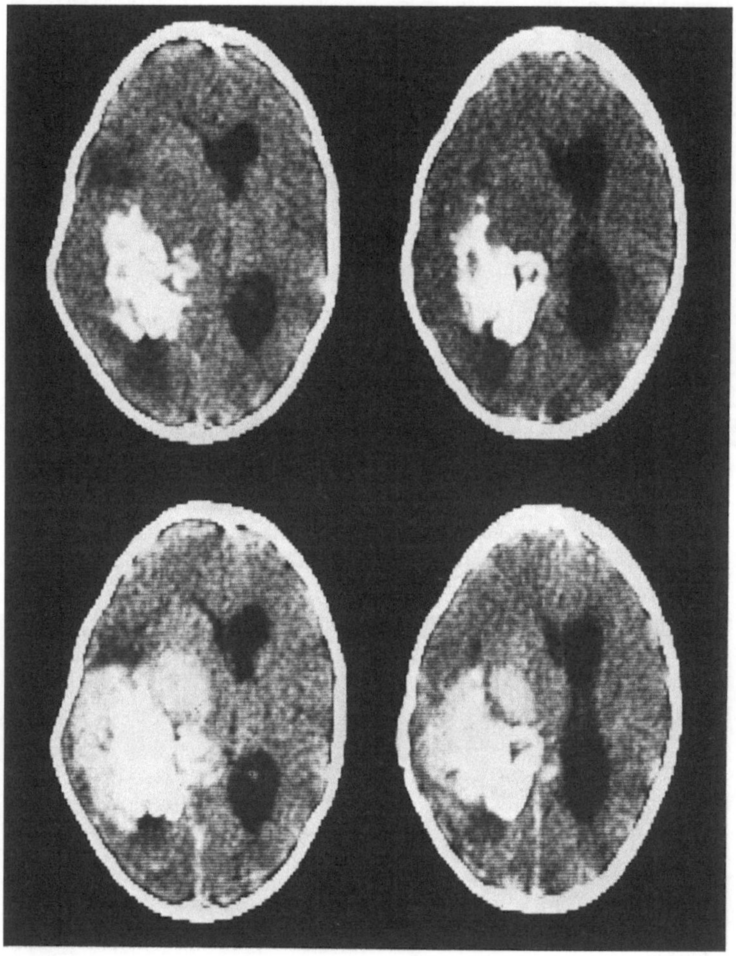

**Fig. D1.158.** Giant tumor with extensive calcification in the left cerebral hemisphere in a 14-year-old girl. Slightly hypodense tumor tissue near the calcification (above) demonstrates strongly positive contrast enhancement (below). Bulging of the vault above the tumor due to slow tumor growth. Definitive histological classification proved impossible, with some portions of the tumor resembling ependymoma and others pilocytic astrocytoma

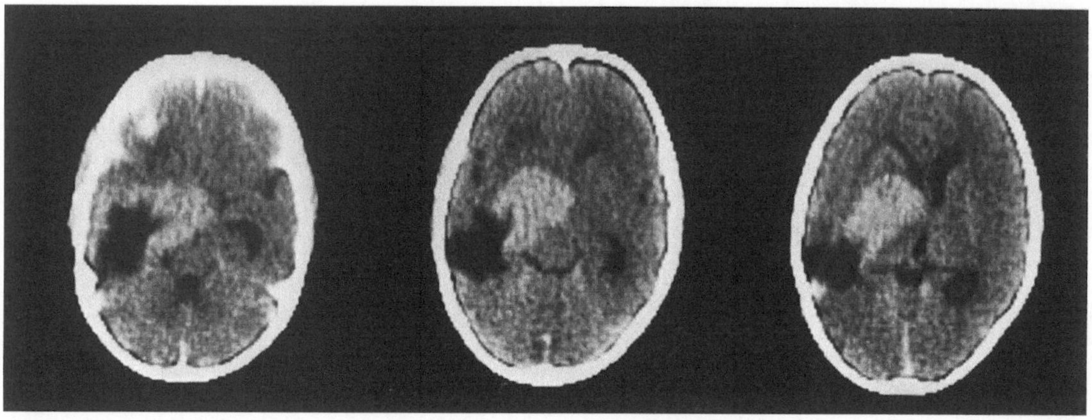

**Fig. D1.159.** Ependymoma of the cerebral hemispheres in a 7-year-old boy with right hemiparesis. Partial removal of the tumor, with a low-density zone following resection. The homogeneous solid portion of the tumor extends to the basal ganglia. Slightly hyperdense values within the tumor in precontrast studies with significant contrast enhancement (postcontrast CT)

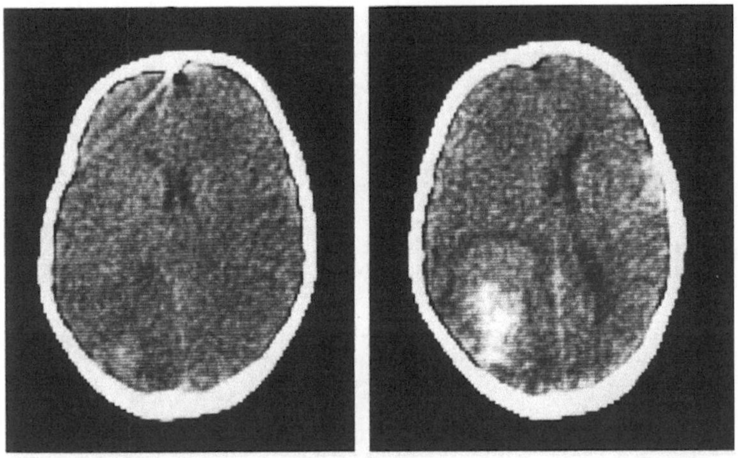

a b

**Fig. D 1.160** a, b. Ependymoma of the cerebral hemispheres in a 9-year-old girl. (**a**) Dec 3, 1975: Status epilepticus. Small slightly hyperdense zone with minimal contrast uptake in the left occipital lobe. Preliminary diagnosis of tumor. (**b**) Follow-up study on Dec 31, 1975 after sudden loss of consciousness: Large space-occupying lesion with high density values at the center suggesting hemorrhage in a tumor in the left occipitoparietal region. Confirmation at operation

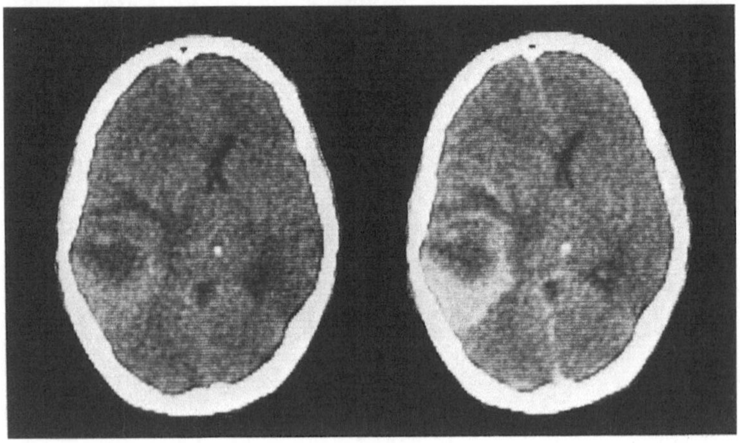

**Fig. D 1.161**. Anaplastic ependymoma with central necrosis and slight perifocal edema at the junction of the temporal, parietal, and occipital lobes in a 20-year-old male. Slightly hyperdense solid tumor in precontrast CT (left) and significant contrast enhancement (right)

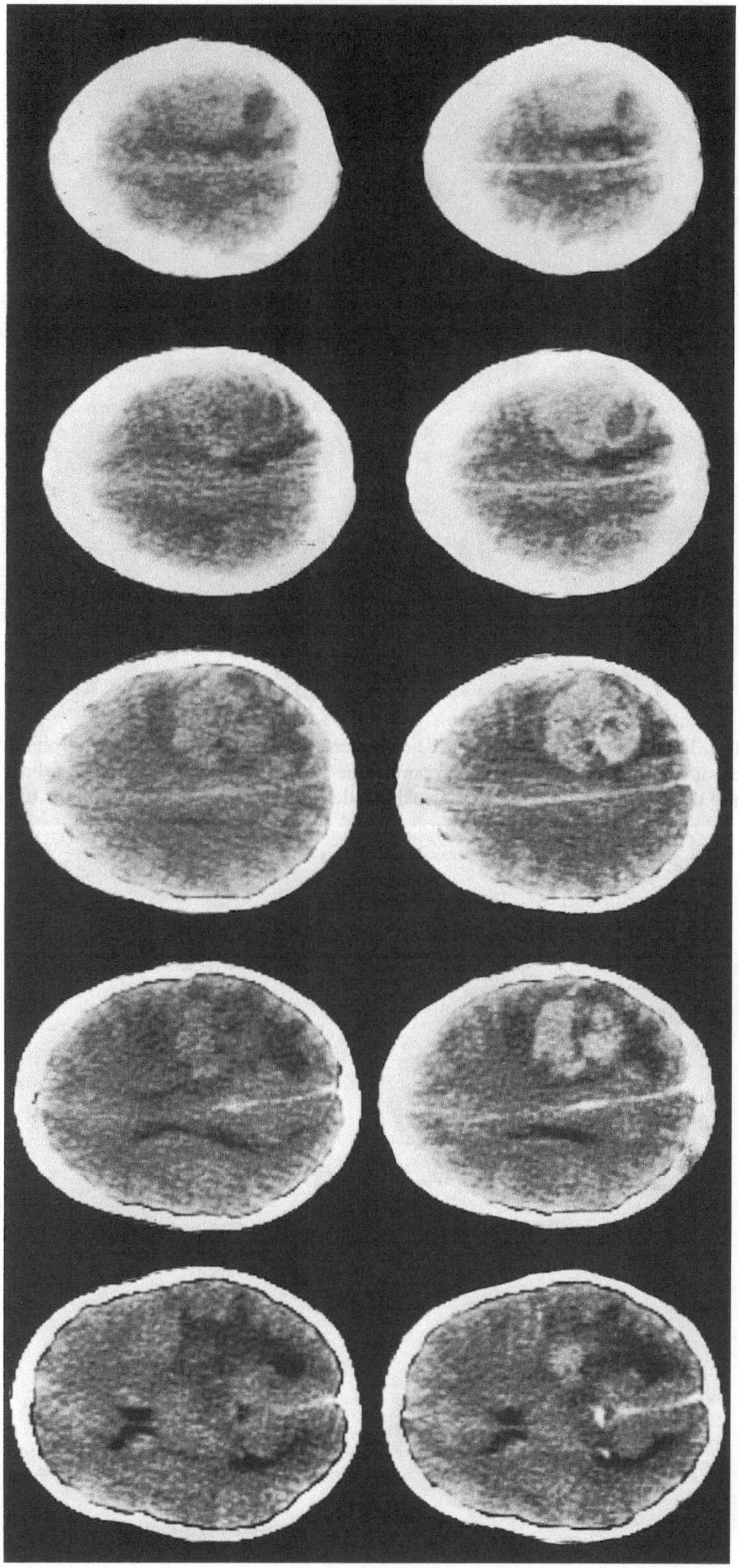

**Fig. D1.162.** Anaplastic ependymoma in the right temporoparietal region with extension to the trigonum in a 21-year-old male. Irregular internal structure of the neoplasm; grade I/grade II perifocal edema. Solid portions of the tumor are isodense or slightly hyperdense in precontrast studies (above) and demonstrate significant contrast enhancement (below)

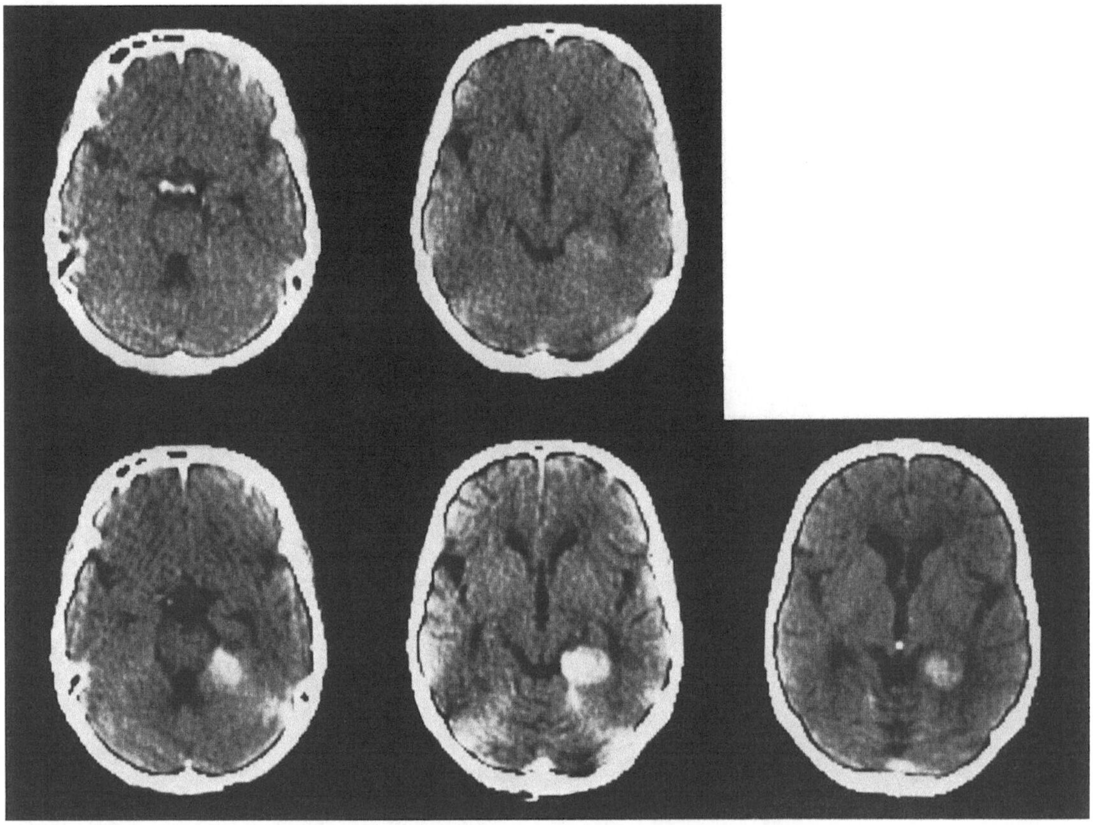

**Fig. D 1.163.** Ependymoma of the cerebral hemispheres at an atypical location deep in the right temporal lobe with extension to the ambient cistern in a 21-year-old female with seizures. Isodense and slightly hyperdense absorption values in precontrast studies (above) and strongly positive contrast enhancement within the tumor (below)

## j) Subependymal Giant Cell Astrocytomas

These tumors are extremely rare intracranial lesions, occurring in 0.4% of tumors in our series, and are usually found in cases of tuberous sclerosis. First signs are usually recognized in childhood and adolescence, with males affected approximately as often as females.

### Typical Location

The tumor is most often found in the lateral ventricles. When located between the foramen of Monro, the septum pellucidum, and the head of the caudate nucleus, the subependymal giant cell astrocytoma may cause occlusion of one or both foramina of Monro with marked hydrocephalus and signs of increased intracranial pressure. These signs may develop very rapidly and lead to an acute life-threatening situation. Patients often suffer from epilepsy and sebaceous adenoma in the face.

Three of 14 subependymal giant cell astrocytomas in our series were not located in the lateral ventricle but rather in the parasagittal region, the left temporal lobe (Fig. D1.170), and the right occipital lobe (Fig. D1.171).

Recurrence of the tumor after total resection has not been observed, and this suggests grade I malignancy.

### Additional Diagnostic Procedures

Other methods usually provide nonspecific evidence, and diagnosis is currently made with the CT scan in conjunction with the other characteristic signs and symptoms described above.

## Computed Tomography (Figs. D1.164–171)

### Precontrast Study

Subependymal giant cell astrocytoma has a characteristic appearance in the plain scan. The tumor is usually located in the anterior horn (Figs. D1.164, 166–169) and demonstrates isodense or slightly hyperdense absorption values. Calcification within the tumor may be observed in a few cases (Fig. D1.169), and intramural calcification of the ventricle wall at a distant location is a typical finding (Figs. C1.166–169).

Since hydrocephalus is almost always present, subependymal giant cell astrocytomas are usually well differentiated from the surrounding CSF, even when the tumor has the same density as normal brain tissue (Fig. D1.164). The tumors are usually approximately 2–3 cm in diameter, but may attain enormous proportions, especially in children with ventriculoatrial shunts (Fig. D1.169b).

### Postcontrast Study

A standard dose of contrast medium results in a mean density increase of 20–30 HU. Maximum density is reached shortly after administration of the contrast medium, while the decrease in absorption is somewhat protracted. Contrast uptake is usually homogeneous since cysts and necrosis are rare.

The marked increase in density after contrast enhancement results in even clearer demarcation of the tumor, with better demonstration of the relations to the head of the caudate nucleus and other adjacent structures.

### Differential Diagnosis

Intraventricular *ependymomas* and *subependymomas* at this location were very rare in our series (Fig. D1.152, 153a). Two *astroblastomas* were found at the same place (Fig. D1.165). Our experience suggests that *plexus papilloma* is usually located in the posterior segments of the lateral ventricle. *Colloid cysts* of the foramen of Monro are never found outside the third ventricle, have higher density values in the precontrast CT, and do not take up contrast media. Colloid cysts are found almost exclusively in adults. Recently we observed a *cavernous hemangioma* at the foramen of Monro (see Fig. D 6.4b, p. 298).

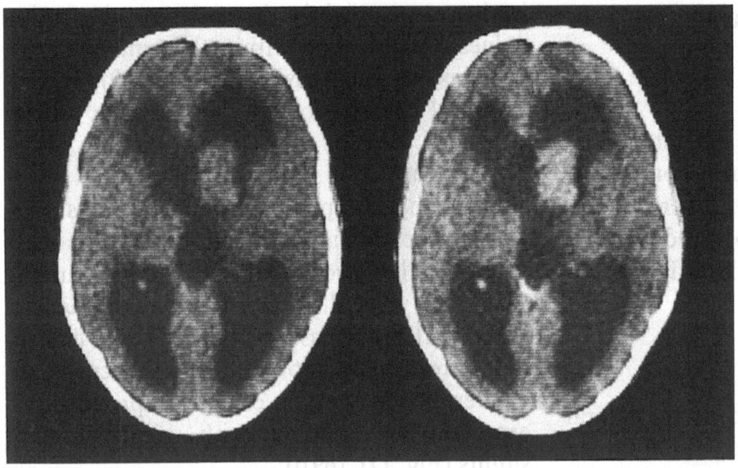

**Fig. D 1.164.** Subependymal giant cell astrocytoma in the right anterior horn between the foramen of Monro and the head of the caudate nucleus in an 11-year-old boy with acute loss of consciousness, probably due to decompensated hydrocephalus. The tumor appears isodense but well delineated by surrounding CSF in the precontrast study (left). Strongly positive homogeneous contrast enhancement (right). Extreme hydrocephalus. Typical location for this type of tumor

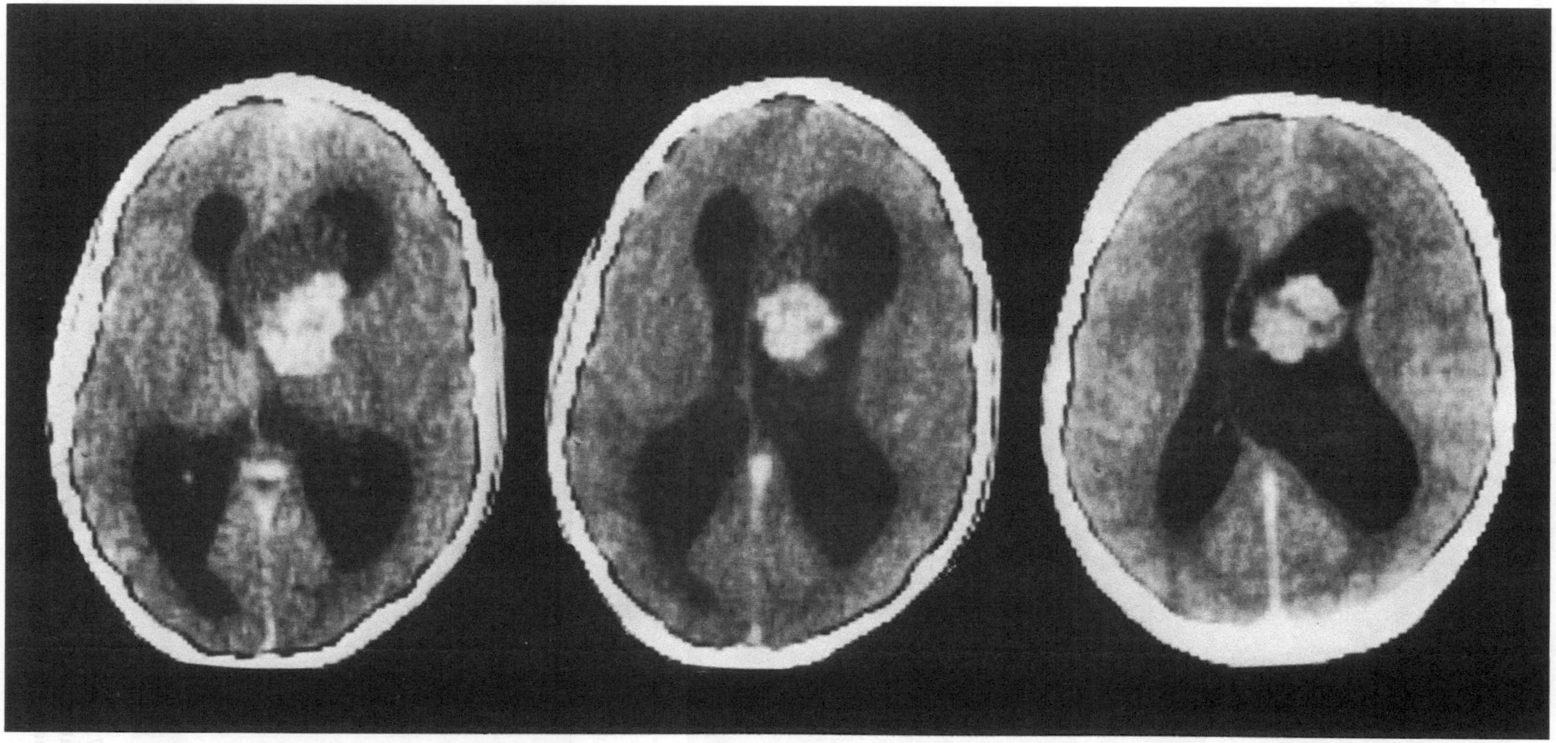

**Fig. D1.165.** Astroblastoma with calcification and a cyst in the right anterior horn between the foramen of Monro, the septum pellucidum, and the head of the caudate nucleus. Extreme hydrocephalus, especially on the right. The pellucid septum is displaced to the left (right). Postcontrast studies. The CT diagnosis was subependymal giant cell astrocytoma. Certain differentiation is not possible if other signs of subependymal giant cell astrocytoma such as calcifications at the ventricular walls or cutaneous alterations (sebaceous adenoma) are absent

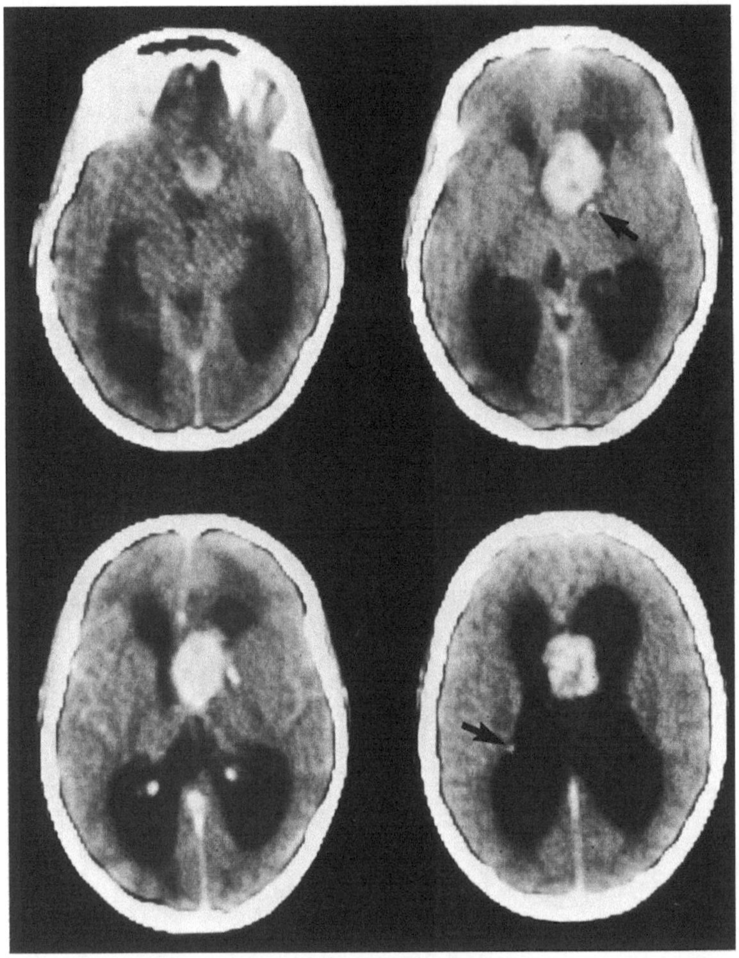

**Fig. D1.166.** Subependymal giant cell astrocytoma at the typical location in the right anterior horn in a 17-year-old patient with tuberous sclerosis. The tumor has caused pronounced hydrocephalus. In addition, one sees two small intramural calcifications (arrows) characteristic of tuberous sclerosis, which is often associated with subependymal giant cell astrocytoma

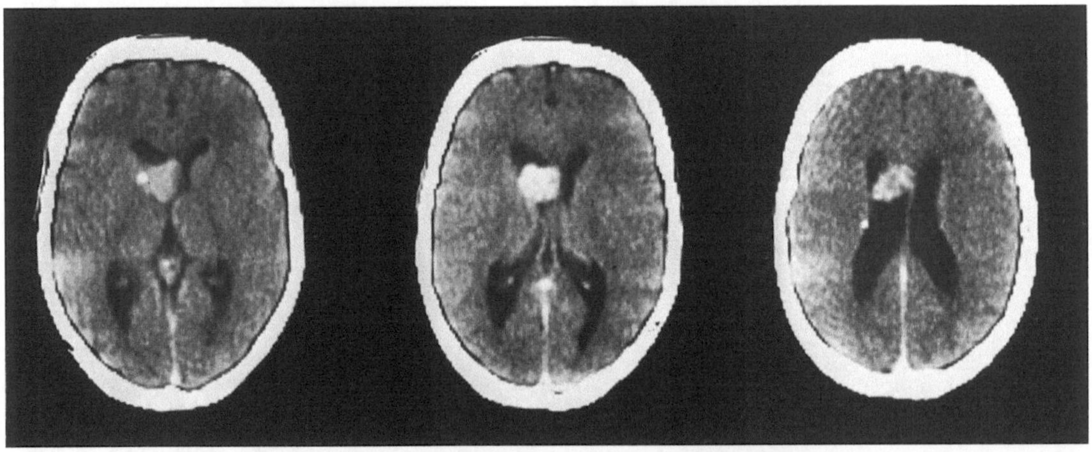

**Fig. D1.167.** Subependymal giant cell astrocytoma at the typical location in the left anterior horn in a 17-year-old girl with characteristic signs of tuberous sclerosis including seizures, sebaceous adenoma, and intraventricular tumor. A small calcification is visible in the corpus region of the left lateral ventricle. Postcontrast CT studies

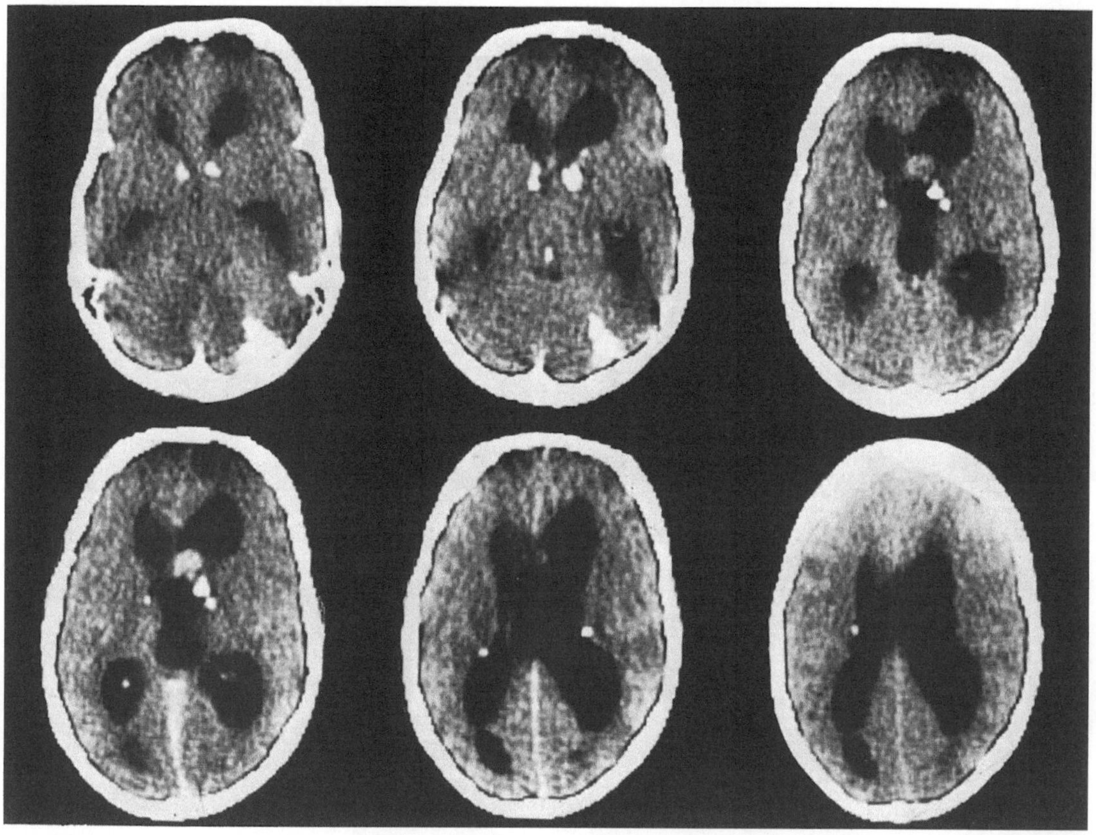

**Fig. D1.168.** Subependymal giant cell astrocytoma with a cyst and calcifications at the right anterior horn in a 17-year-old boy with signs of increased intracranial pressure. Numerous calcifications in the ventricular walls characteristic of tuberous sclerosis

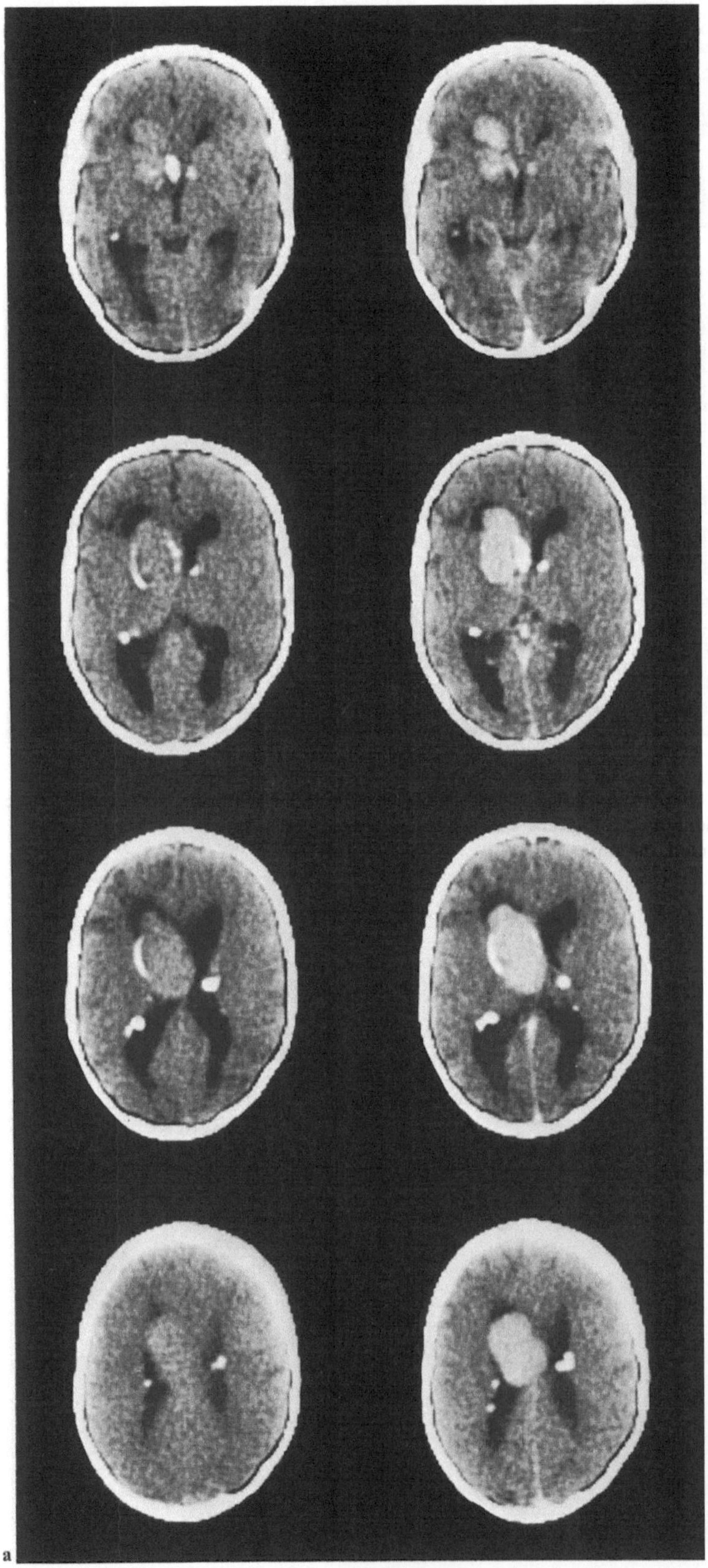

a

**Fig. D1.**169 a, b. Serial CT studies in a $5^1/_2$-year-old girl with subependymal giant cell astrocytoma and tuberous sclerosis. (**a**) Dec 19, 1977: Large tumor at the typical location in the left lateral ventricle between the foramen of Monro, the septum pellucidum, and the basal ganglia. Isodense and hyperdense values (due to calcification) in precontrast studies (left). Numerous calcified tubers on the ventricular walls characteristic of the underlying disease. Significant contrast enhancement (right). (**b**) Nov 28, 1978: Major increase in size of the tumor during the preceding 11 months. No surgical intervention because of extreme mental retardation. Precontrast studies (left) and postcontrast studies (right)

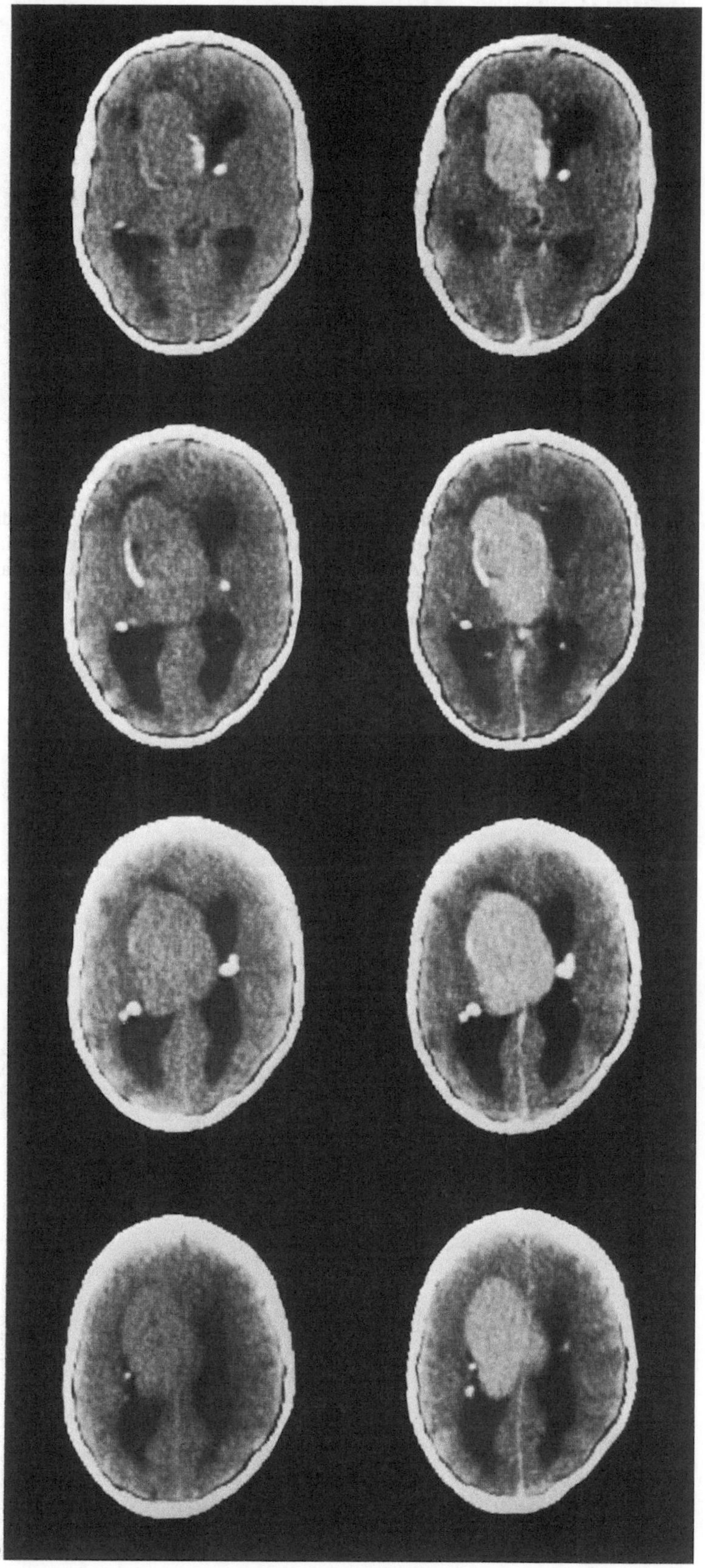

b

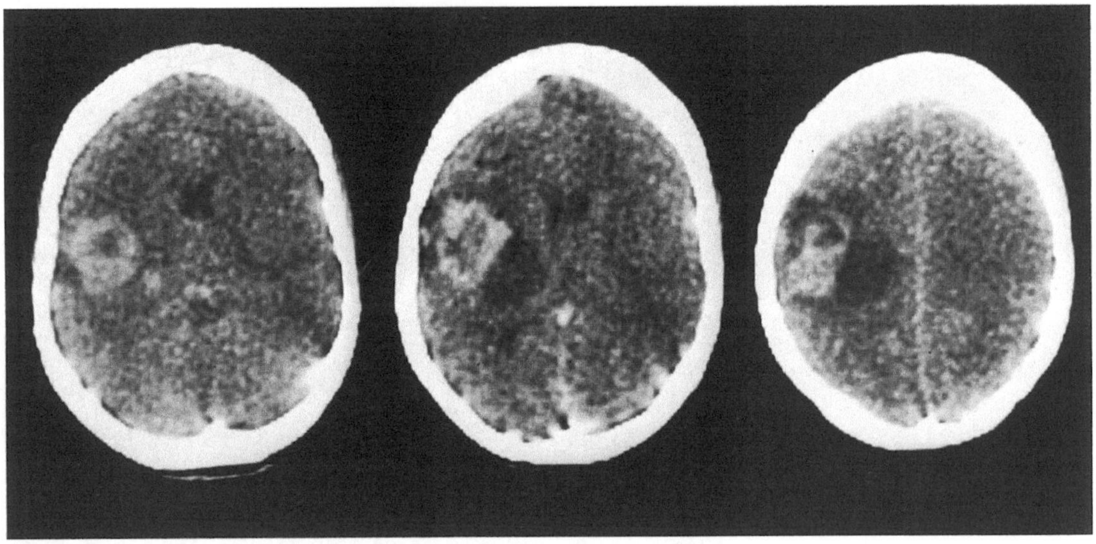

**Fig. D1.170.** Subependymal giant cell astrocytoma in the left temporal lobe in a 24-year-old female. Mixed density values in the precontrast study. An inhomogeneous tumor with a marginal cyst appeared in the postcontrast study. Low density zones within the tumor proved to be cysts at operation. CT studies did not permit a prediction of histological type; uncharacteristic appearance in the CT scan led to the preliminary diagnosis of a rare brain tumor (postcontrast studies)

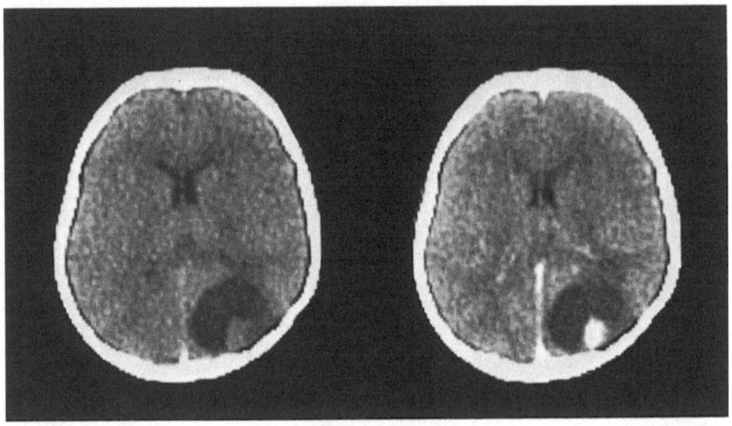

**Fig. D1.171.** Subependymal giant cell astrocytoma in the right occipital lobe of a 14-year-old girl with occasional seizures. Precontrast CT (left) reveals a large hypodense sharply delineated area with a marginal isodense zone which demonstrated strong contrast enhancement in the postcontrast study. A large cyst with a marginal solid tumor nodule the size of a cherry was found at operation. Histological examination provided a diagnosis of subependymal giant cell astrocytoma. Atypical CT finding. Preliminary CT diagnosis: pilocytic astrocytoma

## k) Nerve Cell Tumors

Primary nerve cell tumors are very rare brain neoplasms and comprise 0.5% of all intracranial tumors.

The following tumors, which derive from ganglia and nerve cells, are classified according to degree of malignancy:

1. Dysplastic gangliocytoma (grade I)
2. Ganglioglioma (gangliocytoma) (grade II)
3. Anaplastic ganglioglioma (ganglioneuroblastoma) (grade III)
4. Neuroblastoma (grade IV)

These tumors usually occur in the first 3 decades of life, and males are affected somewhat more frequently than females.

### Typical Locations

Primary nerve cell tumors are most often found in the cerebral hemispheres with a predilection for the medial portion of the temporal lobe, the tuber cinereum, the thalamus, and the midbrain (Zülch 1958). Our studies have shown that these tumors may also occur near the midline in the frontal and parietal lobes (Figs. D1.172–175). Cysts and calcification are common. A dysplastic variant of the tumor is found in the cerebellum, where hyperplastic cerebellar gyri are observed in a circumscribed "blastomatous region" (Zülch 1958, 1980) (Fig. D1.178).

### Characteristic Clinical Findings

Epileptic seizures are the most common findings in neuronal tumors of the cerebral hemispheres and may be evident for years before diagnosis is made. Neurological deficit is rare but may occur in large tumors.

Gangliocytomas in the posterior fossa usually present with signs of cerebellar dysfunction. In two of three cases in our series dysdiadochokinesis and cranial nerve lesions were prominent.

## Computed Tomography (Figs. D1.172–181)

### Precontrast Study

Cysts and calcification found in gangliocytomas and gangliogliomas are readily visible in the plain CT scan (Figs. D1.172–178, 180). The combination of a large cyst and calcified tumor suggests a gangliocytoma or related tumor (Figs. D1.172, 174, 180).

The density of neuroblastomas is usually very similar to that of normal brain tissue.

### Postcontrast Study

Contrast uptake may be found in the solid uncalcified portions of the tumor, but this finding is not obligatory. There is usually little difference between the plain scan and the CT picture following contrast administration.

### Differential Diagnosis

Oligodendrogliomas may present with an appearance similar to that of gangliocytoma in the CT scan, but the presence of large cysts does not favor the diagnosis of oligodendroglioma. Pilocytic astrocytoma is another alternative in differential diagnosis. Calcified cerebellar tumors in adults should always suggest a diagnosis of gangliocytoma. It is not possible to diagnose gangliocytoma in the CT scan if the features described above, especially calcification, are not present (Fig. D1.173).

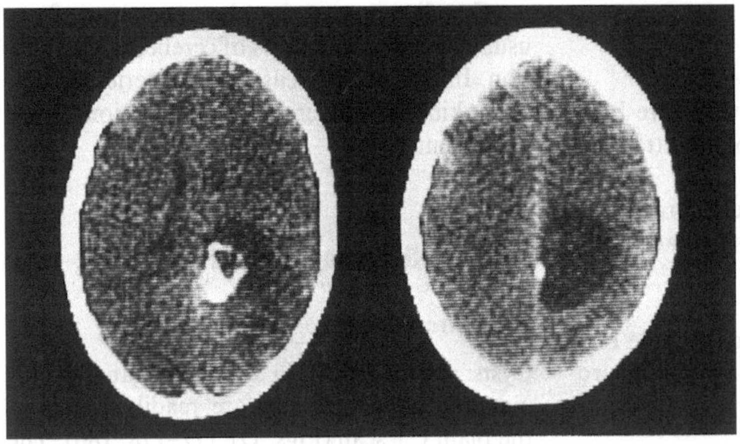

**Fig. D1.172.** Gangliocytoma in the right parietal region adjacent to the interhemispheric fissure in a 51-year-old male with focal seizures. The tumor consists of a small calcified portion and a large cyst. No other tumor in our series produced a similar CT finding (cf. Fig. D1.175)

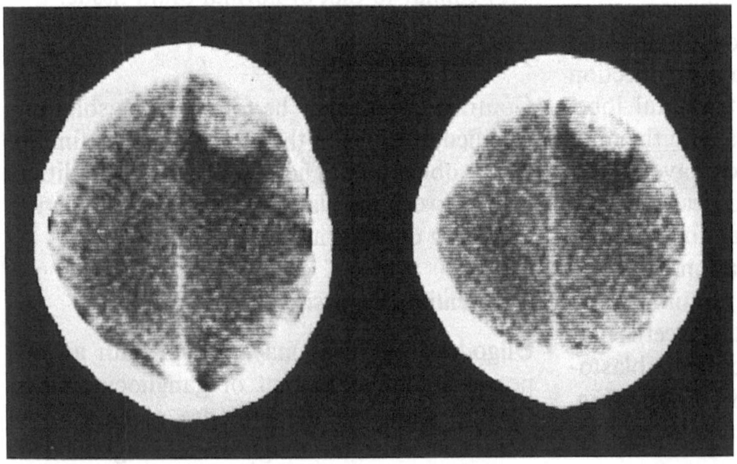

**Fig. D1.173.** Gangliocytoma in the right frontoparietal region in a 37-year-old male. Solid tumor nodule with contrast enhancement within a sharply delineated hypodense zone (representing a cyst). Preliminary diagnosis of meningioma. Postcontrast study

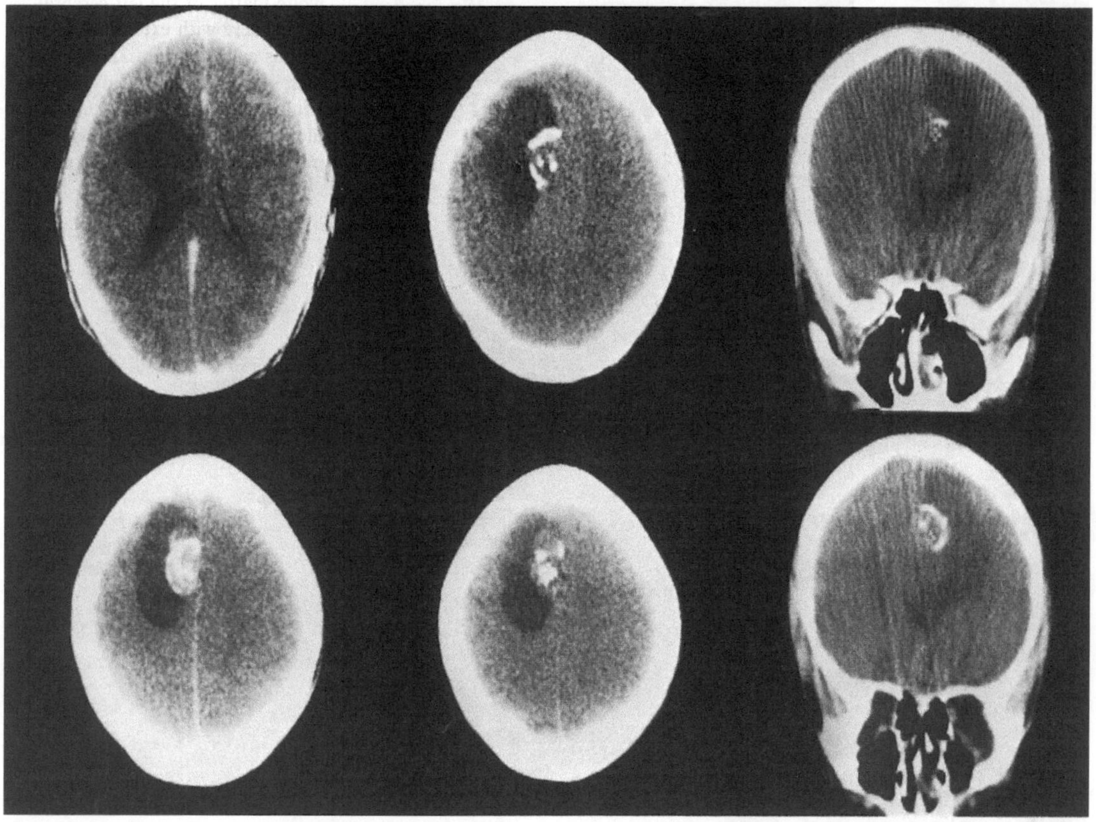

**Fig. D1.174.** Ganglioglioma in the left frontoparietal region in an 18-year-old male. The tumor is composed of solid portions with slight contrast enhancement as well as calcifications located in the wall of a large cyst (postcontrast study). Coronary projections demonstrate extension of the cyst into the cortex of the left cerebral hemisphere (cf. Fig. D1.172). (CT studies courtesy of Dr. Hammer, Department of Radiology, Wagner-Jauregg-Hospital, Linz, Austria)

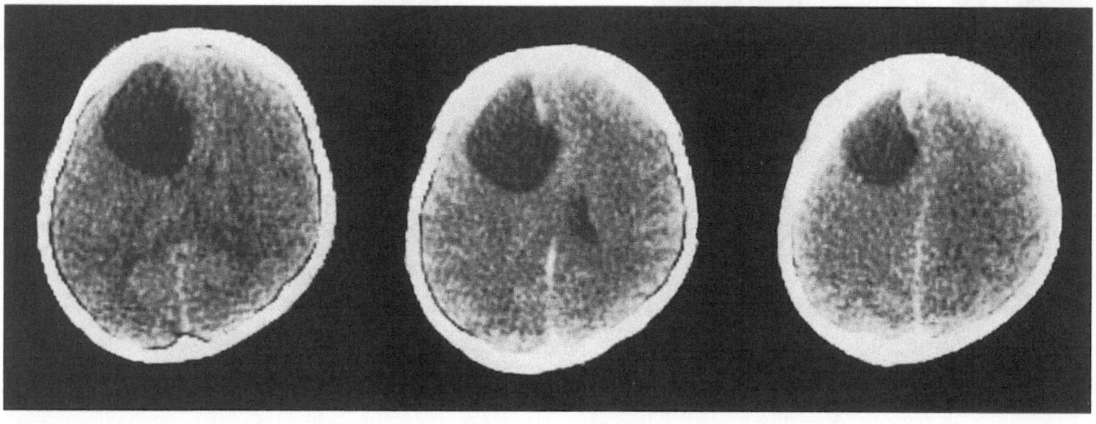

**Fig. D1.175.** Ganglioneuroblastoma in a 27-year-old male with seizures. Solid tumor with positive contrast enhancement at the medial wall of a large cyst (postcontrast studies middle and right). Absorption values of the cyst fluid 19.5 HU

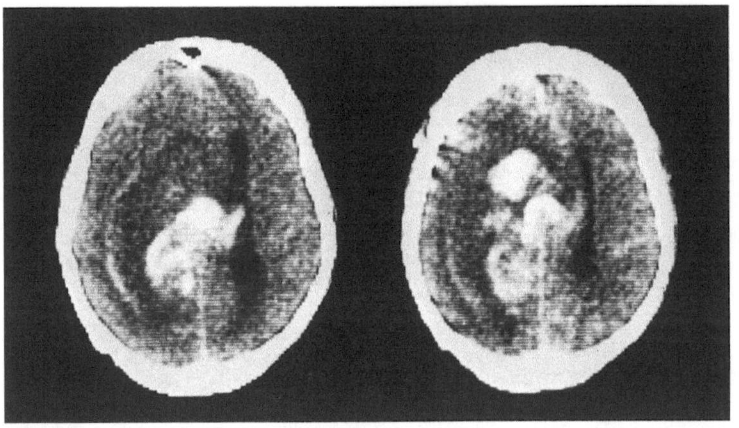

**Fig. D1.176.** Gangliocytoma in the white matter of the left cerebral hemisphere with extension to the corpus callosum in a 32-year-old male with seizures and dysphasia. Multiple partly calcified tumor nodules with significant contrast medium uptake. (Postcontrast studies)

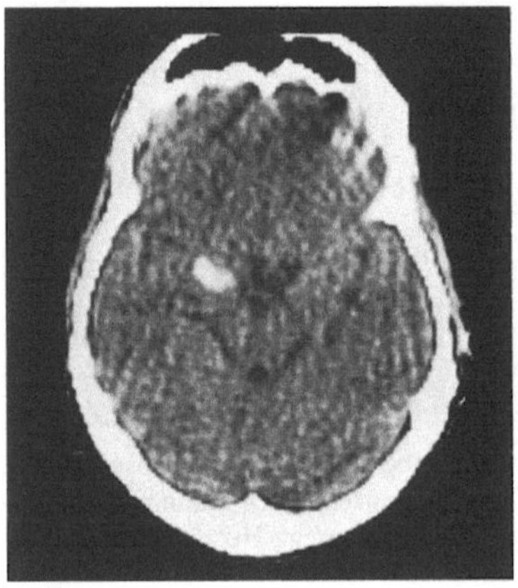

**Fig. D1.177.** Gangliocytoma at the uncus of the left temporal lobe in a 25-year-old male with temporal lobe epilepsy. The CT study reveals a comma-shaped zone of very high density (calcification)

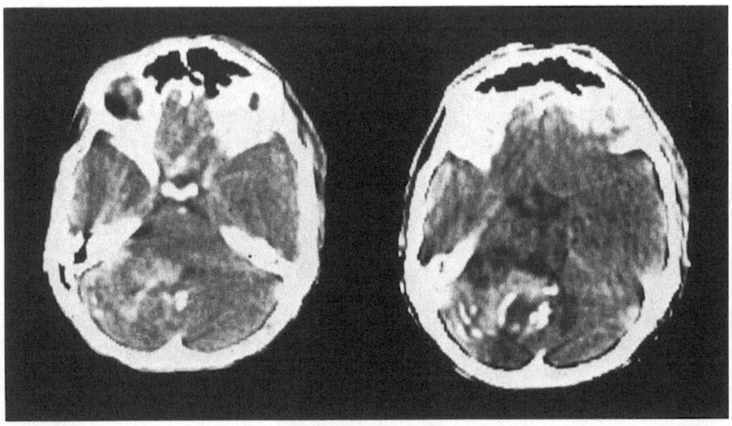

**Fig. D1.178.** Large gangliocytoma in the left cerebellar hemisphere with multiple calcifications and slight contrast enhancement in the solid portions of the tumor. Slight perifocal edema. Thirty-two-year-old male with dyspraxia of the left hand and visual disorders

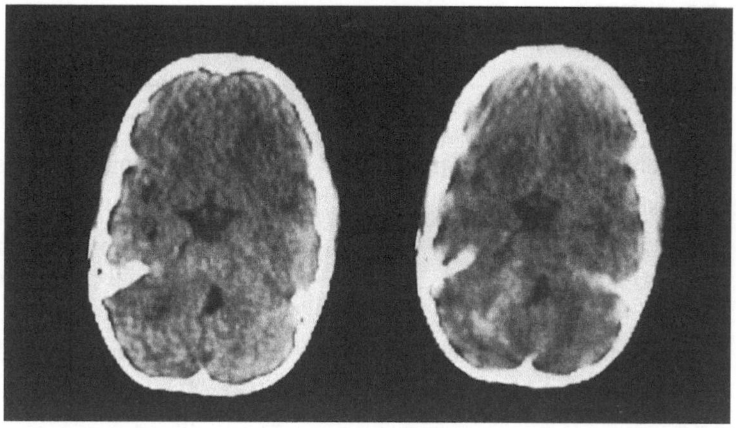

**Fig. D1.179.** Gangliocytoma in the left cerebellar hemisphere in a 7-year-old girl with ataxia and deficits limited to the caudal cranial nerves on the left. Displacement of the fourth ventricle. Isodense and hypodense regions in the precontrast study (left) with inhomogeneous contrast enhancement (right). Prediction of histological type is not possible on the basis of CT studies

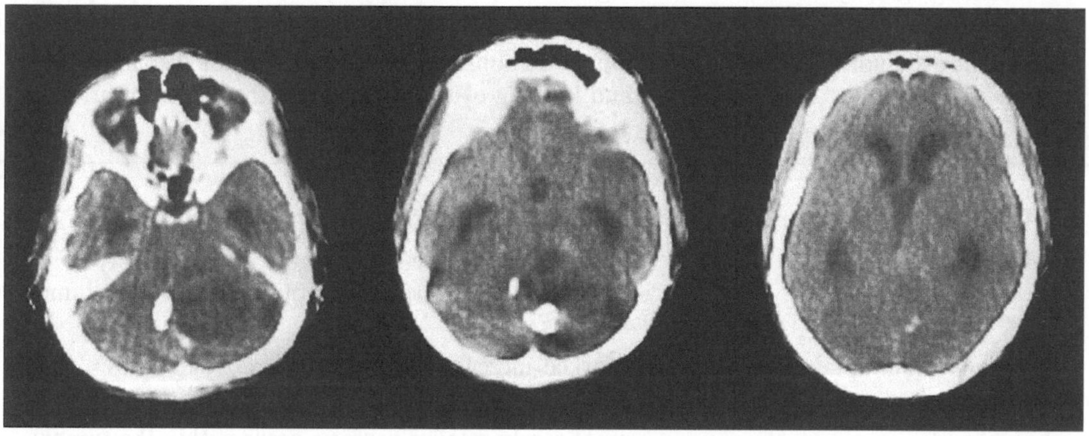

**Fig. D1.180.** Ganglioneuroblastoma in the right cerebellar hemisphere in a 37-year-old male with ataxia and signs of increased intracranial pressure. The neuronal tumor appears as a partly calcified ring structure. The solid uncalcified portions of the tumor demonstrate slight contrast enhancement. Displacement of the fourth ventricle and obstructive hydrocephalus. Postcontrast study

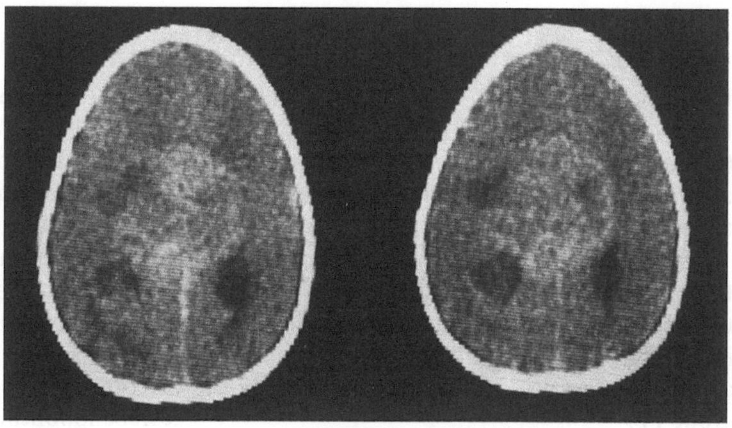

**Fig. D1.181.** Neuroblastoma in the corpus callosum of a 2-year-old boy admitted in coma. Large midline tumor with slight inhomogeneous contrast enhancement. Dilatation of the ventricular system secondary to blockage of the foramen of Monro bilaterally. CT studies do not allow prediction of histological type. Postcontrast study

## l) Medulloblastomas

| | |
|---|---|
| Incidence | 2–6% |
| Characteristic age at diagnosis | First and second decades |
| Sex distribution | Preponderance of males |
| Typical locations | Cerebellar vermis, fourth ventricle, cerebellar hemispheres, caudal brain stem; spreading in all CSF spaces possible |
| Characteristic clinical findings | Headache, vomiting, and ataxia |
| Skull film | Signs of increased intracranial pressure common |
| EEG | Unspecific changes |
| Echoencephalography | Ventricular dilatation in almost all cases |
| Serial brain scintigraphy | Radionuclide uptake in all large tumors |
| Cerebral angiography | Signs of a space-occupying lesion; delicate pathological vessels in some cases; capillary blush |
| Other contrast studies | Direct demonstration of the tumor or displacement and kinking of the aqueduct in the central ventriculogram |
| **Computed Tomography** | |
| Precontrast study | Slightly hyperdense zones in the great majority of cases, isodense zones in exceptional cases with tumor necrosis |
| Contrast medium uptake | Marked increase in density in almost all cases |
| Appearance after contrast enhancement | Homogeneous solid tumor in the majority of cases, more rarely smaller necrotic areas within the tumor; slight perifocal edema in nearly half of cases |
| **Differential Diagnosis** | |
| Pilocytic astrocytoma<br>Ependymoma<br>"Pseudotumor vermis"<br>Cerebellar arteriovenous malformation | |

Frequency of medulloblastoma among all brain tumors ranges from 4.2% (ZÜLCH) to 4.5% (CUSHING) and 6.5% (RINGERTZ). The tumor comprised only 2% of all brain tumors in our collective.

Medulloblastoma is the most common brain tumor in children, with a peak incidence between 5 and 15 years, but it may also occur in adults. Males are affected more than twice as often as females. Malignancy is classified as grade IV.

**Typical Locations**

Medulloblastoma is most often found on the roof of the fourth ventricle and in the vermis of the cerebellum, and the tumor may spread in all directions from this origin. The fourth ventricle may be filled with tumor which may extend through the foramen of Magendie into the cisterna magna and the spinal canal as well as through the foramina of Luschka into the cerebellopontine angle and through the aqueduct to the third ventricle. Presence of tumor in a single cerebellar hemisphere without involvement of the vermis is rare. Medulloblastomas may occasionally originate in the caudal brain stem. The tumor is highly malignant and tends to metastasize to all regions of the CSF space.

The *cerebellar arachnoid sarcoma* described by FÖRSTER and GAGEL is a variant of medulloblastoma with a predilection for the cerebellar hemispheres. RUSSEL and RUBINSTEIN designated the tumor as *desmoplastic medulloblastoma*. Peak incidence occurs somewhat later than in medulloblastoma, and prognosis is considerably more favorable (grade III–IV).

### Characteristic Clinical Findings

Localizing signs such as ataxia and dysdiadochokinesis are almost always accompanied by headache and vomiting, which indicate increased intracranial pressure as a result of disrupted CSF circulation. Torticollis due to irritation of the cervical nerve roots is not uncommon.

### Additional Diagnostic Procedures

Plain skull films, electroencephalograms, and echoencephalography demonstrate nonspecific pathological changes which do not suggest a histological diagnosis. Dynamic brain scintigraphy is capable of demonstrating all large medulloblastomas, and angiography reveals typical indirect signs of a space-occupying lesion of the posterior fossa as well as pathological vessels and a tumor blush in some cases. Ventriculography may demonstrate the solid portion of the tumor in the fourth ventricle.

## Computed Tomography (Figs. D1.182–186, 188, 190–204)

### Precontrast Study

Approximately two-thirds of all medulloblastomas demonstrate hyperdense sharply delineated zones near the fourth ventricle and the vermis of the cerebellum (Fig. D1.183). Mixed density resulting from necrosis or hemorrhage in the tumor may be found in about 20% of all cases (Fig. D1.185a). Solid isodense medulloblastomas are less common and comprise about 10% of cases in our collective (Figs. D1.182, 193).

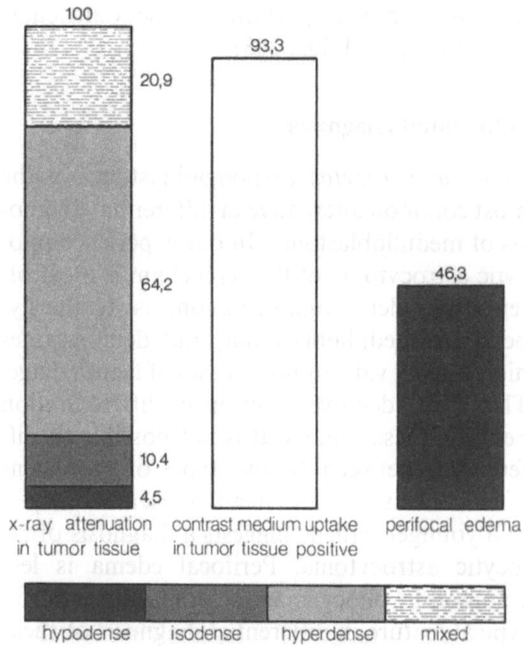


**Fig. D 1.182.** X-ray attenuation, contrast uptake, and frequency of perifocal edema in medulloblastoma (percent)

Hypodense medulloblastomas are exceptional and revealed almost complete necrosis in the two cases which we observed. Very high density results from hemorrhage in the tumor (Fig. D1.194).

Hypodense zones surrounding a medulloblastoma indicate perifocal edema, found in 46% of cases. Cysts are very rare in these tumors (Figs. D1.195, 196).

### Postcontrast Study

Viable portions of the tumor readily accept contrast media, with a resulting increase in density averaging 11–12 HU following a standard dose of contrast medium. Maximum density is attained shortly after administration and is followed by a rapid decline.

Administration of contrast media usually permits clear delineation of the entire tumor. Contrast uptake is generally homogeneous (Figs. D1.183, 184), though necrotic zones produce defects in a few cases (Fig. D1.185, 186). Perifocal edema is more readily visible after contrast enhancement.

Tumor growth in the meninges results in increased density values in all areas of the CSF space affected by the tumor (Fig. D1.192). Enormous metastatic tumors may be found in the supratentorial portions of the ventricular system (Figs. D1.202, 203).

**Differential Diagnosis**

*Pilocytic astrocytoma* (spongioblastoma) is the most common alternative in differential diagnosis of medulloblastoma. In our experience pilocytic astrocytoma of the cerebellum is most often a hypodense tumor, in contrast to the hyperdense medulloblastoma, and demonstrates high density values only in cases of hemorrhage. This is the decisive criterion in differentiation between these tumors. It is not possible to differentiate between the two types of neoplasms after contrast enhancement. Presence of cysts in a younger patient suggests a diagnosis of pilocytic astrocytoma. Perifocal edema is less common in pilocytic astrocytoma but is not a typical feature in differential diagnosis of these tumors. In addition, the typical location of pilocytic astrocytoma is usually lateral rather than medial, as is the case in classic medulloblastoma. Desmoplastic medulloblastomas are always limited to one cerebellar hemisphere.

Density increase after contrast administration is usually maintained for a longer period in pilocytic astrocytoma than in medulloblastoma (Kazner et al. 1977).

It is not always possible to differentiate between *ependymoma* of the fourth ventricle and medulloblastoma. Calcification suggests ependymoma but may also occur in rare cases of medulloblastoma (Fig. D1.192). Contrast uptake is similarly intense. Dorsal displacement of the fourth ventricle due to growth originating on the floor of the rhomboid fossa suggests a diagnosis of ependymoma.

*Pseudotumor vermis* can be a major pitfall in differential diagnosis of medulloblastoma. The vermis of the cerebellum is composed primarily of gray matter and is surrounded by the cerebellar white matter, which has a somewhat lower density. It accepts contrast media to a limited degree (about 4 HU). This phenomenon may simulate a cerebellar tumor (Fig. D1.187). On the other hand, medulloblastoma in an early phase without blockage of CSF circulation may be misdiagnosed as pesudotumor vermis (Fig. D1.188). Obliteration of the right lateral recess of the fourth ventricle in the case at hand led to the diagnosis.

*Stenosis of the aqueduct in combination with pseudotumor vermis* is a special diagnostic problem, since one might assume that the pseudotumor itself is the cause of hydrocephalus. Ventriculography usually clarifies the diagnosis (Fig. F22, 418).

A *cerebellar arteriovenous malformation* with homogeneous contrast uptake may be confused with medulloblastoma or other cerebellar tumors, as was the case in two patients in our series.

*Displacement of parts of the cerebellum into the tentorial hiatus in infants and small children with shunted hydrocephalus may give the impression of a cerebellar tumor* (Fig. D1.189). The cerebellar tissue within the tentorial hiatus is composed primarily of gray matter with higher density than the surrounding structures.

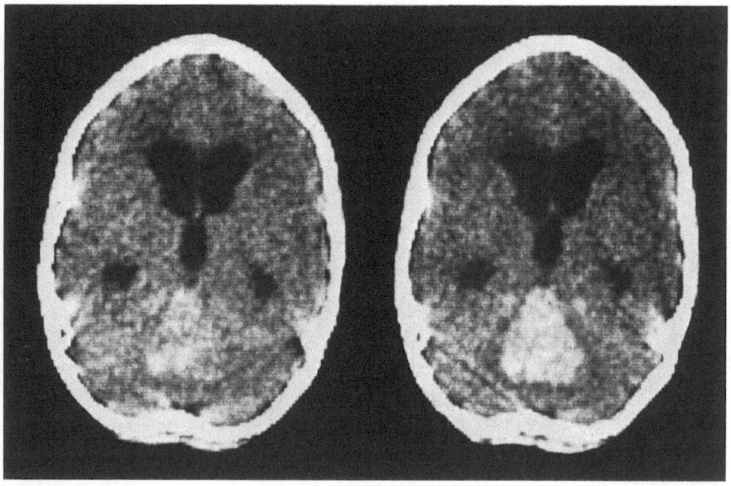

**Fig. D 1.183.** Medulloblastoma of the cerebellar vermis in a 9-year-old child with signs of cerebellar dysfunction. Characteristic CT findings: hyperdense values within the tumor in precontrast studies (left) with strong contrast enhancement (right). Clear delineation of the tumor against the brain stem not possible in this case. Pronounced hydrocephalus

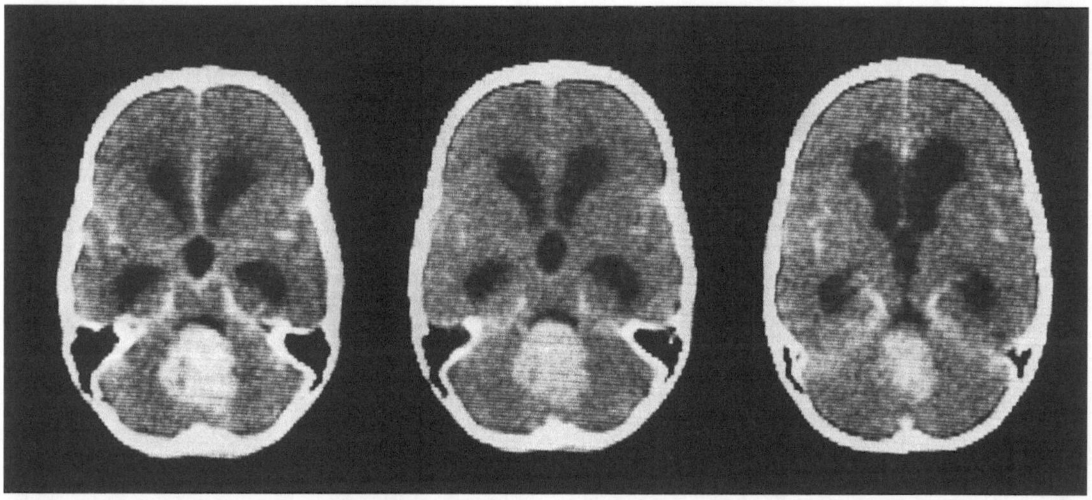

**Fig. D 1.184.** Large medulloblastoma in the cerebellar vermis of a 6-year-old boy. Rather homogeneous contrast enhancement within the tumor, which appeared slightly hyperdense in the precontrast study. Minimal perifocal edema. Good delineation of the tumor against the brain stem due to CSF in the fourth ventricle. Pronounced hydrocephalus. Postcontrast study

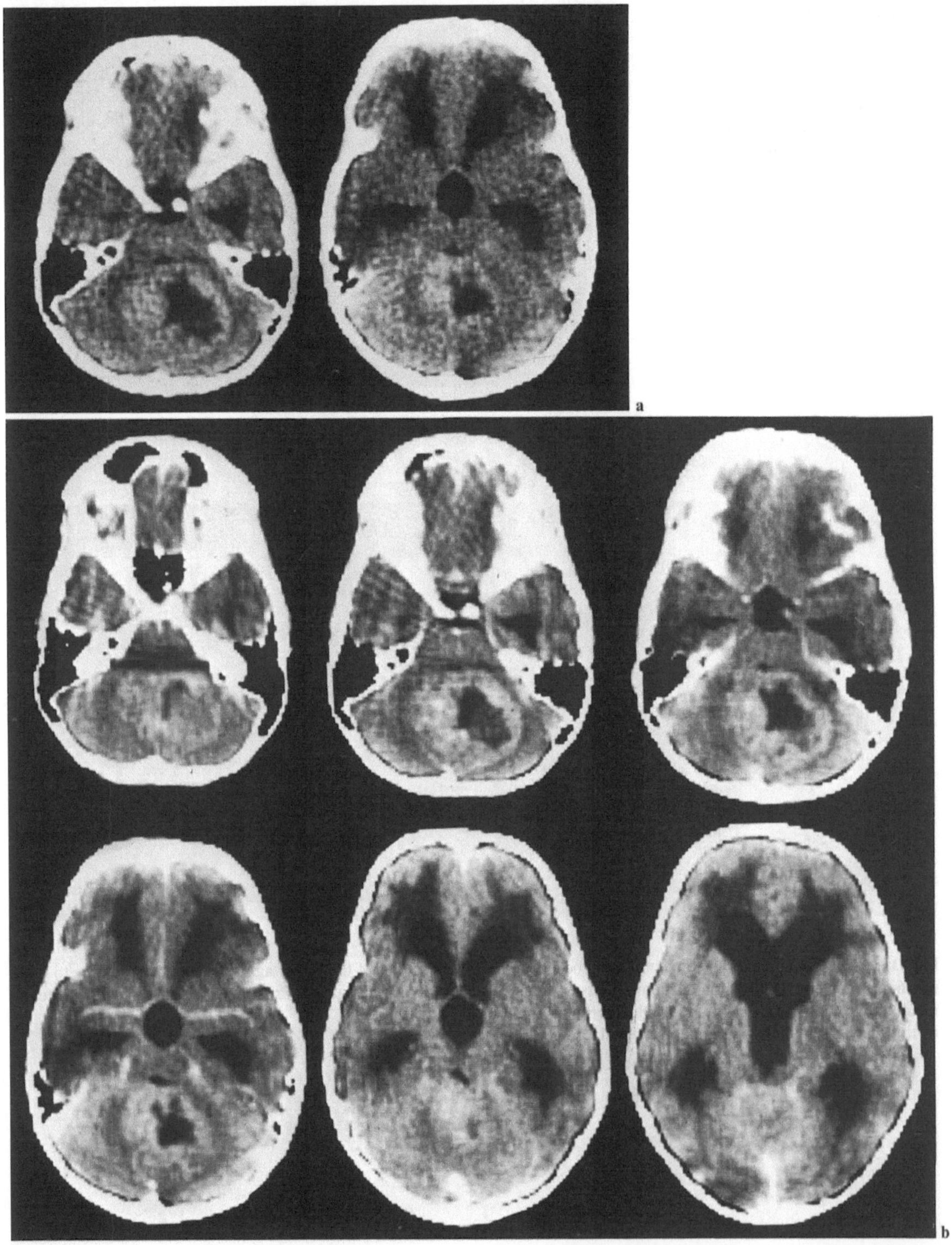


**Fig. D 1.**185 a, b. Very large medulloblastoma in a 7-year-old girl. The tumor originates in the roof of the fourth ventricle and extends far into both cerebellar hemispheres. (**a**) Hyperdense solid tumor in the precontrast study. Large hypodense zone within the tumor as a result of necrosis. A narrow border of CSF delineates the tumor against the brain stem. (**b**) Postcontrast study of the same tumor which takes up contrast material in the viable portions. Extension of the tumor from the foramen magnum to the supracerebellar cistern. Periventricular lucency as a result of obstructive hydrocephalus. Studies made with wide window (200 HU) for optimal demonstration of transependymal CSF penetration. As a result of wide window width contrast enhancement within the tumor seems to be less significant than it usually appears at window widths of 75 or 100 HU

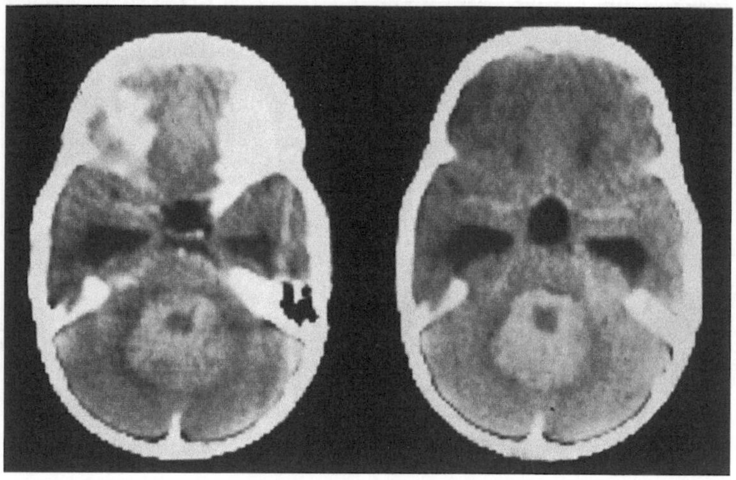

**Fig. D 1.186.** Symmetrically developed medulloblastoma in the cerebellar vermis of a 3-year-old boy with signs of cerebellar dysfunction. Hyperdense values in the precontrast study and positive contrast enhancement with the exception of a small zone of necrosis. Significant compression and flattening of the brain stem. Very limited perifocal edema. Obstructive hydrocephalus. Postcontrast study

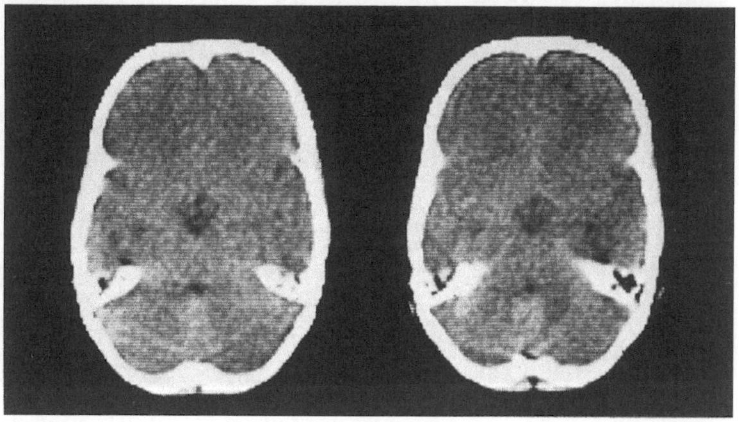

**Fig. D 1.187.** "Pseudotumor vermis" in a 7-year-old boy with signs of cerebellar dysfunction due to inflammation. The postcontrast study (right) creates the impression of a tumor at this location. The mass of gray matter in the region of the vermis cerebelli is responsible for this phenomenon (cf. Fig. D 1.188)

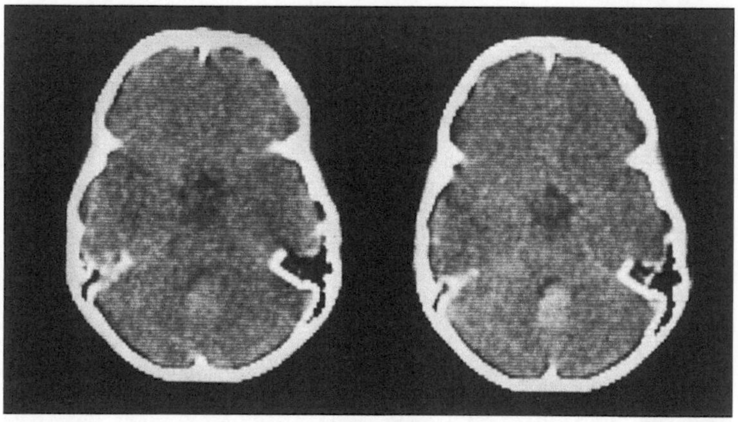

**Fig. D 1.188.** Small medulloblastoma in the roof of the fourth ventricle in an 11-year-old girl with subtle signs of cerebellar dysfunction. Alternatives in differential diagnosis include pseudotumor vermis and medulloblastoma. Asymmetrical dorsal indentation of the fourth ventricle on the right favors a diagnosis of neoplasm

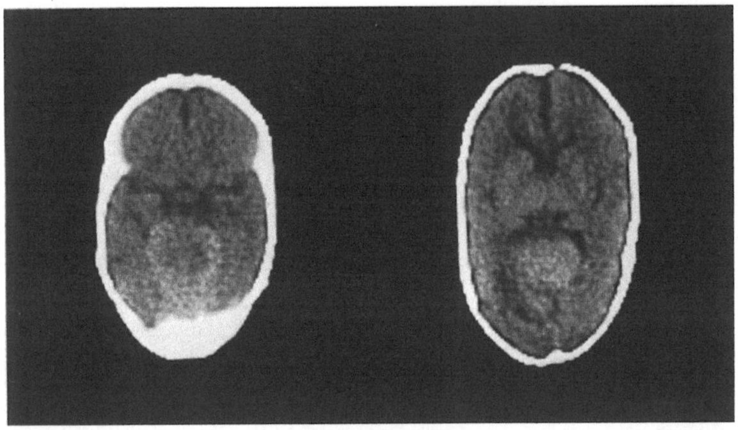

**Fig. D 1.189.** Suspected cerebellar tumor in an 8-month-old infant with a CSF shunt for hydrocephalus. The CSF drainage causes the cerebellum to advance higher into the tentorial hiatus, which produces the impression of a midline or cerebellar tumor. Hyperdense values result from the relatively high proportion of nerve cells in the superior portion of the cerebellar vermis and the cerebellar hemispheres, which are composed predominantly of gray matter

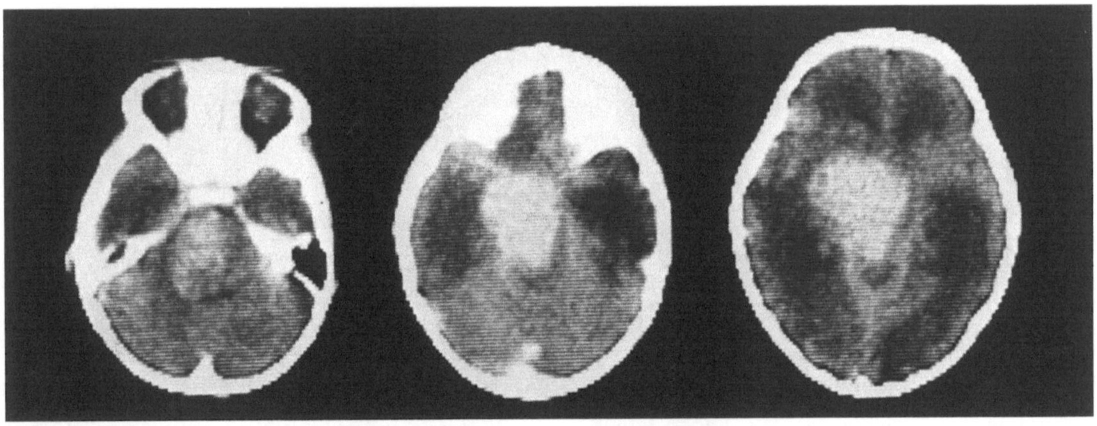

**Fig. D 1.190.** Medulloblastoma of the brain stem with extension to the basal ganglia in a 6-year-old boy. Hyperdense values in the precontrast study and homogeneous contrast enhancement within the tumor. Periventricular lucency due to obstructive hydrocephalus. Postcontrast study

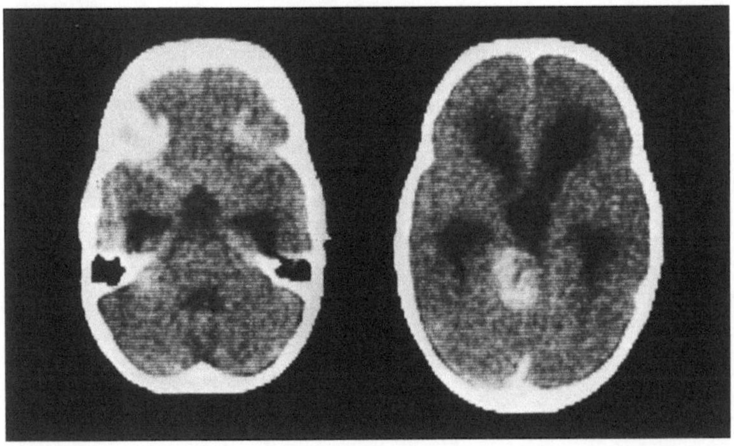

**Fig. D 1.191.** Medulloblastoma in the lamina tecti with extension to the left cerebral peduncle in a 2-year-old child with signs of increased intracranial pressure (right). The posterior fossa appears normal (left). Pronounced hydrocephalus with periventricular lucency secondary to blockage of the mesencephalic aqueduct. Postcontrast study

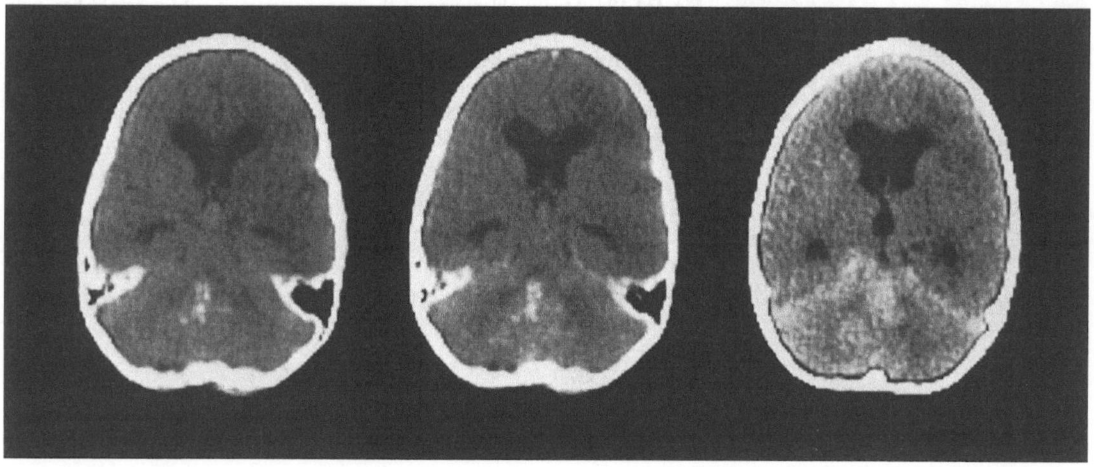

**Fig. D 1.192.** Medulloblastoma with multiple fine calcifications in the cerebellar vermis, meningeal spread, and metastasis in the third ventricle. Precontrast study on the left, postcontrast studies in the middle and on the right. The supracerebellar and ambient cisterns are completely filled with tumor (right). Alternative diagnosis ependymoma

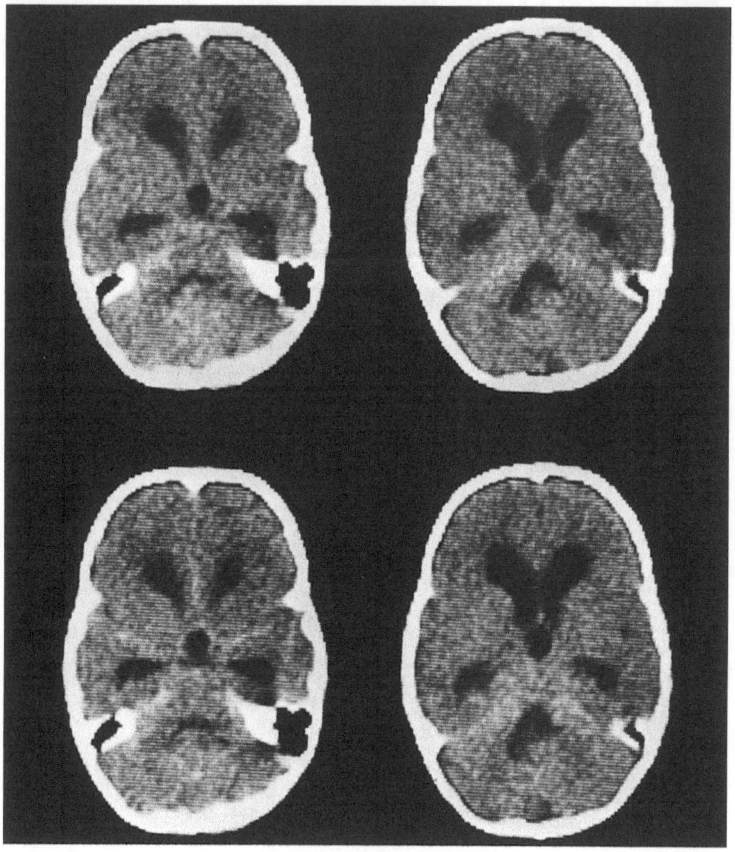

**Fig. D 1.193.** Isodense medulloblastoma in the cerebellar vermis of a 7-year-old boy with signs of cerebellar dysfunction. Absence of contrast enhancement within the tumor is due to recent total necrosis demonstrated at operation. Indentation of the fourth ventricle from the right strongly suggests a diagnosis of neoplasm. Moderate hydrocephalus. Precontrast study (above) and postcontrast study (below)

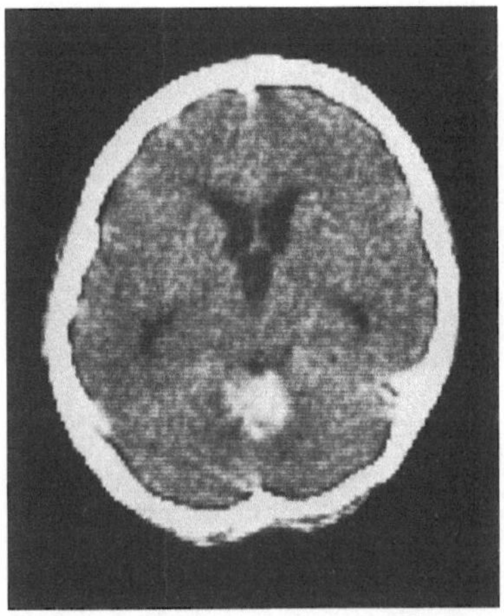

**Fig. D1.194.** Medulloblastoma in the upper vermis in a 14-year-old boy with acute onset of cerebellar dysfunction. A hyperdense zone with density values characteristic of acute hemorrhage is visible in the upper portion of the vermis. A medulloblastoma 3 cm in diameter containing freshly coagulated blood was demonstrated at operation. Similar hematomas may be found in pilocytic astrocytoma and arteriovenous malformation

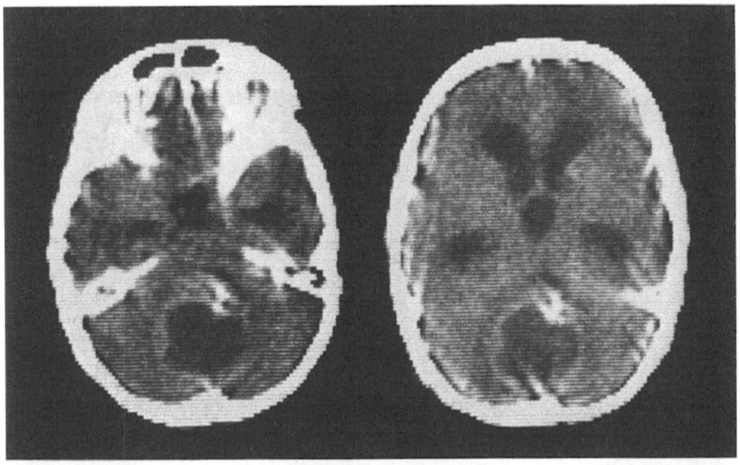

**Fig. D1.195.** Atypical medulloblastoma in the cerebellar vermis of a 9-year-old boy with signs of cerebellar dysfunction. Unusual CT findings including a large centrally located cyst and marginal calcification which might suggest a pilocytic astrocytoma. The solid portion of the tumor was slightly hyperdense in the precontrast study, which argues against a diagnosis of pilocytic astrocytoma and strongly suggests medulloblastoma

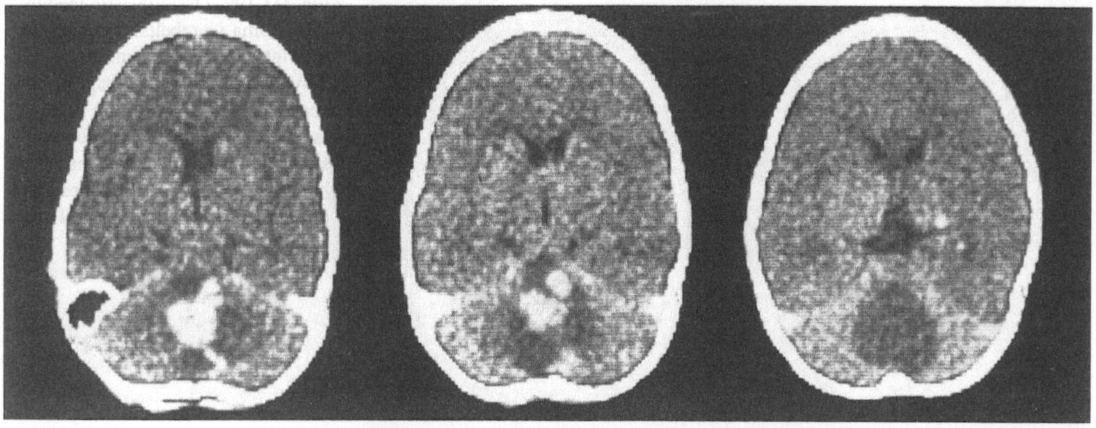

**Fig. D1.196.** Atypical medulloblastoma within a large cyst in a 2-year-old child. Strongly positive contrast enhancement within the tumor, which appeared slightly hyperdense in the precontrast study. Postcontrast study

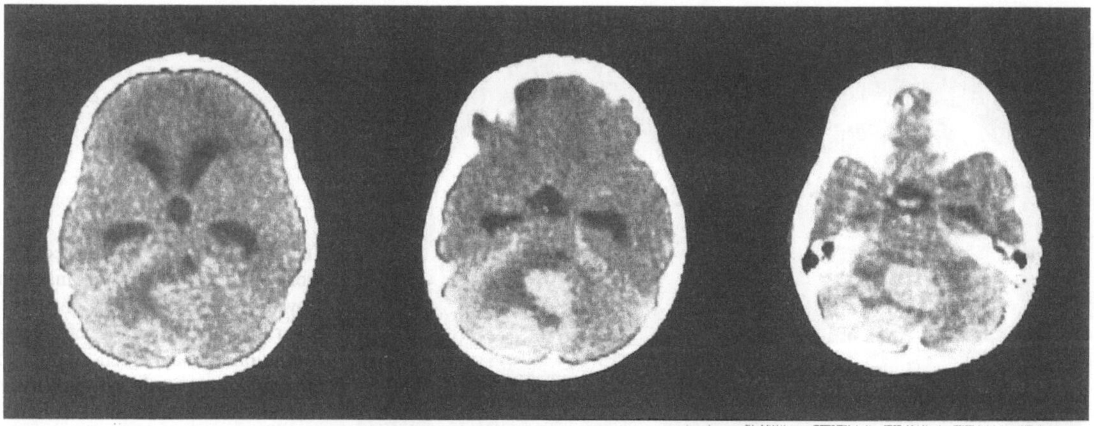

**Fig. D1.197.** Very large desmoplastic medulloblastoma (cerebellar sarcoma) in a 3-year-old boy with signs of cerebellar dysfunction. The tumor extends laterally in the left cerebellar hemisphere, a finding unusual for the typical medulloblastoma. Significant perifocal edema. Slightly hyperdense values in the precontrast study (left) and strongly positive contrast enhancement (middle and right)

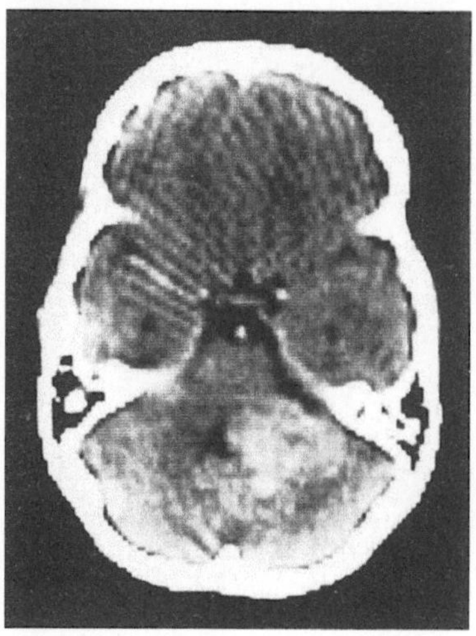

**Fig. D1.198.** Desmoplastic medulloblastoma (cerebellar sarcoma) in a 5-year-old girl with facial nerve palsy and signs of a cerebellar disorder on the right. The tumor extends from the right cerebellopontine angle to the fourth ventricle. Density values typical of medulloblastoma. Postcontrast study

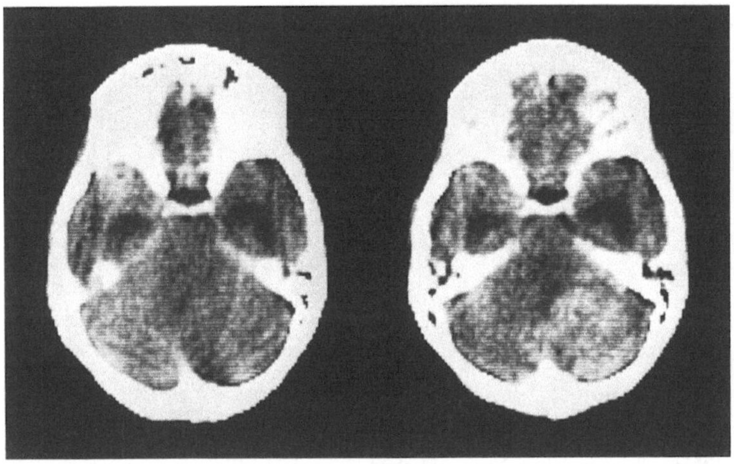

**Fig. D1.199.** Desmoplastic medulloblastoma (cerebellar sarcoma) in the right cerebellar hemisphere of a 29-year-old female with signs of cerebellar dysfunction on the right. Isodense values in the precontrast study (left) and positive contrast enhancement (right). Pronounced hydrocephalus with dilatation of the temporal horns

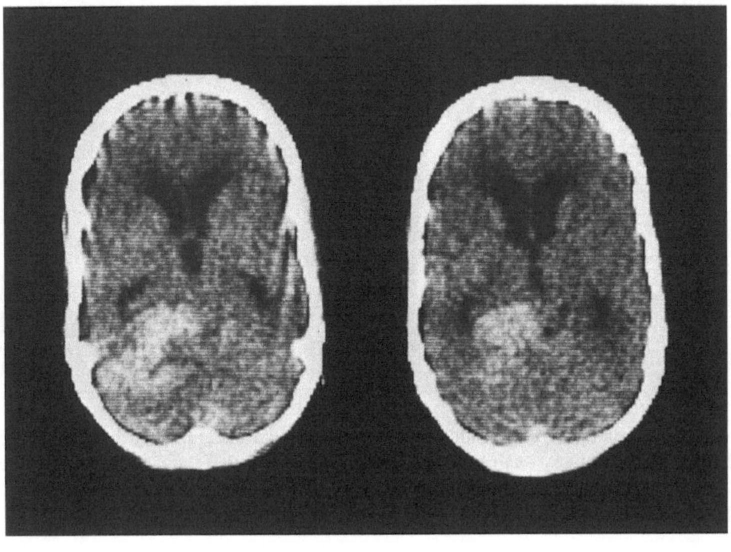

**Fig. D1.200.** Desmoplastic medulloblastoma (cerebellar sarcoma) in a 15-year-old girl with signs of cerebellar dysfunction on the left. Demonstration of a hyperdense tumor in the precontrast study with positive contrast enhancement in the tumor which extends from the left cerebellar hemisphere into the left cerebellopontine angle and the ambient cistern. Pronounced ventricular dilatation. Postcontrast study

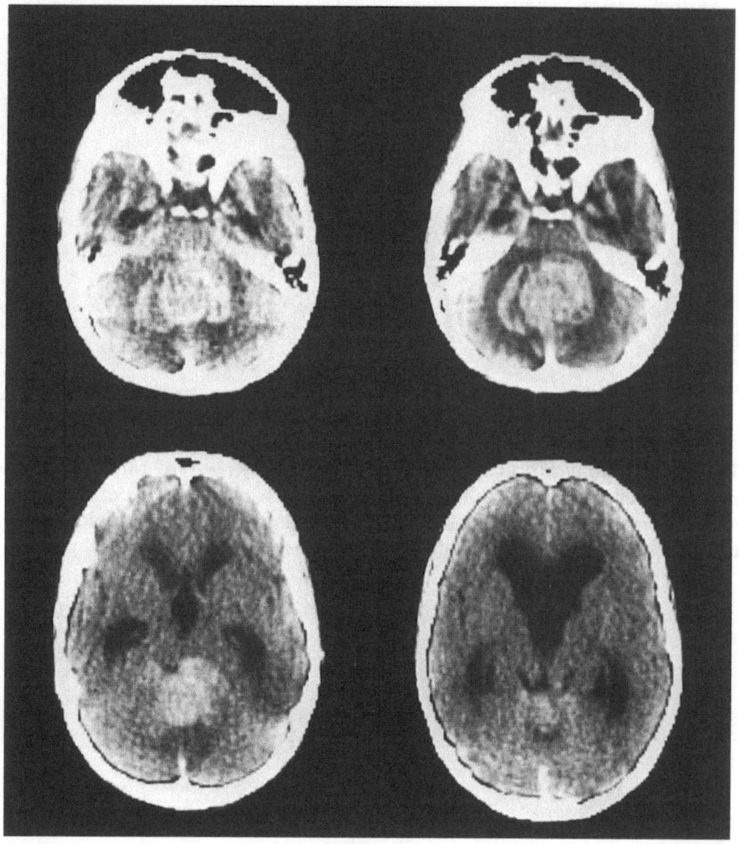

**Fig. D1.201.** Desmoplastic medulloblastoma (cerebellar sarcoma) in a 28-year-old female with ataxia. The precontrast study revealed a hyperdense tumor. Strongly positive contrast enhancement in a large tumor which fills the entire cerebellar vermis. Postcontrast study

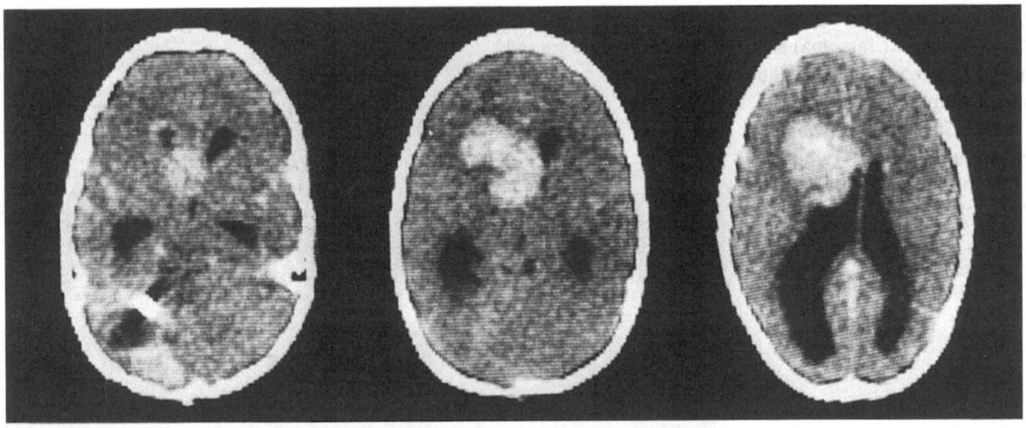

**Fig. D1.202.** Intraventricular metastasis of a previously removed medulloblastoma in a 7-year-old girl. The tumor has almost completely obliterated the left anterior horn and caused hydrocephalus secondary to blockage of the foramina of Monro. There is questionable demonstration of recurrence of the primary tumor in the posterior fossa on the left next to an artifact caused by a metal clip. Postcontrast study

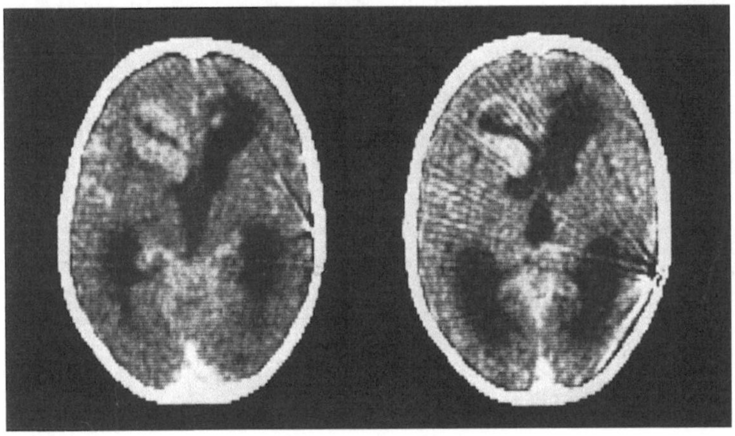

**Fig. D1.203.** Metastatic spread to the meninges and the ventricles following removal of a medulloblastoma in a 10-year-old boy. Strongly positive contrast enhancement in the supracerebellar and ambient cisterns as well as in the walls of the left anterior horn, which is lined with a thick layer of tumor. Spread to the meninges near the left Sylvian fissure. Postcontrast study

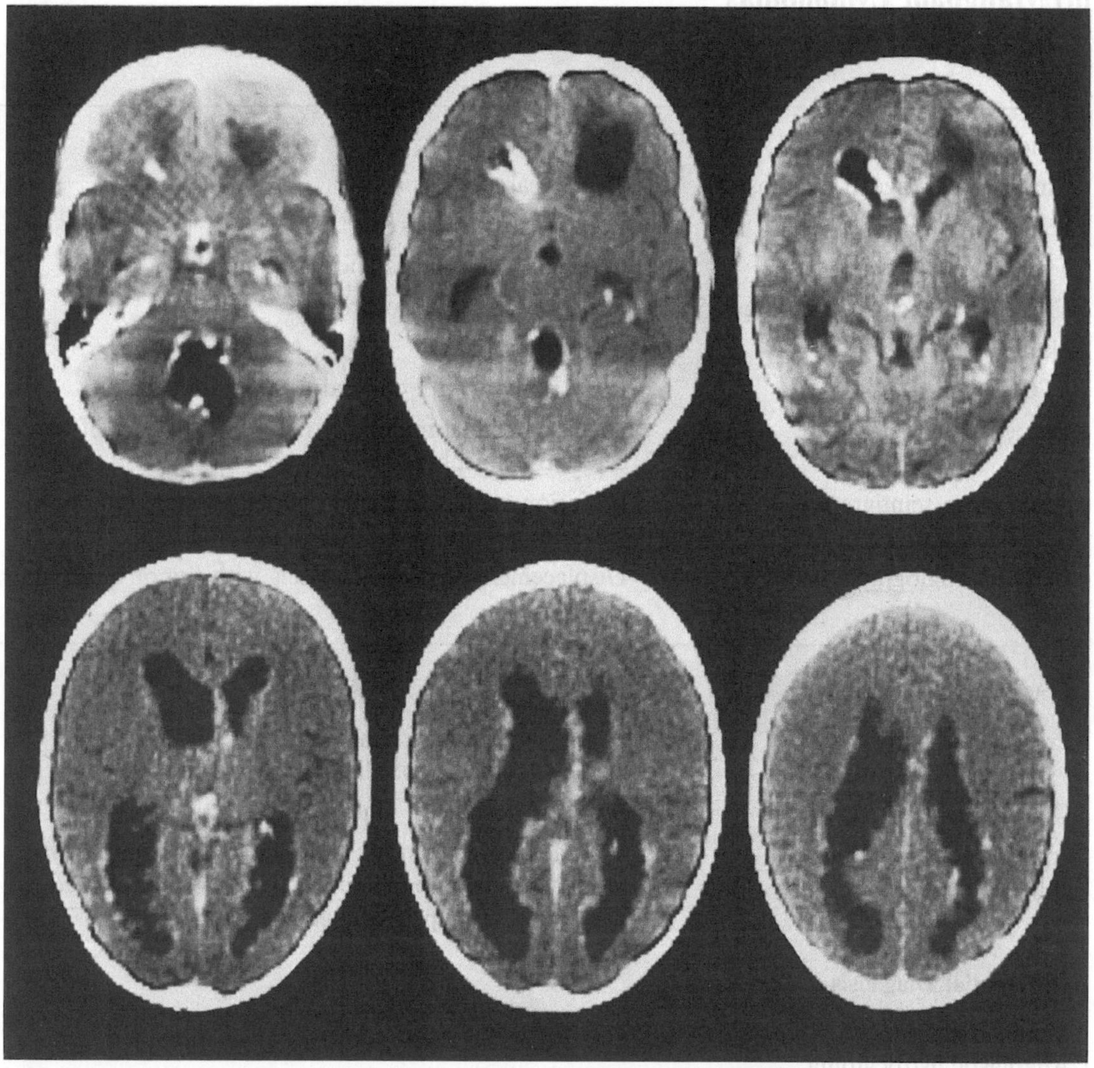

**Fig. D 1.204.** CT studies following removal of a cerebellar medulloblastoma with subsequent irradiation and cytostatic therapy with methotrexate in a 15-year-old boy. Multiple calcifications and knobby structures in the ependyma of the lateral ventricles. Diagnosis of necrotic metastases at the ventricular walls. No histological diagnosis

## m) Malignant Lymphomas

| | |
|---|---|
| Incidence | 0.8–1.5% |
| Characteristic age at diagnosis | 45–65 years |
| Sex distribution | Equal sex distribution |
| Typical locations | Cerebral hemispheres and basal ganglia |
| Characteristic clinical findings | Function of tumor location |
| Skull film | No findings |
| EEG | Focal activity with cortical tumors |
| Echoencephalography | Displacement of midline structures in tumors of the cerebral hemispheres |
| Serial brain scintigraphy | Perfusion similar to that in glioblastomas; radionuclide uptake similar to that in meningiomas |
| Cerebral angiography | Displacement of normal vessels with tumor blush in some cases |
| **Computed Tomography** | |
| Precontrast study | Slightly hyperdense zone common, with isodense zones in some cases; almost always homogeneous |
| Contrast medium uptake | Strongly positive in almost all cases |
| Appearance after contrast enhancement | Well-delineated tumors; differentiation from meningioma may be impossible when tumors are located near the cortex; perifocal edema common |
| **Differential Diagnosis** | |
| Meningioma<br>Anaplastic astrocytoma<br>Metastases<br>Disseminating encephalomyelitis<br>Leukemic infiltrates | |

The term "malignant lymphoma" for certain tumors originating primarily in the brain is relatively new. The group comprises a large number of former diagnoses including *lymphosarcoma, reticulosarcoma, leptomeningeal sarcoma, perivascular sarcoma, perithelial sarcoma, periadventitial sarcoma, diffuse sarcoma, microgliomatosis, diffuse vascular sarcomatosis, and "reticulohistiocytic granulomatous encephalitis."*

These lesions are usually classified as grade III or grade IV tumors.

Reports in the literature place the incidence at 0.8% (Jellinger et al. 1975) and 1.5% (Zimmermann 1975) with a total of 1.2% of all tumors in our collective. Males and females are affected equally, and the disease usually occurs between the ages of 40 and 70 years with peak incidence in the 5th decade.

### Typical Locations

Malignant lymphomas are most often found in the cerebral hemispheres and the basal ganglia, rarely in the brain stem and the cerebellum. Multiple tumors are not uncommon (Figs. D1.216, 219).

**Characteristic Clinical Findings – Additional Diagnostic Procedures**

Presenting signs are a function of location, and the history is usually rather short, ranging from a few weeks to several months. Plain skull films, EEG, and electroencephalography provide nonspecific findings. Serial cerebral scintigraphy is striking, with a perfusion phase resembling that of glioblastomas and radionuclide uptake similar to that in meningiomas.

Cerebral angiography reveals displacement of vascular structures corresponding to the size of the tumor. Small irregular pathological vessels may be demonstrated in some cases.

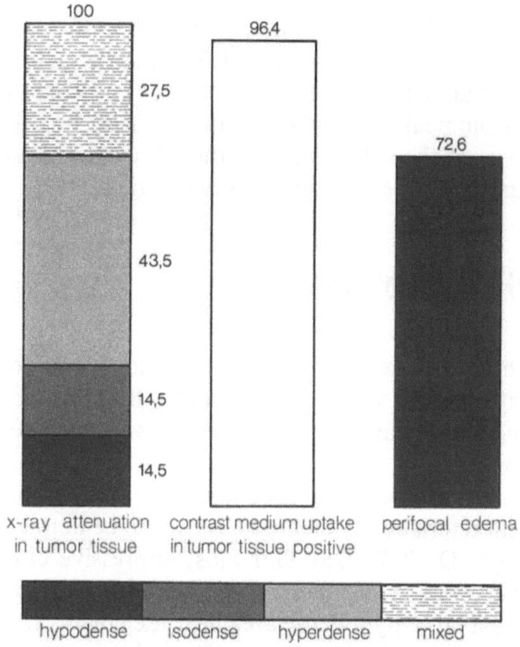


**Fig. D1.205.** X-ray attenuation, contrast uptake, and frequency of perifocal edema in malignant lymphomas and sarcomas (percent)

## Computed Tomography (Figs. D1.205–220)

**Precontrast Study**

Solid tumor nodules have slightly increased density in the plain scan, with mean density values of 38 HU (Figs. D1.206, 212, 214, 216). Diffuse growth produces a hypodense zone as in astrocytomas or brain edema (Fig. D1.218).

**Postcontrast Study**

A homogeneous increase in density averaging 18.6 HU after a standard dose of contrast medium is usually found in solid tumors. This is not the case in diffusely spreading tumors. Maximum density values, somewhat lower than those found in meningioma, are attained shortly after application of the contrast medium, and this is followed by a slow decline in density within 25 min of injection (Kazner et al. 1978).

Solid tumor nodules of malignant lymphomas are visible more clearly after contrast enhancement, and delineation of the tumor in relation to adjacent structures and edema is improved, although still not as distinct as that found in meningioma. Perifocal edema is a common finding (Figs. D1.205, 207–211, 216, 219, 220).

**Differential Diagnosis**

Malignant lymphoma may be confused with *meningioma* when the tumor is located near the convexity (Figs. D1.206–209). However, angiography does not produce the tumor blush typical of meningioma. The indistinct borders observed in many malignant lymphomas were discussed above (Figs. D1.210, 213). Certain differentiation between *anaplastic astrocytoma* and lymphoma in the white matter is not possible in most cases. Differentiation between multiple malignant lymphomas and *intracranial metastases* is impossible with CT alone. The history and other clinical findings aid in diagnosis of *acute disseminating encephalomyelitis* or *leukemic infiltration*. The latter demonstrate hyperdense zones with homogeneous contrast uptake such as that found in meningioma and malignant lymphoma (Figs. D1.221, 222). In other cases the infiltrate may cause prominent edema (Fig. D1.223).

## n) Monstrocellular Sarcomas

These are very rare, highly malignant grade IV tumors without definite histological classification and have been described as xanthomatous glioblastomas or malignant pleomorphic fibrous histiocytomas. They may occur at any age and usually contain cysts.

In the **CT scan** the tumor usually demonstrates a hyperdense zone with a peripheral ring structure after contrast administration (Figs. D1.225, 226). Appearance in the CT scan closely resembles cystic anaplastic or pilocytic astrocytoma, glioblastoma, or abscess. The correct histological diagnosis cannot be made on the basis of the CT scan, even though cystic structures would seem to be characteristic.

The CT appearance of the few *malignant histiocytomas* in our series resembled that in intracranial metastases (Fig. D1.228). Our experience has shown that prediction of the histological diagnosis is not possible from the CT scan.

## o) Histiocytomas

These are extremely rare intracranial tumors with widely varying malignancy. Both benign and malignant histiocytomas have been reported.

Experience with these tumors is limited and characteristic **CT findings** have yet to be defined (Figs. D1.227, 228). Our most impressive case concerned a 48-year-old female with seizures and a large hypodense area near the corpus callosum in the plain CT scan. The lesion accepted contrast medium readily and simulated a meningioma of the falx (Fig. D1.227). The density values of the tumor before and after contrast application did not fit any previously known pattern. At operation a highly vascular soft yellow tumor the size of an apple was found near the corpus callosum, and histological examination provided the diagnosis of benign histiocytoma.

## p) Histiocytosis X

Histiocytosis X rarely involves intracranial structures. It is most often found near the hypothalamus and the chiasma in rare cases of intracranial location. Visual and endocrine disorders are the most prominent clinical findings, and narcolepsy is sometimes observed.

The **CT scan** reveals a slightly hyperdense zone which partially or completely fills the opticochiasmatic cistern (Fig. D1.230). Contrast application results in a homogeneous, slightly blurred but very intense increase in absorption in the tumor tissue, which may resemble malignant lymphoma (Figs. D1.229–231). This makes a diagnosis of pituitary adenoma or suprasellar meningioma quite unlikely, while pilocytic astrocytoma and ectopic pinealoma (germinoma) are possibilities in differential diagnosis. Malignant lymphomas at this location are very rare.

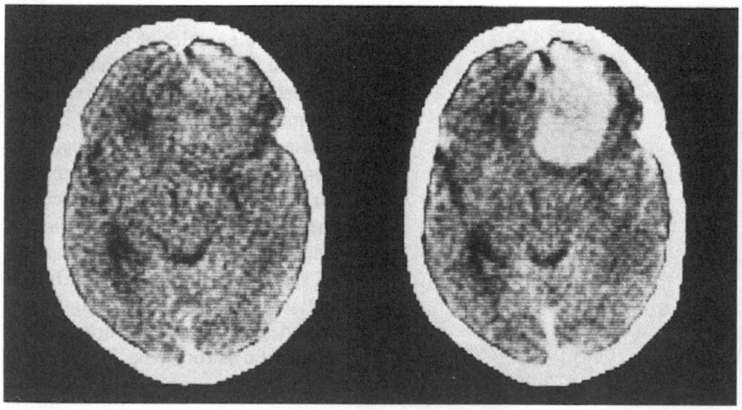

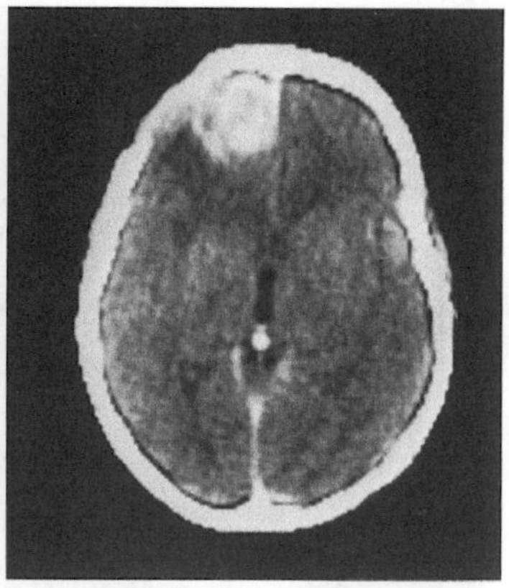

▲

Fig. D1.206. Malignant lymphoma in the right frontal lobe of a 69-year-old female with headache and organic brain syndrome. The precontrast study (left) shows slightly hyperdense values in comparison with adjacent normal brain tissue (18.6 EMI units). Strongly positive contrast enhancement (right). Differentiation between lymphoma and meningioma is not possible with computed tomography alone

▲

Fig. D1.207. Malignant lymphoma in the left frontal lobe in a 63-year-old female with dysphasia and an organic brain syndrome. Recurrence after resection of a primary cerebral lymphoma at the same location. Demonstration of a slightly hyperdense tumor in precontrast studies with strong contrast enhancement and extensive perifocal edema which attains the right frontal lobe. CT findings similar to those in meningioma. Postcontrast study

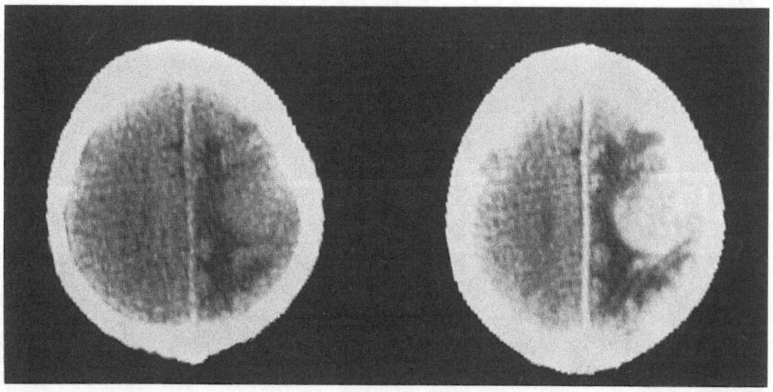

Fig. D1.208. Malignant lymphoma in the right parietal region in a 79-year-old female. Density values similar to those in meningioma. Differentiation between the two requires angiography. Precontrast study (left) and postcontrast study (right)

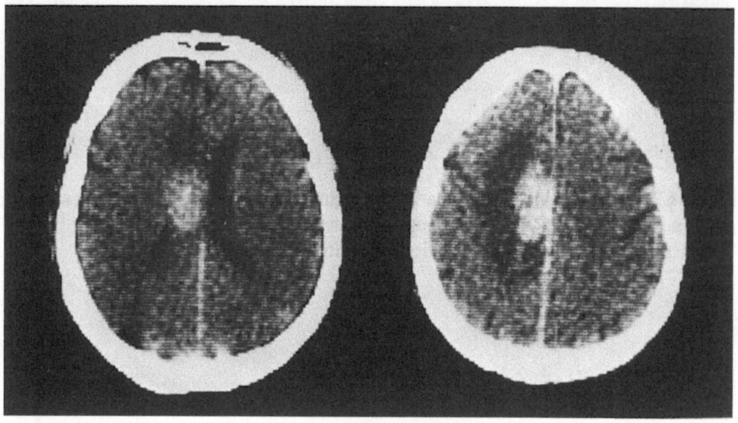

Fig. D1.209. Malignant lymphoma in the left parietal region at the falx cerebri. Location of the tumor suggested a diagnosis of meningioma. The CT scan does not allow further differentiation

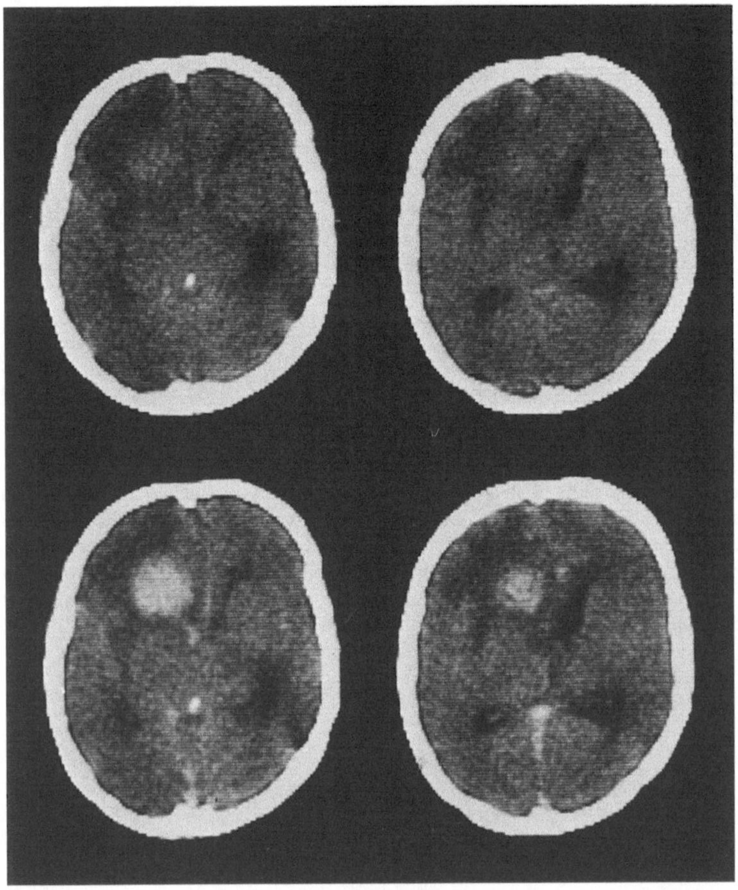

**Fig. D1.210.** Malignant lymphoma in the white matter of the left frontal lobe in a 50-year-old patient with headache and an organic brain syndrome. The tumor is slightly hyperdense and barely visible in the precontrast study (above) but demonstrates positive contrast enhancement (below). Demarcation from adjacent edematous brain tissue not as sharp as in meningiomas. Differential diagnosis of the CT findings includes malignant lymphoma and anaplastic astrocytoma

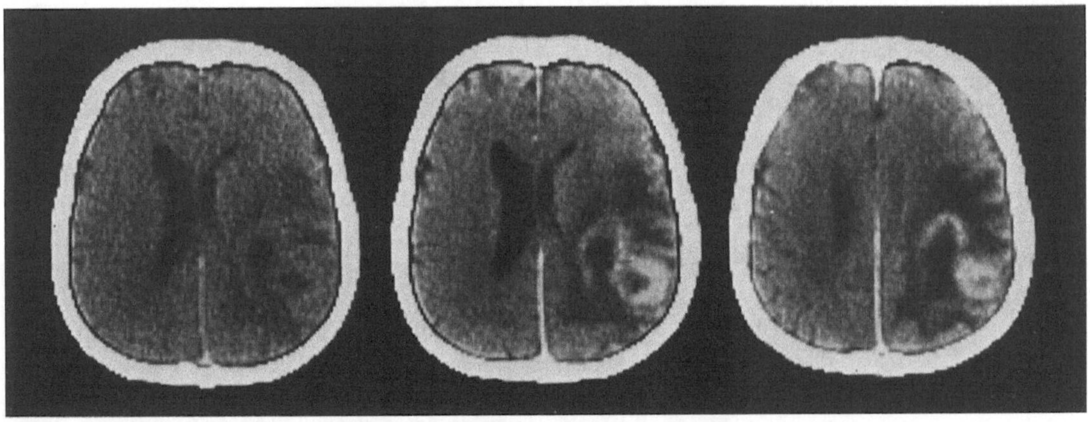

**Fig. D1.211.** Malignant lymphoma in the right parietal region in a 65-year-old male. Unusual appearance with an "open ring" following administration of contrast medium. Precontrast study (left) and postcontrast studies (middle and right)

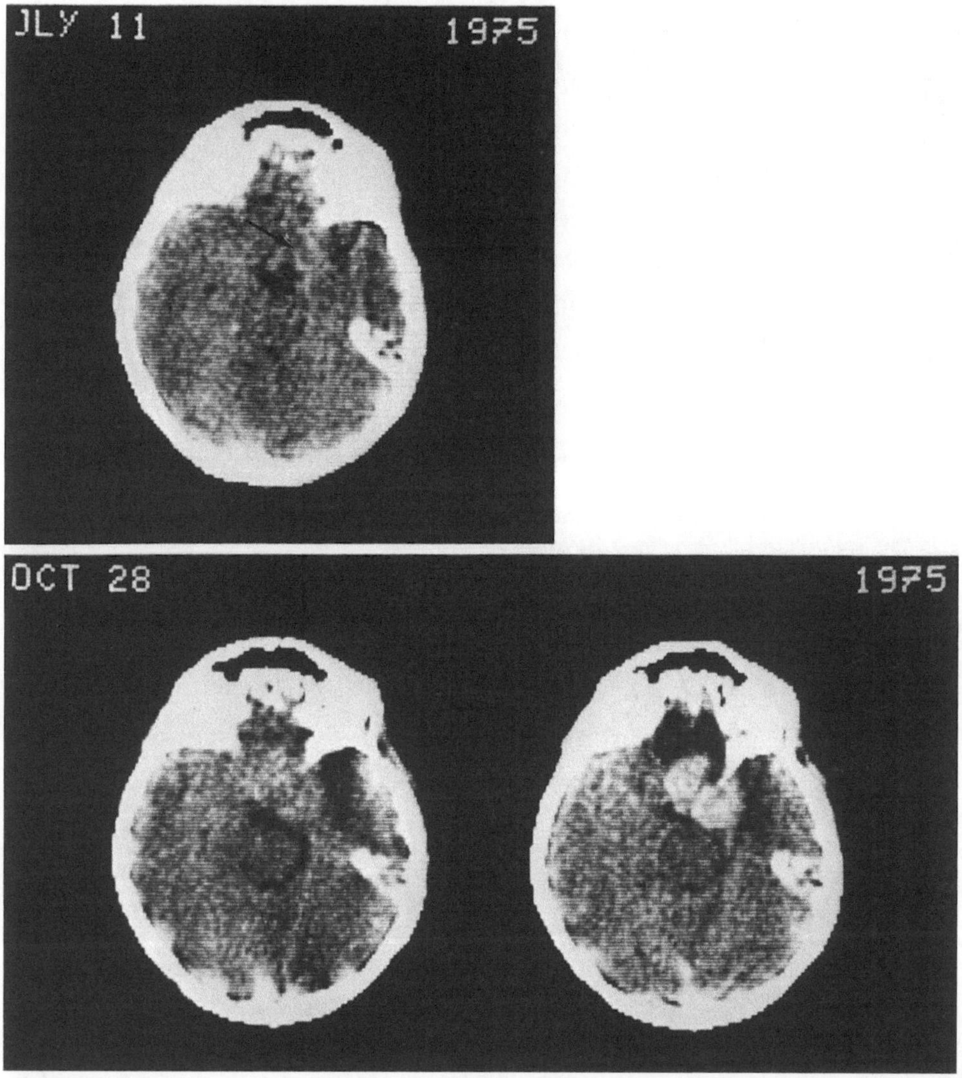


**Fig. D1.212.** Follow-up studies of malignant lymphoma in the suprasellar region. July 11, 1975: 49-year-old patient with paresis of the right third cranial nerve. Small zone with contrast enhancement in the right parasellar region (arrow). Granulation tissue was removed from the vicinity of the third cranial nerve at operation. Histological examination revealed no evidence of tumor. Second CT examination on Oct 28, 1975 after development of right trigeminal neuralgia: large multinodular space-occupying lesion in the suprasellar region with extension to the right. Histological diagnosis of centroblastic lymphoma

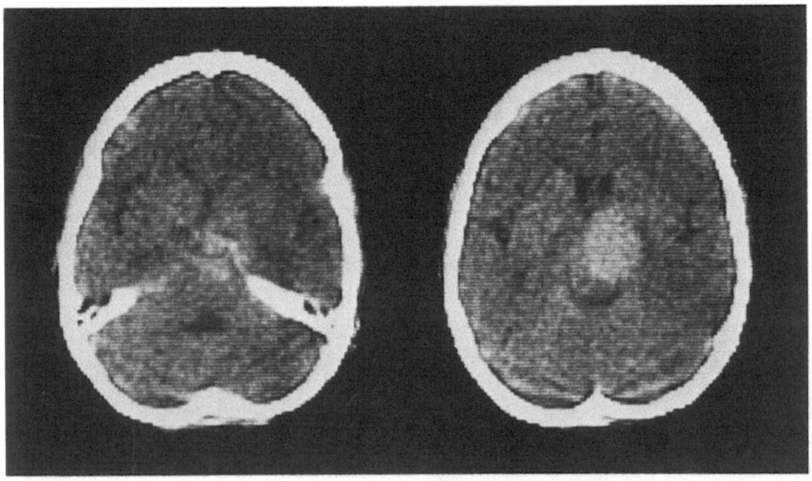

a

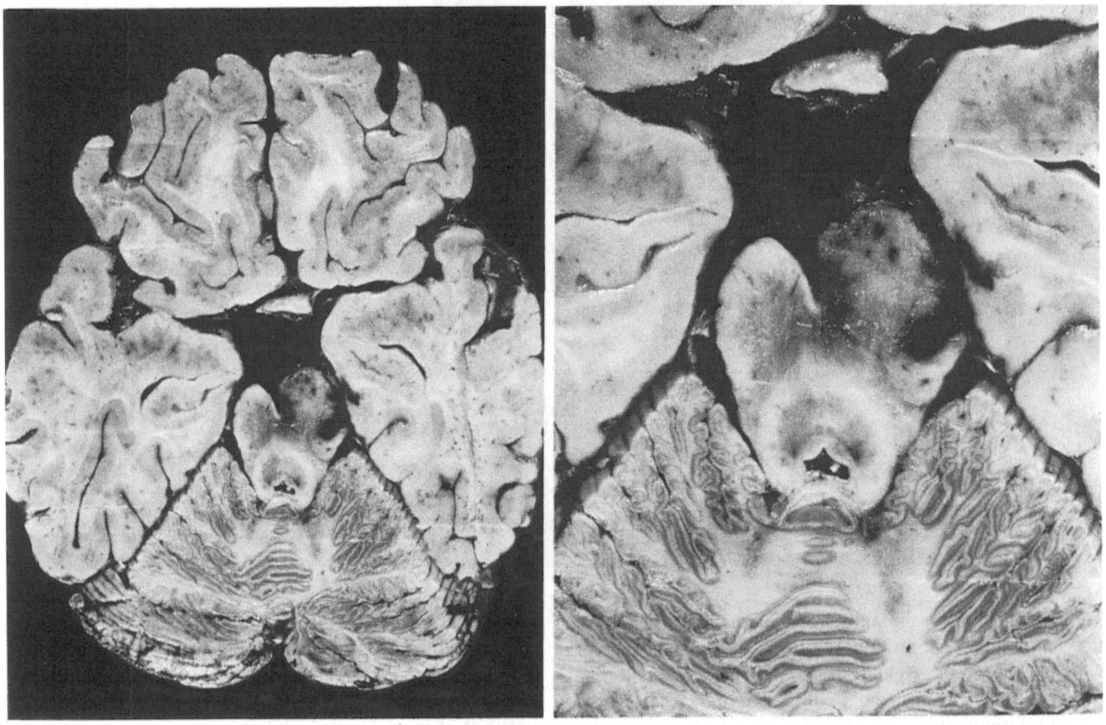

b

**Fig. D1.213** a, b. Malignant lymphoma in the right cerebral peduncle and thalamus in a 41-year-old female with vertigo, diplopia, and third nerve palsy. (**a**) Space-occupying lesion with positive contrast enhancement at the floor of the right middle fossa with extension to the right thalamus and midbrain. CT finding suggests a diagnosis of basal meningioma or malignant lymphoma. Histological examination after biopsy confirmed the diagnosis of malignant lymphoma. Death occurred 4 weeks later. (**b**) Autopsy specimen: distension of the right cerebral peduncle. Microscopic demonstration of tumor in the basal ganglia bilaterally, especially on the right. Diffuse tumor growth

**Fig. D1.214.** Malignant lymphoma in the right cerebellar hemisphere in a 52-year-old man with signs of cerebellar dysfunction on the right. Precontrast studies (above) demonstrate a hyperdense space-occupying lesion in the right cerebellar hemisphere. Strongly positive contrast enhancement (below). Initial diagnosis of meningioma in the posterior fossa. A soft intracerebellar tumor was found at operation. Histological diagnosis of lymphoblastic lymphoma

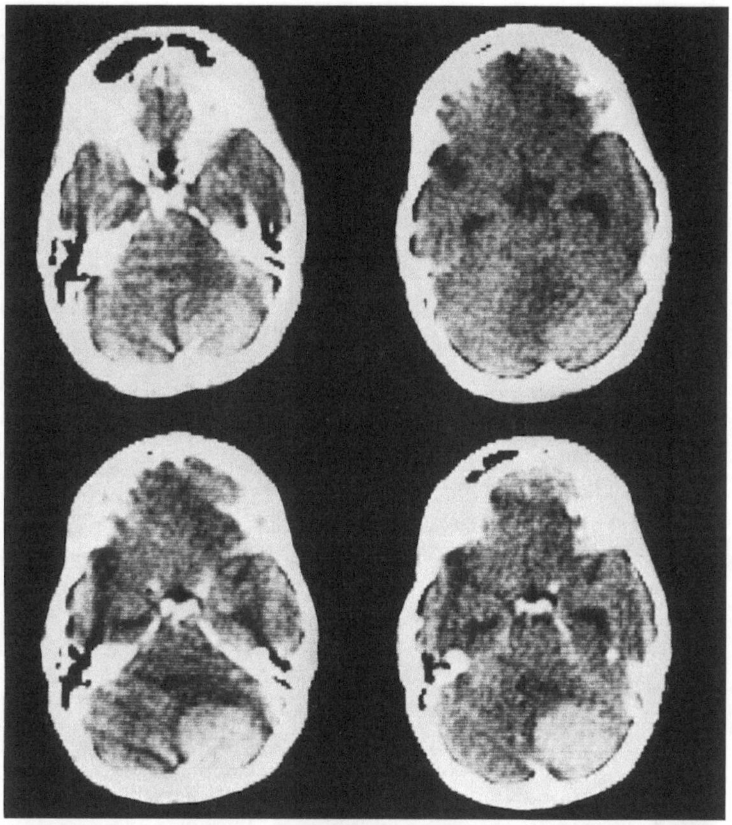

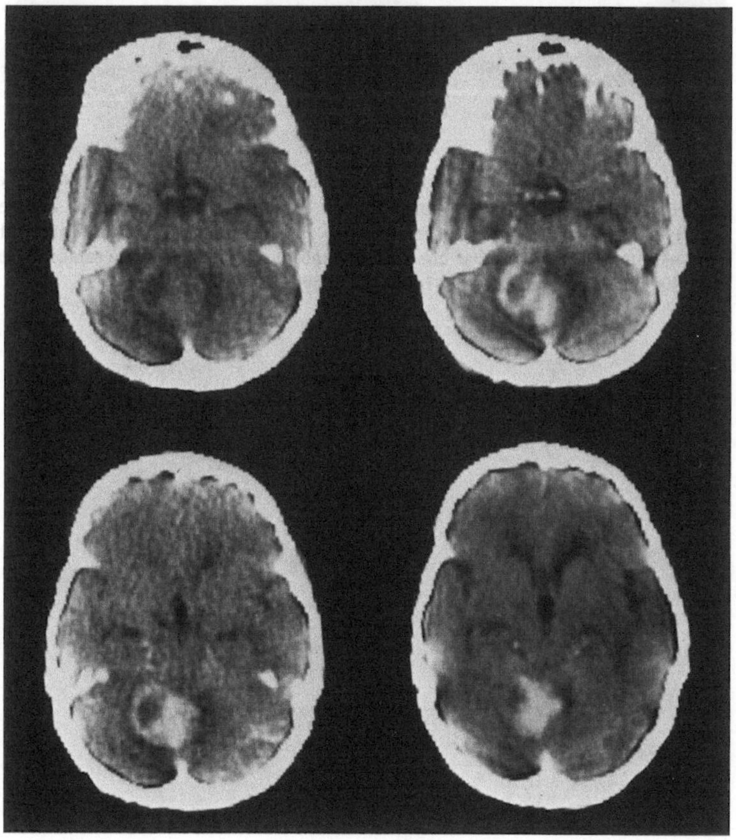

**Fig. D1.215.** Malignant lymphoma (centroblastic-centrocytic lymphoma) in the cerebellar vermis and the left cerebellar hemisphere in a 51-year-old female with signs of cerebellar dysfunction. Precontrast study reveals a tumor with isodense and hypodense portions (above left). Strongly positive contrast enhancement in viable tumor tissue with appearance of an open ring structure

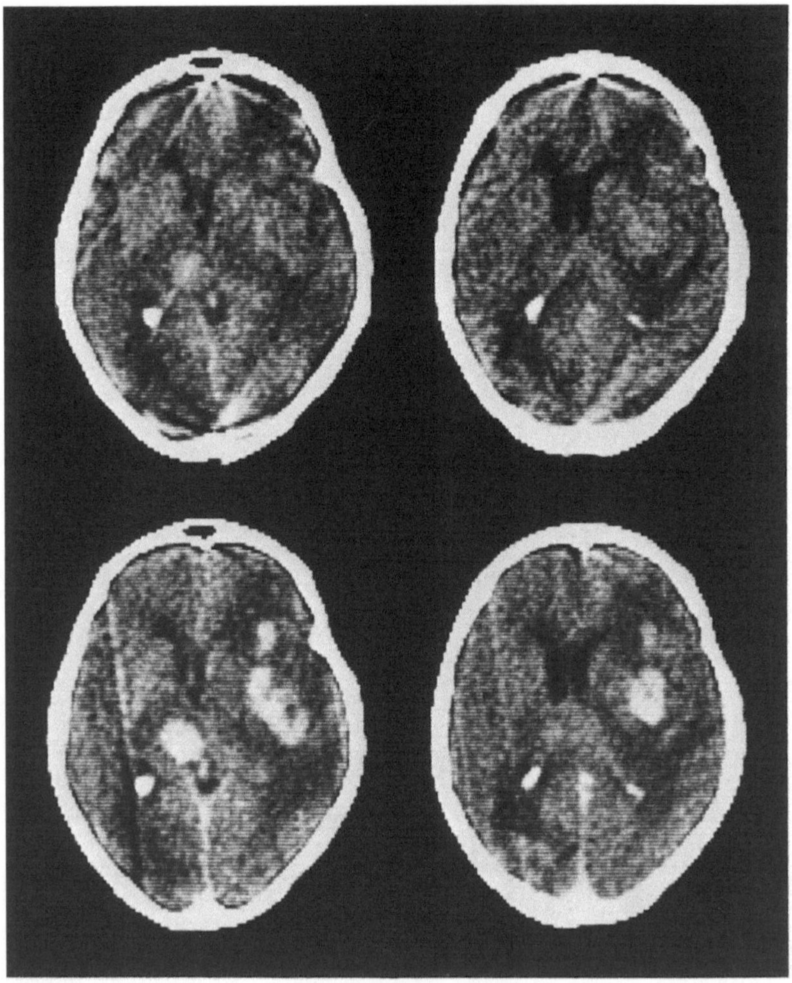

a

**Fig. D1.216** a–c. Multiple malignant lymphomas in a 63-year-old female. (**a**) The lesions appear isodense or slightly hyperdense in the precontrast study (above) and demonstrate strongly positive contrast enhancement (below). Extensive perifocal edema. Initial CT diagnosis: multiple metastases of an unknown primary tumor. (**b**) The multiple tumor nodules are barely visible in the brain section corresponding to the CT scan. (**c**) Enlargement of (**b**) showing the tumor nodules more clearly

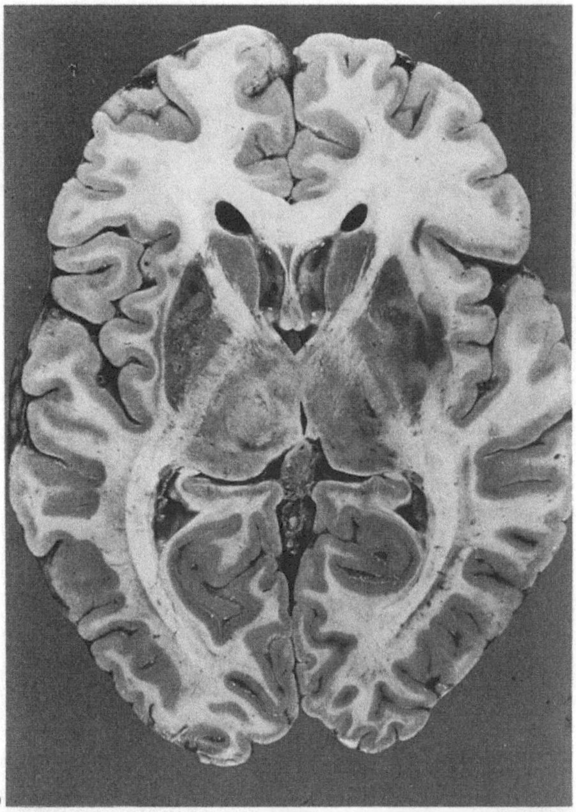

b

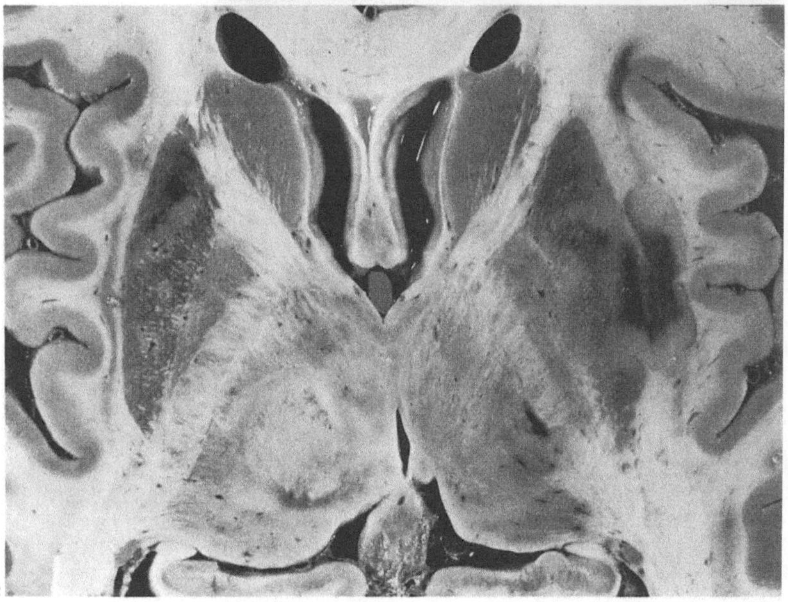

c

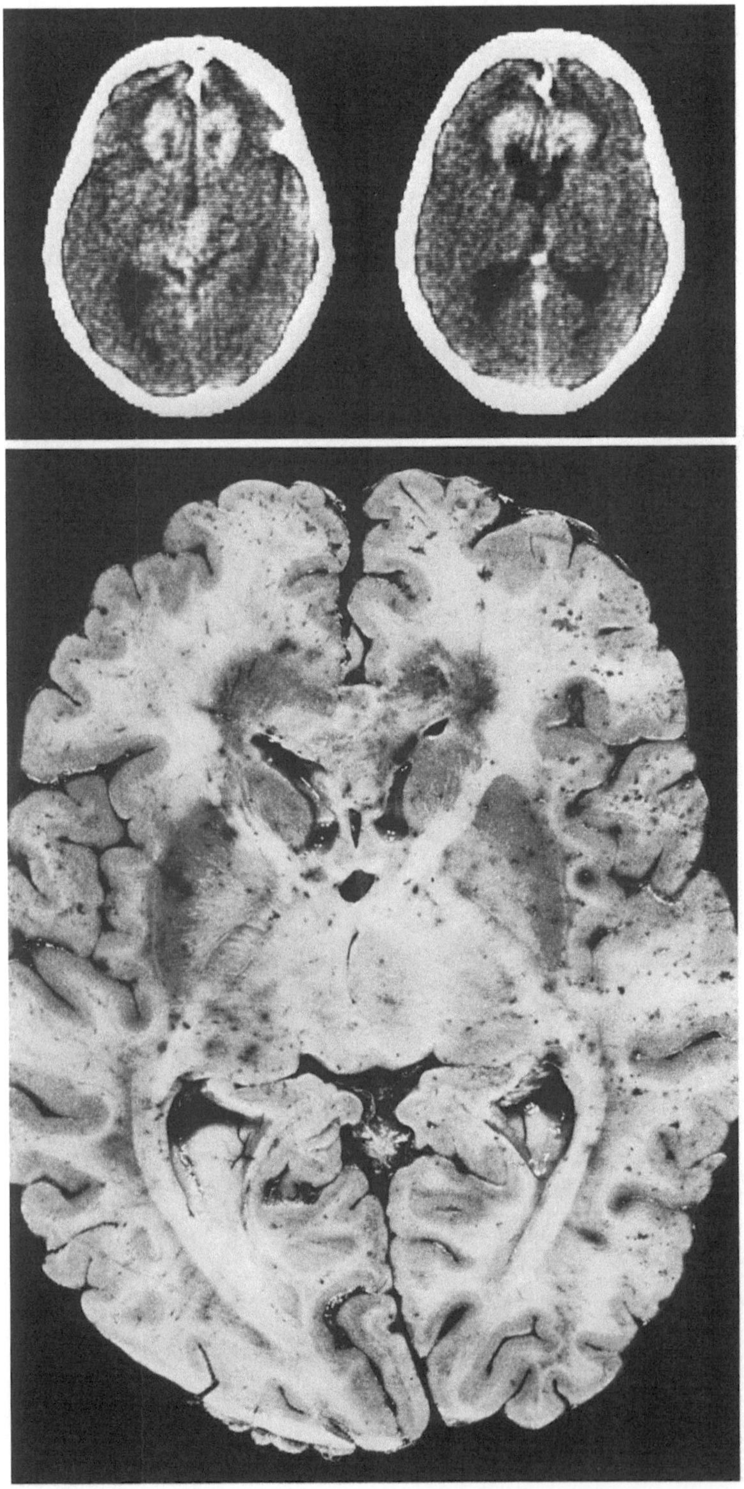

a

b

**Fig. D1.217** a, b. Malignant lymphoma in a 59-year-old female with headache, progredient left hemiparesis, and an organic brain syndrome. (**a**) Demonstration of multiple tumors bilaterally in the basal ganglia and the quadrigeminal region as well as periventricular growth of the tumor. Initial diagnosis of butterfly glioma or malignant lymphoma. Death occurred 4 weeks after CT examination. (**b**) Brain section demonstrating growth pattern of the tumor corresponding to the CT slices. Histological diagnosis: lymphoplasmacytoid lymphoma

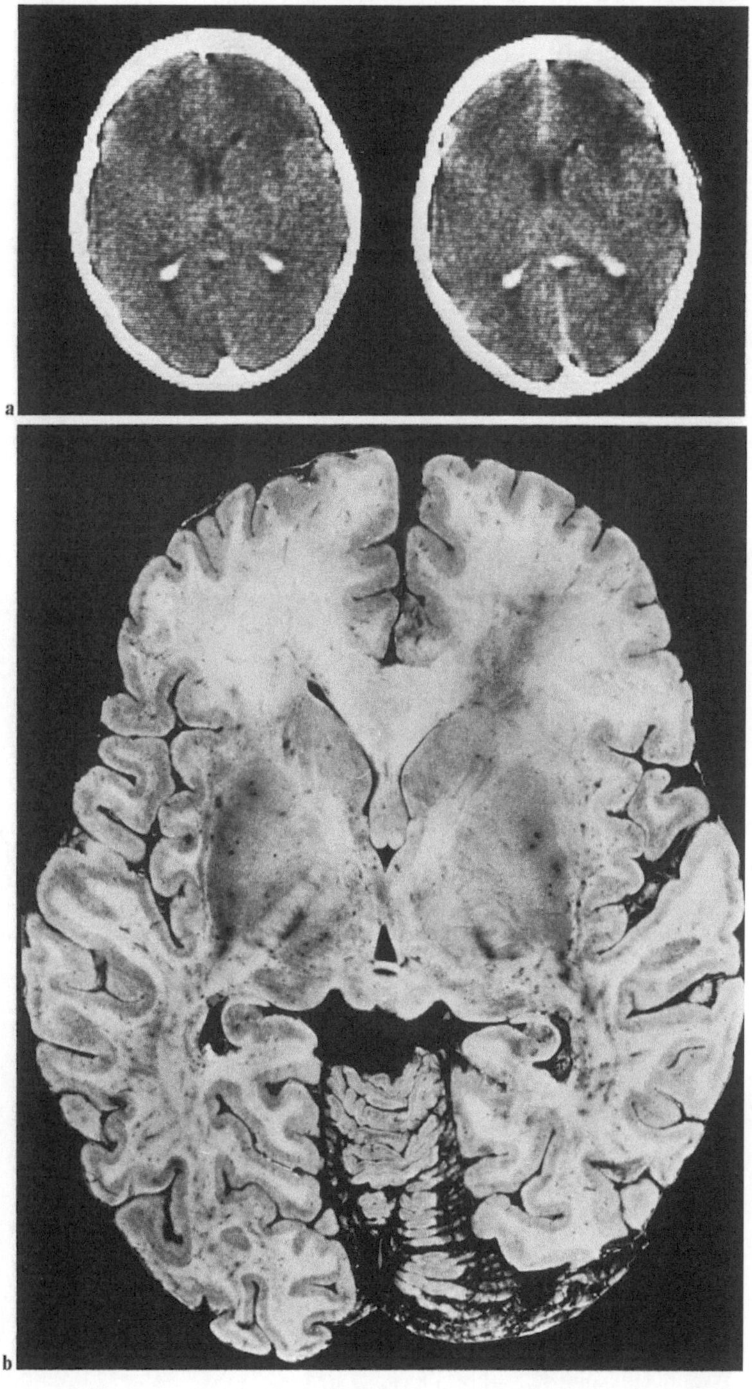

**Fig. D 1.218** a, b. Diffusely growing malignant lymphoma in a 55-year-old male with acute loss of consciousness which lasted until death. (**a**) CT studies reveal low density in both frontal lobes; no contrast medium uptake visible. (**b**) At autopsy a diffusely growing tumor with distension of the anterior corpus callosum and diffuse increase in the volume of both frontal lobes was found. (Brain section courtesy of Priv.-Doz. Dr. GISELA EBHARDT, Neuropathological Institute, Free University of Berlin)

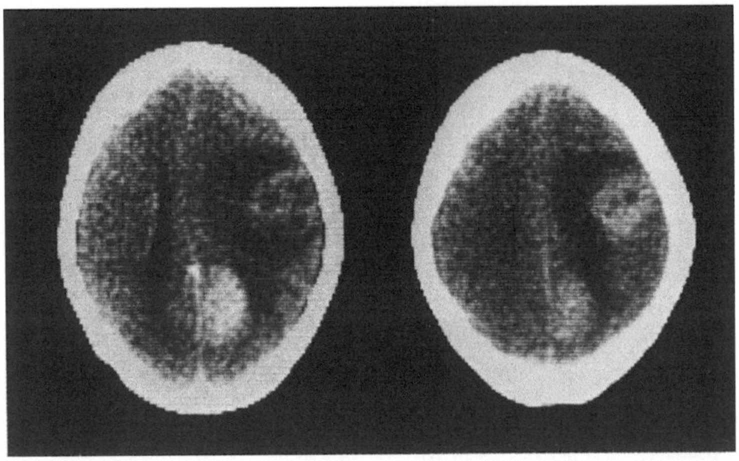

**Fig. D1.219.** Multifocal malignant lymphoma (lymphoblastic type) in a 39-year-old female with progredient weakness in the left hand for 3 months. The tumors, though different in appearance, are both slightly hyperdense in the precontrast study and demonstrate positive contrast enhancement. Preliminary diagnosis of multifocal glioblastoma or multiple metastases. Postcontrast study

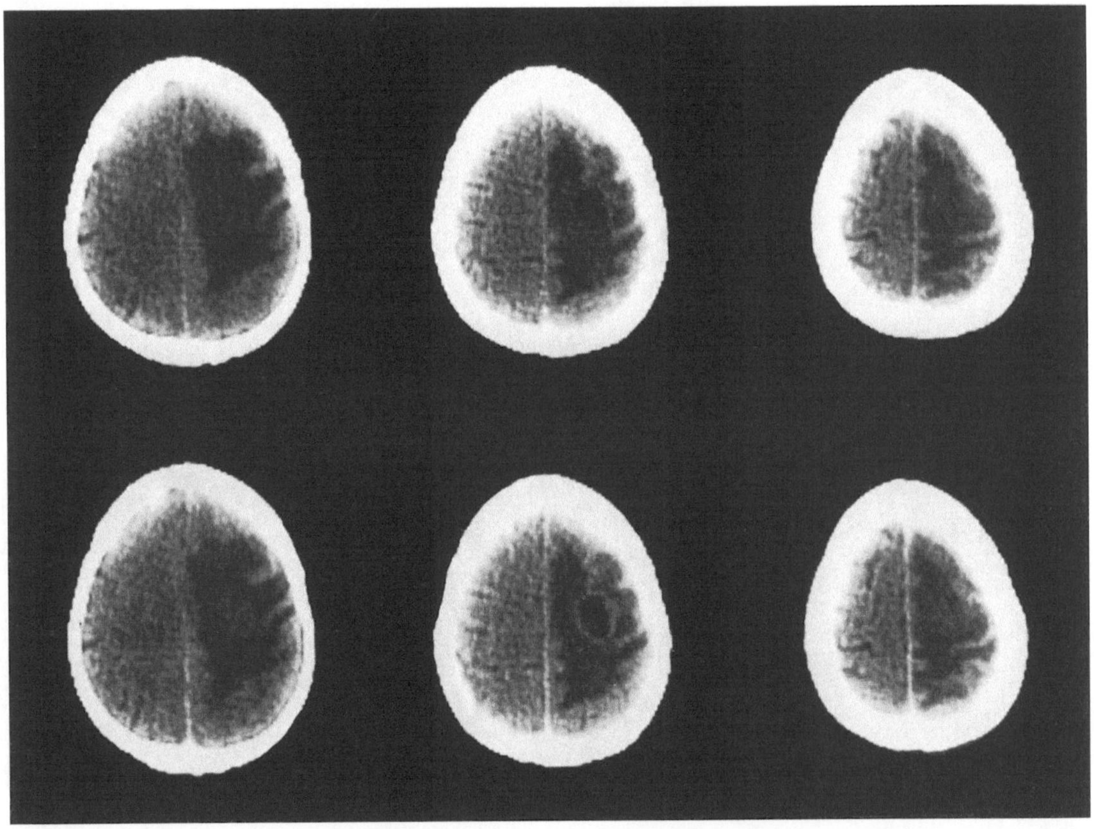

**Fig. D1.220.** Metastasis of a malignant lymphoma in the right parietal lobe of a 51-year-old female who had undergone resection of a malignant inguinal lymphoma 9 years previously. The precontrast study shows an extensive hypodense region (above) while the postcontrast study demonstrates a delicate ring figure that suggested an initial diagnosis of malignant glioma. Histological examination of the tumor led to a diagnosis of malignant lymphoma

**Fig. D 1.221.** Leukemic infiltrate in the right cerebellar hemisphere with bone destruction in a 15-year-old girl undergoing chemotherapy of acute lymphoblastic leukemia. The precontrast study demonstrates a hyperdense zone and perifocal edema in the cerebellum as well as obstructive hydrocephalus (above). The postcontrast study demonstrates a further increase in density (below)

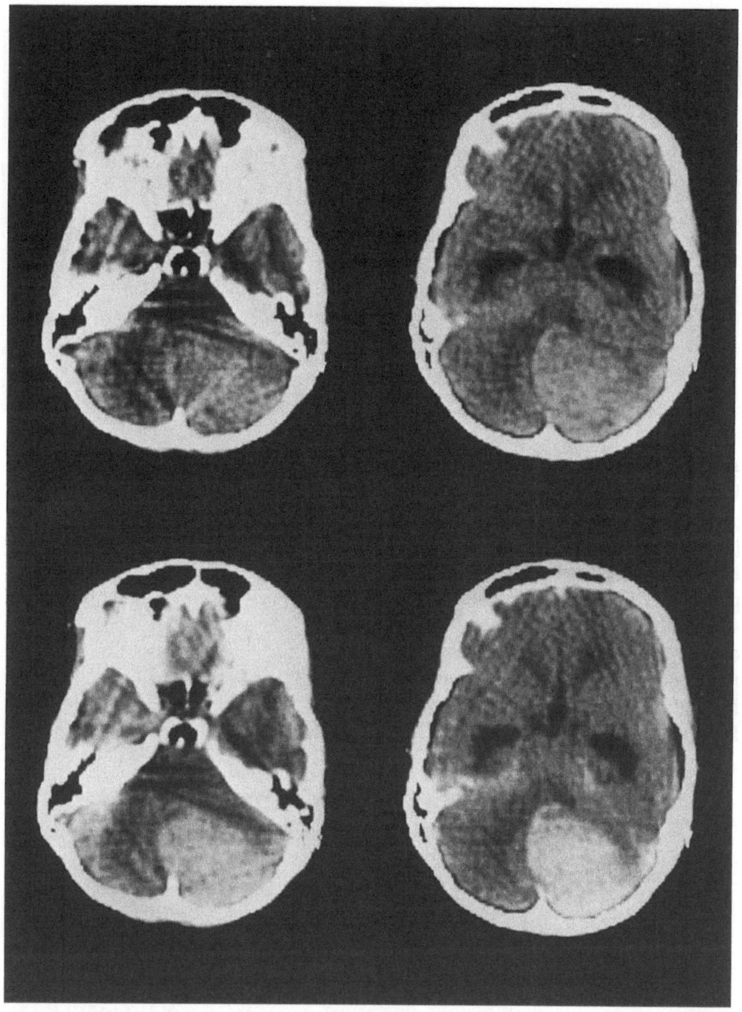

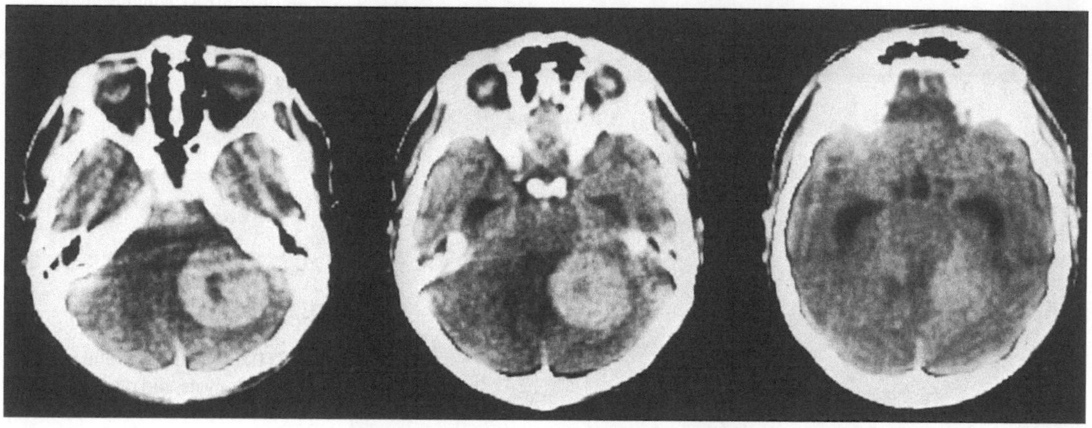

**Fig. D 1.222.** Leukemic infiltrate in the right cerebellar hemisphere with extension to the cerebellopontine angle and the right ambient cistern in a 22-year-old male undergoing chemotherapy of acute myeloblastic leukemia. The caudal slices demonstrate a sharply delineated lesion with central necrosis while high cerebellar slices show indistinct borders due to infiltration of the meninges by tumor. (Slightly hyperdense tumor in precontrast studies; all figures are postcontrast studies)

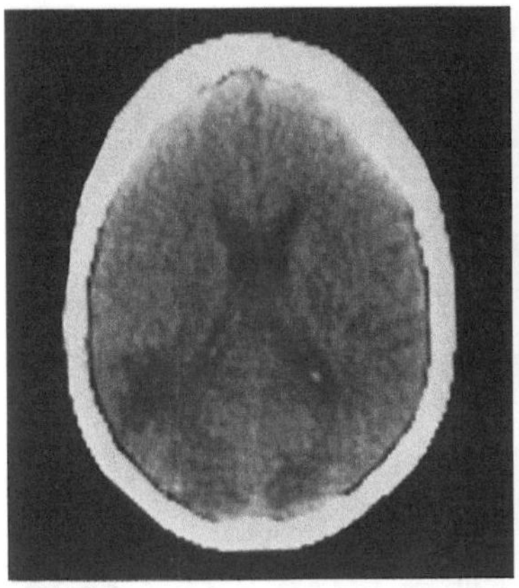

▲
**Fig. D1.223.** Hodgkin lymphoma (lymphogranulomatosis) in the left occipital lobe in a 53-year-old female with generalized lymphogranulomatosis. The lymphoma itself is slightly hyperdense and surrounded by perifocal edema. A low-density zone in the white matter of the right occipital lobe may also represent infiltration with lymphogranulomatosis. Precontrast study

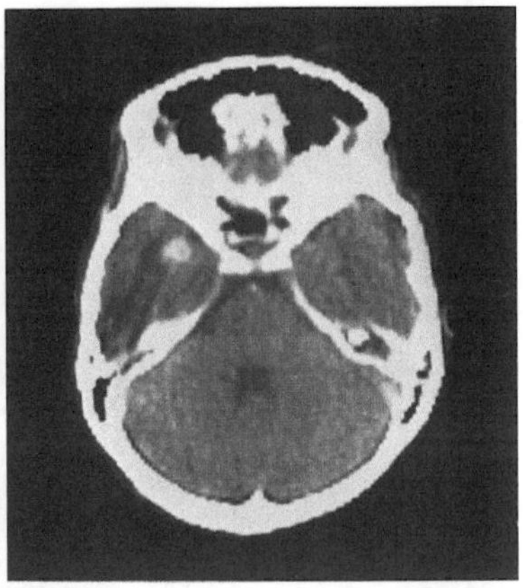

▲
**Fig. D1.224.** Cerebral manifestation of multiple myeloma with a lesion in the mediobasal segments of the left temporal lobe. Postcontrast study. Tumor appeared slightly hyperdense in precontrast studies (45-year-old female with plasmocytoma)

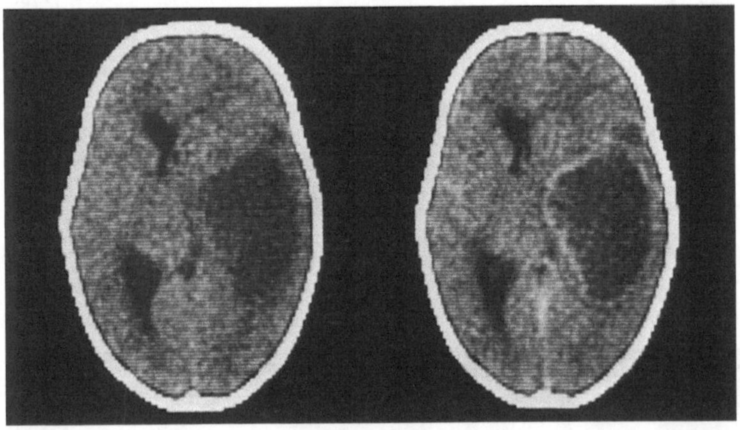

**Fig. D1.225.** Large monstrocellular sarcoma in the right temporal region of a $2^1/_2$-year-old child. The precontrast study shows a large hypodense zone (left). Administration of contrast medium was followed by demonstration of a narrow marginal zone of contrast enhancement (right). Ependymoma or brain abscess were the preliminary diagnoses of the CT scans

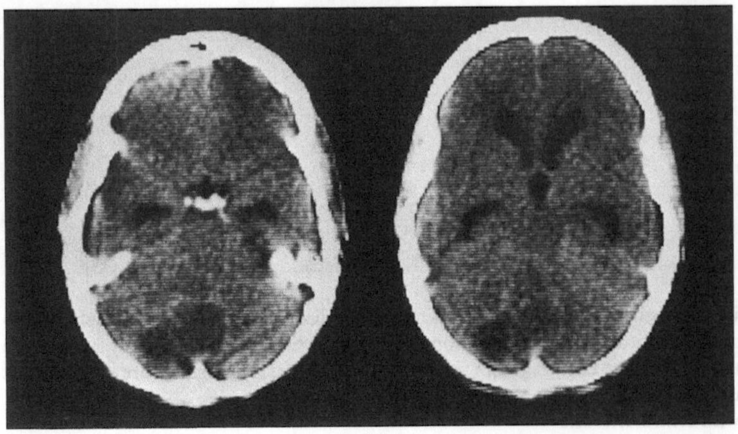

**Fig. D1.226.** Monstrocellular sarcoma with cysts and slight marginal contrast enhancement within the upper segment of the cerebellar vermis and the left cerebellar hemisphere in a 29-year-old male. Density values within the cyst are much higher than those of CSF, which indicates high protein content. Postcontrast study

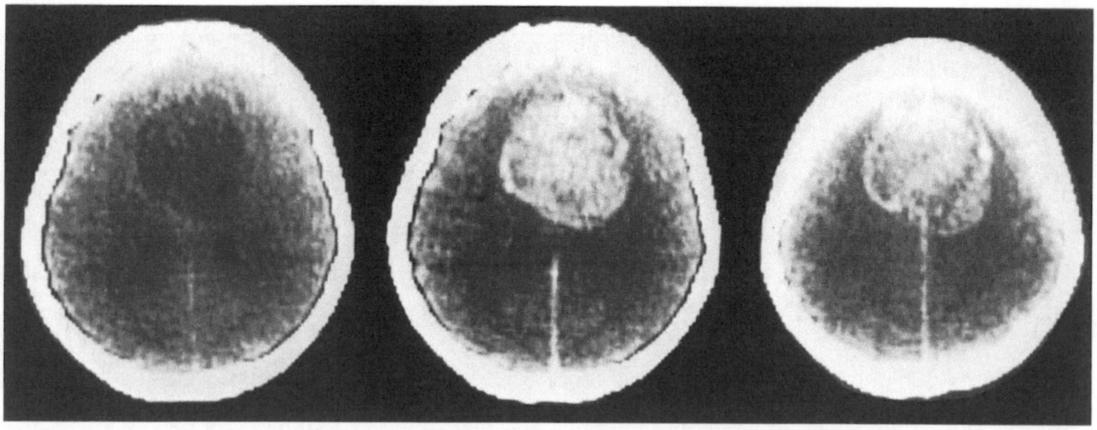

**Fig. D1.227.** Histiocytoma in a 48-year-old female with a short history of seizures. The tumor is clearly hypodense in the precontrast study (left), while the postcontrast scan demonstrates a strong but inhomogeneous increase in density resulting in a picture similar to that found in falx meningioma (middle and right). At operation neoplastic tissue was found on both sides of the falx in the interhemispheric fissure and the callosal cisterns. The tumor was well demarcated, yellow in color, and similar to neurinoma in consistency

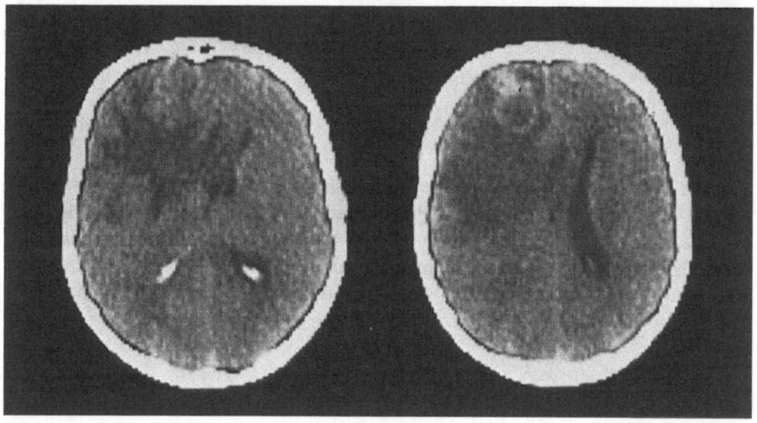

**Fig. D1.228.** Malignant histiocytoma with extensive perifocal edema in the left frontal lobe of a 46-year-old male. The tumor appears as combination of ring and solid tumor nodule. Differentiation from a metastasis is not possible. Precontrast study on the left, postcontrast study on the right

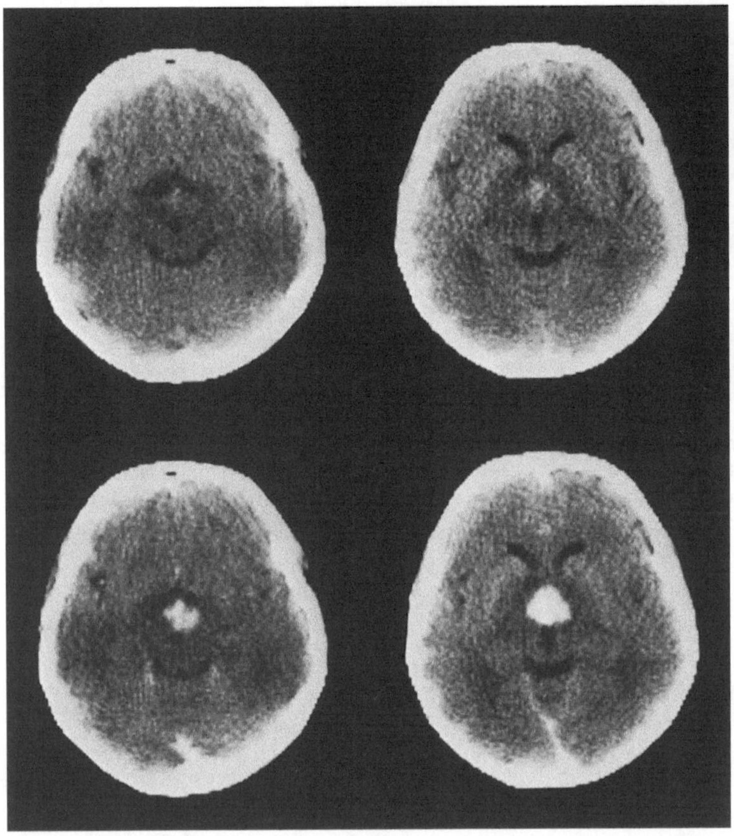

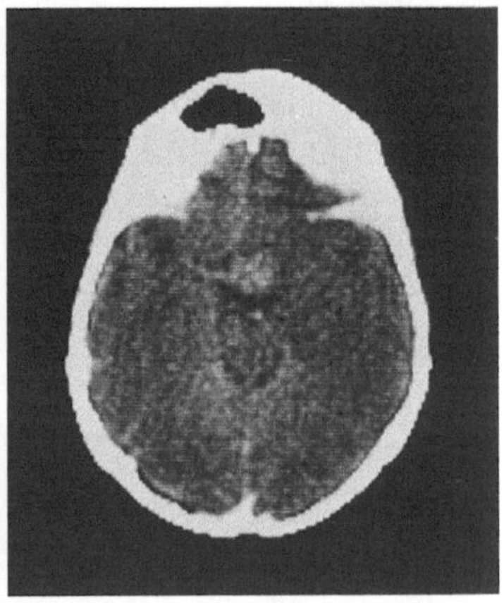

**Fig. D1.229.** Histiocytosis X in the region of the chiasma and the hypothalamus in a 52-year-old male with visual disorders and endocrine abnormalities. Slight contrast enhancement within the tumor, which has filled the chiasmatic cistern and spread to the suprasellar region. Differentiation from a pilocytic astrocytoma at the same location is not possible, though age at diagnosis argues against pilocytic astrocytoma

**Fig. D1.230.** Histiocytosis X at the optic chiasm and the hypothalamus in a 33-year-old female with narcolepsy. Precontrast studies demonstrate a slightly hyperdense tumor with perifocal edema (above). Strongly positive contrast enhancement. The tumor has involved the region of the chiasma and the hypothalamus. Enormous distension of the optic chiasma was found at operation. Biopsy led to a diagnosis of histiocytosis X

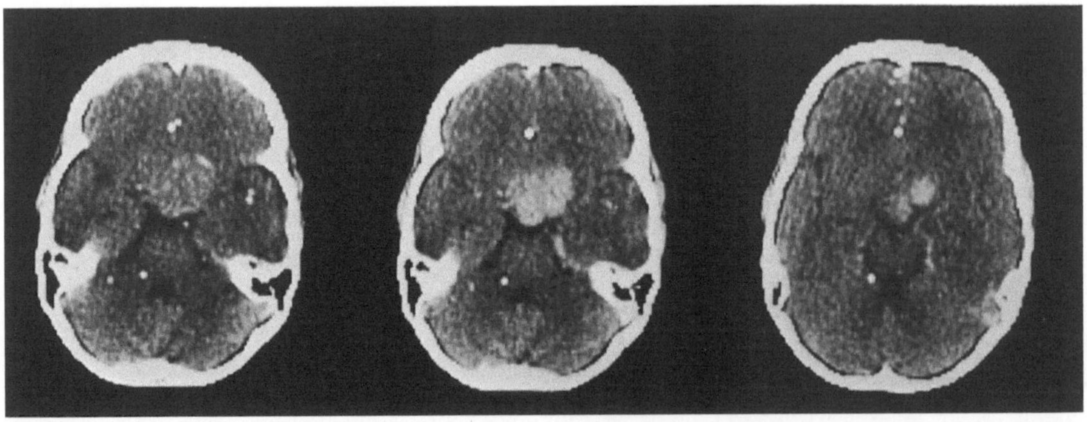

**Fig. D1.231.** Histiocytosis X in the optic chiasma and the hypothalamus in a 14-year-old girl. The precontrast study shows a clearly hyperdense lesion which fills the entire chiasmatic cistern and has spread far into the suprasellar region (left). The postcontrast study reveals positive contrast enhancement and demonstrates two separate tumor nodules. Initial diagnosis of pituitary adenoma. The small white flecks represent drops of contrast medium following myelography

## q) Plexus Papillomas

| | |
|---|---|
| Incidence | 0.3–0.6% |
| Characteristic age at diagnosis | Children and adolescents; adults in middle age |
| Sex distribution | Equal sex distribution |
| Typical locations | Fourth ventricle and lateral ventricles (in the region of the trigonum), rarely third ventricle |
| Characteristic clinical findings | Signs of increased intracranial pressure |
| Skull film | Secondary signs of increased pressure; calcification of the tumor in some cases |
| EEG | Uncharacteristic |
| Echoencephalography | Ventricular dilatation |
| Serial brain scintigraphy | Radionuclide uptake demonstrable only in large tumors |
| Cerebral angiography | Diffuse homogeneous tumor stain |

**Computed Tomography**

| | |
|---|---|
| Precontrast study | In most cases slightly hyperdense, sometimes partly calcified intraventricular lesion |
| Contrast medium uptake | Strongly positive |
| Appearance after contrast administration | Solid intraventricular tumor nodule with knobby surface |

**Differential Diagnosis**

Ventricular meningioma
Subependymal giant cell astrocytoma
Ependymoma
Fourth ventricle: pilocytic astrocytoma and – in very rare cases – solid angioblastoma

This tumor originates in the choroid plexus and is usually benign (grade I) with rare malignant forms (grade III, plexus carcinoma).

Zülch and Cushing both reported finding plexus papilloma in 0.6% of intracranial tumors, while Olivecrona reported 0.3%. The tumor comprised 0.4% of our series with an approximately equal distribution between males and females. Experience has shown that there is a peak in early childhood and another in middle age.

### Typical Locations

Plexus papilloma is found – in decreasing order of frequency – in the fourth ventricle, the lateral ventricle, especially near the trigonum, in the third ventricle, and in the cerebellopontine angle.

### Characteristic Clinical Findings

Signs of increased intracranial pressure caused by obstruction of CSF circulation as well as by increased production of CSF by the tumor are characteristic. Hydrocephalic deformation of the skull results when the tumor occurs in infants.

### Additional Diagnostic Procedures

Plain skull films, EEG, and echoencephalography generally produce nonspecific findings. Radionuclide accumulation may be found in large tumors.

Angiography often reveals a diffuse homogeneous tumor blush.

## Computed Tomography (Figs. D1.232–237)

### Precontrast Study

Plexus papilloma appears as an isodense or slightly hyperdense lesion which is entirely surrounded by CSF when the tumor lies in the ventricle (Figs. D1.232, 235). Varying degrees of calcification may be observed (Figs. D1.232, 234), but cysts are very rare (Fig. D1.237a). When the tumor is located in the trigonum, it may be accompanied by significantly reduced density in the adjacent brain tissue, a result of both edema and penetration of CSF into the brain tissue (Figs. D1.236, 237a). Dilatation of the temporal horn may also be observed in such cases (Fig. D1.236, 237b).

### Postcontrast Study

The tumor is highly vascular and accepts contrast media readily, with an increase in absorption comparable to that found in meningioma. Contrast enhancement is usually homogeneous (Figs. D1.233, 235–237).

The strong increase in density results in even better delineation of the tumor against the surrounding CSF and brain tissue. A knobby surface is often demonstrated (Figs. D1.232, 233, 235, 236).

### Differential Diagnosis

*Meningiomas of the lateral ventricles* usually have a smoother surface than does plexus papilloma. All patients with meningioma in our series were older than 25 years of age, while all cases of plexus papilloma of the lateral ventricles involved children and adolescents with one exception.

*Subependymal giant cell astrocytoma* usually originates near the foramen of Monro at the head of the caudate nucleus and is therefore easily differentiated from plexus papilloma, which has never been found at this location. The same considerations apply to *ependymomas* of the lateral ventricle, which usually occur near the foramen of Monro.

Pilocytic astrocytomas (Fig. D1.115) and ependymomas (Figs. D1.147, 148) may also be found surrounded by CSF in the fourth ventricle, but the surface of these tumors is usually smoother than that of plexus papilloma, with the exception of ependymomas on the floor of the fourth ventricle. Location and form of plexus papilloma in the cerebellopontine angle are so characteristic that hardly another lesion deserves consideration as a possible alternative diagnosis (Fig. D1.234).

Angioblastoma may occur within the fourth ventricle in rare cases, and the appearance in CT scans may resemble that found in plexus papilloma.

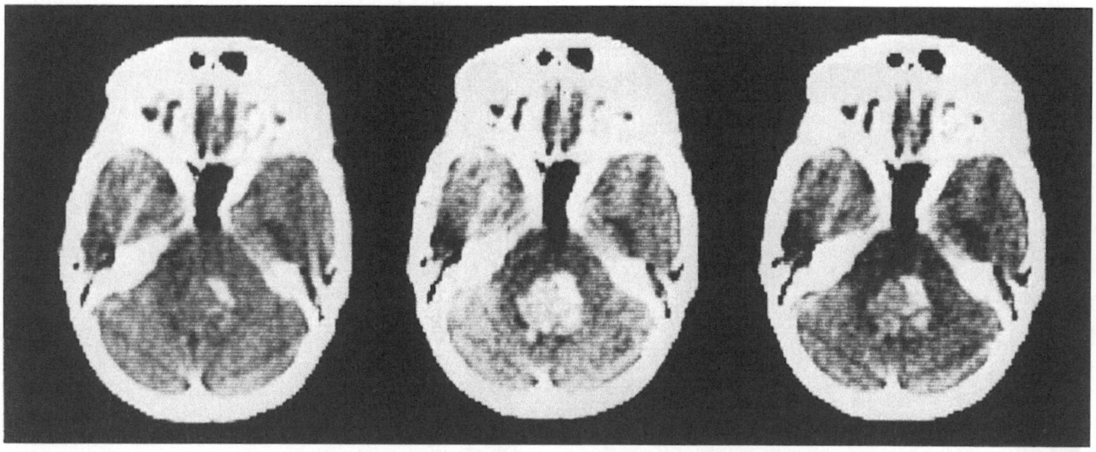

**Fig. D1.232.** Plexus papilloma in the fourth ventricle of a 53-year-old female with signs of increased intracranial pressure. The precontrast study reveals an isodense tumor with marginal calcification (left). The lesion is surrounded on all sides by CSF. The postcontrast study shows strongly positive contrast enhancement (middle) with a rapid decrease of density values within 20 min (right). The knobby surface of the tumor suggested a diagnosis of plexus papilloma

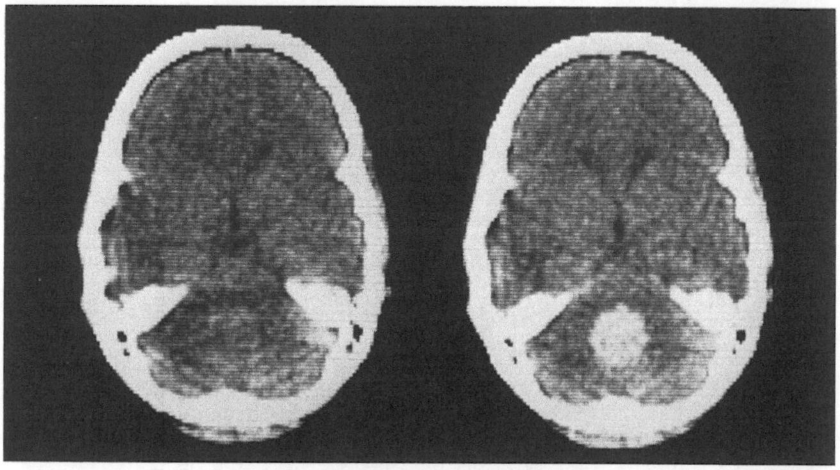

**Fig. D1.233.** Plexus papilloma in the fourth ventricle of a 37-year-old female. The tumor is barely visible in the precontrast study (left) but demonstrates strongly positive contrast enhancement (right). Knobby surface

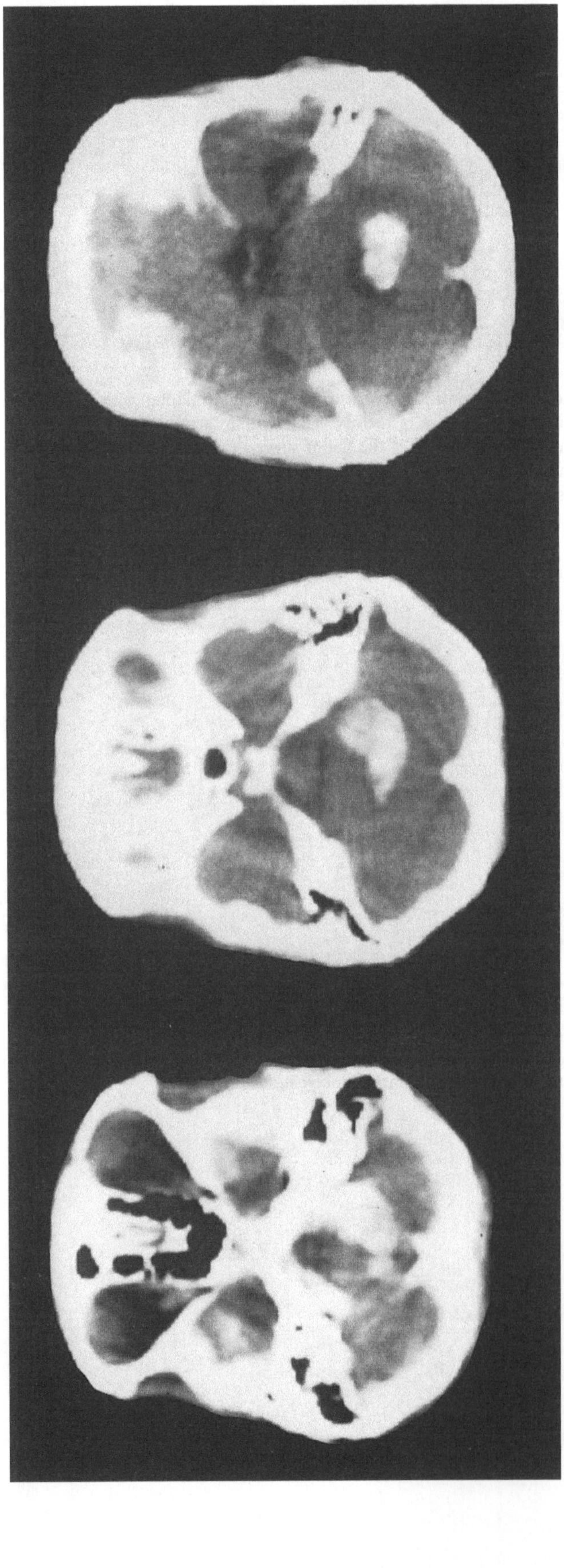

**Fig. D 1.234.** Calcified plexus papilloma extending from the right cerebellopontine angle into the fourth ventricle. The tumor originates in the choroid plexus at the foramen of Luschka (34-year-old female with signs of a lesion in the cerebellopontine angle)

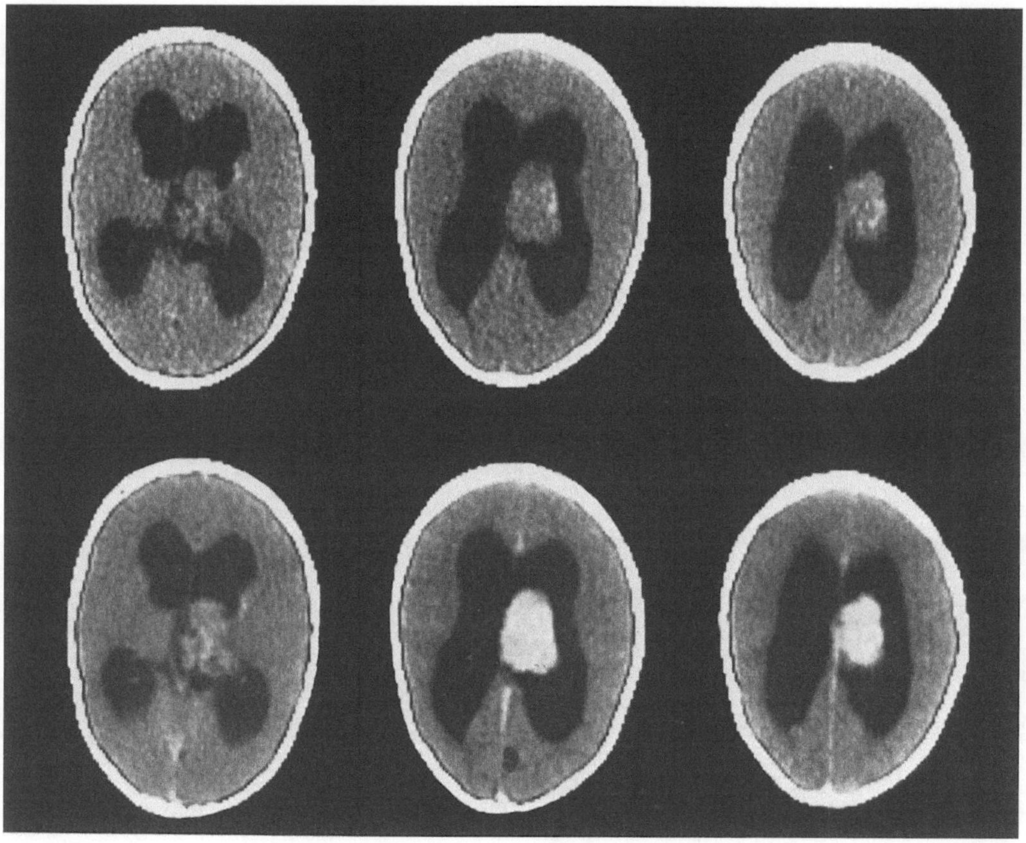

**Fig. D1.235.** Plexus papilloma in the cella-media portion of the right lateral ventricle in a 2-year-old child with hydrocephalus. The precontrast study (above) demonstrates a predominantly isodense tumor with fine speckled calcification. Postcontrast studies (below) show strongly positive contrast enhancement in the tumor, which is located entirely within the dilated lateral ventricle. The irregular surface of the tumor is most apparent in the postcontrast series

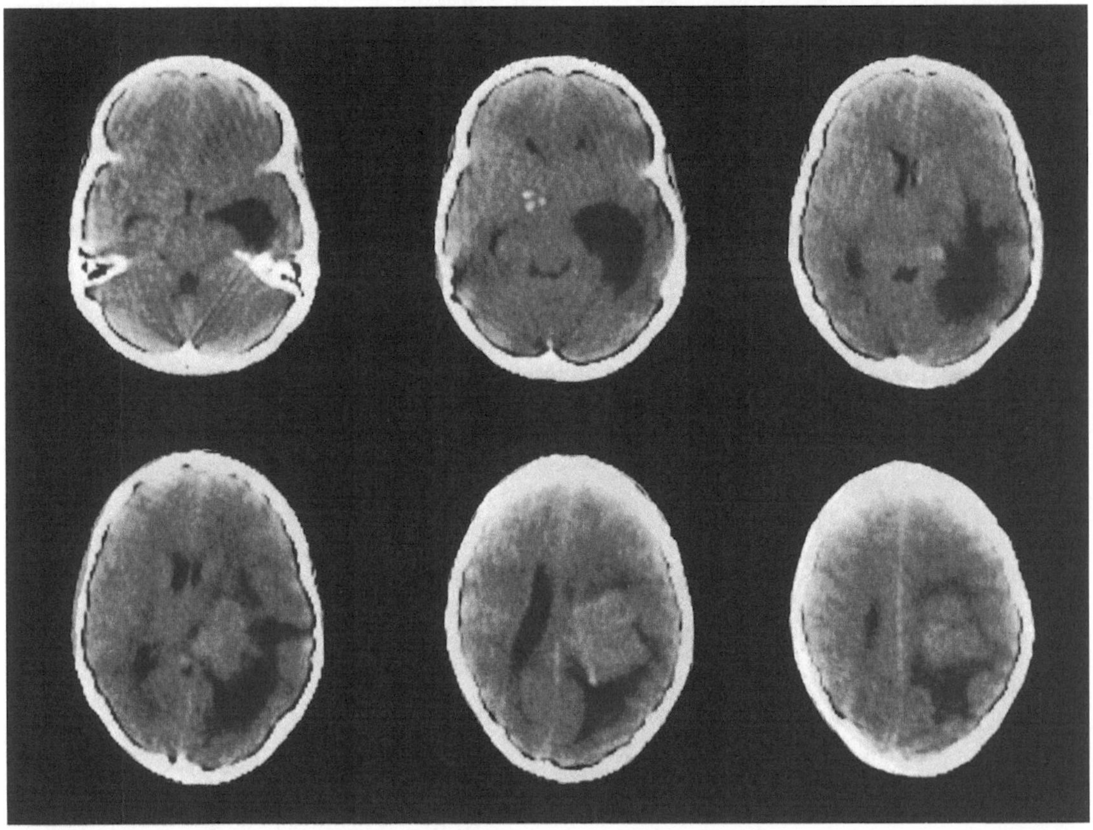

**Fig. D 1.236.** Plexus carcinoma in the trigonum of the right lateral ventricle with dilatation of the right inferior horn and penetration of CSF into surrounding brain tissue (lower series). The tumor is hyperdense and lobulated in the precontrast study. No contrast studies as a result of iodine allergy. Specks of calcification in the left basal ganglia are an incidental finding.

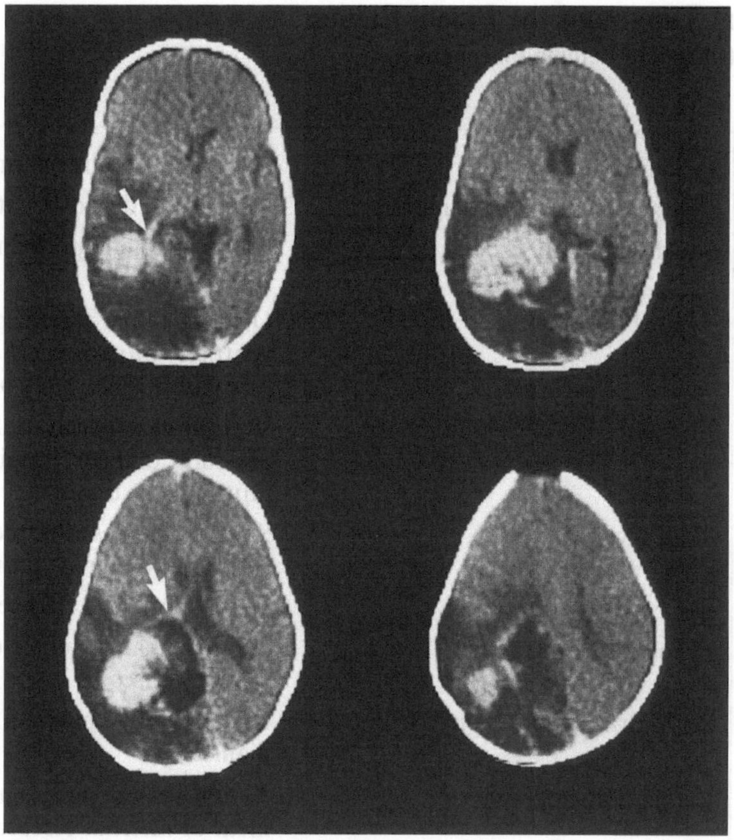

**Fig. D1.237a.** Plexus papilloma in the region of the left trigonum and the posterior horn in a 4-month-old infant with rapid skull enlargement, especially on the left. The anatomical relations between the cystic tumor and the choroid plexus are evident in the CT scans on the left (arrows). Penetration of CSF into brain tissue, simulating perifocal edema

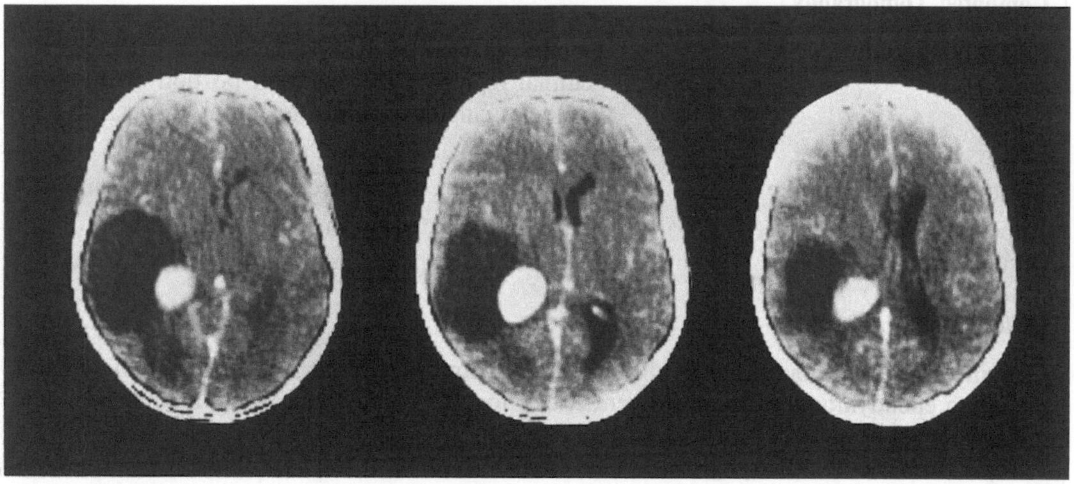

b

**Fig. D1.237b.** Plexus papilloma the size of a walnut in the left trigonum of a 25-year-old female. The tumor has caused obstruction of the left lateral ventricle with enormous dilatation of the left temporal horn, which resembles a cyst. The tumor was hyperdense in the precontrast study and readily accepted contrast media (all figures are postcontrast studies).

## r) Tumors of the Pineal Region
**(Including Ectopic Pinealomas)**

| | |
|---|---|
| Incidence | 0.5% of all brain tumors |
| Characteristic age at diagnosis | Children and adolescents; rarely in adults |
| Sex distribution | Males affected approximately twice as frequently as females |
| Typical locations | Quadrigeminal region, posterior section of the third ventricle; infundibulum and fourth ventricle in very rare cases of *ectopic tumor* |
| Characteristic clinical findings | Vertical gaze paralysis. Signs of increased intracranial pressure; diabetes insipidus and visual disorders in infundibular tumors |
| Skull film | Signs of increased intracranial pressure; separation of sutures in children; pronounced gyric impressions |
| EEG | Uncharacteristic changes |
| Echoencephalography | Hydrocephalus; tumor-echo complex in the midline in many cases |
| Serial brain scintigraphy | Radionuclide uptake in tumors larger than 1.5 cm in diameter |
| Cerebral angiography | Tumor vessels rare; signs of hydrocephalus; displacement of internal cerebral veins |

**Computed Tomography**

| | |
|---|---|
| Precontrast study | Round isodense or hypodense zone in the quadrigeminal region or the posterior portion of the third ventricle; calcification not uncommon; occlusive hyodrocephalus |
| Contrast medium uptake | Positive except in calcified portions of the tumor |
| Appearance after contrast enhancement | Sharply delineated hyperdense solid tumors |

**Differential Diagnosis**

Genuine pineal tumors cannot be differentiated from other tumors occurring in this region, including ependymoma of the third ventricle, pilocytic astrocytoma of the lamina tecti, and metastases
Ectopic forms: craniopharyngioma, pilocytic astrocytoma of the hypothalamus (infundibuloma)
Metastasizing medulloblastoma may result in pictures similar to those in germinoma

Genuine pineal tumors are either grade I–III **pineocytomas** (pinealocytomas) or grade IV **pineoblastomas** (pinealoblastomas), both exceedingly rare.

The **germinoma,** the most common tumor of the pineal region, is a grade II–III germinal cell tumor histologically unrelated to the pineal gland.

Tumors of the pineal region make up 0.5%–0.7% of all intracranial tumors, with clear predominance in males. The tumors are most often found in children and adolescents but may also occur in adults. Typical location is the roof of the midbrain and the pineal body. Other *germinomas, originating in the infundibulum* (Figs. D1.245, 246), were previously designated ectopic pinealomas. Ectopic pineocytomas may occur in the fourth ventricle (Fig. D1.251).

*Pinealomas may metastasize in the CSF pathways,* which results in spinal, meningeal, and ventricular tumors.

A number of other tumors and malformations may be observed in the **pineal region,** including *pilocytic astrocytoma of the roof of the midbrain, ependymoma in the posterior portion of the third ventricle, meningioma at the tentorial hiatus, teratoma, epidermoid and dermoid cyst, lipoma of the lamina tecti, arachnoid cyst of the quadrigeminal cistern, aneurysm of the vein of Galen, and metastasis.*

### Characteristic Clinical Findings

The primary indicators of tumors in the pineal region are signs of increased intracranial pressure resulting from blockage of CSF circulation at the third ventricle and the aqueduct as well as vertical gaze paralysis (Parinaud syndrome).

### Additional Diagnostic Procedures

Plain skull films often reveal secondary signs of increased intracranial pressure with enlargement of the sella. The calcified pineal body may lie in the midline but the calcified figure is considerably enlarged in pinealoma. Echoencephalography shows dilatation of the lateral ventricles and a tumor-echo complex in the midline in many cases. Larger tumors accumulate radionuclides, while the EEG demonstrates nonspecific changes.

Angiography shows displacement of the posterior choroidal vessels as well as elevation and flattening of the internal cerebral vein.

Ventriculography reveals varying degrees of ventricular dilatation as well as a filling defect in the posterior portion of the third ventricle caused by the tumor.

## Computed Tomography (Figs. D1.238–251)

### Precontrast Study

Pineal tumors are highly cellular and appear isodense or slightly hyperdense in the precontrast study. Calcification may occur, and cysts have been observed after radiation therapy (Fig. D1.238).

### Postcontrast Study

All genuine pineal tumors demonstrate intense contrast uptake unless complete calcification is present. This allows exact determination of tumor size and delineation from adjacent structures.

Contrast uptake is usually homogeneous; ring structures are very rare.

Increased density values in the cortex and contrast uptake in the cisterns may be observed when the meninges are involved (Fig. D1.239). Spread to the ventricles may result in the latter being entirely filled with tumor (Fig. D1.244), a phenomenon most often observed in the anterior horns.

### Differential Diagnosis

*CT findings similar to those in pinealoma may also appear in pilocytic astrocytoma, ependymoma, meningioma of the tentorial hiatus, and in metastasis.* It may be impossible to differentiate among these tumors in some cases. Cysts are most often seen in pilocytic astrocytomas. Diagnosis of an *aneurysm of the vein of Galen,* which is located in the same region, usually presents no problem because this lesion is very large and shows strong contrast enhancement; demonstration of large draining veins in the CT scan confirms the diagnosis (Fig. F72. p. 450).

Hypodense tumors and malformations in this region are shown on pages 312, 313, 332, 333 and 426.

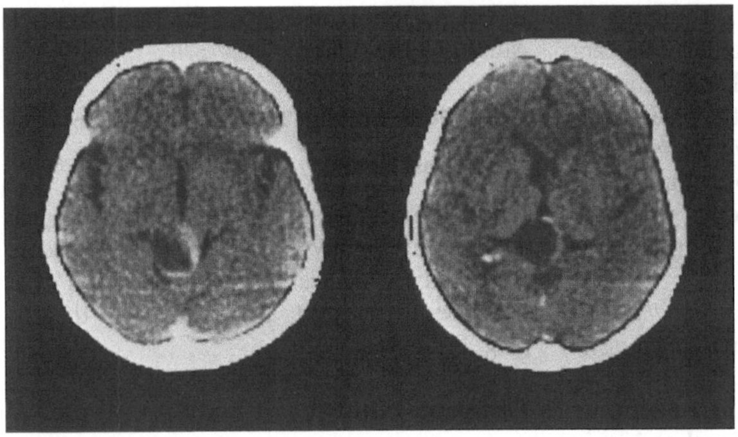

**Fig. D1.238.** Pineocytoma in the quadrigeminal region with a ring of contrast enhancement and a central cyst. Previous radiation therapy. The tumor was slightly hyperdense and demonstrated homogeneous contrast uptake before irradiation. (42-year-old patient with Parinaud syndrome)

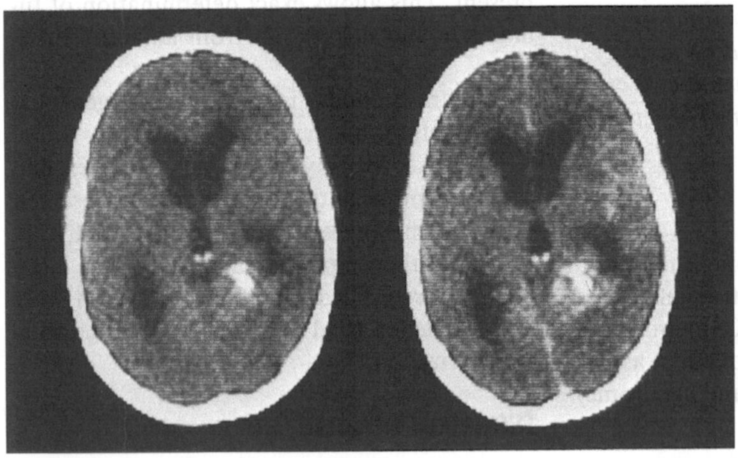

**Fig. D1.239.** Pineoblastoma in a 34-year-old man. The tumor originated in the pineal body and has extended primarily to the region of the right trigonum. Tumor tissue isodense to slightly hyperdense with some calcification in the precontrast study (left) and significant contrast uptake (right). Delicate contrast uptake near the Sylvian fissure due to meningeal infiltration by the tumor

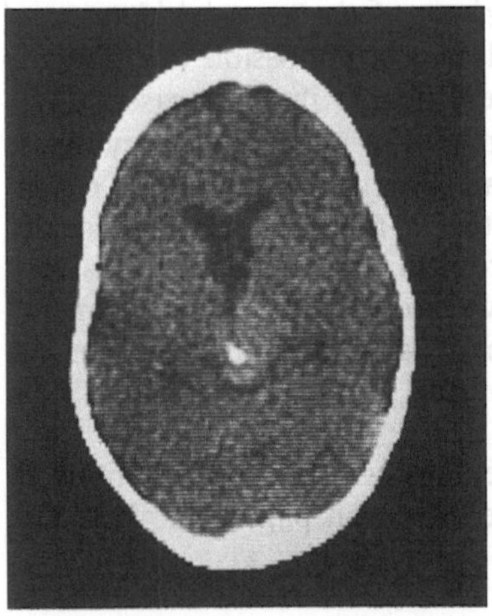

**Fig. D1.240.** Germinoma of the pineal region with extension to the right thalamus in a 21-year-old patient (precontrast study)

▶

**Fig. D1.241.** Germinoma of the pineal region in a 22-year-old man. Postcontrast studies on the right. The series on the left consists of vertical reconstructions demonstrating the anatomical relations of the tumor to both the tentorium and the cisterns. (Reconstructions made with Somatom and provided courtesy of Prof. Dr. LISSNER, Radiology Department, Universität München)

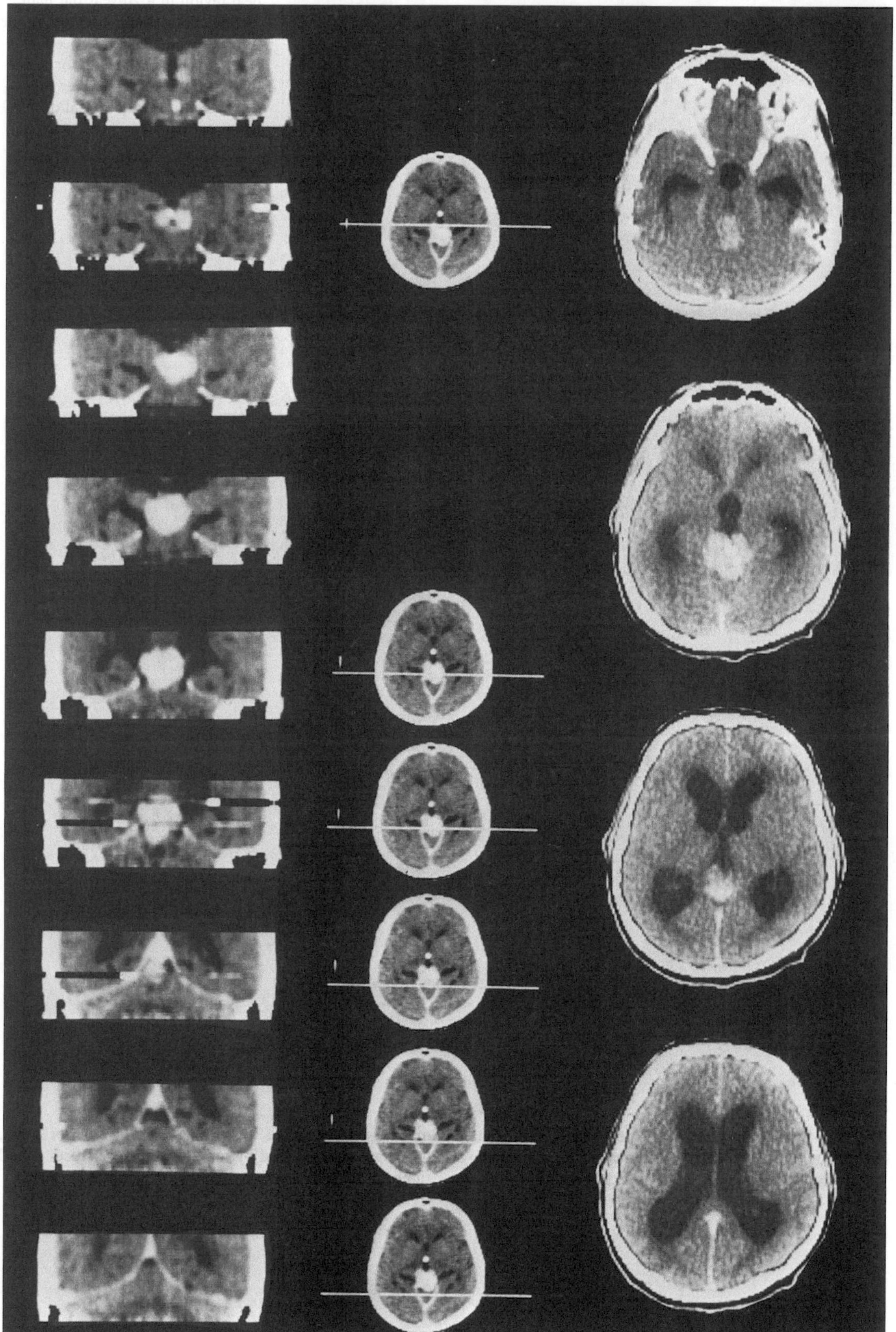

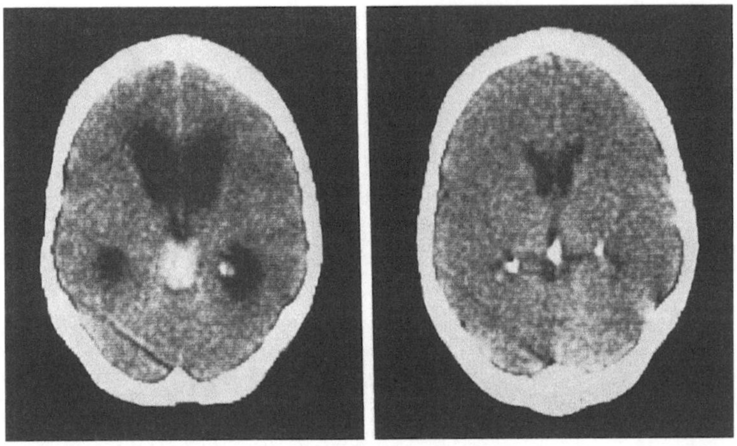

**Fig. D1.242.** Germinoma of the pineal region in a 20-year-old man. Strong contrast enhancement in the tumor. Pronounced hydrocephalus (left). No evidence of tumor in follow-up studies 2 years later following irradiation with a total dose of 6,000 rad (right)

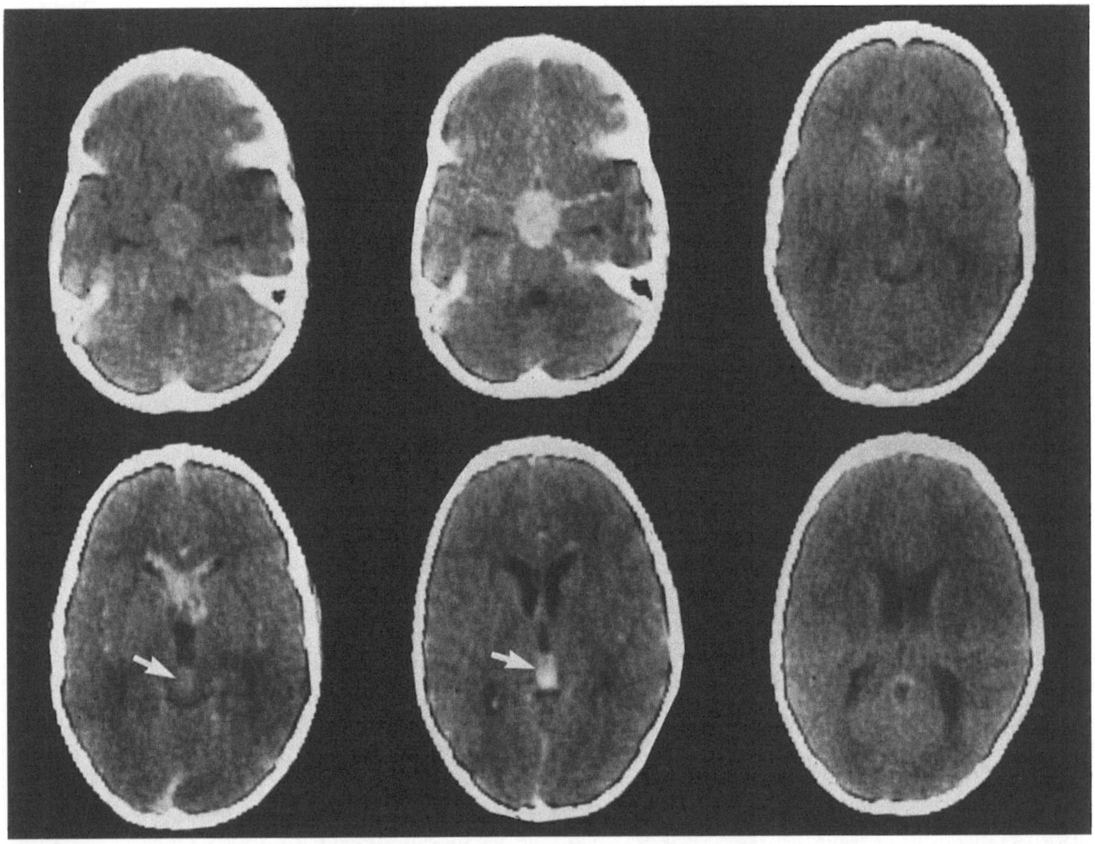

**Fig. D1.243.** Germinoma of the pineal region with ectopic growth and intraventricular metastases in a 12-year-old boy. CT studies demonstrate a large spherical tumor in the chiasmatic cistern as well as tumor masses in the anterior horns, which are entirely filled by tumor in the lower slices. Small tumor in the pineal region (arrow). (Postcontrast studies)

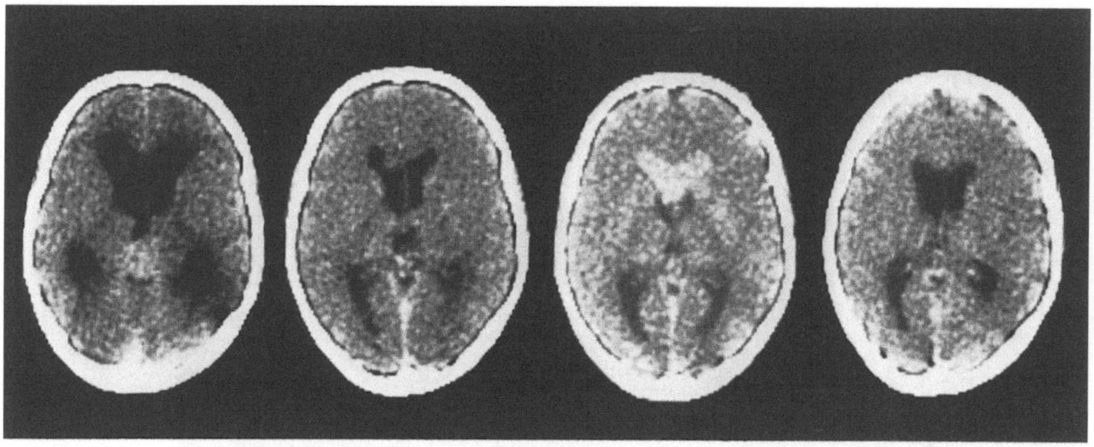

a b c d

**Fig. D 1.244** a–d. Serial studies in a 21-year-old female with a pineal tumor and intraventricular metastases (no histological diagnosis). (**a**) First CT examination on Jan 8, 1976: hyperdense tumor in the pineal region with indentation of the third ventricle and pronounced hydrocephalus. (**b**) Follow-up study on April 22, 1976 after therapy with 5,000 rad: the tumor in the pineal region is no longer clearly identifiable. Metastasis at the wall of the left anterior horn. (**c**) Follow-up study on May 24, 1976: both anterior horns are entirely filled with tumor which demonstrates strong contrast enhancement. (**d**) Follow-up study on Sept 20, 1976, after an additional course of radiation therapy with 6,000 rad, documents the disappearance of all tumor tissue

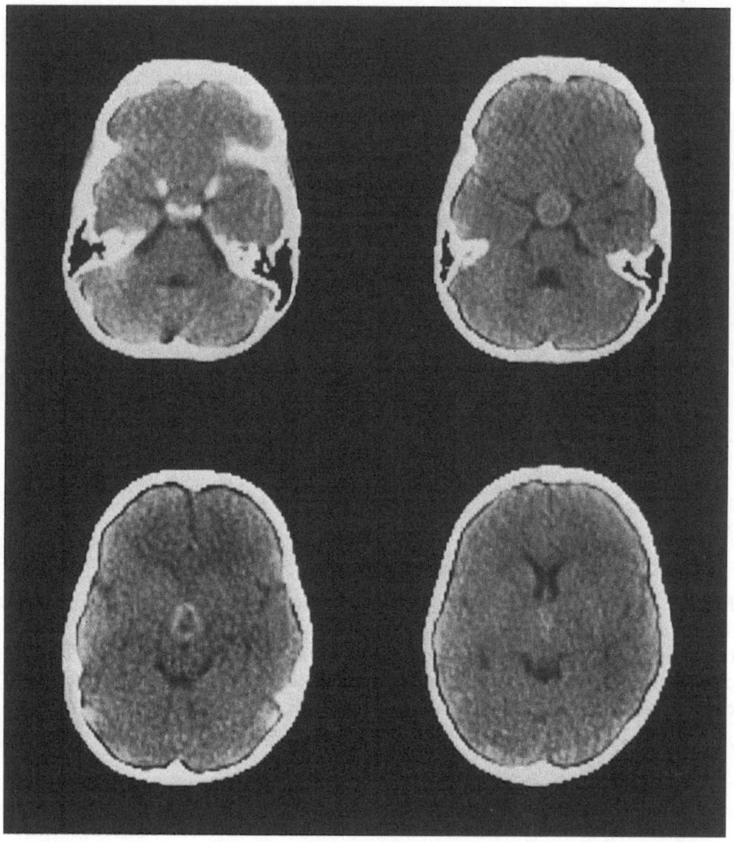

**Fig. D 1.245.** Ectopic pinealoma (germinoma) in the suprasellar region with contrast enhancement especially pronounced in the capsule of the tumor in a 5-year-old girl. Postcontrast study

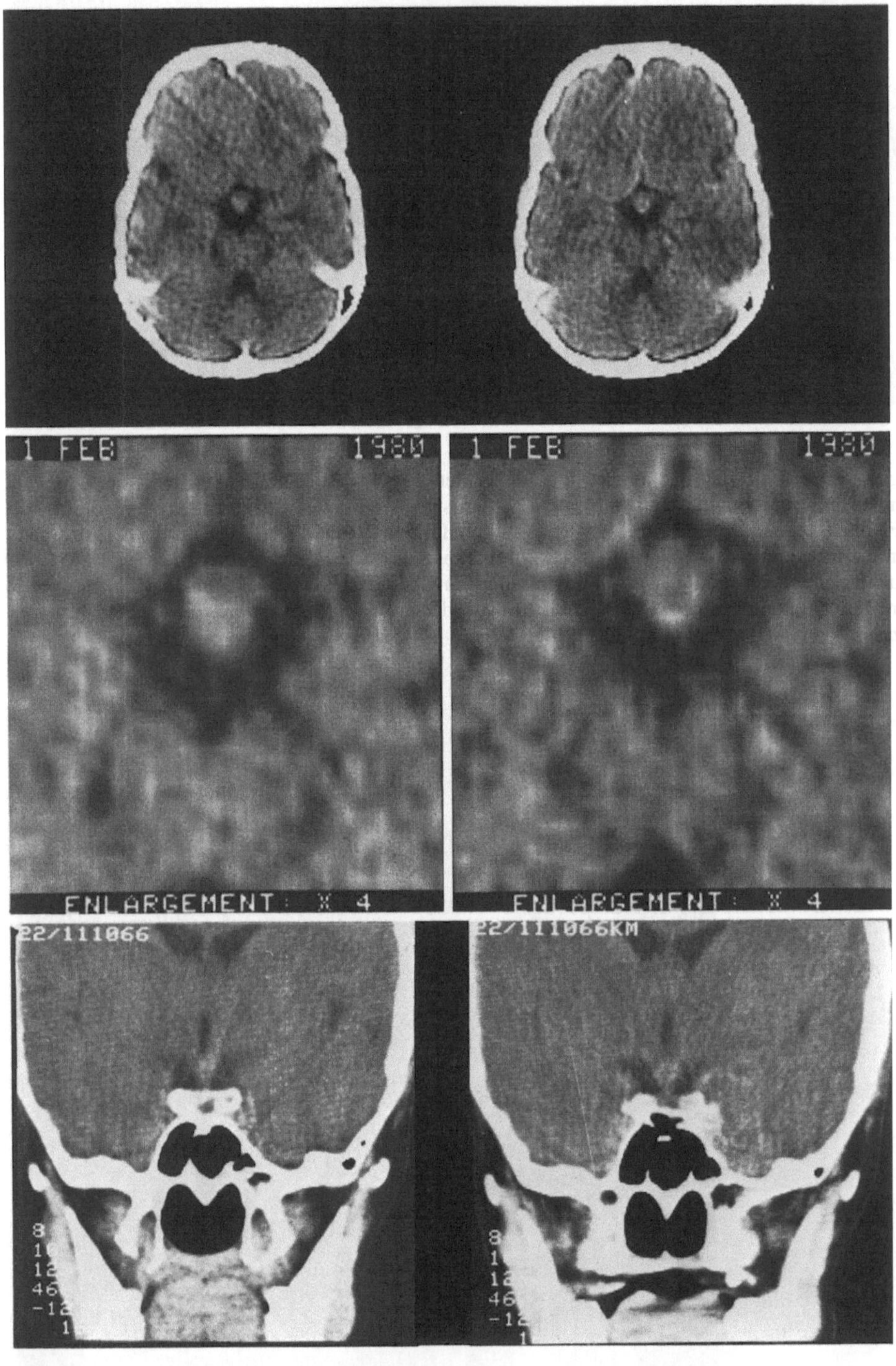


**Fig. D1.246.** Ectopic pinealoma (germinoma) in the pituitary stalk in a 13-year-old boy with diabetes insipidus. The tumor appears as a hyperdense zone in the opticochiasmatic cistern. (Middle: enlargement of the region of interest. Postcontrast study). Coronary slices provide conclusive demonstration of tumor location in the pituitary stalk. (Coronary slices made with Somatom 2 and provided courtesy of Prof. Dr. Witt, Radiology Department, Rudolf-Virchow-Krankenhaus, Berlin)

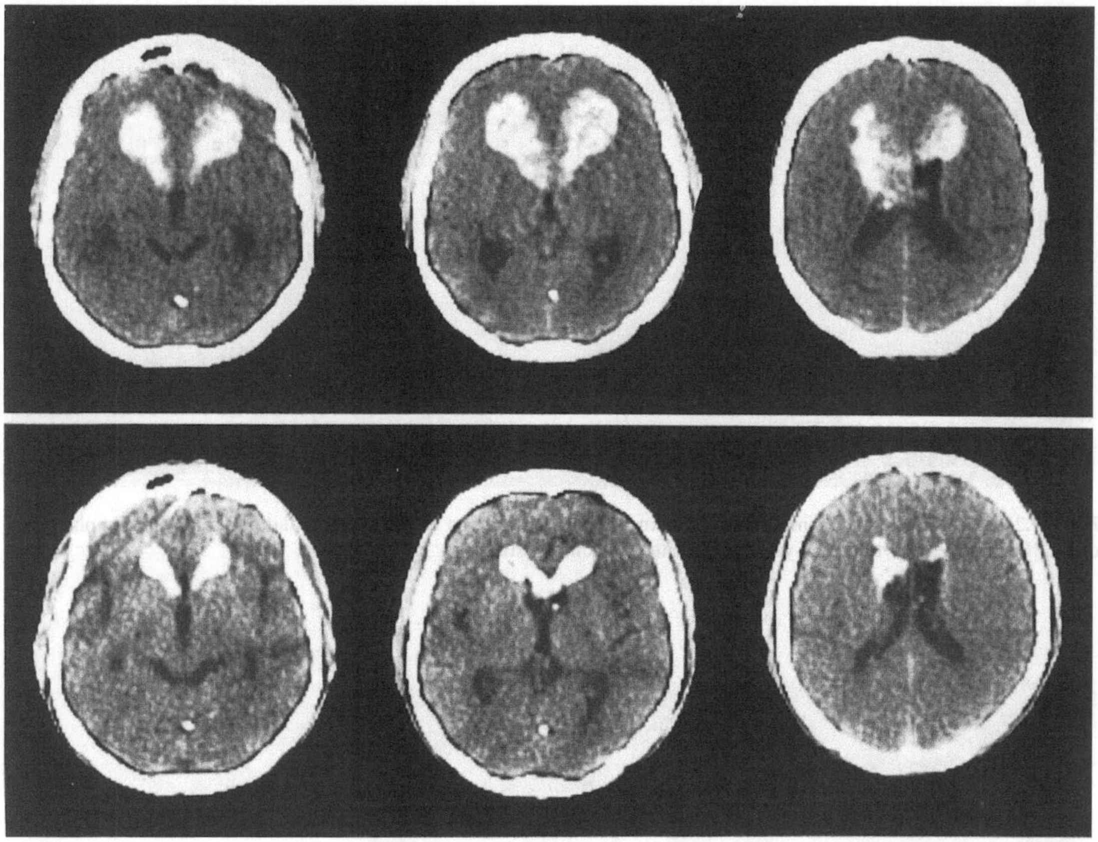

**Fig. D 1.247.** Serial CT studies of a spinal and intraventricular germinoma in a 19-year-old patient presenting with signs of a spinal cord disorder. After resection of a spinal tumor classified as germinoma, cranial CT studies were performed, although no signs of an intracranial lesion were present. The anterior horns were filled with strongly hyperdense tumor which did not take up contrast media (upper series). Follow-up studies 4 months later demonstrated a significant reduction in the size of the tumor after irradiation with 6,000 rad (lower series)

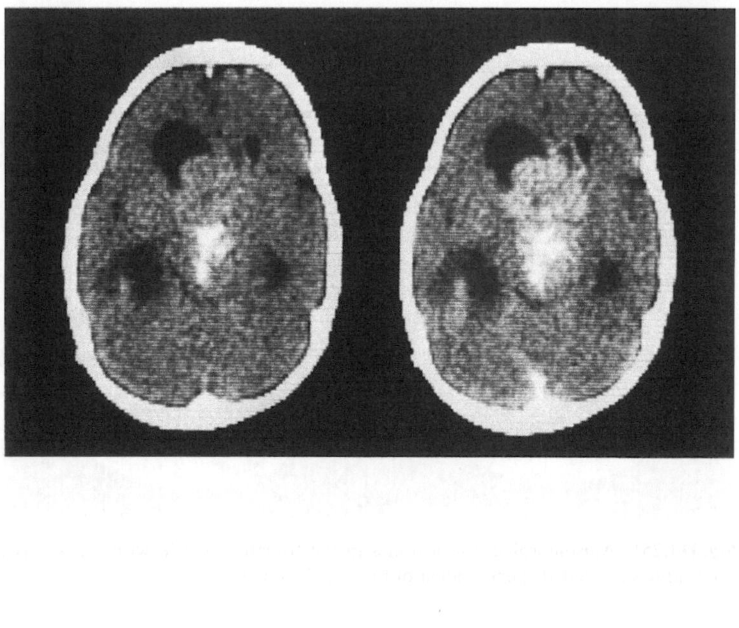

**Fig. D 1.248.** Malignant mixed cellular embryonal tumor originating in the pineal region and extending through the third ventricle to both anterior horns in a 2-year-old boy. The tumor appears hyperdense with calcification in the precontrast study (left) and demonstrates strong contrast enhancement (right)

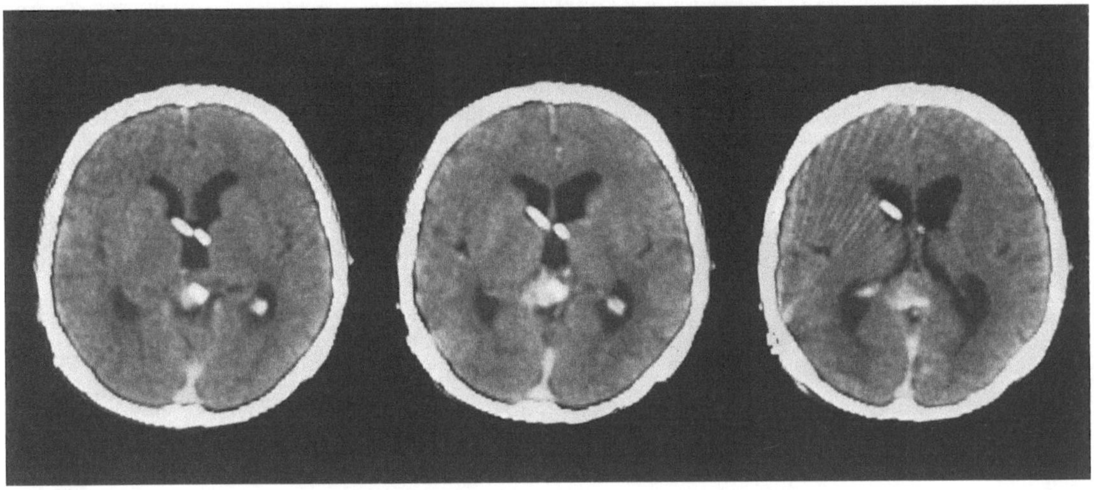

**Fig. D1.249.** Partially calcified pineal tumor of unknown histological type 15 years after radiation therapy and implantation of a CSF shunt. Pineocytoma? 54-year-old patient. Postcontrast study

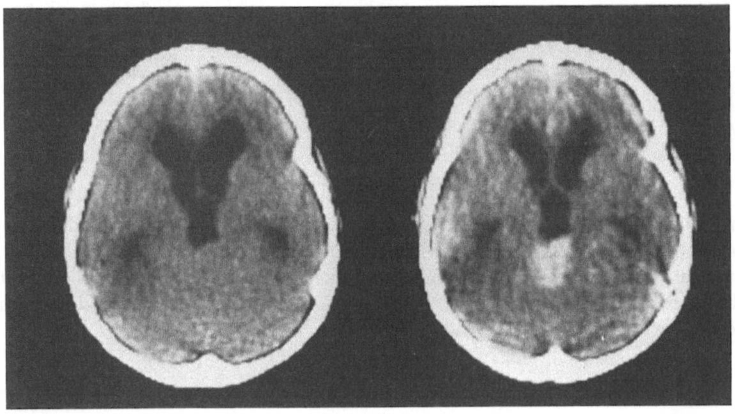

**Fig. D1.250.** Isodense pineal tumor with strong contrast uptake in a 54-year-old female with Parinaud syndrome and signs of increased intracranial pressure; occlusive hydrocephalus. No histological diagnosis

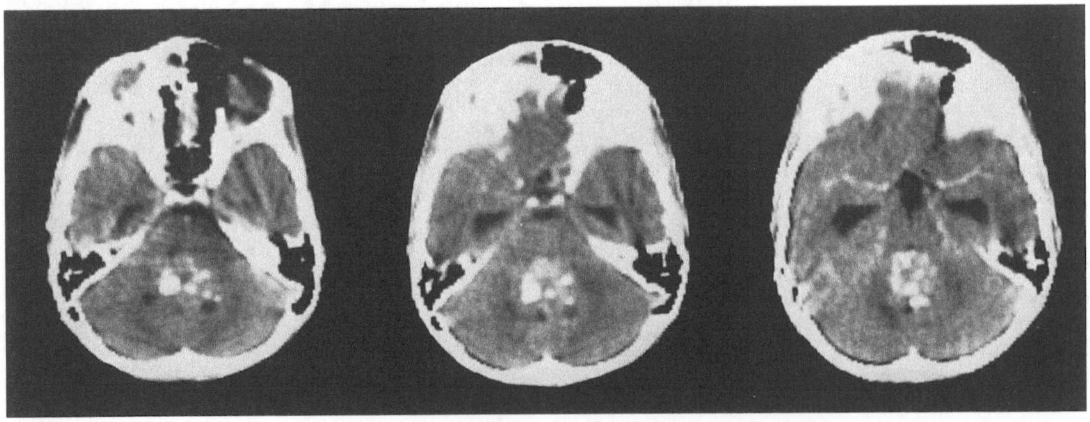

**Fig. D1.251.** Anisomorphic pineocytoma in the fourth ventricle with numerous calcifications in a 15-year-old boy. The CT findings suggested ependymoma of the fourth ventricle

# 2. Meningeal Tumors

## a) Meningiomas

| | |
|---|---|
| Incidence | 14–18% |
| Characteristic age at diagnosis | 35–70 years |
| Sex distribution | Almost twice as common in females |
| Typical locations | Parasagittal region, falx cerebri, convexity, entire base of the skull, posterior fossa, tentorium, and lateral ventricles |
| Characteristic clinical findings | Neurological deficits and seizures as a function of tumor location |
| Skull film | Hyperostosis, bone destruction, dilated vascular canals, secondary signs of increased intracranial pressure |
| EEG | Pathological findings related to tumor location |
| Echoencephalography | Displacement of midline structures or ventricular dilatation (related to location of the tumor) |
| Serial brain scintigraphy | Typical pattern in many cases: Intense radionuclide uptake diminishing from early to delayed scans |
| Cerebral angiography | Displacement of intracranial vessels; typical tumor staining |

**Computed Tomography**

| | |
|---|---|
| Precontrast study | Mostly homogeneous slightly hyperdense tumor zone, rarely isodense area, with calcification in 10%–20%, surrounded by hypodense areas (edema) in many cases |
| Contrast medium uptake | Strongly positive except in totally calcified meningiomas |
| Appearance after contrast enhancement | Homogeneous sharply delineated tumors closely related to the meninges and the skull vault or base; moderate perifocal edema common |

**Differential Diagnosis**

*Convexity and Falx*

Metastasis
Malignant lymphoma
and (rarely) glioblastoma or anaplastic astrocytoma

*Suprasellar Region and Anterior Fossa*

Pituitary adenoma
Pilocytic astrocytoma
Aneurysm of the carotid artery
Chordoma
Chondroma
Metastasis of carcinoma and malignant lymphoma in rare cases

Continuation

*Middle Fossa*

Trigeminal neurinoma
Gangliocytoma
Pilocytic astrocytoma
Aneurysm of the carotid artery
Chondroma

*Posterior Fossa*

Acoustic neurinoma
Metastasis
Solid hemangioblastoma
Malignant lymphoma
Aneurysm
Glomus tumor and chordoma of the clivus

*Ventricles*

Plexus papilloma
Colloid cyst (third ventricle)

Meningiomas are among the most common intracranial tumors. CUSHING reported finding meningiomas in 13.4% of all tumors in his series, while ZÜLCH found 16.6% and OLIVECRONA 18.2%. Meningiomas made up 15.9% of tumors in our collective.

Peak incidence occurs between the ages of 36 and 70 years, though meningioma may also occur in younger patients. Females are affected almost twice as often as males.

Meningiomas derive from the arachnoid mater and initially displace brain tissue and the pia mater. Tumor growth disturbs venous circulation and may result in ischemic necrosis of the cerebral cortex with penetration of the tumor to the white matter. This is always accompanied by brain edema.

Meningiomas are generally slow-growing benign (grade I) tumors. Anaplastic variants with a tendency to more rapid growth were observed in 5% of cases in our series.

Meningiomas tend to recur if in toto resection is not possible, as may be the case near the base of the skull.

**Typical Locations**

Close proximity to the meninges and the skull bone are characteristic of meningioma. Typical locations in diminishing order of frequency are the parasagittal region in the anterior, middle, and posterior segments of the sagittal sinus, the cerebral falx, the convexity, the olfactory groove, the tuberculum sellae, the medial and lateral sphenoid wings, Meckel's cave, the tentorium, the cerebellopontine angle, the clivus, and the craniocervical junction.

Meningiomas may also develop in the choroid plexus of the third and lateral ventricles in rare cases.

Multiple tumors have been observed. In some of these cases diffuse seeding – designated as meningiomatosis – may have taken place, which most often occurs in CNS manifestations of neurofibromatosis. Aside from tumor knobs or nodules, meningioma may also show superficial (en plaque) growth, a form most often observed in osteoplastic meningioma of the sphenoid bones. Meningiomas may invade adjacent bone, resulting in visible thickening of the vault. The tumors also invade the orbits and the paranasal sinuses in rare cases.

**Characteristic Clinical Findings**

Clinical findings vary with the location of the tumor. The patient may present with acute cerebral ischemia or with seizures, very common in meningioma of the convexity. Severe organic brain syndromes are observed in meningioma of the olfactory groove and the frontotemporal region of the dominant hemisphere.

Sphenoid wing meningiomas may produce swelling of the temporal region and exophthalmus, while tumors at the base of the skull cause cranial nerve lesions. Meningiomas of the posterior fossa often result in signs of chronic increase in intracranial pressure as well as cerebellar symptoms.

### Additional Diagnostic Procedures

Plain skull films reveal pathological findings in almost half of cases of meningioma. Thickening of the vault or the base of the skull at the origin of the tumor (enostosis) is the most common finding. Osteoplastic sphenoid meningiomas may be diagnosed in the plain skull film.

Spiculae – fine columns of bone oriented at right angles to the surface of the skull – may be observed if meningioma penetrates the skull vault.

Dilatation of the vascular canals in the vault results from increased blood flow to the tumor with hypertrophy of the meningeal vessels.

Intracranial meningiomas may demonstrate extensive calcification visible on the plain skull film. Changes secondary to increased intracranial pressure, especially in the sella contour, are often found.

The EEG frequently shows focal activity in supratentorial meningiomas. Echoencephalographic findings vary with the location of the tumor and may be normal in parasagittal tumors which often do not cause a midline shift.

All large meningiomas exhibit intense radionuclide uptake which is demonstrable early in the arterial phase and persists well into the venous phase. Static brain scans show intense radionuclide activity in the early phase with a subsequent rapid decrease in activity. These criteria are so characteristic that they permit a diagnosis of meningioma with brain scintigraphy.

Meningiomas may be served by both the external and the internal carotid arteries. Selective demonstration of each is necessary in order to define the full extent of the tumor. Angiographic findings are characteristic, with large afferent vessels and a homogeneous capillary phase. In contrast to glioblastomas, arteriovenous fistulas are quite rare, and very early venous filling does hardly occur. Findings of a sharply delineated tumor – sometimes consisting of several knobs – large hypertrophic branches of the external carotid artery, and a homogeneous tumor blush persisting until the end of the venous phase are typical of meningioma and may be regarded as pathognomonic.

## Computed Tomography (Figs. D2.1–81)

### Precontrast Study

The vast majority of meningiomas (74.7%) appears as a homogeneous zone of increased density in the plain CT scan (Fig. D1.2–4). Calcification may be found within the tumor in 10%–20% of cases (Fig. D2.5). Some tumors are entirely calcified, especially at infratentorial locations (Figs. D2.6–9). The osteoplastic sphenoid wing meningioma is a special form of meningioma (Fig. D2.10).

Of the meningiomas in our series, 14.4% were isodense in the precontrast study (Figs. D2.11, 12). Such tumors may be overlooked if perifocal edema or signs of a mass lesion are not present. This was true of almost 40% of isodense meningiomas in our experience. Ten percent of meningiomas demonstrate mixed

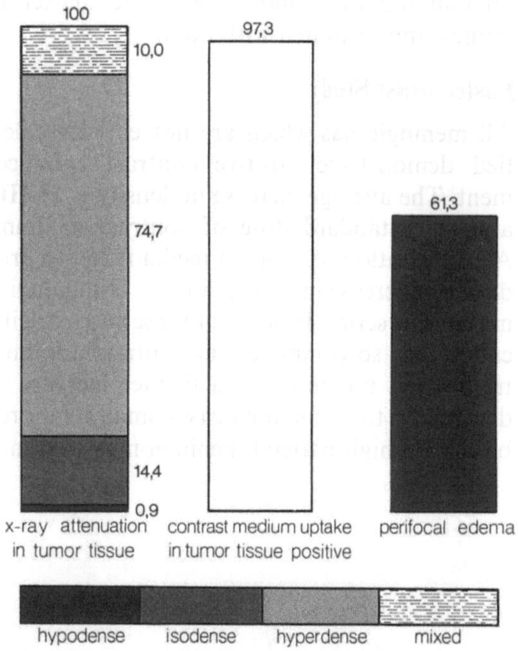


**Fig. D2.1.** X-ray attenuation, contrast medium uptake, and frequency of edema in meningiomas (percent)

density other than calcification within hyperdense tumors. Mixed density is most often found in tumors with cysts or other regressive changes (Figs. D2.13–17). Cysts may occur within the tumor or outside the tumor at its margin (Figs. D2.15–17). Meningiomas rarely appear as hypodense lesions in the precontrast study (0.8%) (Figs. D2.18, 19).

A diagnosis of meningioma is supported by demonstration of *hyperostosis at the origin of the tumor* (Figs. D2.20, 21). Thickening of the skull vault caused by the tumor may be found in some cases (Fig. D2.22).

*Perifocal edema* is a common finding in meningioma (61.3%), and it delineates the tumor exactly in the precontrast study (Fig. D2.14). Exceptions are temporobasal and high parietal meningiomas, which often demonstrate the edema but not the tumor itself. Meningiomas in the Sylvian fissure may cause *blockage of CSF circulation in the insular cisterns* (Fig. D2.24). The low density zone between a meningioma and surrounding brain tissue does not always represent perifocal edema, but may in some cases represent a *thin fluid layer*. Analysis of density values in such areas reveals Hounsfield numbers that are much lower than those usually found in brain edema. At operation one finds pale yellow fluid between the surface of the meningioma and the edematous brain tissue surrounding the tumor. The white matter is spongy and saturated with fluid.

## Postcontrast Study

All meningiomas which are not entirely calcified demonstrate positive contrast enhancement. The average increase in density is 18 HU after the standard dose of contrast medium. Administration of contrast media failed to produce an increase in density in 3% of meningiomas in our series. In some of these cases calcification was so complete that contrast administration did not result in a further increase in density. In the remaining cases small temporobasal and high parietal meningiomas were not demonstrated because interference from bony structures and artifacts did not allow direct demonstration even after contrast enhancement.

Maximum increase in X-ray attenuation is observed immediately after contrast injection. A rapid decrease in density occurs within the first half hour of contrast administration.

A homogeneous increase in density is characteristic of meningioma. As a result contrast administration allows significant improvement in delineation of the tumor, especially in isodense meningiomas. The tumor usually has a well-defined border and smooth surface with round, oval, or segmented knots of tumor tissue. The tumors are always related to the meninges or the skull bone, except in cases of ventricular meningioma. Malignant meningiomas and tumors with diffuse "en plaque" growth may have irregular and blurred borders.

Enhancement of the falx or the tentorium demonstrates the relations of tumor and meninges in some cases. Coronary sections are sometimes better suited to this purpose and are indispensable for demonstration of small tumors growing at the base of the middle cranial fossa (Fig. D2.25). Cysts and other regressive changes are best demonstrated after contrast enhancement. A ring structure is sometimes observed in such meningiomas, and this may result in confusion with other ring-like lesions (1.5% of meningiomas) (Fig. D2.26).

Vassoulithis and Ambrose (1979) tried to establish a more differentiated correlation between CT findings and histological subgroups of meningioma, such as the transitional, fibroblastic, angioblastic, and syncytial types. Analysis of 102 cases of meningioma showed some degree of correlation, though our experience indicates that a reliable prediction of histological subtype cannot be made with the CT scan. Failure to demonstrate typical CT criteria of the meningioma suggests aggressive and destructive growth and a diagnosis of malignant meningioma (see p. 249).

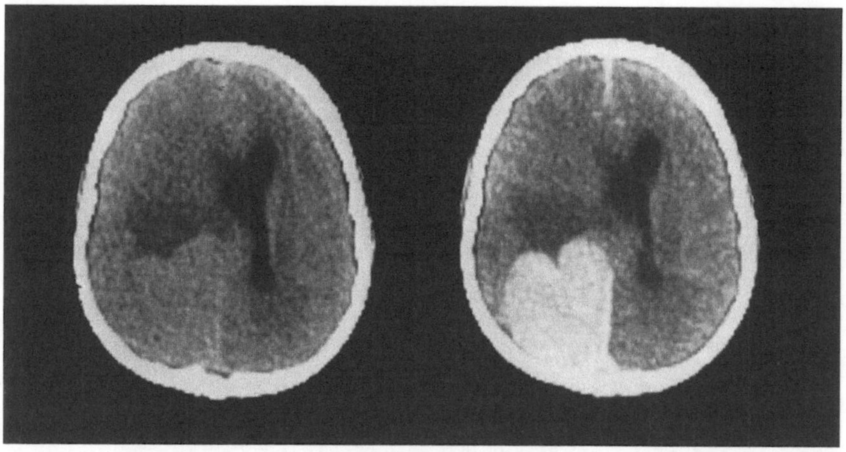

**Fig. D2.2.** Parasagittal meningioma in the posterior third of the sagittal sinus in a 35-year-old man. The tumor appears slightly hyperdense in the precontrast study (left). The outline of the tumor is visible against the perifocal edema at the anterior margin of the lesion. There is strong homogeneous contrast enhancement (right)

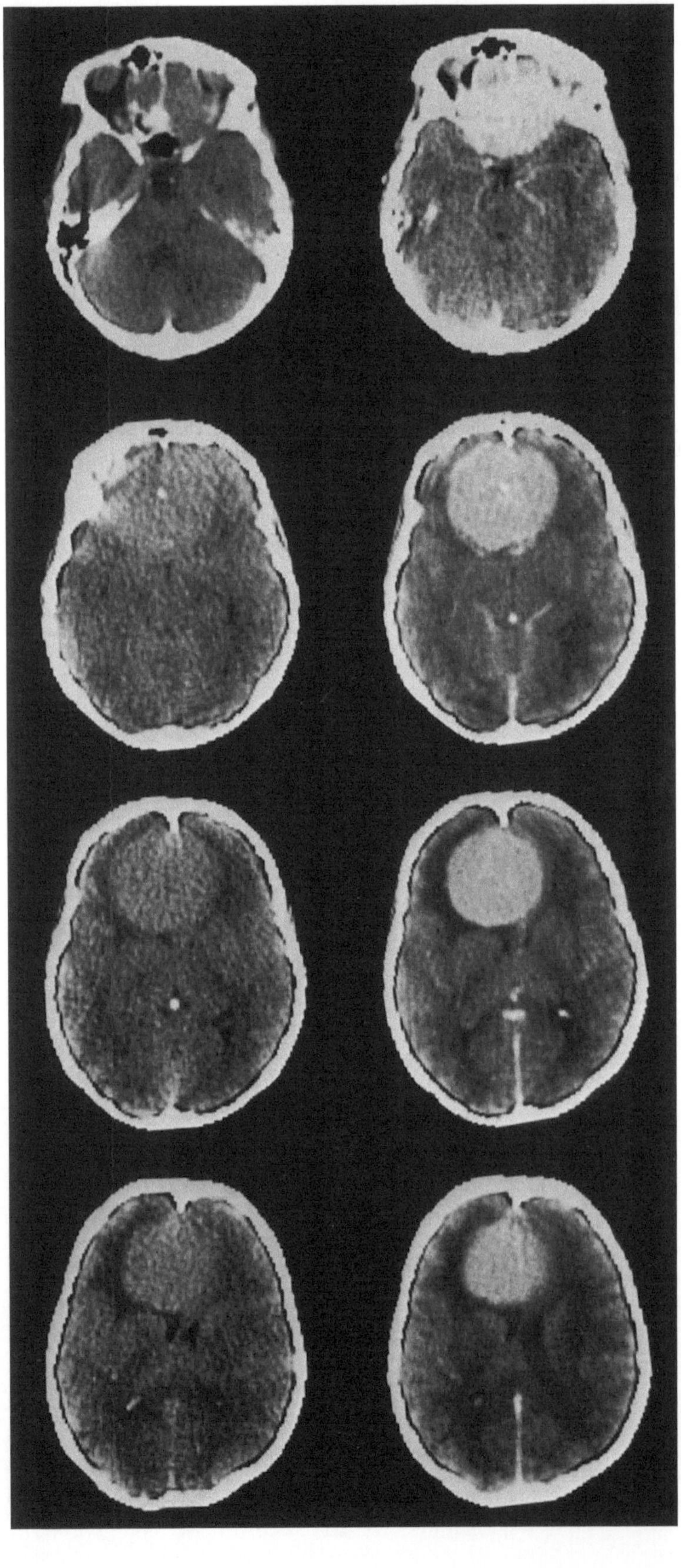

**Fig. D2.3.** Large olfactory groove meningioma in a 45-year-old man with frontal headache and a disorder of the sense of smell. The tumor appears hyperdense in precontrast studies (series on the left). Small central calcification and frontal lobe edema, more pronounced on the left. The tumor has caused dorsal displacement of the anterior horns. Strong contrast uptake (series on the right)

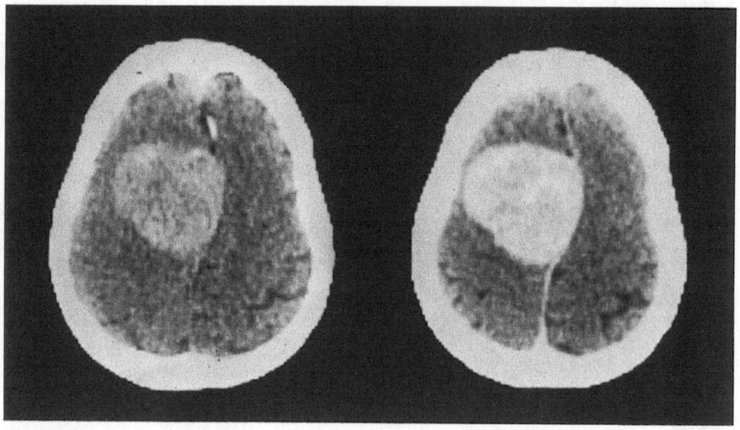

**Fig. D2.4.** Meningioma in the lower third of the falx cerebri. Hyperdense values in the precontrast study with further increase in density in post-contrast studies (right). Significant displacement of the middle section of the falx to the right. (61-year-old female)

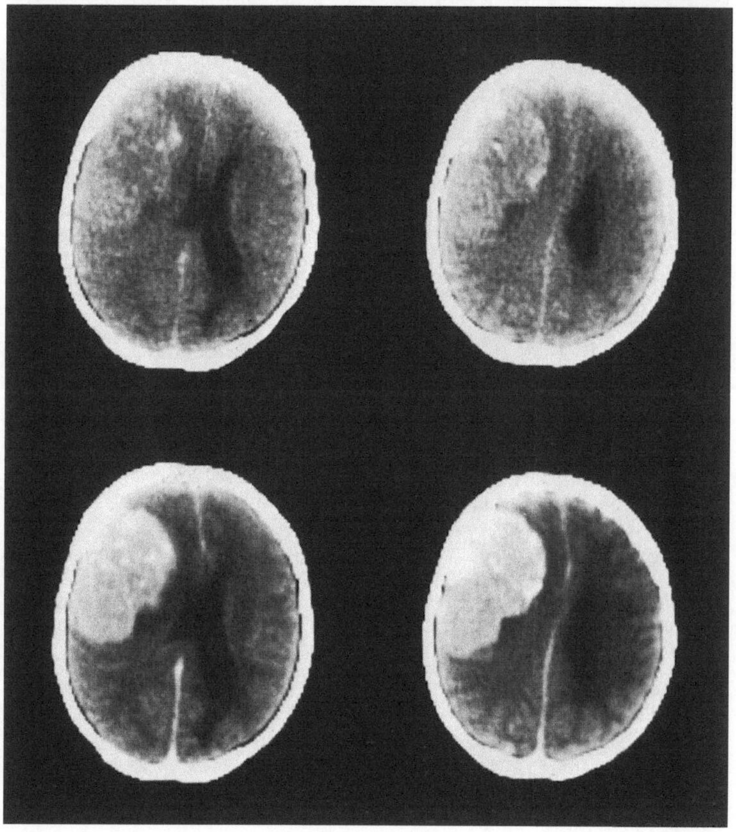

**Fig. D2.5.** Large meningioma of the convexity in the left frontoparietal region with inhomogeneous attenuation values in the precontrast study. Numerous calcified specks (upper pair). Intensive homogeneous contrast enhancement resulting in clear demarcation of the tumor (lower pair). Signs of intracranial mass effects with displacement of the ventricles and the falx in the lower and middle segments

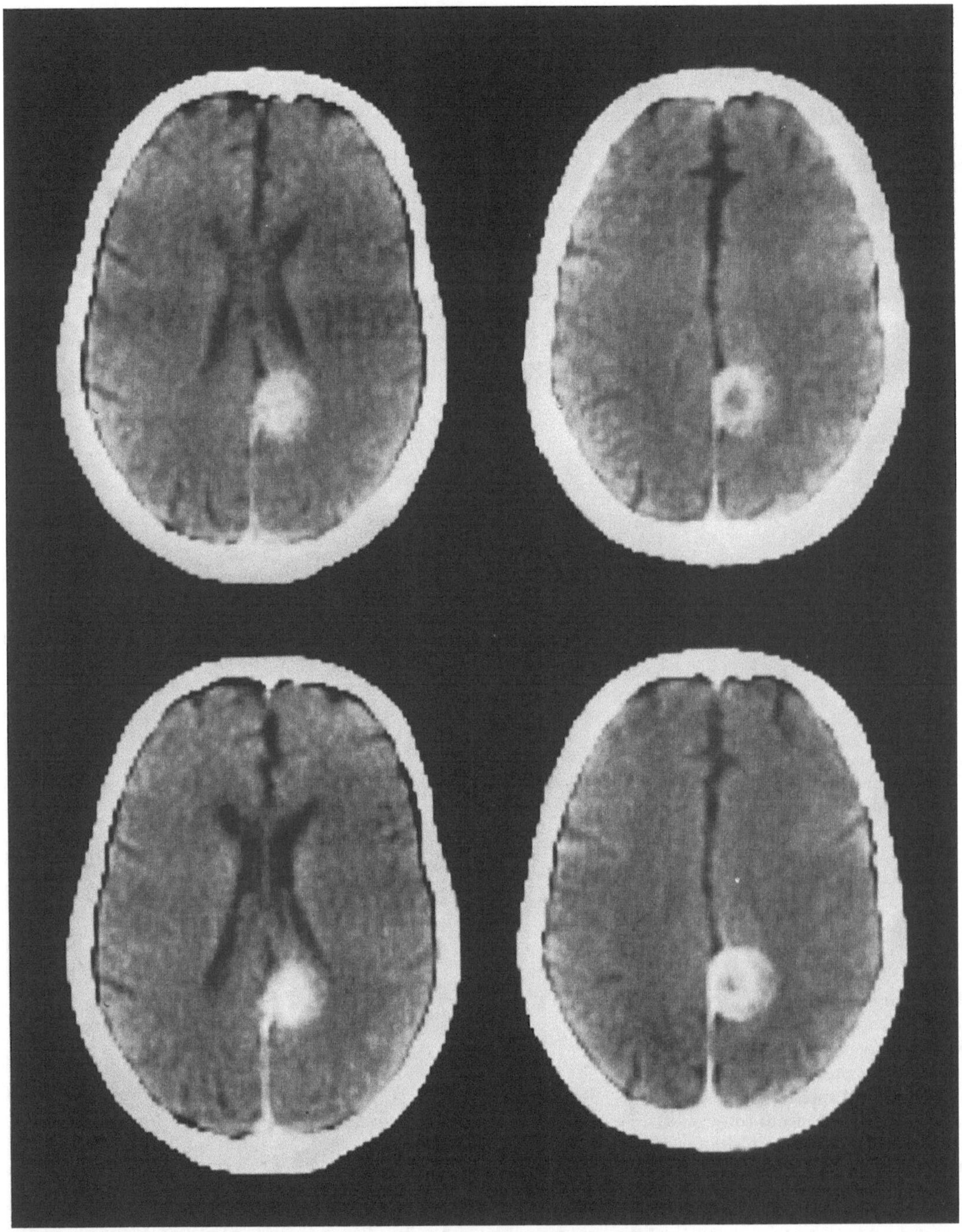

**Fig. D2.6.** Small partially calcified meningioma on the lower border of the falx. The tumor demonstrates very high attenuation values in precontrast studies (above) with limited contrast medium uptake (below)

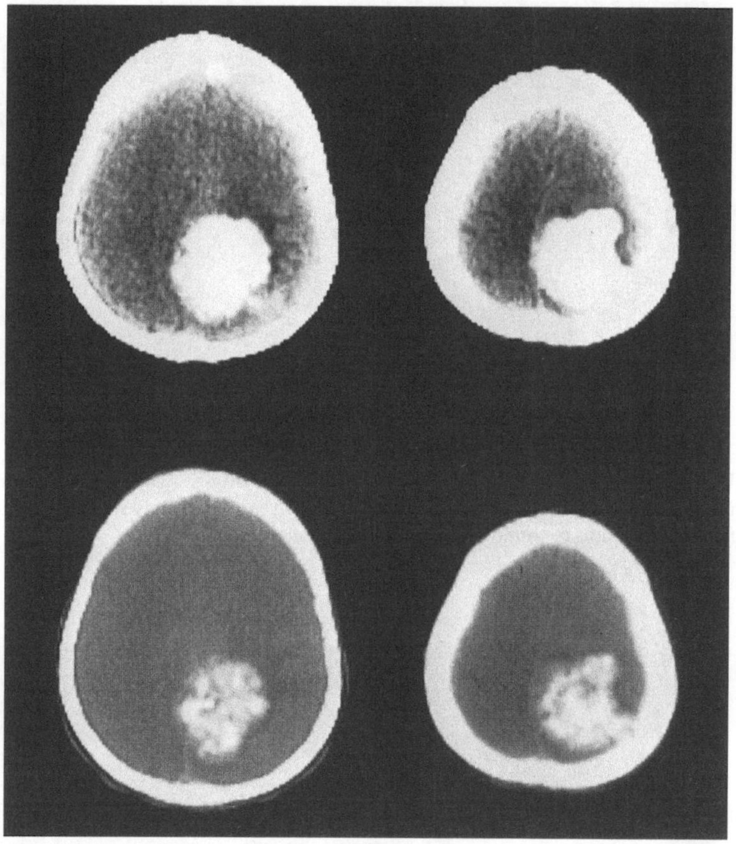

**Fig. D2.7.** Highly calcified parasagittal meningioma at the junction of the middle and posterior thirds of the superior sagittal sinus in a 54-year-old female. Enlargement of window width (400 HU) allows more differentiated demonstration of the calcified figures within the tumor (lower pair)

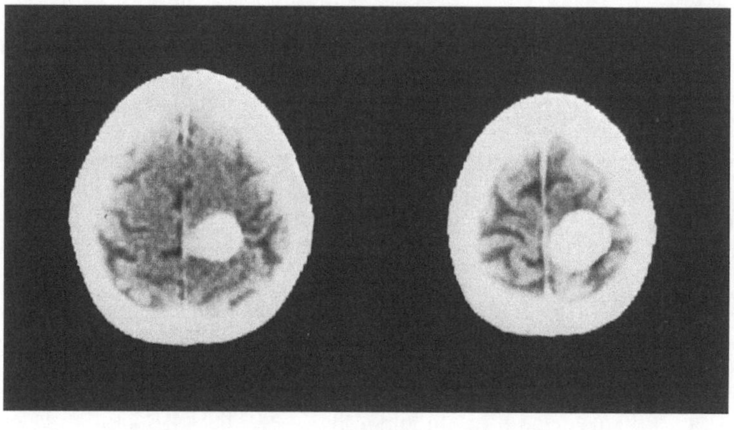

**Fig. D2.8.** Entirely calcified meningioma in the middle third of the superior sagittal sinus in a 73-year-old patient. Width of the sulci is normal for the age of the patient. The sulci have not been obliterated by the tumor. No evidence of perifocal edema. Precontrast study

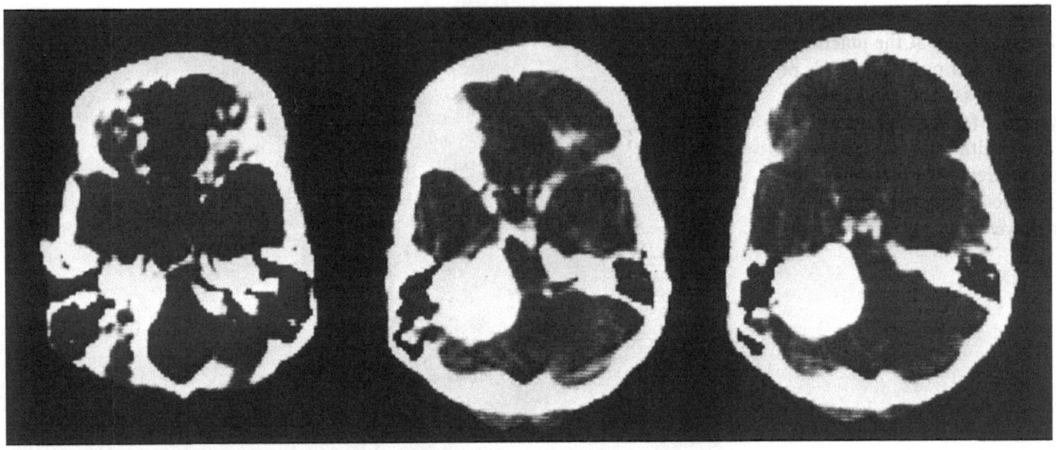

**Fig. D2.9.** Entirely calcified subtentorial meningioma originating at the left cerebellopontine angle in a 64-year-old female. Variation in window width and level demonstrates the extent of calcification within the tumor. All slices show only structures with bone density

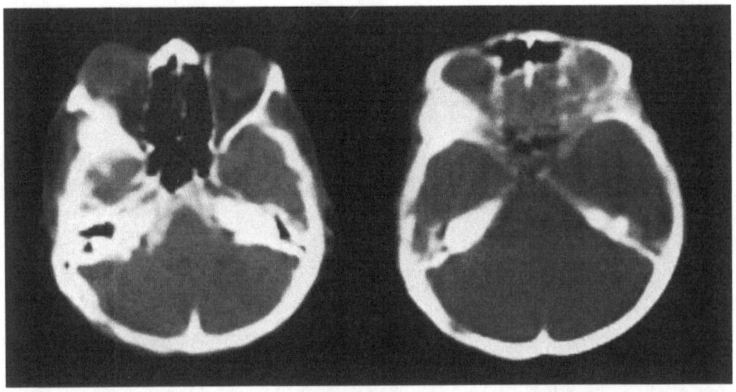

**Fig. D2.10.** Osteoplastic meningioma of the left sphenoid wing in a 65-year-old patient. Proptosis has occurred secondary to massive dilatation and thickening of the sphenoid wing by the tumor. CT diagnosis is possible only if the base of the skull is symmetrically positioned in the CT scanner

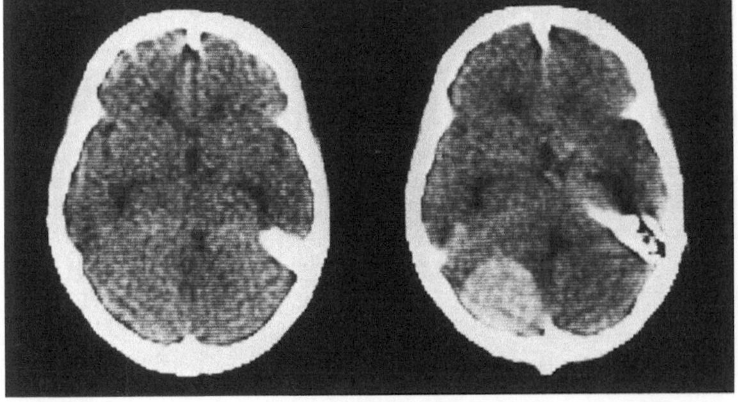

**Fig. D2.11.** Infratentorial meningioma above the left cerebellar hemisphere in a 60-year-old patient. The tumor is isodense in precontrast studies; slight perifocal edema and displacement of the fourth ventricle suggest its presence (left). Clear demonstration of the spherical sharply demarcated tumor after contrast enhancement (right)

**Fig. D2.12.** Isodense suprasellar meningioma in a 61-year-old patient. The tumor is visible as a solid figure projecting into the chiasmatic cistern in the precontrast study (left). Strong contrast uptake (right)

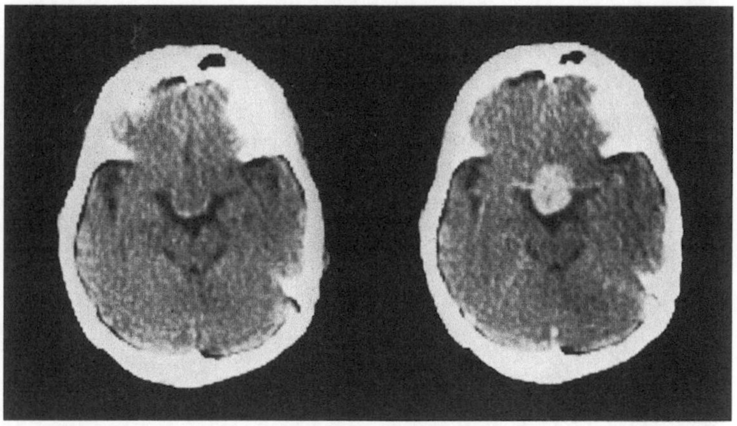

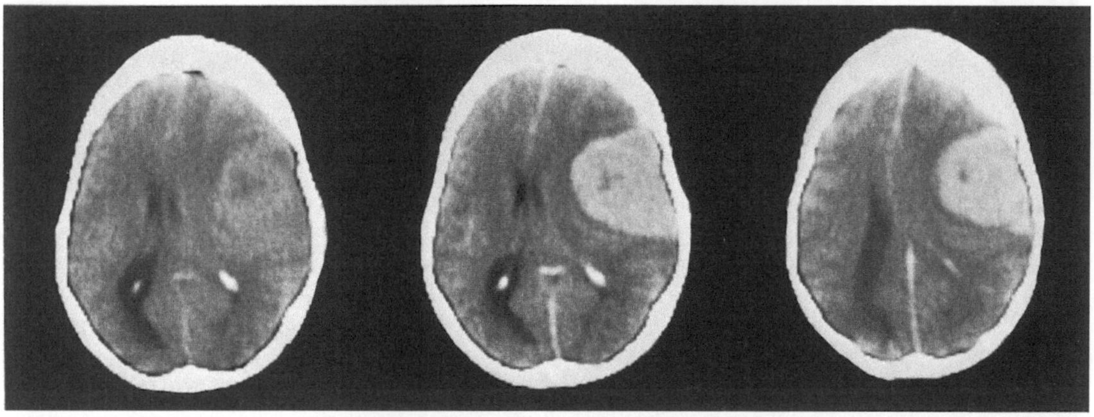

**Fig. D2.13.** Large meningioma on the convexity at the spurs of the right sphenoid wing in a 26-year-old man. The tumor demonstrates both hypodense and slightly hyperdense attenuation values in the precontrast study (left). Contrast enhancement reveals a small eccentrically located hypodense zone resulting from regressive changes within the tumor (right)

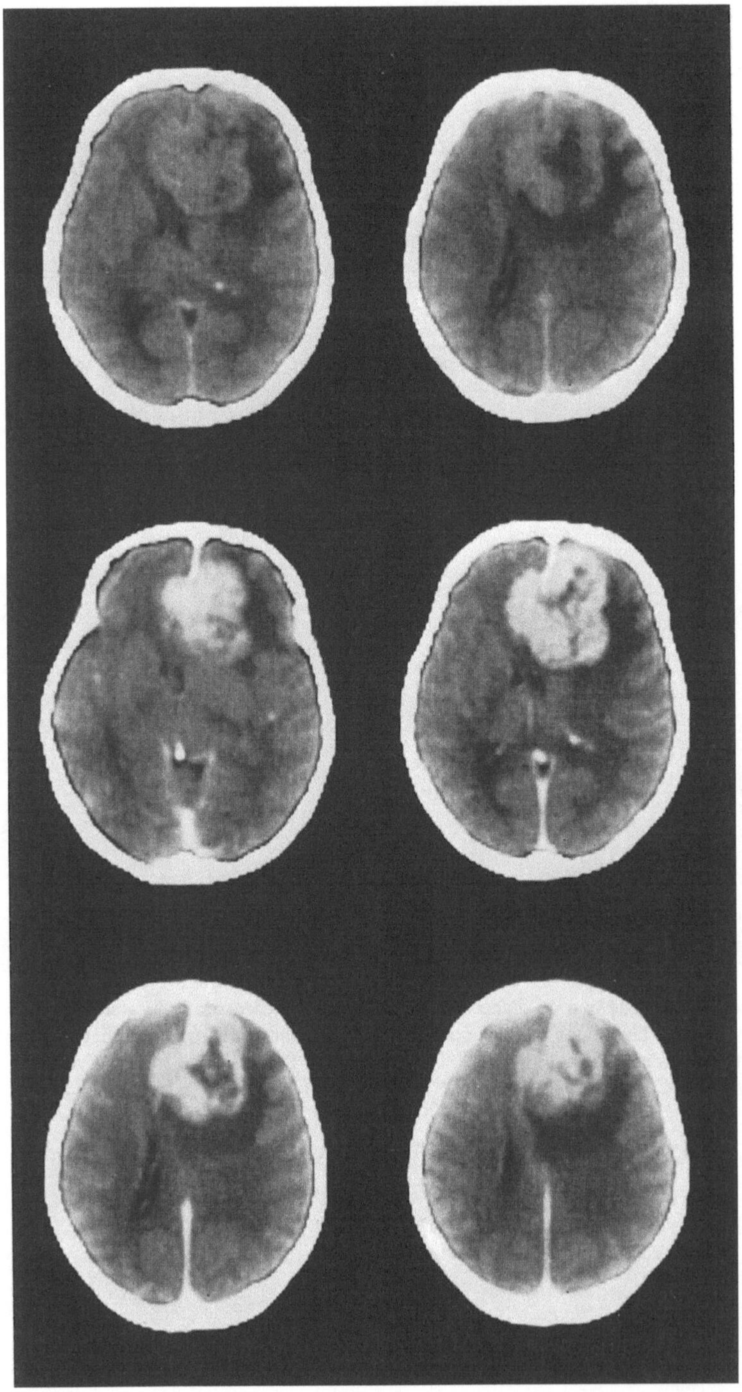

**Fig. D2.14.** Falx meningioma in the anterior third of the superior sagittal sinus with extension to the left. Sharp delineation of the isodense and hypodense tumor by perifocal edema in the precontrast study (upper pair). Contrast enhancement demonstrates regressive change more clearly in the characteristically knobby tumor (middle, below). (53-year-old patient)

**Fig. D2.15** a, b. Atypical meningioma with a cyst in the right frontoprecentral region in a 71-year-old patient. (**a**) Postcontrast studies demonstrate a mixed density tumor with solid portions near the skull vault and a cyst with delicate ring enhancement and sedimentation effect in its posterior part (upper pair). Hyperostosis initially suggested a diagnosis of meningioma. (All CT scans postcontrast studies). (**b**) Surgical specimen with a large marginal cyst

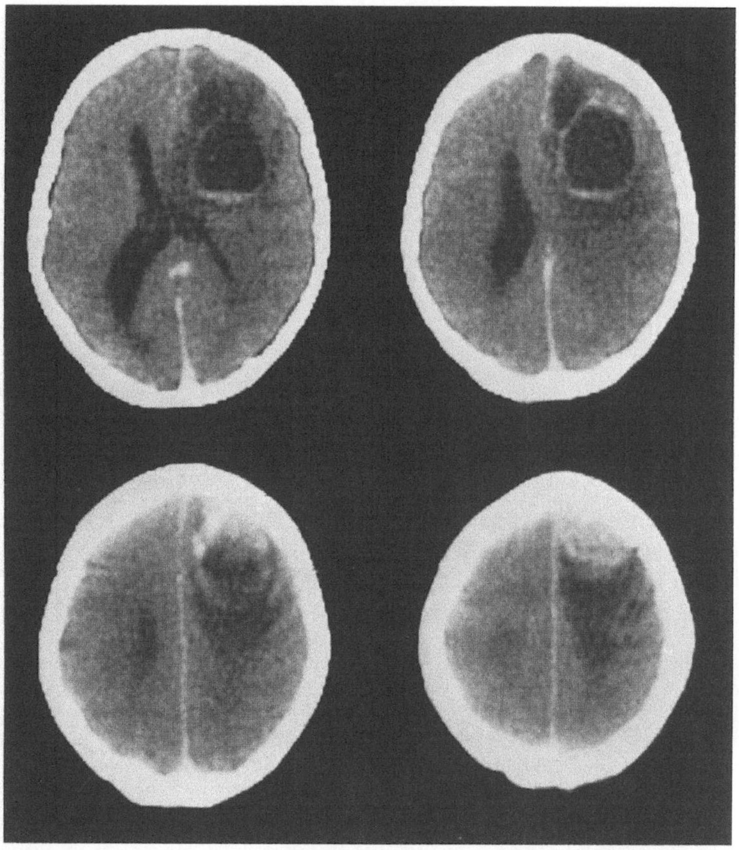

a

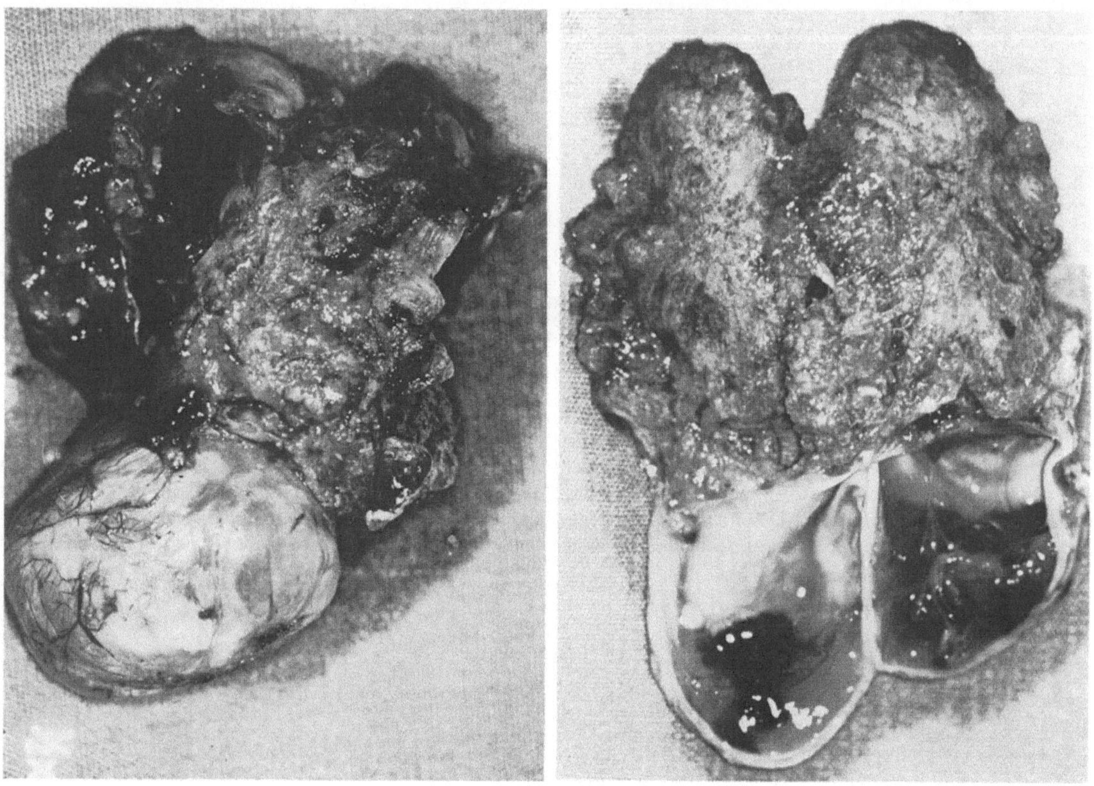

b

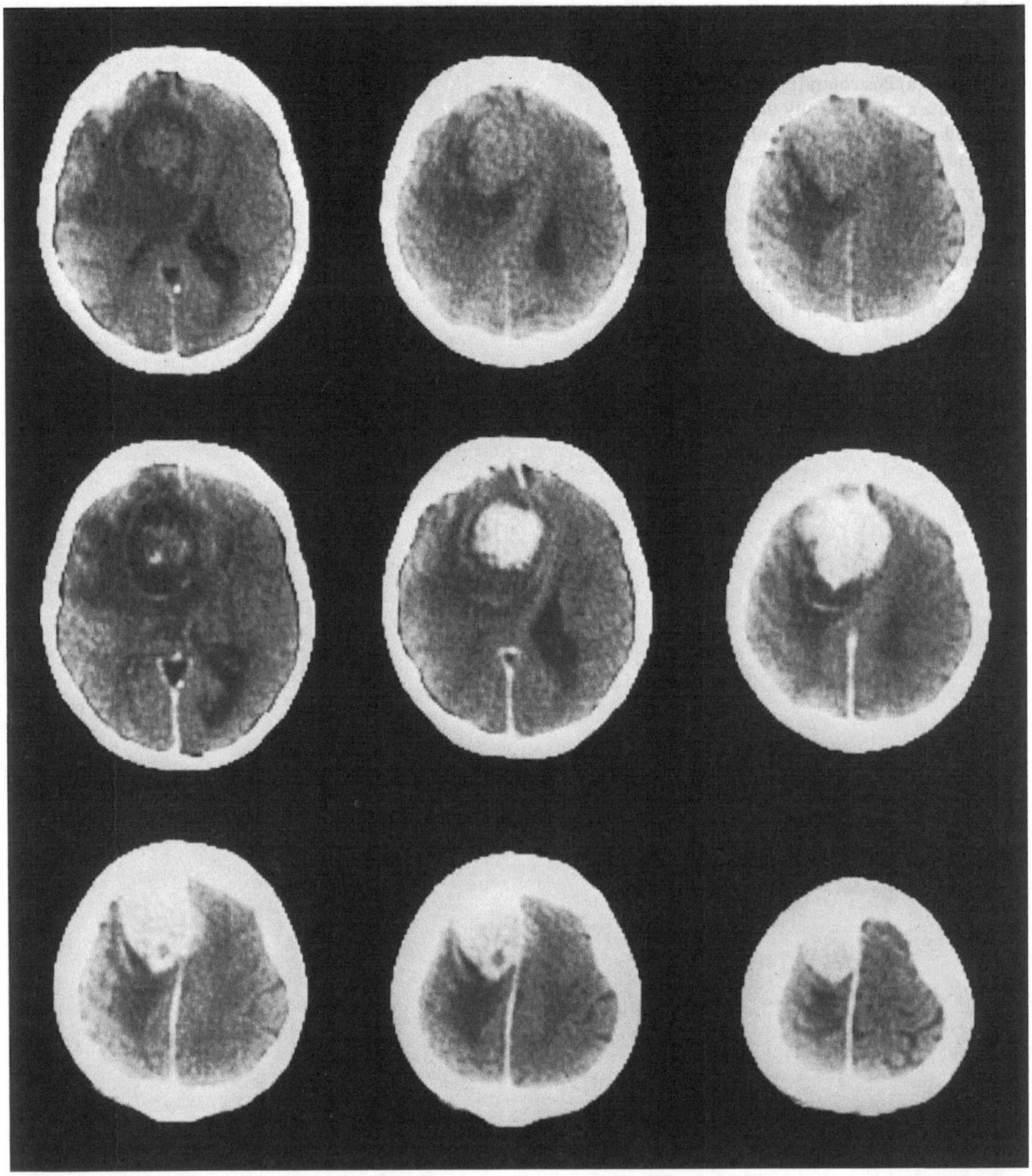

**Fig. D2.16.** Atypical falx meningioma in the anterior third of the superior sagittal sinus in a 67-year-old female. Precontrast studies reveal isodense and hypodense values (upper series). Contrast enhancement shows the true extent of the tumor (middle and lower series). Despite atypical appearance, a diagnosis of meningioma was possible on the basis of location between the vault and the falx cerebri as well as homogeneous contrast medium uptake in the solid portions of the tumor. The rosette figures in the lower segments of the tumor suggest extensive regressive change (middle row, left, and middle). Pronounced displacement of intracranial structures. Grade II to grade III perifocal edema

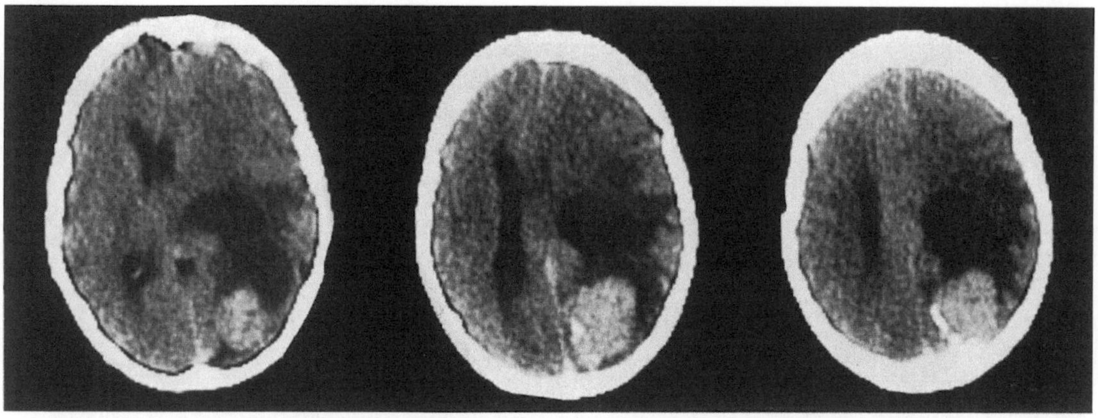

**Fig. D2.17.** Meningioma on the convexity in the occipital region in a 45-year-old man with left homonymous hemianopsia. Solid hyperdense tumor with marginal calcification, hyperostosis of the vault above the lesion, and a sharply demarcated hypodense zone representing a cyst at the anterior margin of the tumor; grade II perifocal edema. Major displacement of midline structures, especially near the septum pellucidum (postcontrast studies)

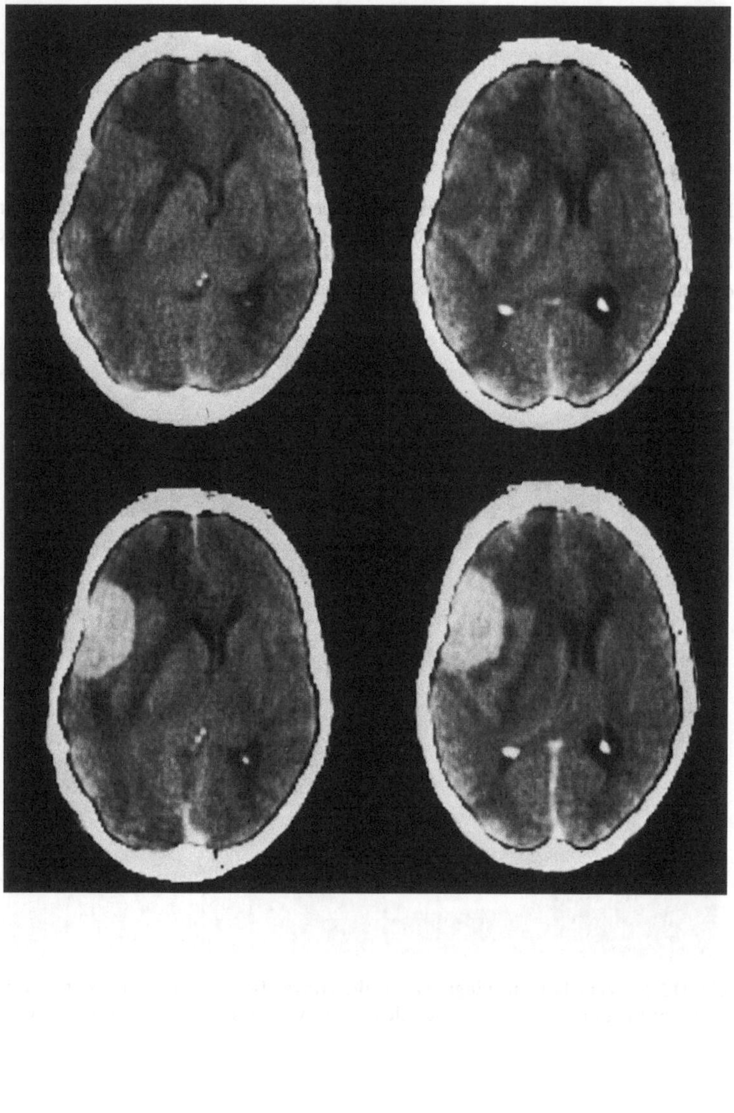

**Fig. D2.18.** Hypodense meningioma of the convexity in the left frontotemporal region. The true extent of the tumor is not evident in precontrast studies despite pronounced perifocal edema (upper series). Contrast enhancement produces findings typical of meningioma (lower series). Thirty-seven-year old male with a 4-year history of psychiatric disorders terminating in dysphasia

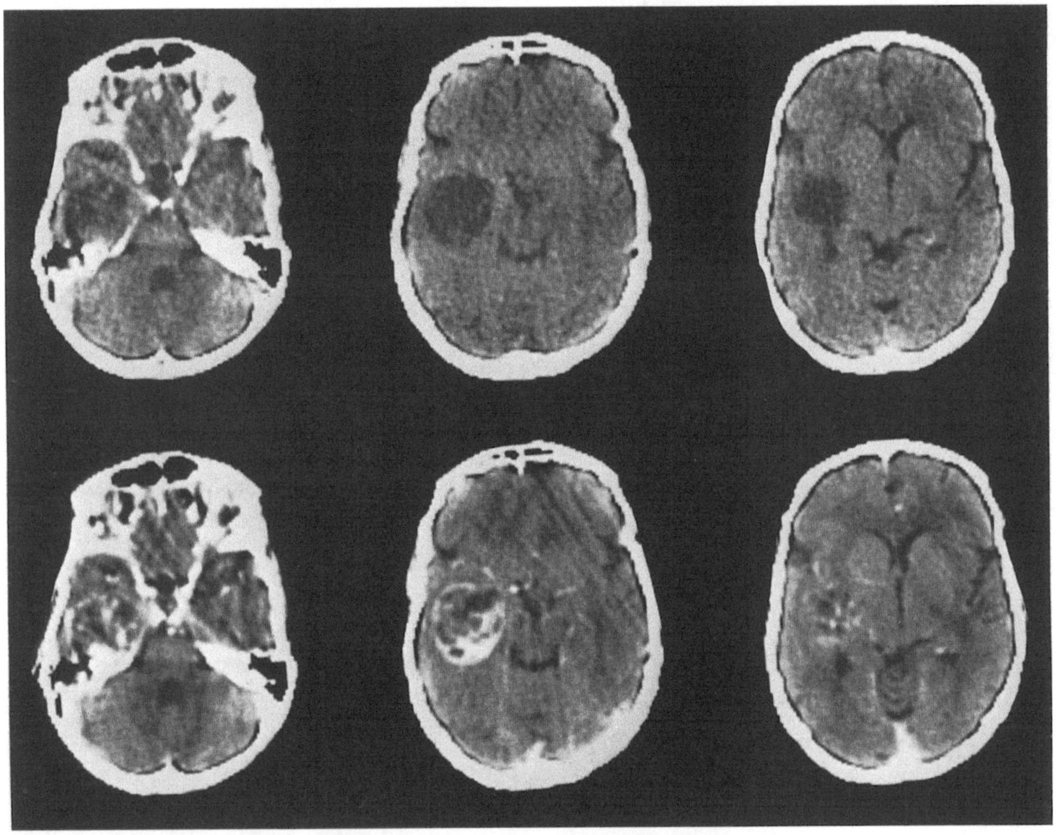

**Fig. D2.19.** Hypodense meningioma at the base of the middle fossa on the left in a 59-year-old male (upper series). Contrast medium administration results in inhomogeneous contrast uptake (lower series). The smooth borders of the tumor suggest meningioma as the most likely diagnosis. Lower density values at the center of the lesion due to regressive change

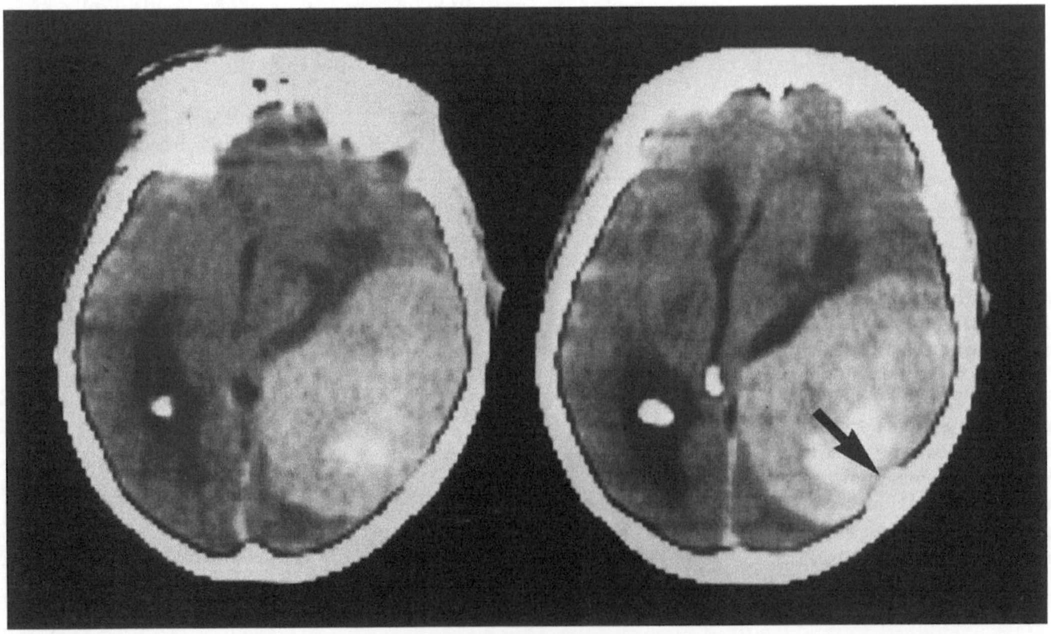

**Fig. D2.20.** Very large meningioma on the convexity in the right temporo-parieto-occipital region with enostosis at the origin of the tumor (arrow). Large calcification within the tumor opposite the enostosis. (Postcontrast studies)

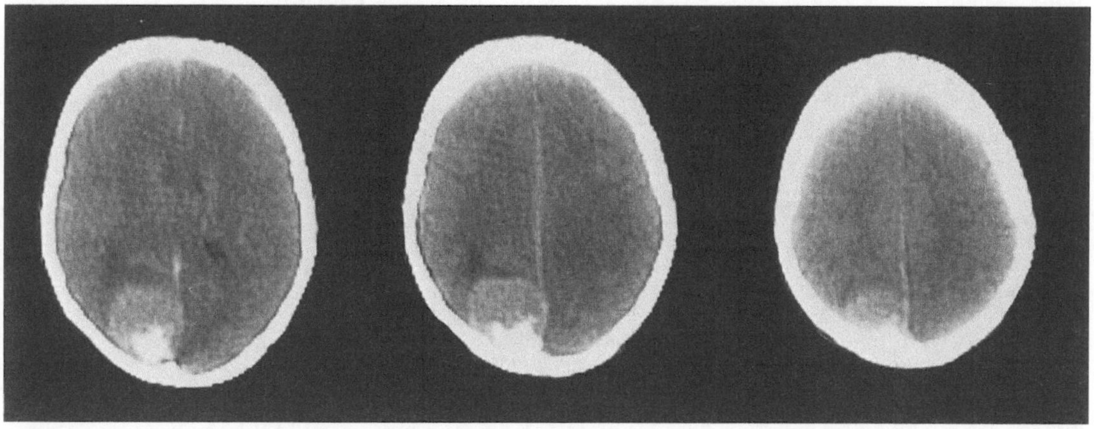

**Fig. D2.21.** Left parasagittal meningioma in the posterior third of the superior sagittal sinus in a 51-year-old female. Marked enostosis of the vault with calcification in the contiguous portions of the tumor. Slight contrast within the meningioma due to wide window (200 HU)

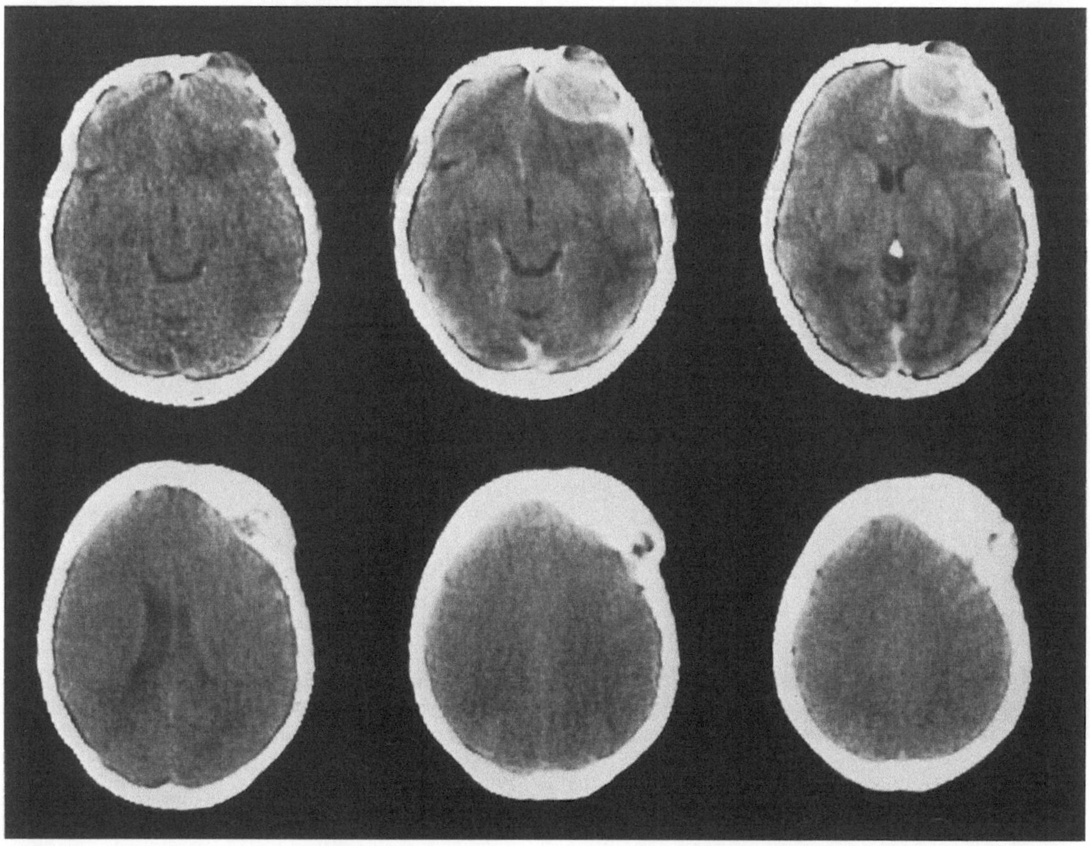

**Fig. D2.22.** Right frontal meningioma with distension of the vault and penetration of bone by soft tumor tissue in the right frontal region. Portions of the tumor extending into the intracranial cavity are only demonstrated after contrast enhancement (upper series, middle, and right). Findings typical of meningioma

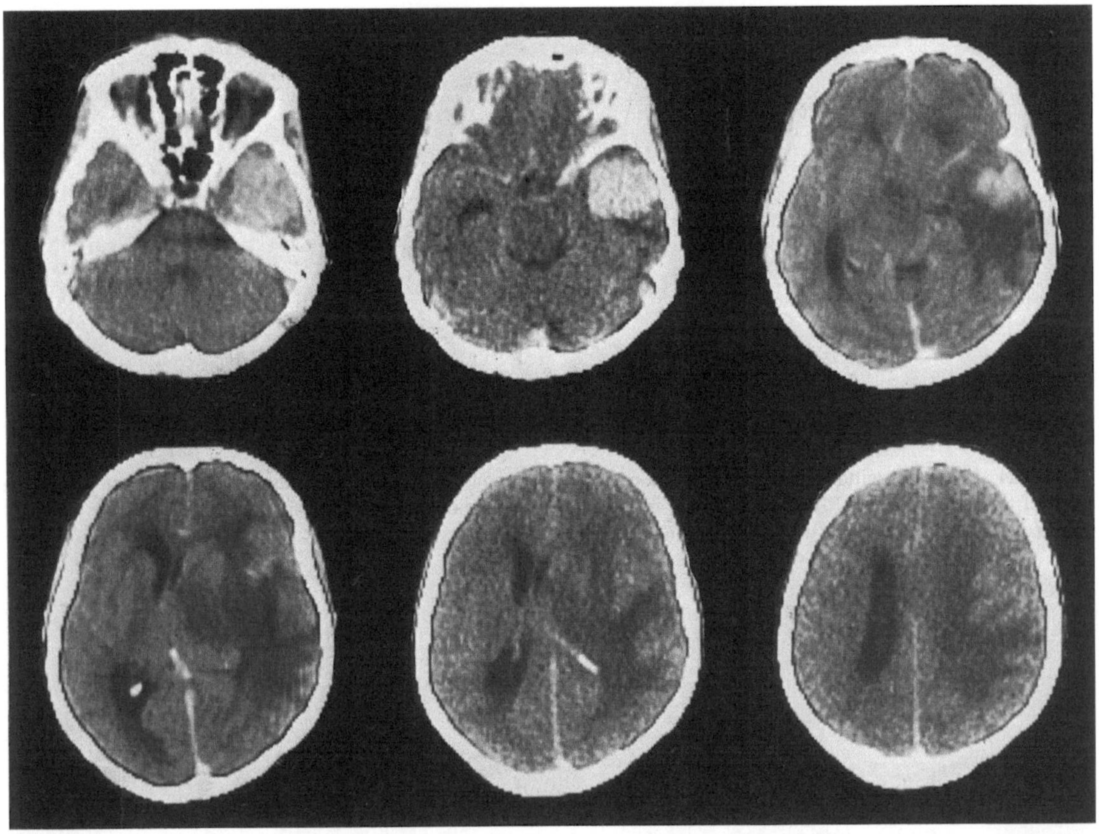

**Fig. D2.23.** Meningioma at the base of the middle fossa on the right in a 59-year-old patient. The tumor itself was not demonstrated in precontrast studies, though edema extending throughout the right cerebral hemisphere suggested the presence of a space-occupying lesion. Findings typical of meningioma with strong homogenous contrast enhancement and direct contact with the base of the skull. Postcontrast studies

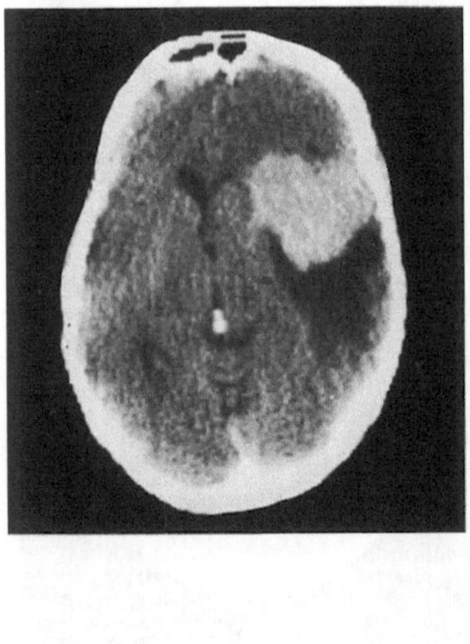

**Fig. D2.24.** Meningioma of the right convexity near the Sylvian fissure in a 46-year-old patient. A large hypodense zone which proved to be the dilated insular cistern delineates the posterior border of the tumor

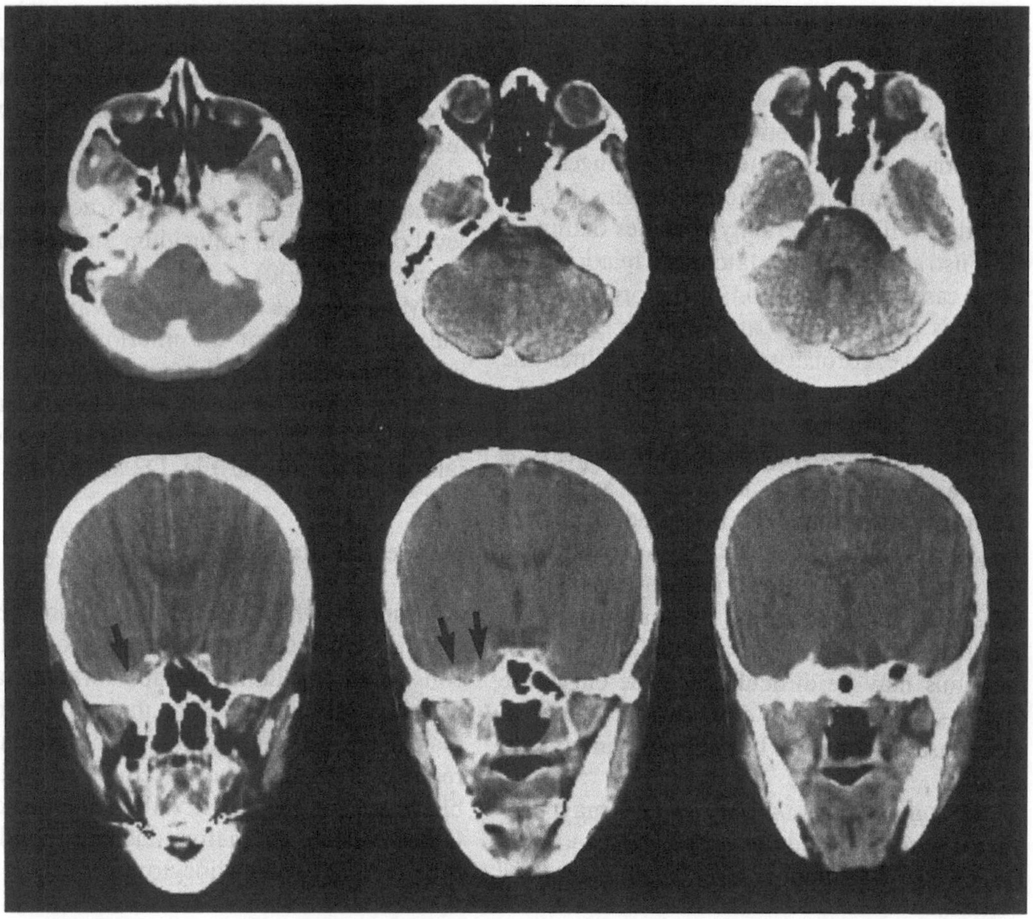

**Fig. D 2.25.** Meningioma with superficial growth (meningioma en plaque) in the middle fossa on the right in a 52-year-old patient. Horizontal scans do not reveal the extent of the tumor (upper series). The tumor is well delineated from the base of the skull in coronary slices (arrows)

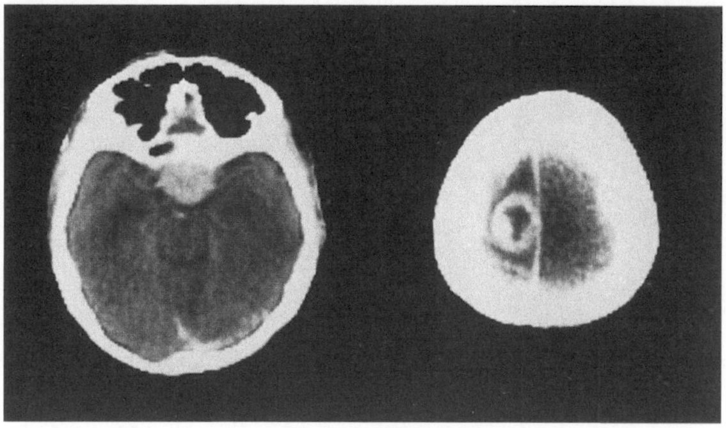

**Fig. D 2.26.** Multiple meningiomas in a 77-year-old female. The meningioma at the tuberculum sellae shows homogeneous contrast enhancement, while the tumor in the left parasagittal region demonstrates a ring figure suggesting a diagnosis of glioblastoma or metastasis. Both tumors proved to be meningiomas at operation

## Meningiomas of the Falx and the Parasagittal Area

CT findings alone are often insufficient for exact differentiation between parasagittal meningiomas which originate in the meninges next to the sinus and meningiomas originating on the falx itself. Angiography provides definitive demonstration of the anatomical relations. In a few cases demonstration of the origin of the tumor is possible only at operation. As mentioned above, coronary scans are sometimes the best means of demonstrating the anatomical relations of the tumor.

*Parasagittal meningiomas* may appear as small as a cherry or as large as an apple and are most often found in the middle third of the sagittal sinus, less often in the anterior third, and rarely in the posterior segment (Figs. D2.27–29). Demonstration of small meningiomas between the anterior and middle thirds of the sinus may be difficult since the curvature of the skull vault may obscure the tumor. In these cases coronary CT studies provide the diagnosis.

*Meningiomas of the falx cerebri* may produce a variety of findings in the CT scan (Figs. D2.30–36). The tumors may be unilateral or bilateral, and small contralateral extensions are easily demonstrated with CT (Fig. D2.31). Symmetrical and bilateral tumor growth is more likely at lower positions on the falx. Tumors originating in the anterior segments of the falx may attain enormous size and cause extreme displacement of brain structures at the level of the septum pellucidum and the anterior horns (Fig. D2.30).

Meningiomas originating low on the falx in the middle third of the inferior sagittal sinus may block CSF circulation and cause hydrocephalus when the tumor attains sufficient size (Figs. D2.35, 36; cf. meningiomas of the tentorial hiatus, p. 240 and Fig. D2.80, p. 248).

### Differential Diagnosis

All tumors which demonstrate homogeneous contrast enhancement in these regions must be considered, including intracerebral metastasis in the parasagittal region, malignant lymphomas, and grade III gliomas. Meningiomas with regressive changes may be confused with glioblastomas or metastases with ring structures. Other possible alternatives include chondroma, tuberculoma, and histiocytoma.

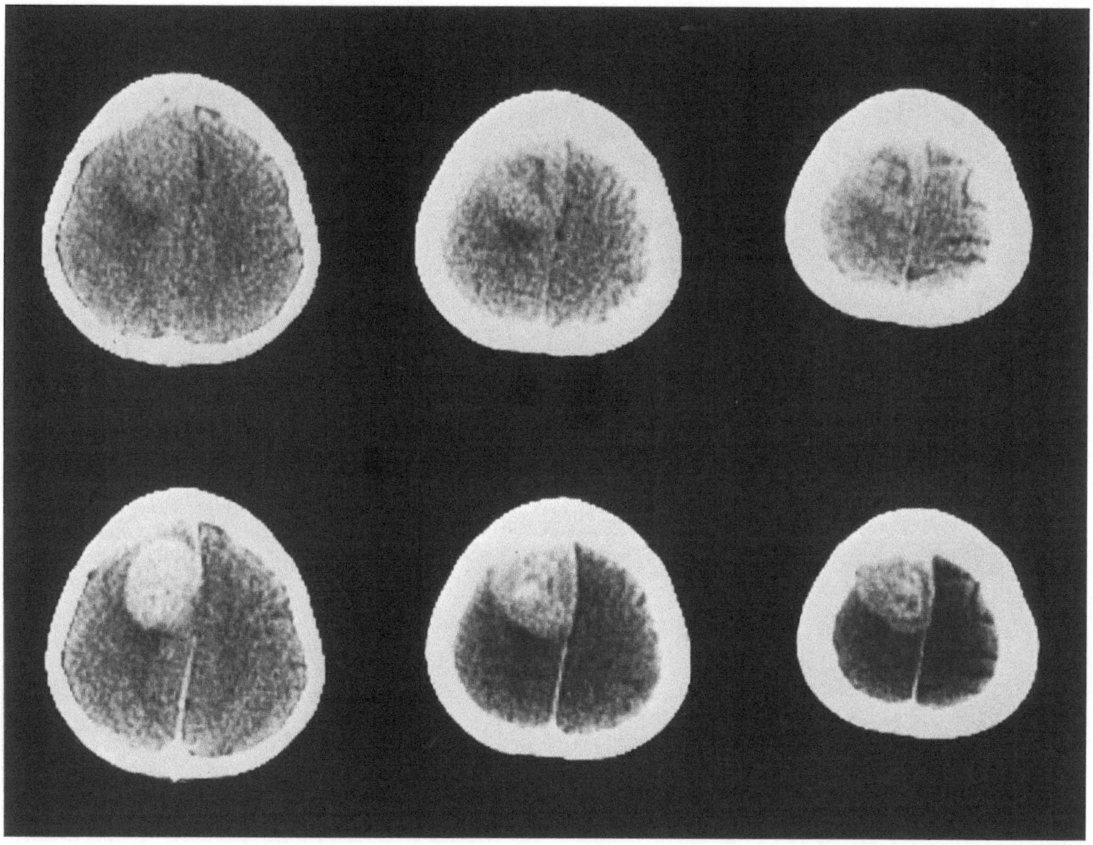

**Fig. D2.27.** Parasagittal meningioma at the junction of the anterior and middle thirds of the superior sagittal sinus in a 58-year-old female. Most of the tumor has slightly hyperdense values with an isodense and hypodense region at its center in precontrast studies (above). Strong contrast enhancement (below). Regressive alterations result in inhomogeneous appearance of the tumor in postcontrast studies. The tumor is in contact with the falx over a wide area. Slight displacement of the falx and minimal perifocal edema. CT studies do not reveal whether the tumor originates in the falx or the dura mater above the convexity in the parasagittal area

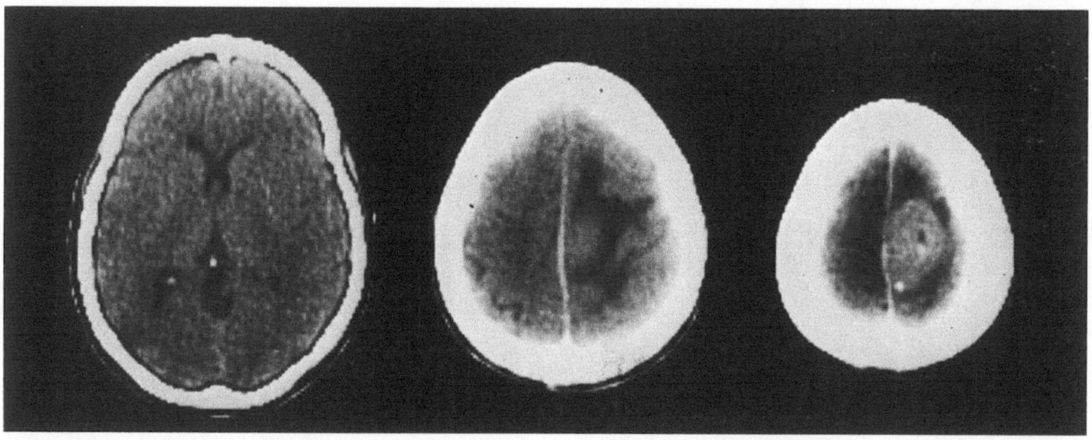

**Fig. D2.28.** Parasagittal meningioma on the right in the middle third of the superior sagittal sinus in a 48-year-old female. Fine calcified specks within the tumor which is surrounded by grade I to grade II edema. No mass effect in the ventricular plane (left)

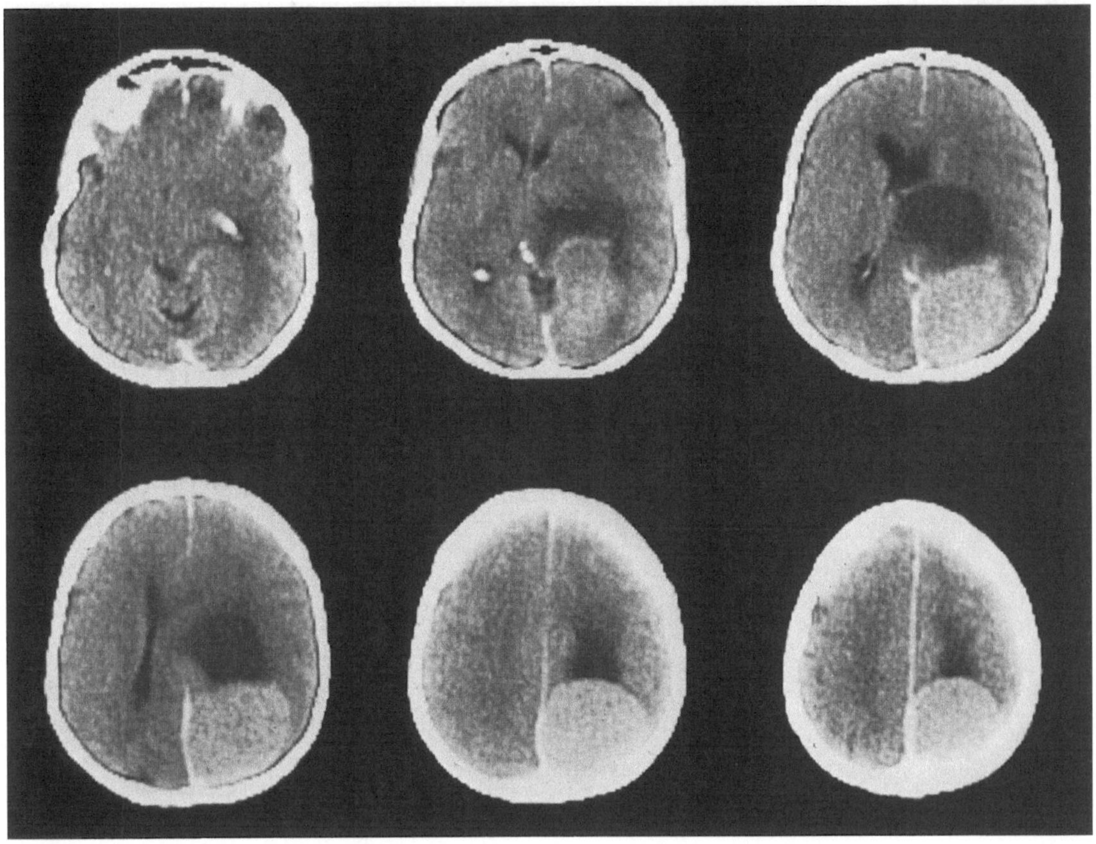

**Fig. D2.29.** Parasagittal meningioma in the posterior third of the superior sagittal sinus on the right in a 67-year-old patient. Large tumor with strong homogeneous contrast medium uptake at the angle of the falx and the convexity. The anterior border of the tumor is formed by a large cyst, demonstrated as a sharply delineated hypodense zone. Slight perifocal edema. Ventral displacement of the choroid plexus in the right lateral ventricle (above left). Postcontrast study

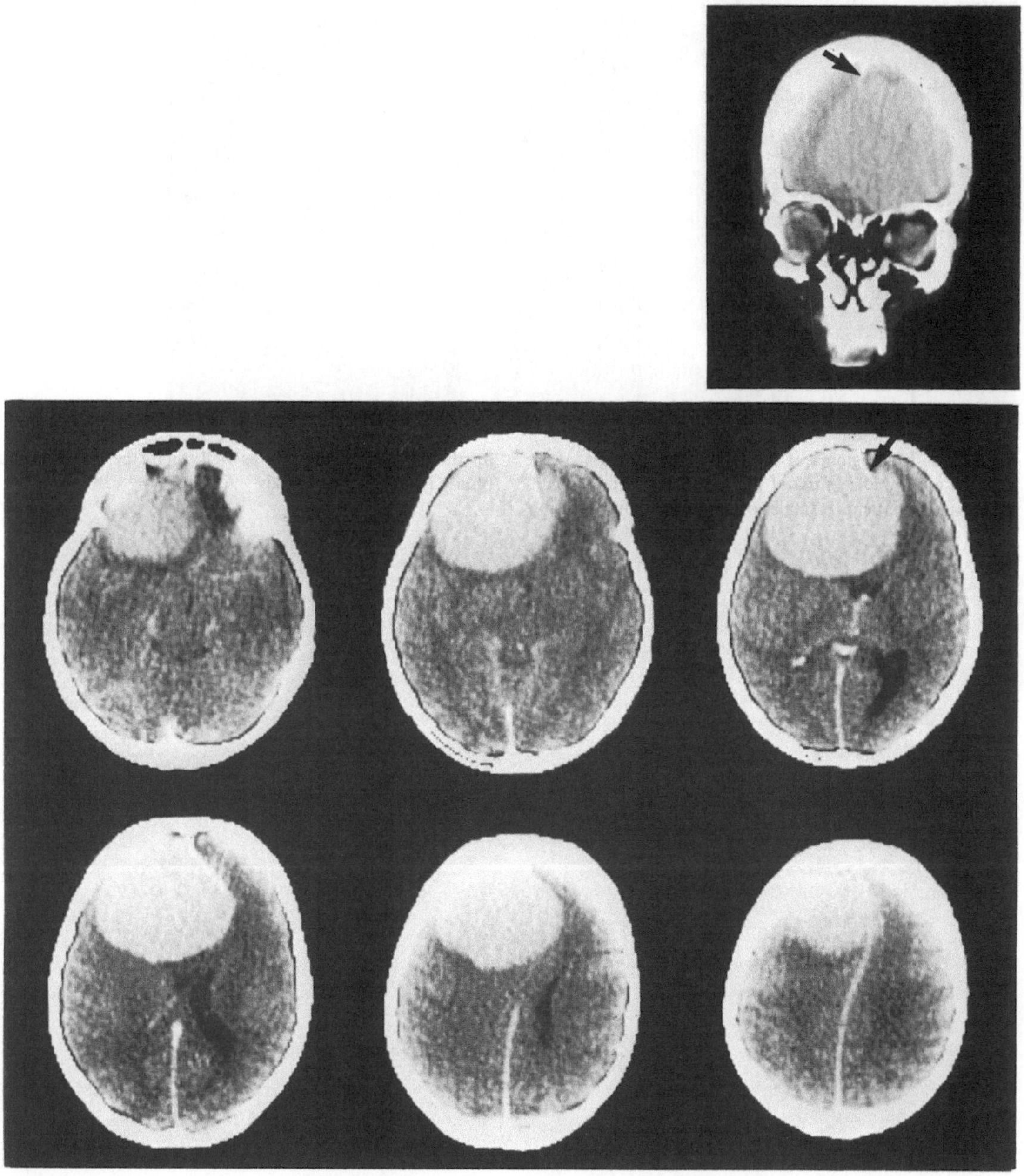

**Fig. D2.30.** Large meningioma originating in the anterior portion of the falx and located primarily in the left frontal region of a 49-year-old female. The tumor demonstrates homogeneous contrast uptake. The anatomical relations to the falx, which appears to be oriented obliquely, are clearly visible (arrow). Coronary slices also show the tumor's relations to the falx (arrow). The lesion also extends to the base of the anterior fossa. Major displacement of the falx to the right in its anterior segment (below right). Postcontrast study

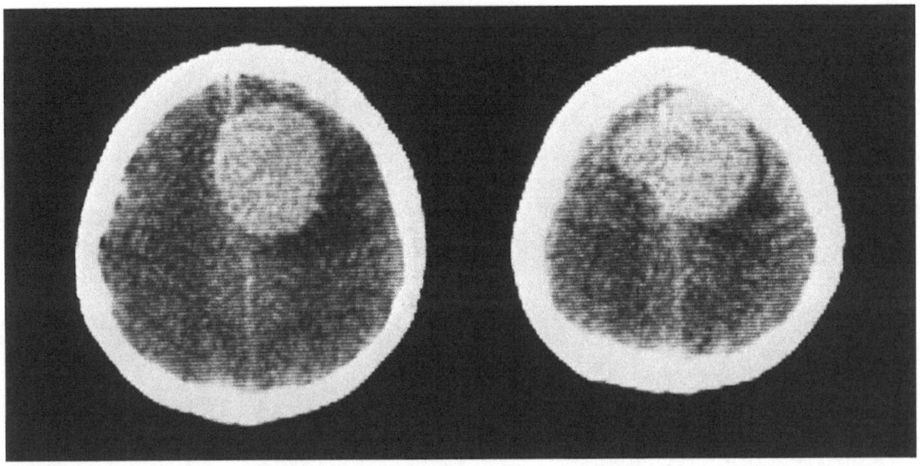

**Fig. D2.31.** Meningioma of the falx at the junction of the anterior and middle thirds of the superior sagittal sinus in a 34-year-old patient. A small portion of the tumor is visible on the left side of the falx as well. Slight perifocal edema (grade I). Postcontrast study

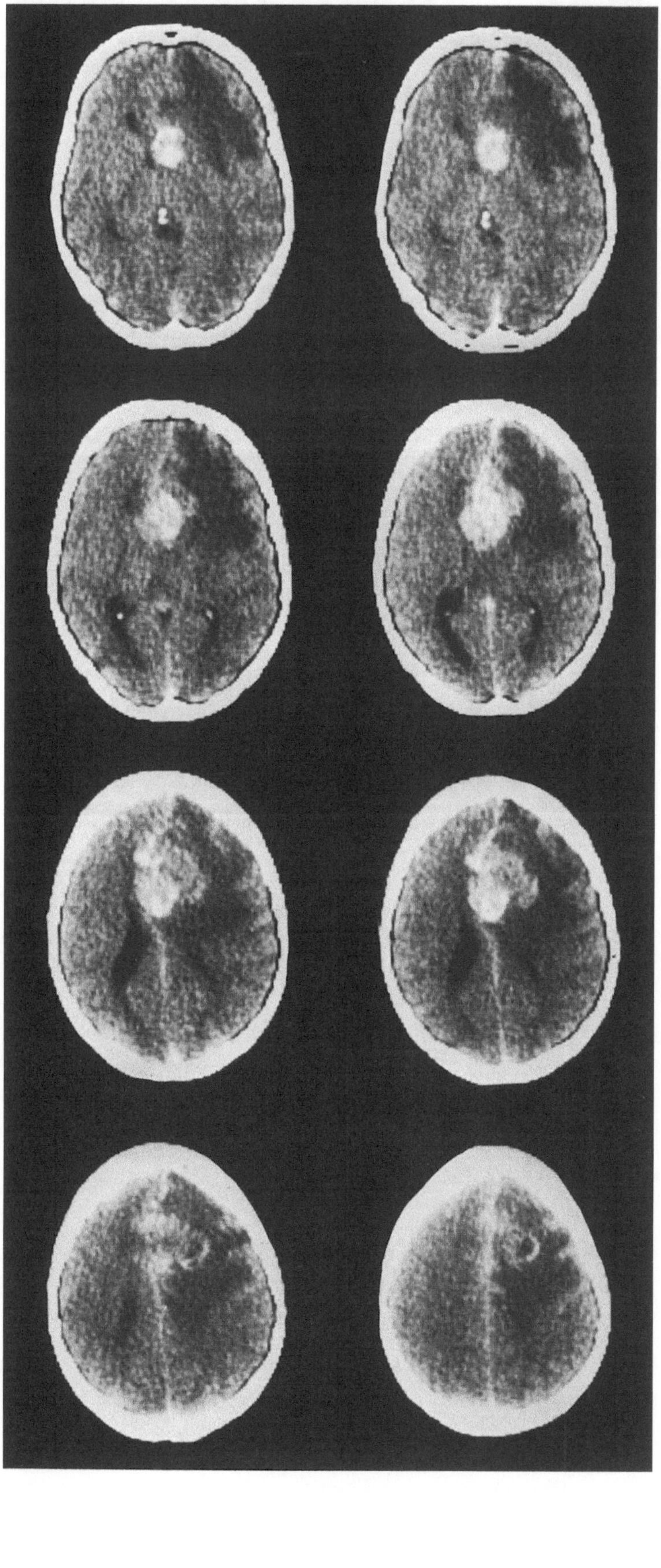

**Fig. D2.32.** Tumor initially diagnosed as atypical meningioma and later as malignant histiocytoma originating at the lower border of the falx. Slight contrast medium uptake in a very inhomogeneous tumor. Extensive perifocal edema (grade II to grade III). Definitive classification of the tumor is not possible on the basis of CT findings. Left, precontrast studies; right, postcontrast studies. Tumor recurrence within 10 months, similar CT appearance. Final histological diagnosis: malignant angioblastic meningioma

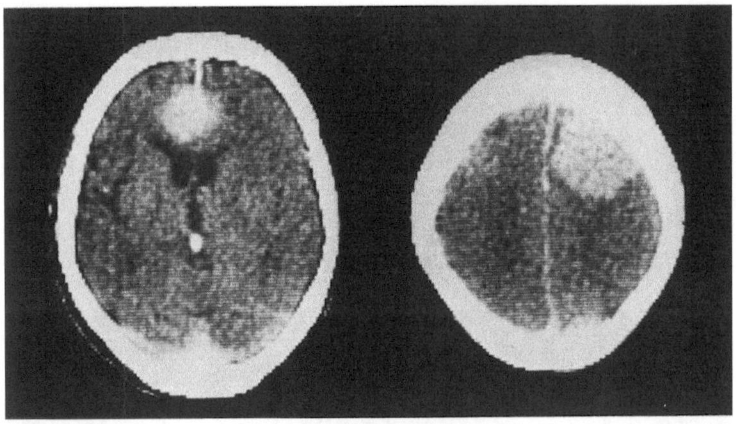

**Fig. D 2.33.** Multiple meningiomas in a 75-year-old patient. Small meningioma at the inferior border of the falx in the anterior third of the sagittal sinus (left). Larger meningioma on the convexity in the right precentral area. Homogeneous contrast enhancement in both tumors. Postcontrast study

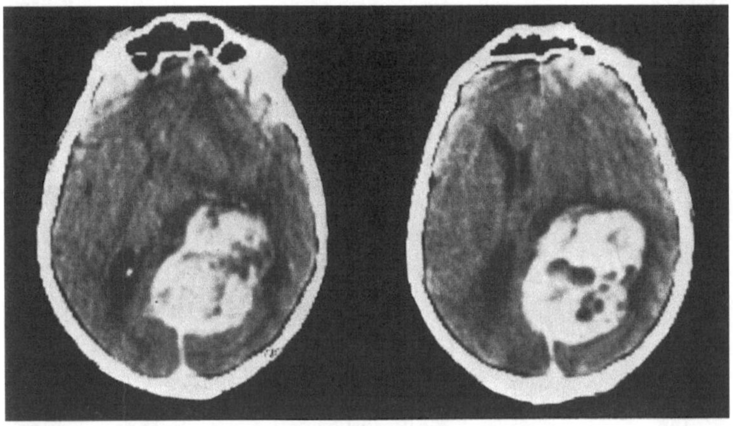

**Fig. D 2.34.** Extremely large meningioma originating at the inferior border of the falx with extension predominantly to the right; typical configuration. Low density zones at the center due to regressive changes. Anatomical relations to the falx clearly demonstrated with CT. Postcontrast study

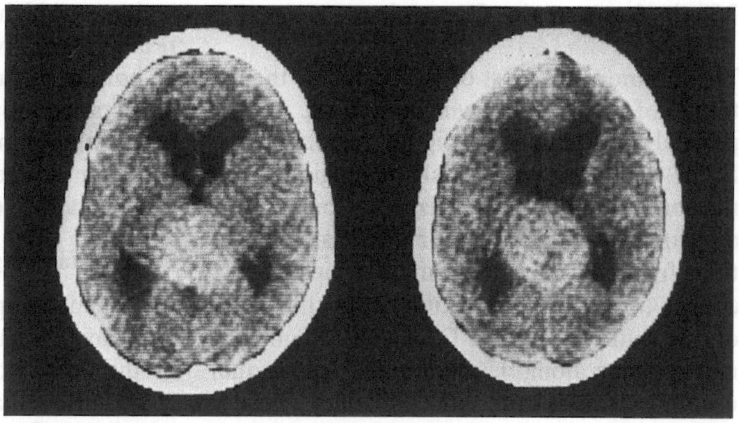

**Fig. D2.35.** Meningioma at the inferior border of the falx in a 47-year-old female. Pronounced dilatation of the lateral ventricles secondary to blockage of the CSF pathways in the third ventricle and the aqueduct (precontrast studies)

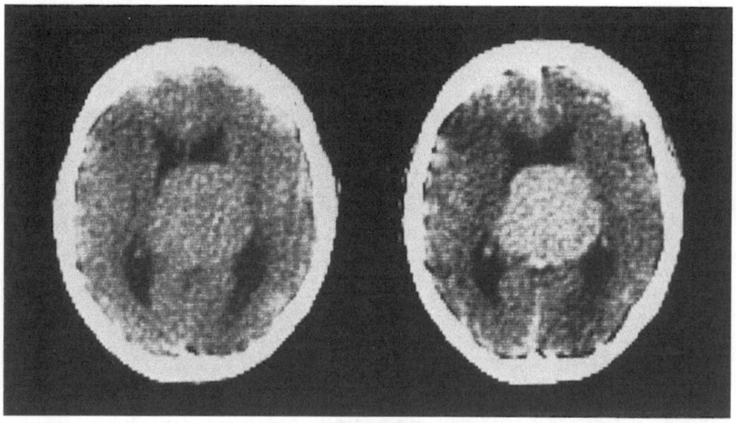

**Fig. D2.36.** Meningioma at the inferior border of the falx at the level of the corpus callosum in a 36-year-old female. Slight dilatation of the lateral ventricles due to compression of the third ventricle from above. Hyperdense attenuation values in precontrast studies (left), strong homogeneous contrast enhancement (right)

## Meningioma at the Convexity

These tumors are most often located at the extremes of the sphenoid wing and in the frontoparietal and temporo-occipital regions (Figs. D2.37–43). Even very small meningiomas on the convexity may cause seizures. Contrast administration is necessary for demonstration of these frequently isodense tumors, which usually appear as hemispherical knots with their base on the skull vault (Figs. D2.44–45). Meningiomas growing along the dura mater (en plaque) usually demonstrate an indistinct border against the convexity and are associated with considerable brain edema (Fig. D2.46). Meningiomas which penetrate the skull vault may result in massive hyperostosis and disruption of bony structures (Fig. D2.47). Simultaneous intracranial growth may also be observed. Coronary studies may demonstrate relations to the tentorium in meningiomas located on the occipital convexity (Fig. D2.49).

### Differential Diagnosis

Malignant lymphomas at superficial locations may have the same appearance as meningiomas of the convexity in CT scans (Figs. D1.206–209). Differentiation between meningioma and a large calcified oligodendroglioma may be difficult in some cases.

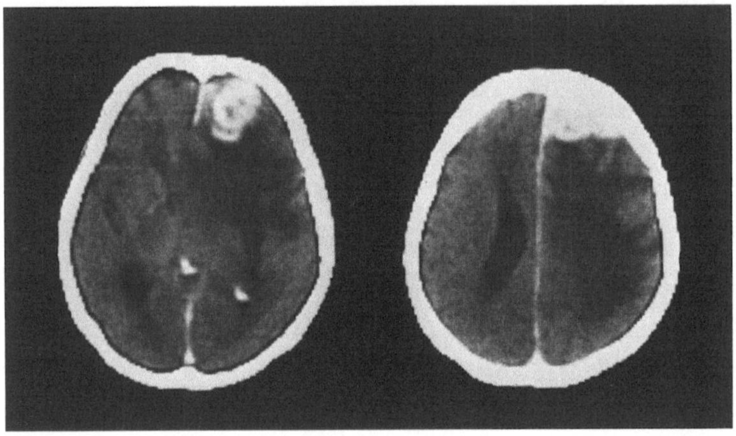

**Fig. D2.37.** Meningioma at the right frontal convexity in a 63-year-old female. Unusually pronounced brain edema (grade III) causing major displacement of midline structures (postcontrast studies)

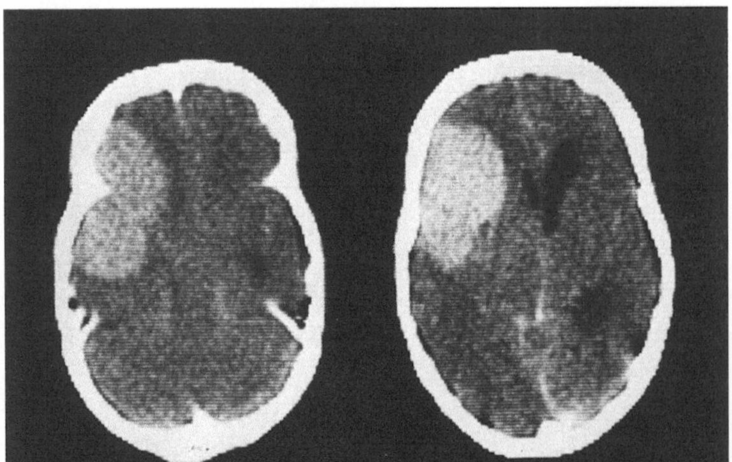

**Fig. D2.38.** Left frontotemporal meningioma at the extremities of the sphenoid wing in a 53-year-old female. Strong homogeneous contrast enhancement in the sharply delineated tumor. No perifocal edema, slight mass effect. Postcontrast study

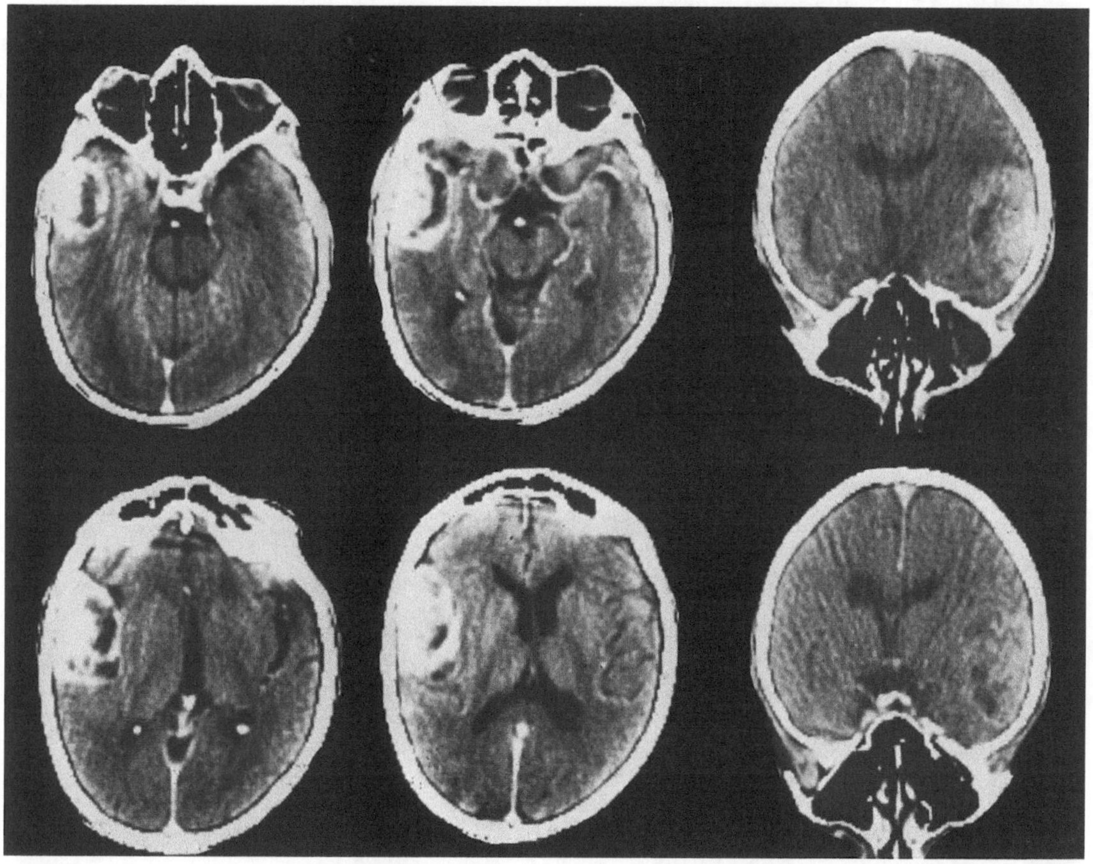

**Fig. D2.39.** Meningioma at the left temporal convexity in a 46-year-old female. Strong contrast uptake in the sharply delineated tumor, which has a marginal defect resulting from regressive change. No perifocal edema and little displacement of midline structures. Narrowing of the ambient cistern on the left due to incipient herniation of the uncus. Coronary slices show the extent of the tumor from cephalad to caudad as well as its relations to the convexity. Postcontrast studies

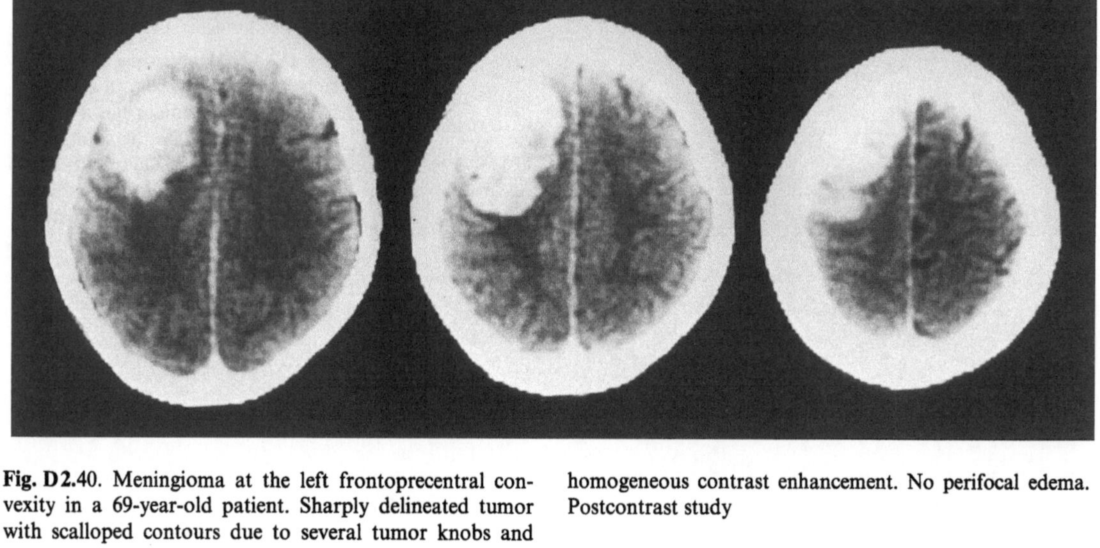

**Fig. D2.40.** Meningioma at the left frontoprecentral convexity in a 69-year-old patient. Sharply delineated tumor with scalloped contours due to several tumor knobs and homogeneous contrast enhancement. No perifocal edema. Postcontrast study

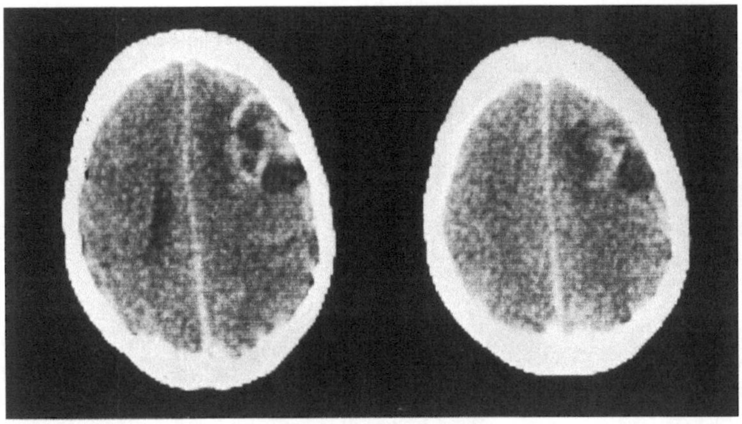

**Fig. D2.41.** Atypical meningioma at the right frontal convexity in a 55-year-old patient. Inhomogeneous density pattern due to extensive regressive change. Initial CT diagnosis of malignant glioma

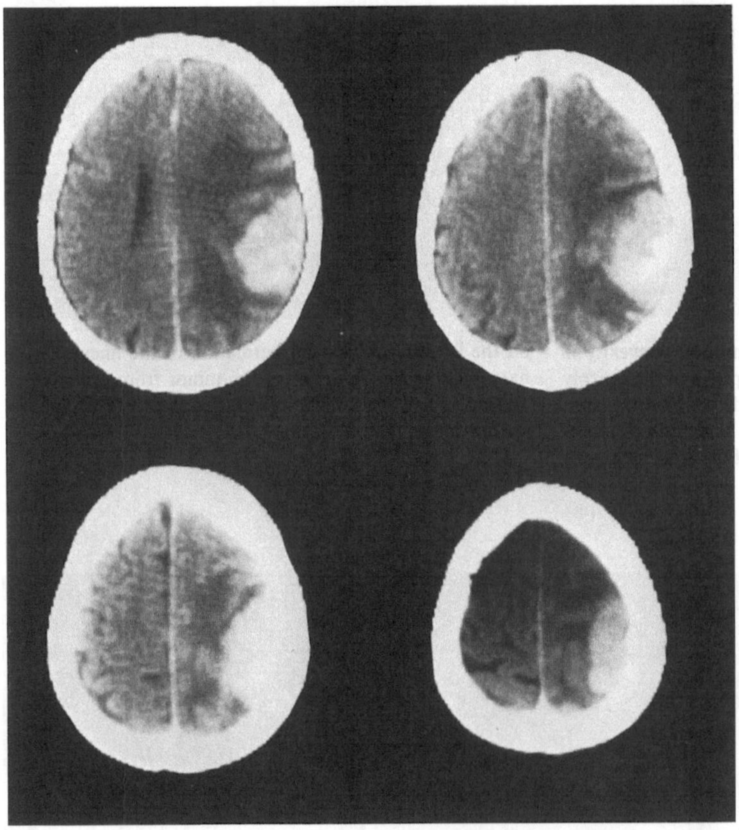

**Fig. D2.42.** Meningioma at the right parietal convexity in a 70-year-old female. The tumor has a large area of contact with the vault. Knobby surface of the tumor, which is well delineated from normal brain tissue by perifocal edema. (Postcontrast study)

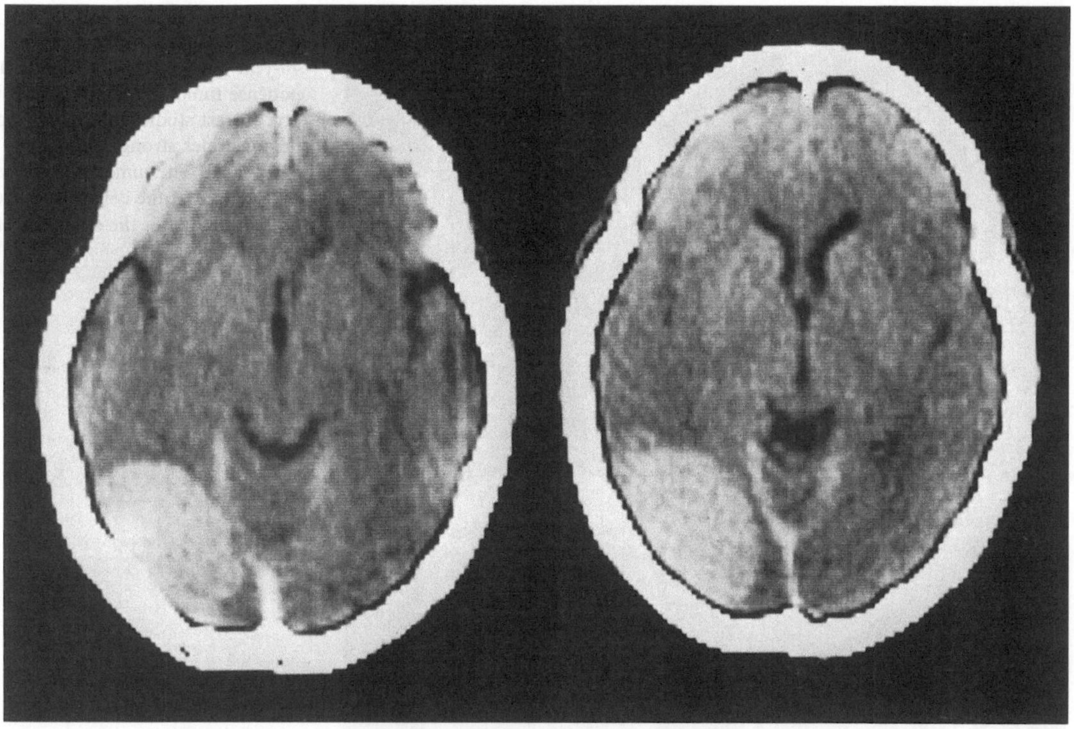

**Fig. D2.43.** Meningioma at the left occipital convexity in a 52-year-old patient. Thickening of the vault above the tumor (left), which excludes the tentorium as a point of origin of the tumor. Postcontrast study

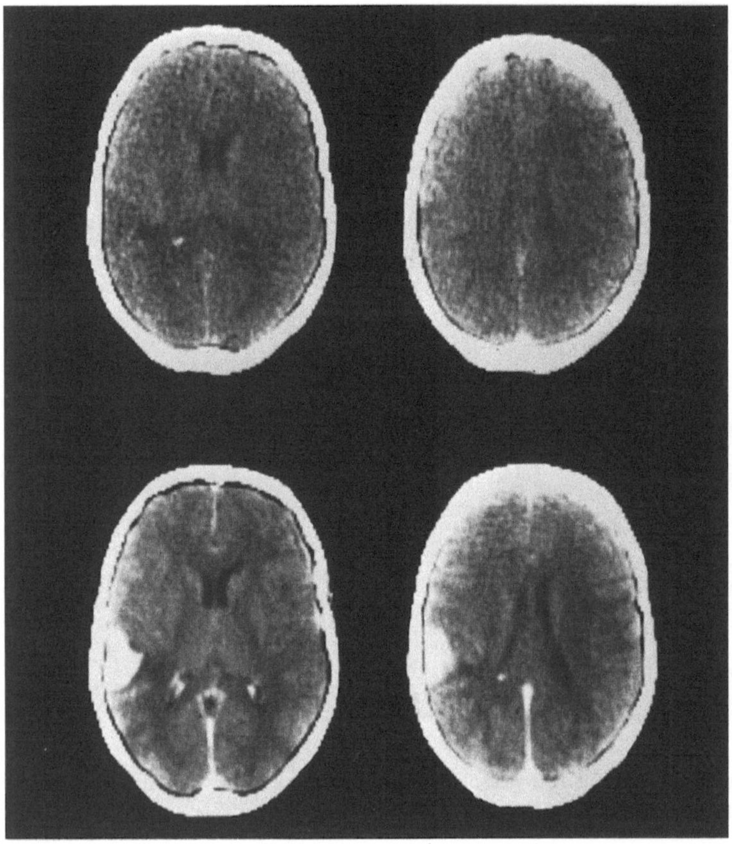

**Fig. D2.44.** Small meningioma at the left temporal convexity in a 40-year-old female. The slightly hypodense tumor is scarcely visible in precontrast studies (above left) and demonstrates strong contrast enhancement. The tumor's broad base on the dura at the convexity leaves little doubt as to the diagnosis of meningioma

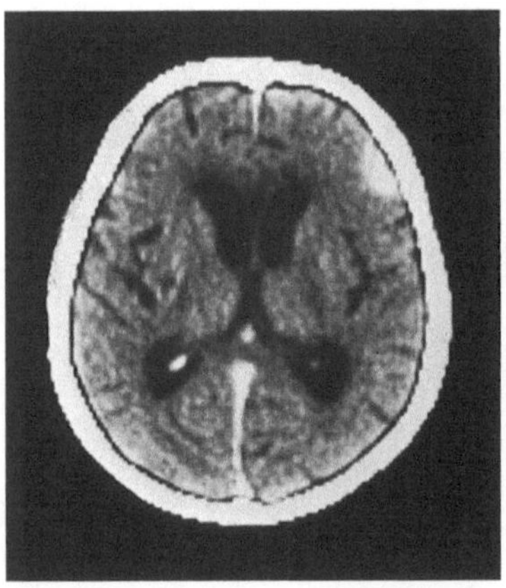

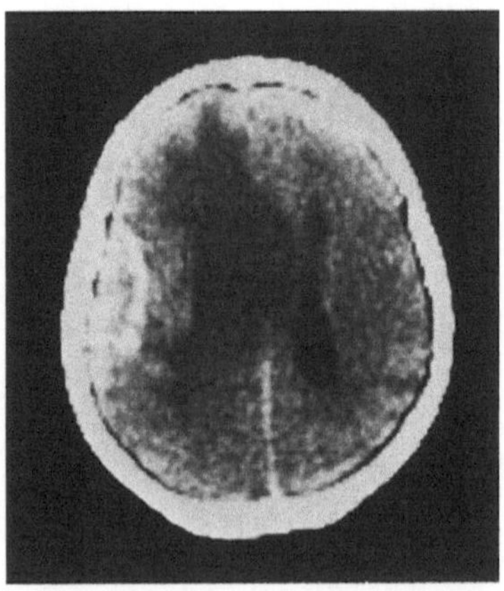

▲ **Fig. D2.45.** Small meningioma at the right frontolateral convexity with no mass effect in a 67-year-old patient. The lesion is demonstrated only with contrast enhancement

▲ **Fig. D2.46.** Meningioma with extensive superficial spread (meningioma en plaque) at the left convexity in a 52-year-old male. The tumor demonstrates laminary calcification and an irregular border against normal brain tissue. Very pronounced brain edema (grade III). Calcification makes a diagnosis of meningioma most likely. Postcontrast study

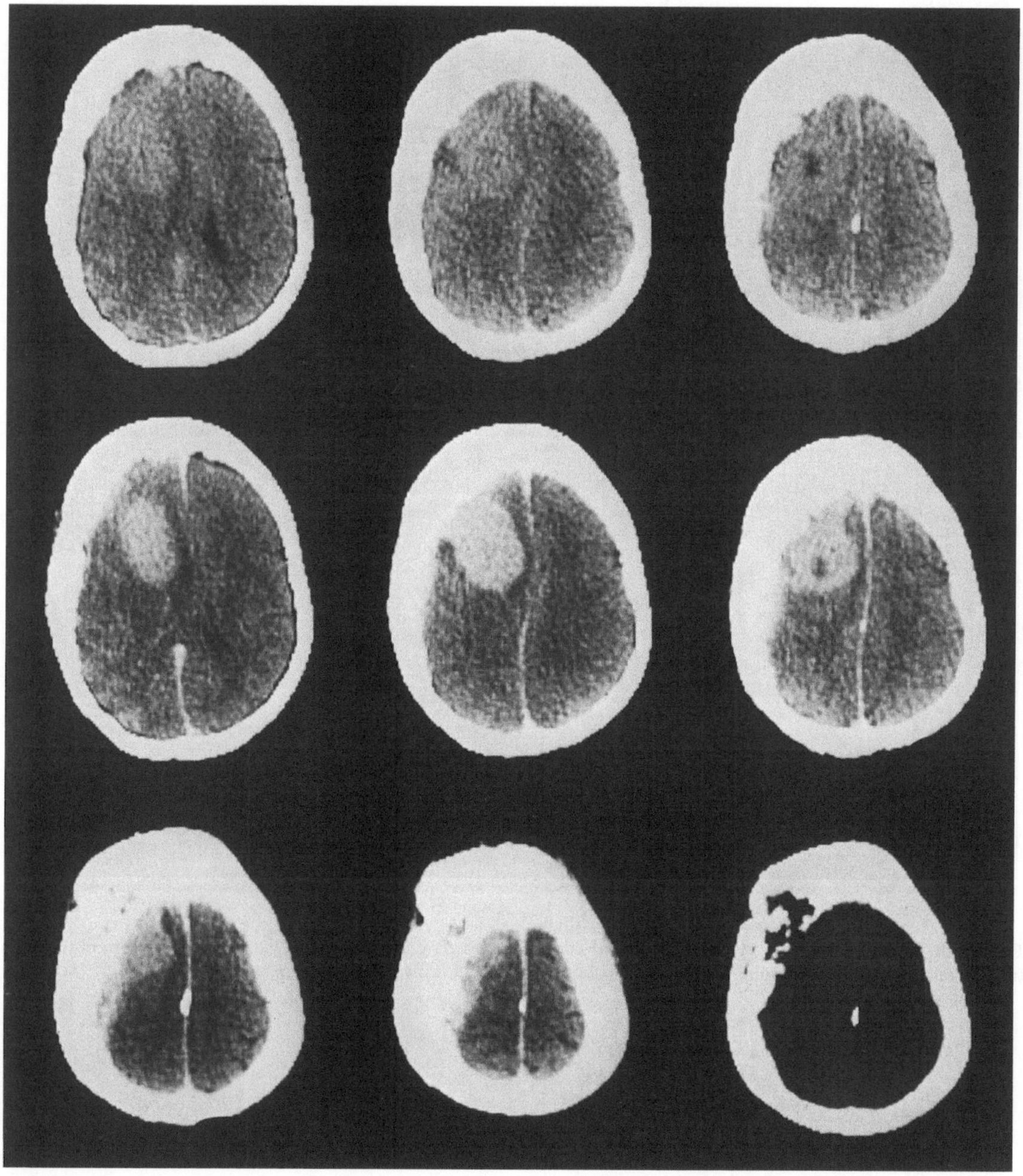

**Fig. D2.47.** Meningioma at the left frontal convexity with involvement of the vault, which is distended over a large area. The intracranial portions of the tumor appear isodense and slightly hyperdense in precontrast studies (upper series) and demonstrate strong contrast enhancement (middle series). Extensive superficial spread of the tumor is evident in higher slices (below left and middle). In addition to osteoplastic growth, bone destruction is present as well, which is demonstrable with appropriate adjustment of the window level. 67-year-old female

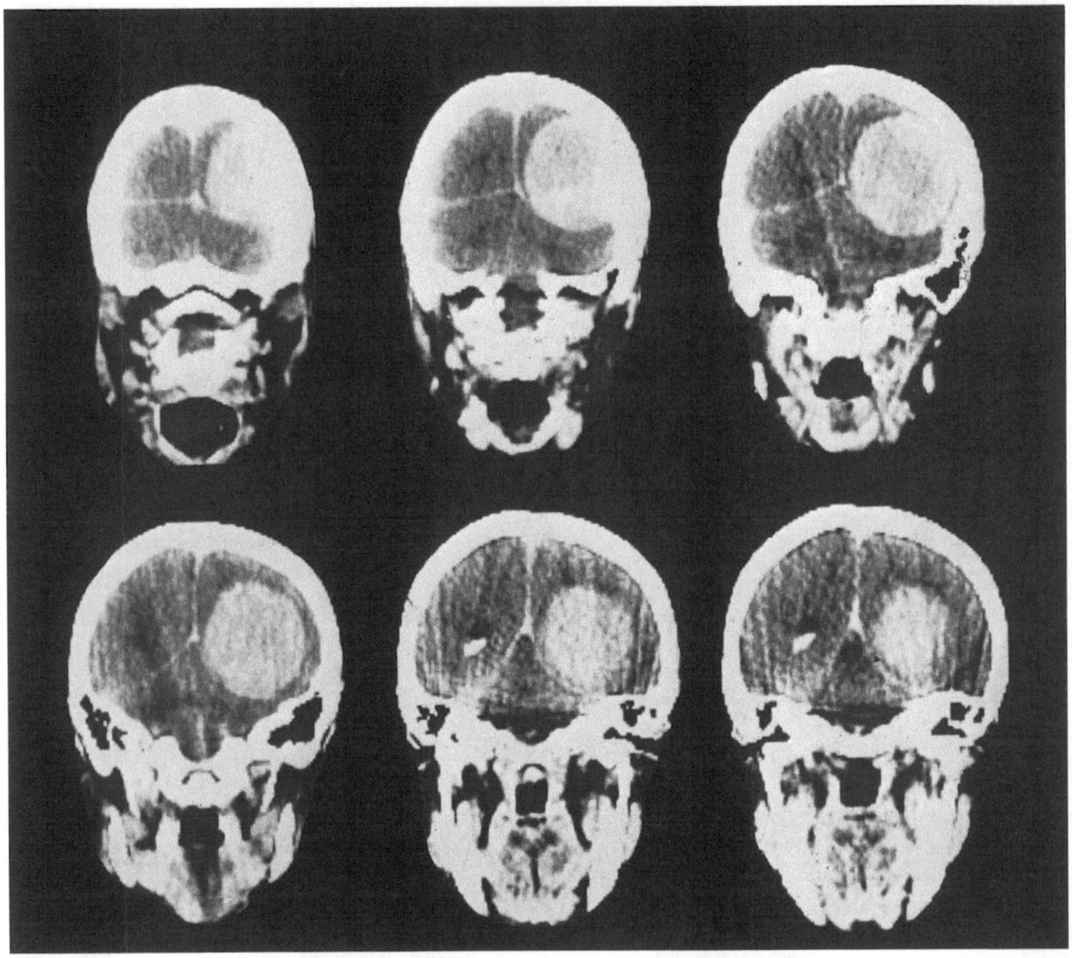

**Fig. D2.48.** Large meningioma at the left occipital convexity in a 65-year-old patient. Coronary slices demonstrate the tumor's relations to the tentorium, which is indented and displaced downward. Postcontrast study

## Meningiomas of the Anterior Cranial Fossa

*Frontobasal meningiomas* have a very characteristic appearance in the CT scan, with round or oval tumor nodules up to the size of an apple accompanied by edema of the white matter in both frontal lobes. Edema is not demonstrated in very large meningiomas of the olfactory groove if the tumor compresses the white matter completely. Coronary CT scans demonstrate the broad attachment of the tumor at the base of the anterior fossa, and thickening of the sphenoid plane is often visible. The tumor may sometimes extend to the ethmoid sinuses, and calcification is common (Figs. D2.3, 49). Unilateral meningiomas in the frontobasal region originate in the meninges (arachnoid mater) at the base of the skull next to the olfactory groove or above the roof of the orbit (Figs. D2.51, 52).

*Suprasellar meningiomas* appear in the CT picture within the opticochiasmatic cistern and extend toward the front (Fig. D2.53).

Large tumors may cause blockage of the foramina of Monro or show extension to the retrosellar region (Figs. D2.54, 55). These meningiomas usually originate near the tuberculum sellae or on the sphenoid plane. Tumors originating on the dorsum sellae extend to the suprasellar region and the clivus (Fig. D2.54).

### Differential Diagnosis

Meningiomas of the olfactory groove present no problems in differential diagnosis.

Suprasellar meningiomas may be misinterpreted as pituitary adenomas in the CT scan. Conventional radiological studies of the sella and evidence of endocrine disorders provide certain differentiation between the two (see Fig. D4.30, p. 285). Other tumors found in this region may occasionally have the same appearance as meningioma in the CT scan. Large aneurysms in the suprasellar region usually demonstrate intramural calcification and/or very intense contrast enhancement (Figs. F60, 61, p. 443, 444).

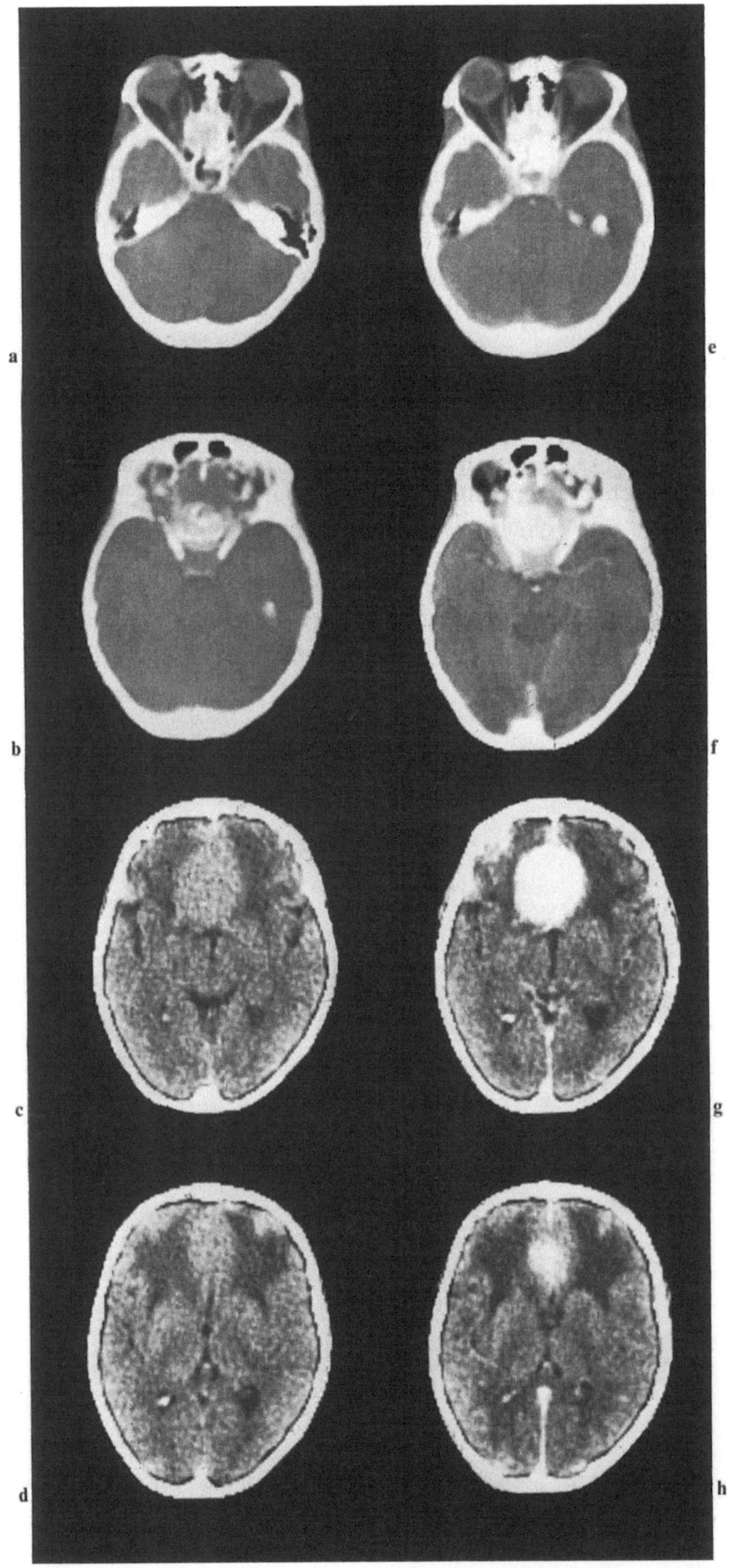


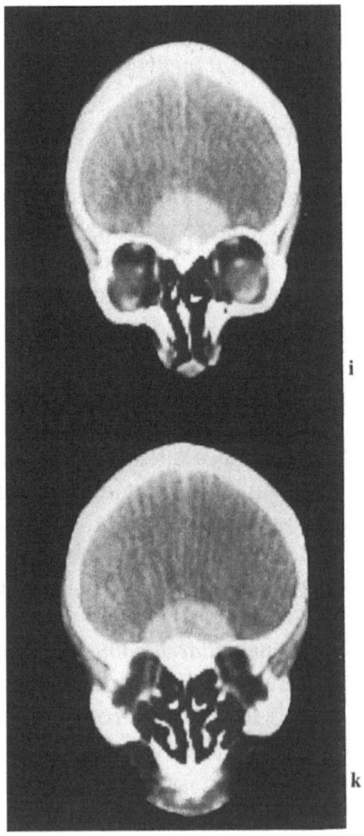


**Fig. D2.**49 a–k. Olfactory groove meningioma in a 62-year-old patient. Precontrast studies demonstrate partial calcification in the basal portions (**a, b**) and isodense and slightly hyperdense attenuation values in the rest of the tumor (**c, d**). Strong contrast enhancement in the solid portions of the tumor (**f–h**). Characteristic bilateral edema in the white matter of the frontal lobes. Origin of the tumor in the olfactory groove is evident in both horizontal and coronary projections. Pronounced thickening of the sphenoid plane (**k**)

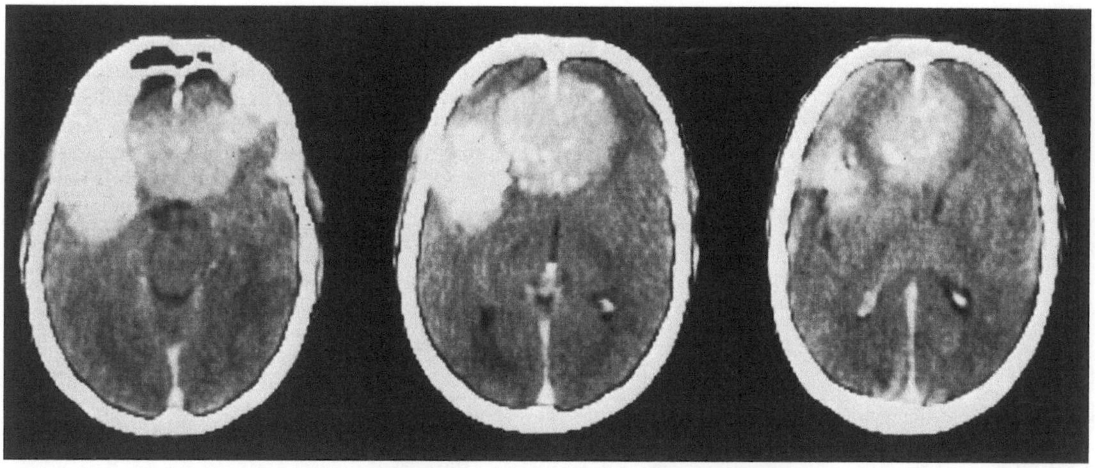

**Fig. D2.50.** Multiple partially calcified meningiomas. Large frontobasal meningioma in the midline with numerous calcified flecks, demonstrating contact with the falx. Immediately adjacent on the left is a highly calcified meningioma originating in the sphenoid wing. The anterior horns are compressed with dorsal and slight right lateral displacement. Postcontrast study

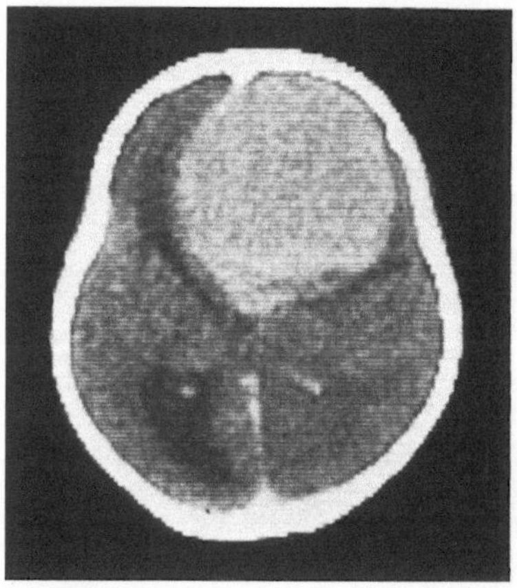

▲

**Fig. D2.51.** Giant frontal meningioma originating in the anterior fossa on the right in a 72-year-old female. Sharply delineated tumor with homogeneous contrast enhancement, typical of meningioma

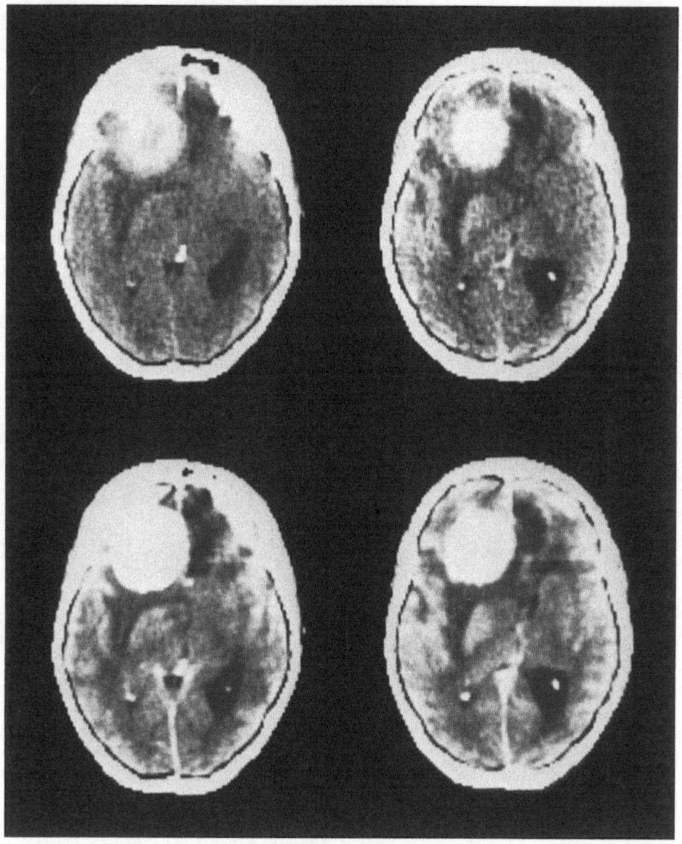

▲

**Fig. D2.52.** Meningioma in the left frontobasal region with extensive calcification (above, precontrast study). Contrast enhancement reveals the full extent of the tumor (below). Significant displacement of the ventricular system to the right in the region of the septum pellucidum. The edema has the typical funnel configuration. Dilatation of the right occipital horn secondary to midline shift with blockage of the CSF passages

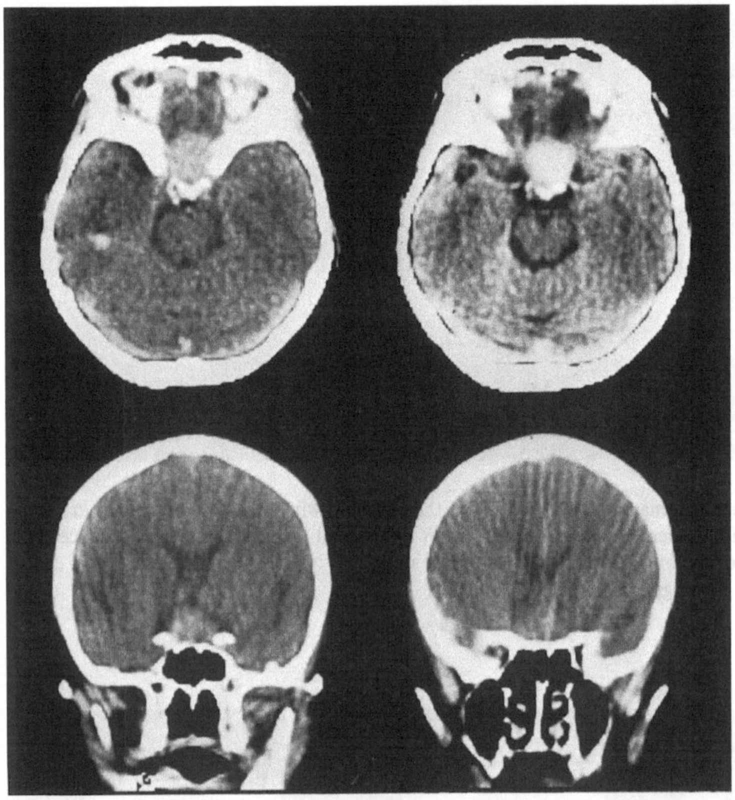

**Fig. D2.53.** Meningioma of the tuberculum sellae in a 59-year-old female. The tumor appears hyperdense in precontrast studies (above left) and demonstrates a further increase in density with contrast enhancement (above right). The CT findings are similar to those in pituitary adenoma. The chiasmatic cistern is almost completely filled with tumor. Coronary slices show that the tumor has a broad base on the sphenoid plane (below)

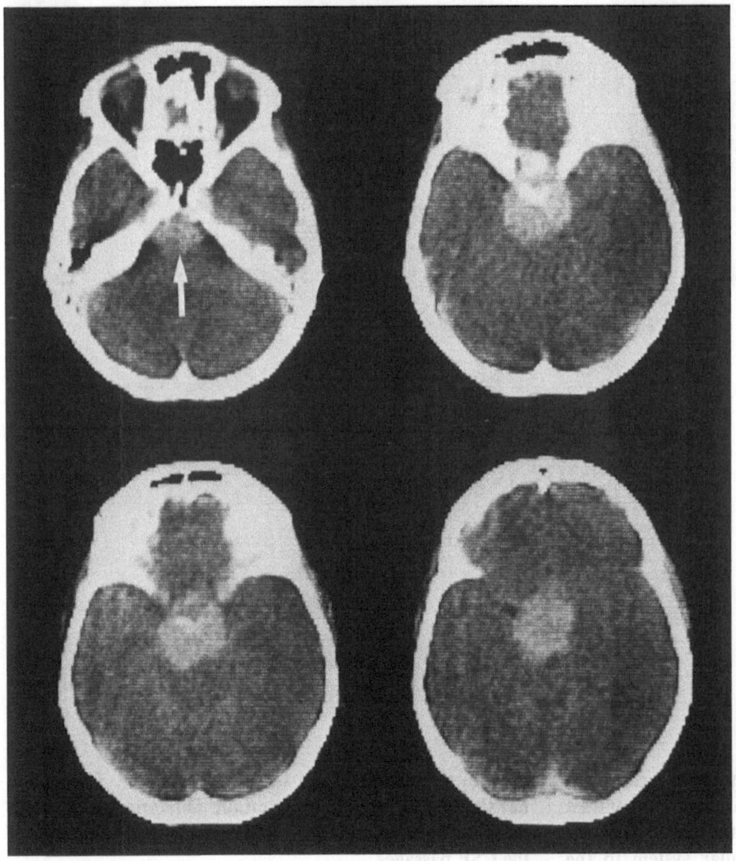

**Fig. D2.54.** Suprasellar meningioma in a 55-year-old female. The tumor originates on the dorsum sellae and extends to the suprasellar region and the posterior fossa along the clivus (arrow). Postcontrast study

**Fig. D2.55.** Recurrence of suprasellar meningioma with extension in both the retrosellar and suprasellar regions, resulting in blockage of the foramina of Monro. This has caused hydrocephalus, more pronounced on the left, as well as periventricular lucency at the anterior and posterior horns on the left. Postcontrast study

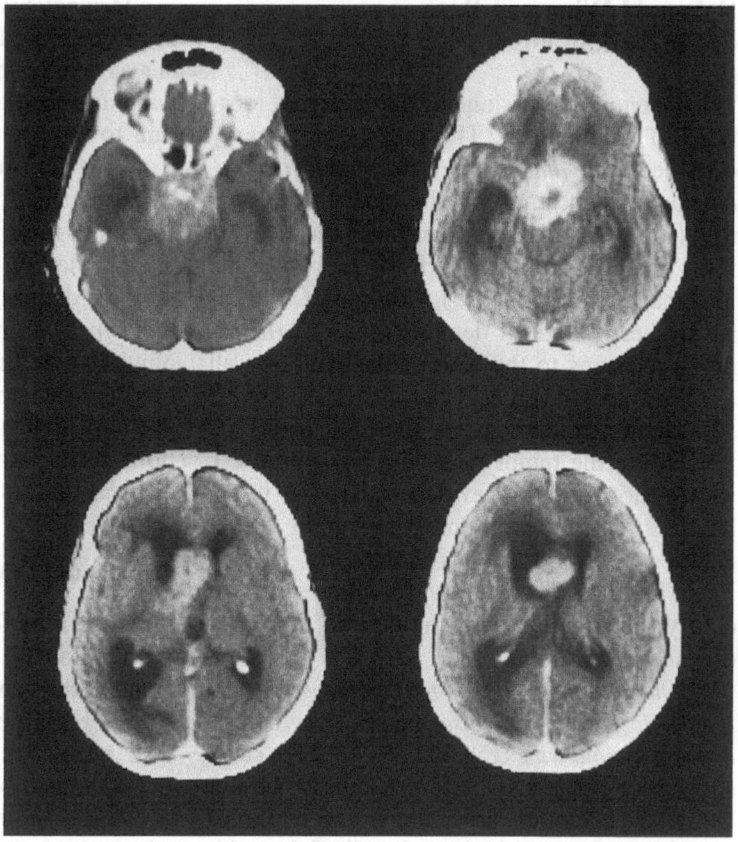

## Sphenoid Wing and Base of the Middle Fossa

The sphenoid ridge is one of the preferred locations of meningioma. The tumors are usually classified as *medial or lateral sphenoid wing meningiomas,* depending on the origin of the tumor (Figs. D2.56–61). Extension to the anterior fossa and even to the posterior fossa is possible in some cases (Fig. D2.59). Coronary CT studies are best suited for demonstration of the tumor's relations to the base of the skull as well as of medial and vertical extension (Figs. D2.57, 59). Demonstration of the internal carotid artery within the tumor mass in a horizontal CT slice is not definitive evidence that the vessel has been entirely surrounded by tumor tissue, as our own experience has shown (Fig. D2.58). Even angiographic studies sometimes fail to clarify the situation with the desired degree of diagnostic certainty.

*Sphenoid meningiomas may demonstrate osteoplastic growth and cause extreme hyperostosis of the sphenoid wing* (Fig. D2.10). In these cases soft tumor tissue may be found anterior to and below the temporal pole, under the temporal muscles, and along the lateral wall of the orbit (Fig. G4, p. 468). Portions of meningiomas with superficial (en plaque) growth may escape CT detection.

*Meningiomas at the base of the middle fossa* are rare (Figs. D2.19, 23). Tumors near Meckel's cave may spread anteriorly to the sphenoid wing and medially over the edge of the tentorium to the brain stem and the posterior fossa. Contrast CT studies show very strong contrast enhancement at the ipsilateral border of the tentorium in these cases (Figs. D2.62, 63).

Painstaking evaluation of CT scans is necessary for demonstration of small *parasellar meningiomas* near the base of the skull (meningioma of the cavernous sinus) since these tumors often spread along the inner surface of the dura mater. Coronary and orbital projections have proved valuable in demonstration of these tumors (Figs. D2.25, 64).

### Differential Diagnosis

Other tumors found in the region include noncystic pilocytic astrocytoma of the medial portion of the temporal lobe. Neurinoma of the third cranial nerve and gangliocytoma must also be excluded. A partially calcified chondroma may also simulate a basal meningioma.

*Large carotid aneurysms may resemble meningiomas in CT scans* (Fig. F64, p. 445). Partial thrombosis of such an aneurysm results in a characteristic target pattern in CT studies (Fig. F67, p. 446).

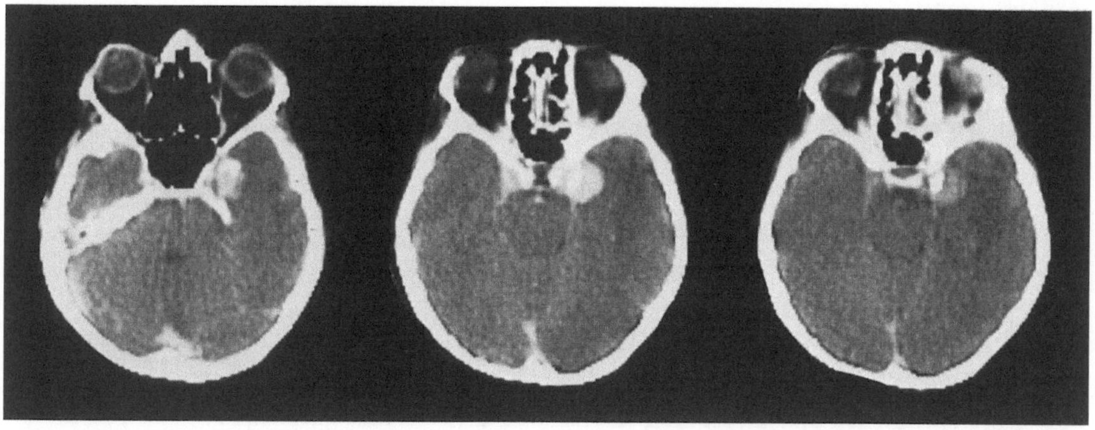

**Fig. D2.56.** Small medial sphenoid wing meningioma on the right in a 57-year-old female. The tumor is slightly hyperdense in precontrast studies and demonstrates very strong contrast enhancement. CT studies do not reveal the tumor's relations to the internal carotid artery. Perifocal edema in the right temporal lobe. Postcontrast study

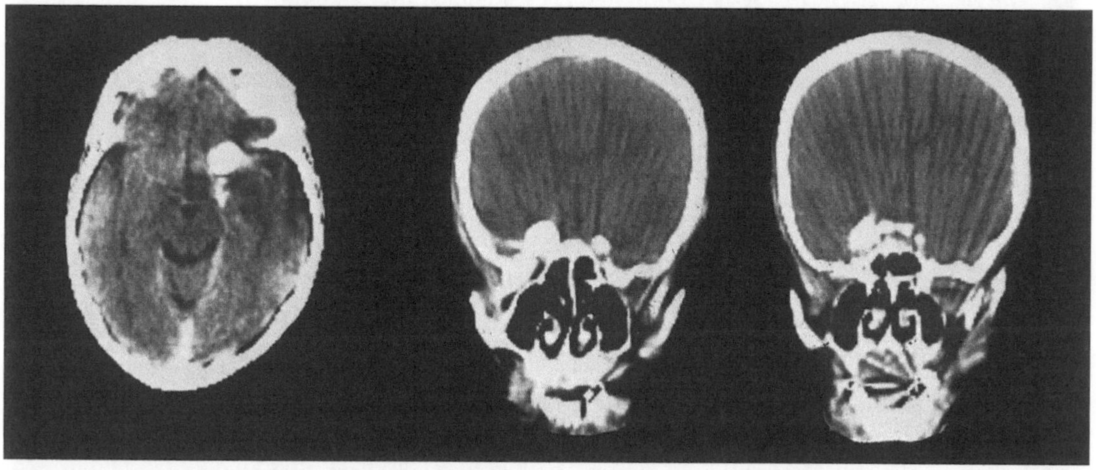

**Fig. D2.57.** Small calcified meningioma located medially on the sphenoid wing in a 70-year-old patient, demonstrated in both horizontal and coronary projections. Postcontrast study

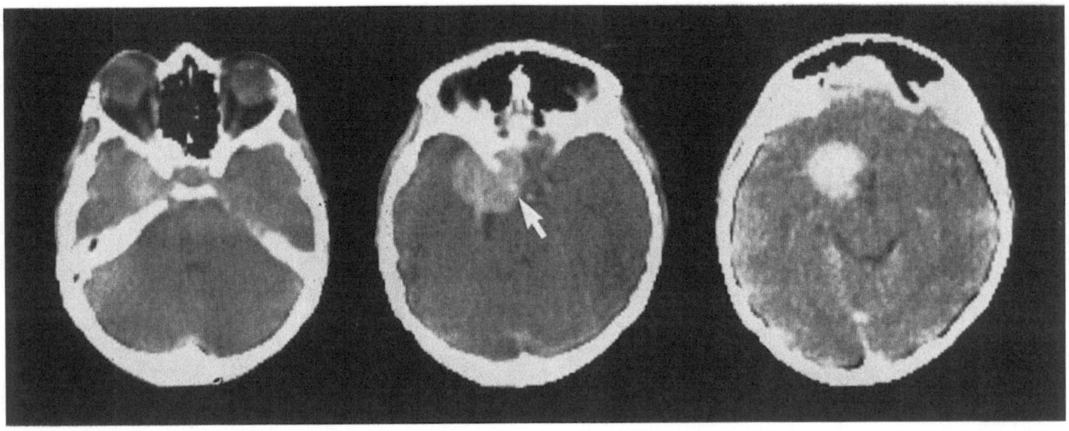

**Fig. D2.58.** Medial sphenoid wing meningioma on the left in a 57-year-old female. Studies with a window width of 200 HU demonstrate the internal carotid artery in orthograde projection on the left within the tumor (arrow). At operation the artery was found immediately adjacent to the tumor. Postcontrast study

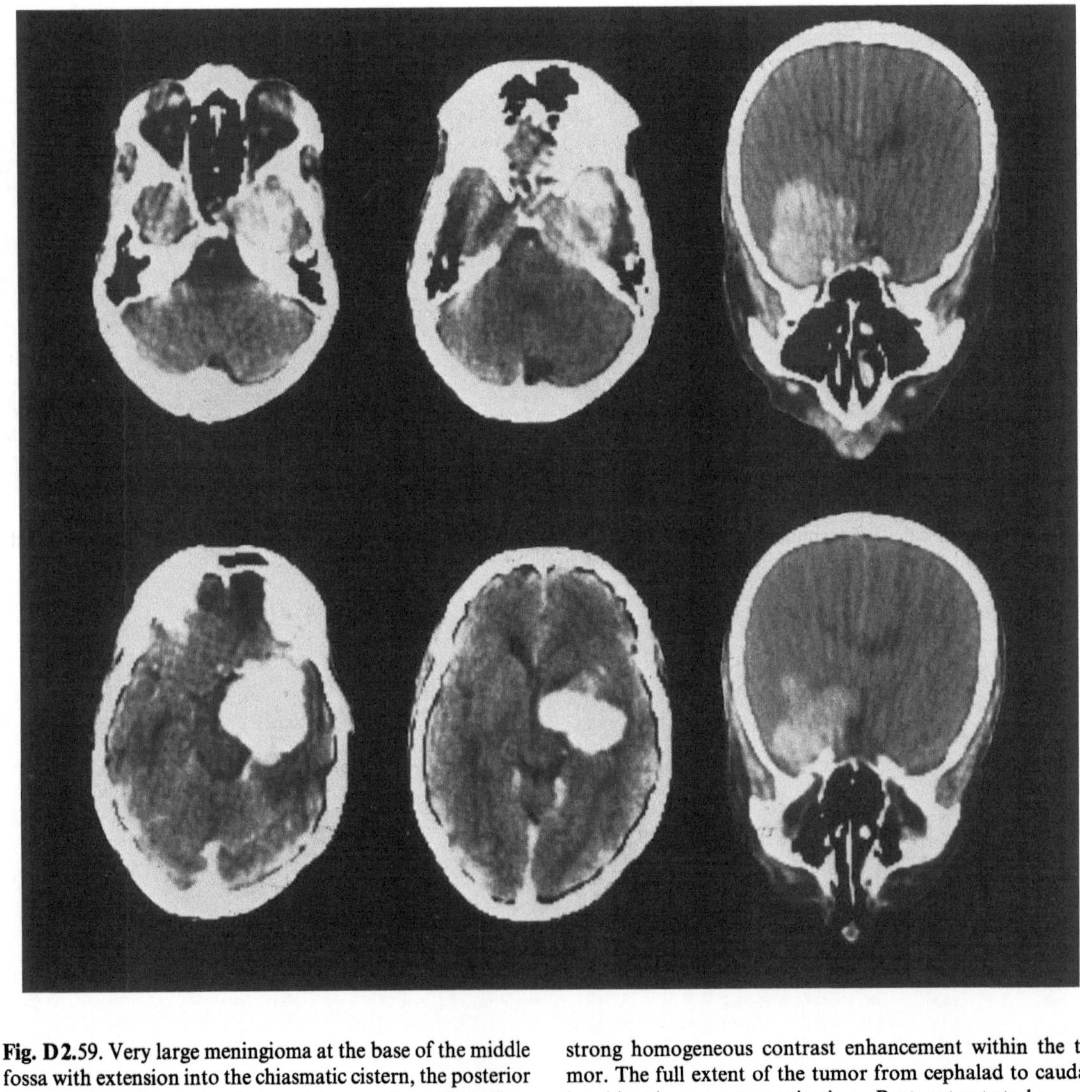

**Fig. D2.59.** Very large meningioma at the base of the middle fossa with extension into the chiasmatic cistern, the posterior fossa, and the basal ganglia in a 50-year-old patient. Very strong homogeneous contrast enhancement within the tumor. The full extent of the tumor from cephalad to caudad is evident in coronary projections. Postcontrast study

**Fig. D2.60.** Large sphenoid wing meningioma on the right in a 71-year-old female. The tumor demonstrates strong contrast enhancement with defects due to regressive change. Very extensive perifocal edema. Herniation of the uncus on the right with compression of the brain stem (arrows). The patient presented with left hemiparesis and disorder of consciousness. Postcontrast study ►

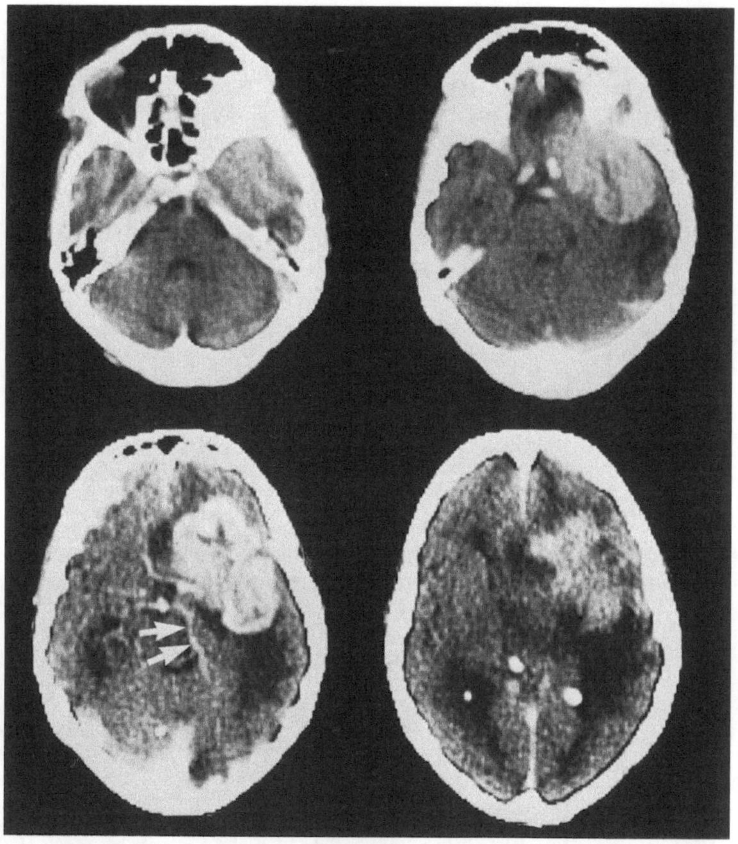

**Fig. D2.61.** Medial sphenoid wing meningioma on the right in a 64-year-old female. The tumor extends far to the left as well as to the suprasellar region and the posterior fossa with significant compression of the brain stem. Grade II perifocal edema in the right hemisphere. Postcontrast study

▼

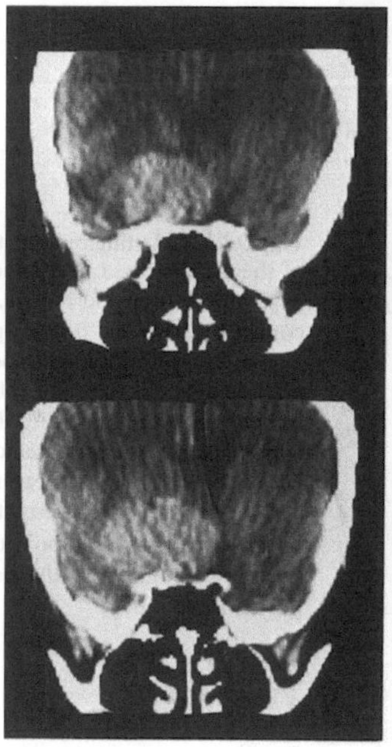

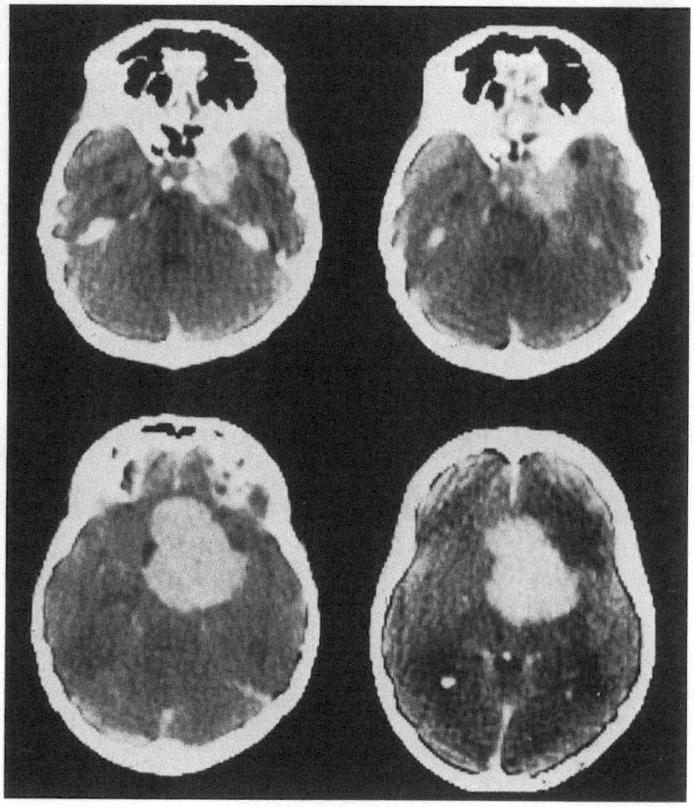

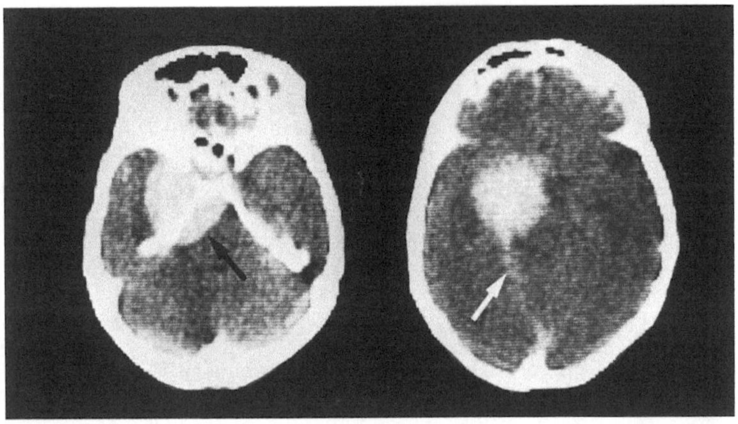

**Fig. D2.62.** Meningioma originating in the dura mater above Meckel's cave with extension across the margin of the tentorium into the posterior fossa (black arrow). Postcontrast studies demonstrate strong contrast medium uptake in the margin of the tentorium behind the tumor (white arrow). Postcontrast study

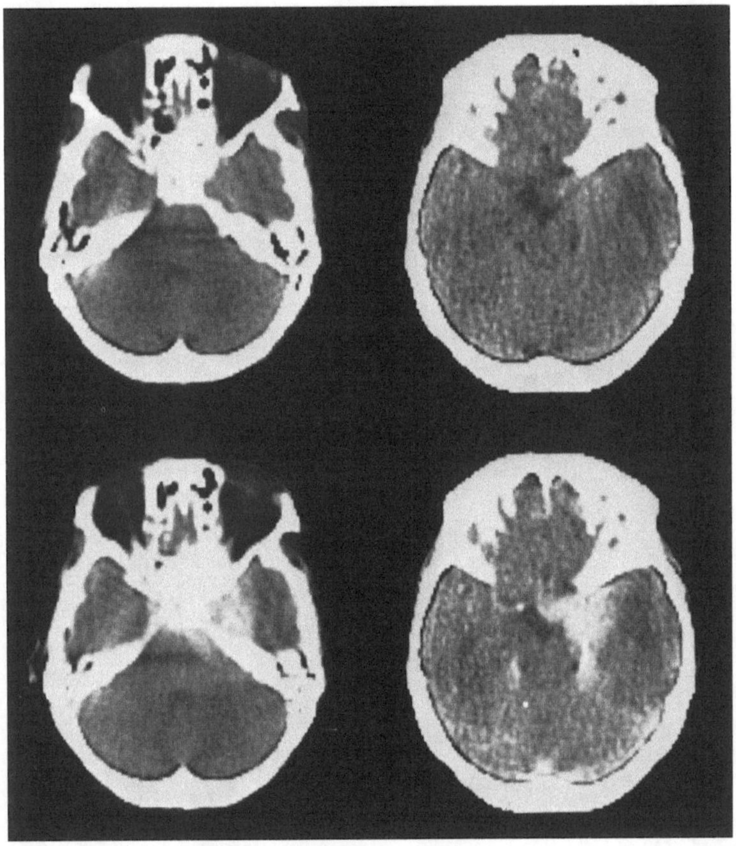

**Fig. D2.63.** Meningioma at the base of the middle fossa near Meckel's cave in a 55-year-old female. In precontrast studies the tumor appears as a defect within the opticochiasmatic cistern on the right (above right). Postcontrast studies demonstrate strong contrast enhancement within the tumor which extends across the margin of the tentorium into the right cerebellopontine angle (above, precontrast study; below, postcontrast study)

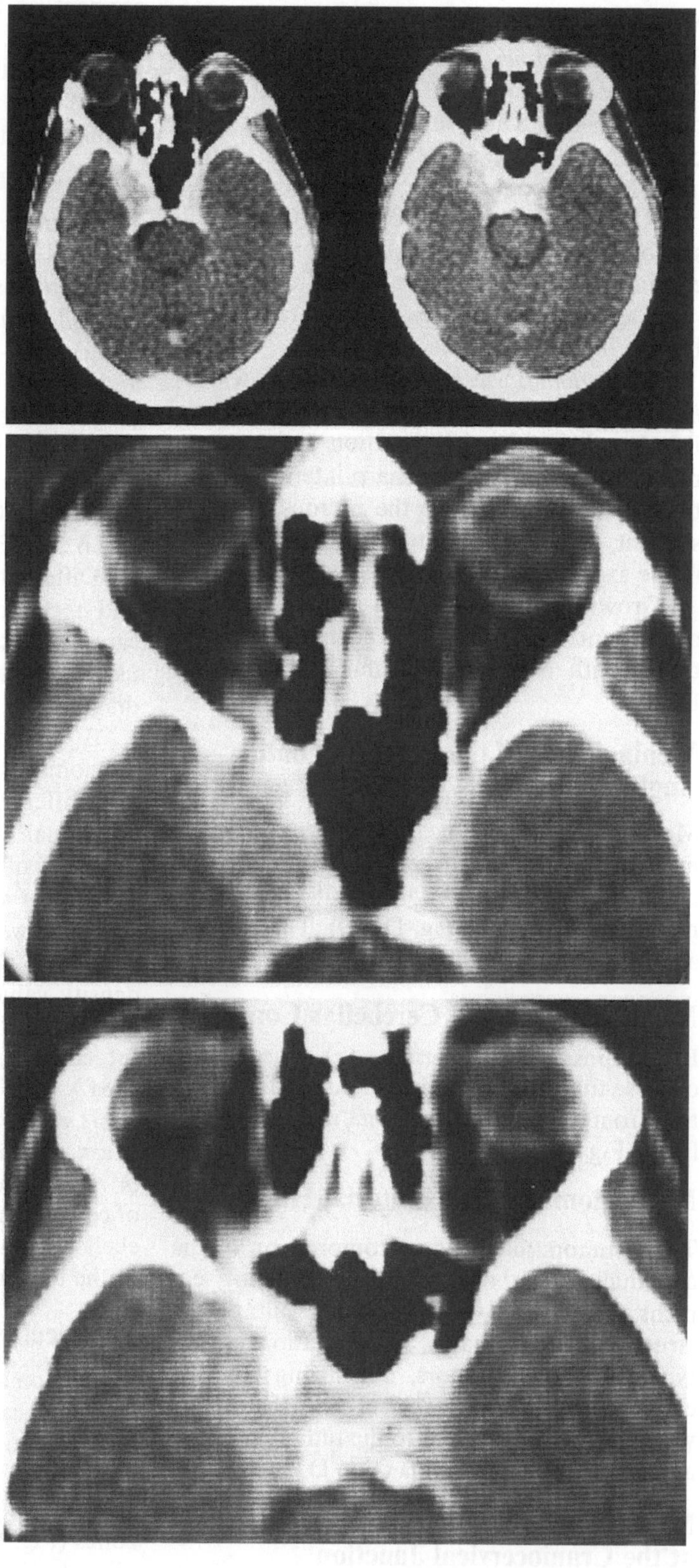

**Fig. D2.64.** Meningioma of the cavernous sinus and the cavum Meckeli on the left with penetration of the left orbit in a 40-year-old patient with proptosis and neurological deficits of the third and fifth cranial nerves. The tumor demonstrates en plaque growth and appears as dilatation of the cavernous sinus, which also takes up contrast medium. The intraorbital portions of the tumor are also demonstrated. Postcontrast study

## Tentorial Meningiomas

Meningiomas originating in the tentorium may demonstrate *either rostral or caudal extension or a combination of both* (Figs. D2.66–69). Coronary CT studies are usually necessary for demonstration of the exact relations to the tentorium. Meningiomas which apparently project into the supratentorial space in horizontal CT sections may prove to be infratentorial tumors causing circumscribed elevation of the tentorium, as coronary studies demonstrate (Figs. D2.75, 76).

*Meningiomas which lie directly on the tentorium may simulate intracerebral tumors* (Fig. D2.67). Infratentorial location of a meningioma is suggested by sharp lateral delineation of the tumor above the petrous bone. A straight, diagonal lateral tumor border is visible in the axial CT scan (Figs. D2.70, 72, 73).

Growth of a meningioma around the edge of the tentorium, creates an identation of the tumor with a typical "comma" shape (Fig. D2.68).

## Meningiomas of the Cerebellopontine Angle

Meningiomas located near the internal acoustic meatus are designated cerebellopontine angle meningiomas (Figs. D2.70, 71, 78). These tumors tend to calcify (Fig. D2.79). The internal acoustic meatus is not widened.

## Meningiomas at the Cerebellar Convexity

It is impossible to determine the exact origin of these tumors in the CT scan, and differentiation from tentorial meningioma may prove difficult (Figs. D2.74, 77).

## Meningiomas of the Tentorial Hiatus

These tumors may lead to compression of the aqueduct from above and of the posterior segment of the third ventricle with resultant obstructive hydrocephalus. This location is also typical of pineal tumors, but strong contrast enhancement at the edge of the tentorium, which is directly adjacent to the tumor, suggests a diagnosis of meningioma (Fig. D2.80).

## Meningiomas of the Clivus and at the Craniocervical Junction

It is difficult to visualize these tumors in axial CT projections. Studies in the plane of the foramen magnum may occasionally reveal a small segment of the tumor on the ventral side of the foramen. With modern CT scanners including reformatted pictures the clear demonstration of such tumors no longer poses diagnostic problems (Fig. D2.65).

### Differential Diagnosis

It is scarcely possible to mistake a large infratentorial meningioma for any other tumor. A large circumscribed *malignant lymphoma* and a *cerebellar sarcoma* (desmoplastic medulloblastoma) both appeared similar to meningioma and caused diagnostic problems in our series (Figs. D1.199, 214).

*Glomus tumors* near the cerebellopontine angle may resemble meningioma, but characteristic destruction of bone allows differentiation (see p. 344, 390, 391).

Differentiation between *acoustic neurinoma* and meningioma may be difficult in certain cases. Clinical and audiometric examinations usually provide adequate information for the diagnosis.

A solid *angioblastoma* may simulate a meningioma, and CT findings do not permit certain differentiation (Fig. D5.10). History and additional clinical findings usually aid in the diagnosis of *metastasis* in this region. Large *aneurysms of the basilar artery with lateral extension* are always sharply delineated and spherical or oval in shape. They demonstrate very high density values after contrast enhancement unless partial thrombosis has occurred. Intramural calcification may also be found (see p. 448 f.).

*It may not be possible to differentiate between chordoma and meningioma of the clivus in the CT scan* (Fig. D7.8). The same is true of calcified meningioma and **osteoma** of the cerebellopontine angle, since the absorption values of the two entities may be identical.

## Ventricular Meningiomas

Meningiomas in the lateral ventricles are usually located near the trigonum with close relations to the choroid plexus. They appear as large, round or oval, homogeneous, and sharply delineated isodense or hyperdense zones (Fig. D2.81). The temporal horn may be dilated. Calcification near the medial surface of the tumor usually represents the displaced glomus of the choroid plexus. Meningiomas are rarely observed in the third ventricle and originate in the plexus in the roof of the third ventricle.

## Differential Diagnosis

Plexus papillomas must always be considered in the differential diagnosis of tumors located in the lateral ventricle near the trigonum. The age of the patient at diagnosis is usually decisive, however, since plexus papillomas are found primarily in children and adolescents, while meningiomas of the lateral ventricles occur almost exclusively in adults.

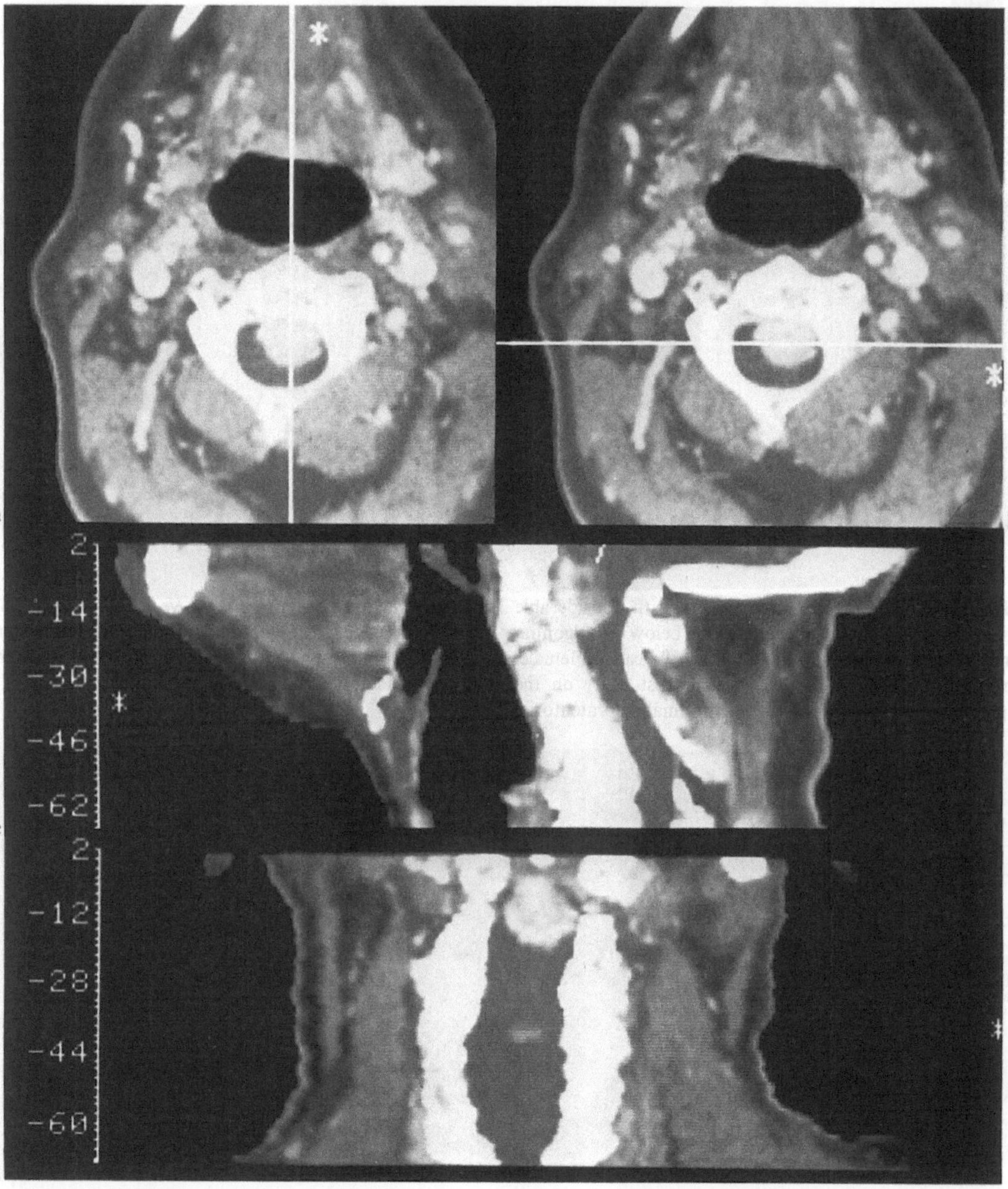


**Fig. D2.65** a–d. Meningioma at the craniocervical junction extending from the foramen magnum to C2. (**a, b**) Conventional slices reveal the tumor with strong contrast enhancement at a ventral location in the spinal canal. (**c, d**) The reformatted pictures represent the planes indicated by the white line in slices **a** and **b**, showing the true extent of the meningioma in the upper segments of the spinal canal. (Courtesy of JAMES C. HIRSCHY, M.D., New York, N.Y., USA; General Electric CT/T 8800)

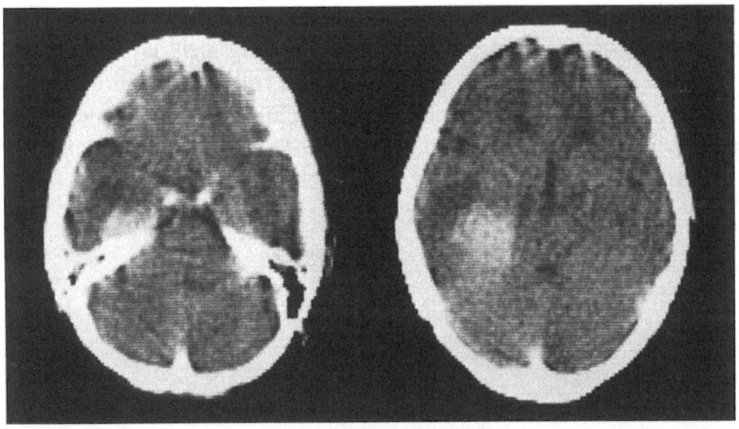

**Fig. D2.66.** Meningioma originating in the tentorium at a supratentorial location on the left in a 60-year-old female. Sharp linear demarcation of the tumor at its medial border points to the origin of the lesion (right). Postcontrast study

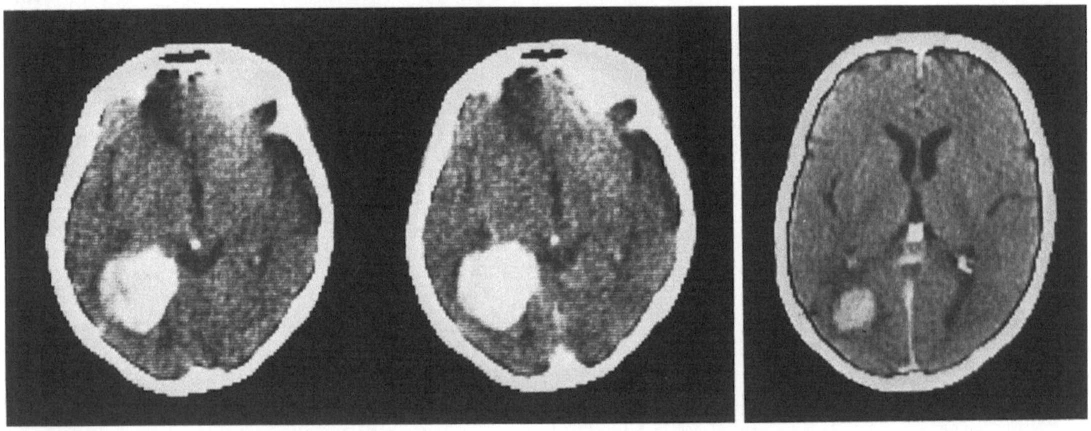

**Fig. D2.67.** (**a**) Tentorial meningioma with considerable calcification at a supratentorial location below the trigonum and the occipital lobe on the left in an 80-year-old female. Precontrast study on the left, postcontrast study on the right; little contrast enhancement. (**b**) Small supratentorial meningioma on the left in a 66-year-old patient. Slight space-occupying effect with obliteration of the left posterior horn. The tumor appears to be an intracerebral lesion, and its origin is not demonstrated in horizontal scans

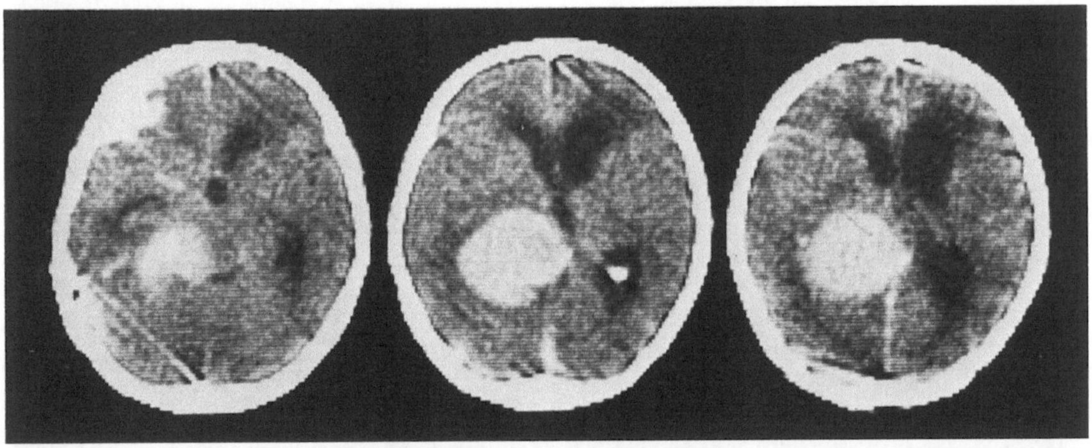

**Fig. D2.68.** Tentorial meningioma on the left in a 71-year-old female. The tumor extends around the margin of the tentorium, with the greater portion of the tumor in a supratentorial location causing displacement of the third ventricle and the aqueduct leading to hydrocephalus and periventricular lucency. The small comma-shaped figure in the picture on the left represents the portion of the tumor extending into the posterior fossa across the tentorial hiatus, resulting in obliteration of the ambient cistern. Postcontrast study

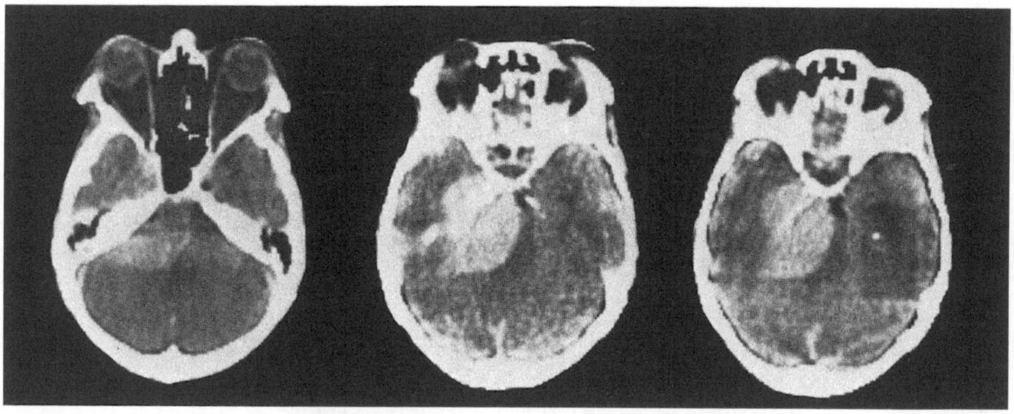

**Fig. D2.69.** Very large meningioma at the left cerebellopontine angle with extension to the clivus, the dorsum sellae, and the middle fossa in a 55-year-old patient. There is significant compression and extreme displacement of the brain stem to the right. Postcontrast study

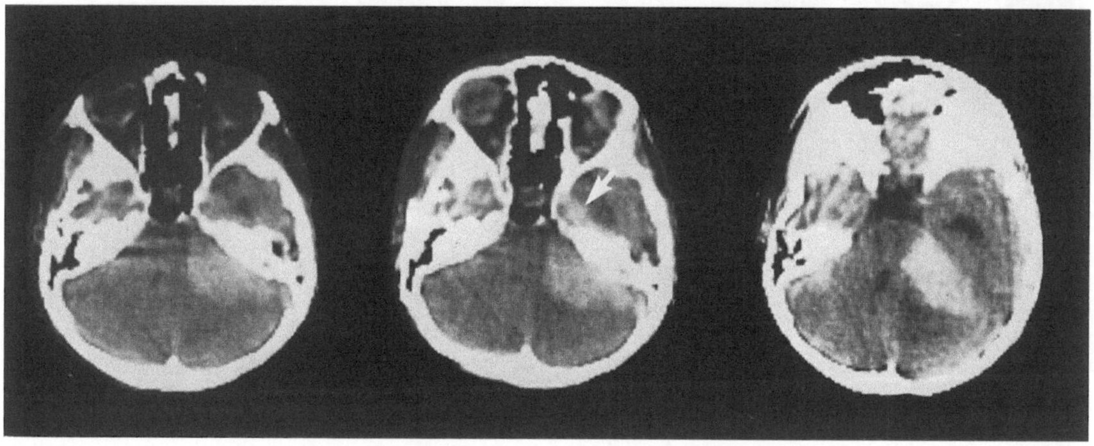

**Fig. D2.70.** Meningioma with superficial extension at the right cerebellopontine angle in a 50-year-old female. Sharp oblique demarcation of the tumor at the junction of the tentorium and the pyramids, which demonstrates an infratentorial origin. Small portion of the tumor in the middle fossa (arrow). Postcontrast study

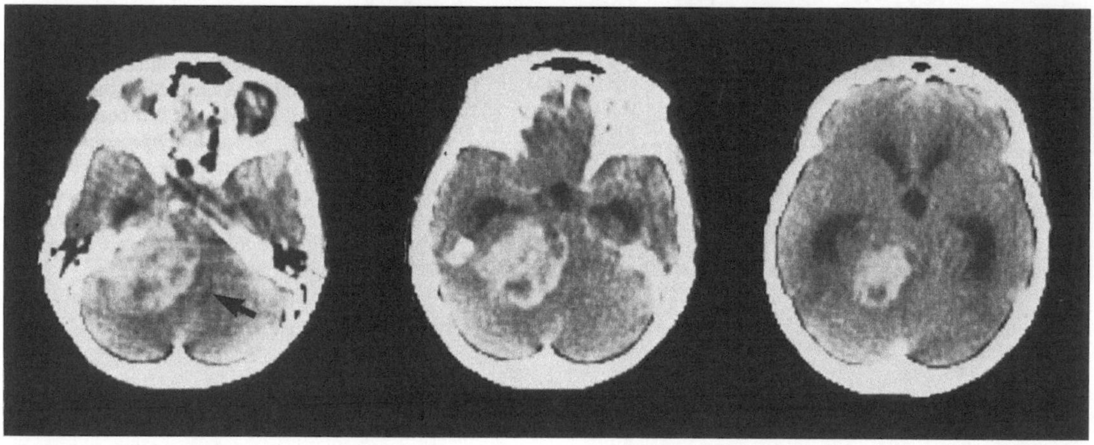

**Fig. D2.71.** Large meningioma with regressive change in the left cerebellopontine angle in a 50-year-old patient. Compression and displacement of the aqueduct and the fourth ventricle (arrow) with obstructive hydrocephalus. Postcontrast study

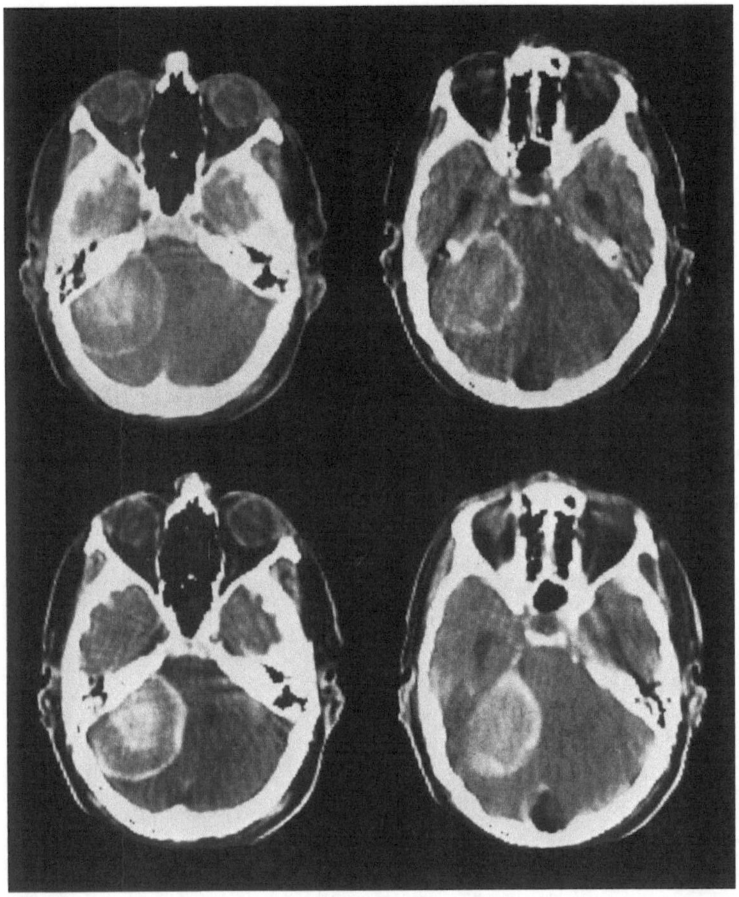

**Fig. D2.72.** Infratentorial meningioma at the margin of the pyramids on the left with atypical CT findings in a 65-year-old man. The texture of the tumor results from fine marginal and central calcification. Sharp oblique demarcation of the tumor at the tentorium in higher projections. Above, precontrast studies; below, postcontrast studies. Slight contrast enhancement

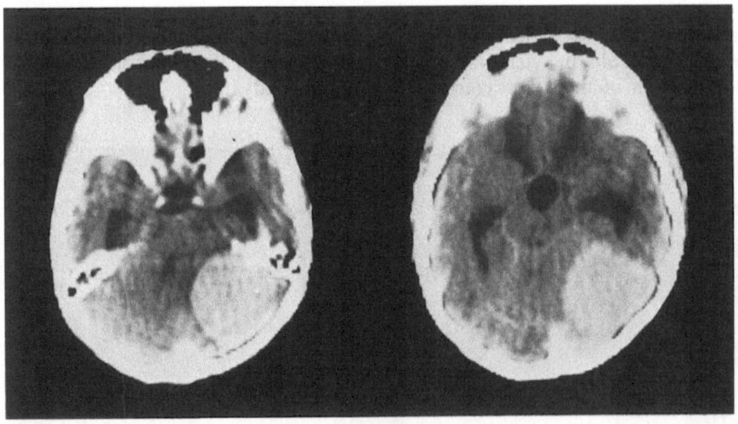

**Fig. D2.73.** Large infratentorial meningioma on the right at the angle of the petrous and occipital bones. Strong homogeneous contrast enhancement in the sharply demarcated tumor, which has displaced the fourth ventricle, resulting in obstructive hydrocephalus. Postcontrast study

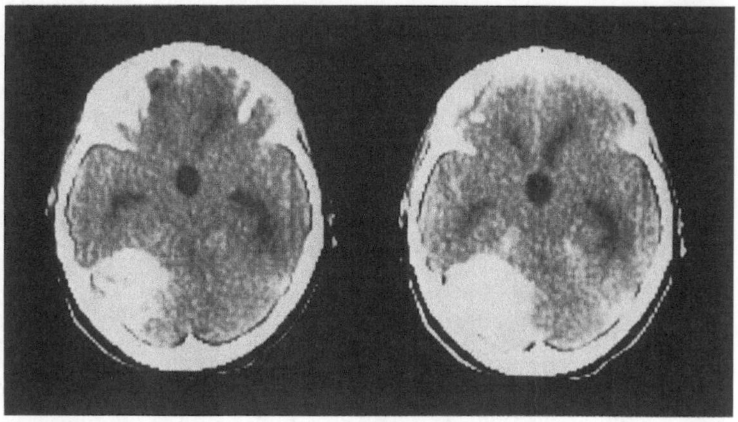

**Fig. D2.74.** Partially calcified infratentorial meningioma on the left at the junction of the petrous and occipital bones. The solid noncalcified portions of the tumor appear isodense in precontrast studies (left). Contrast enhancement demonstrates the full extent of the tumor (right). Fifty-one-year-old female with signs of cerebellar dysfunction on the left

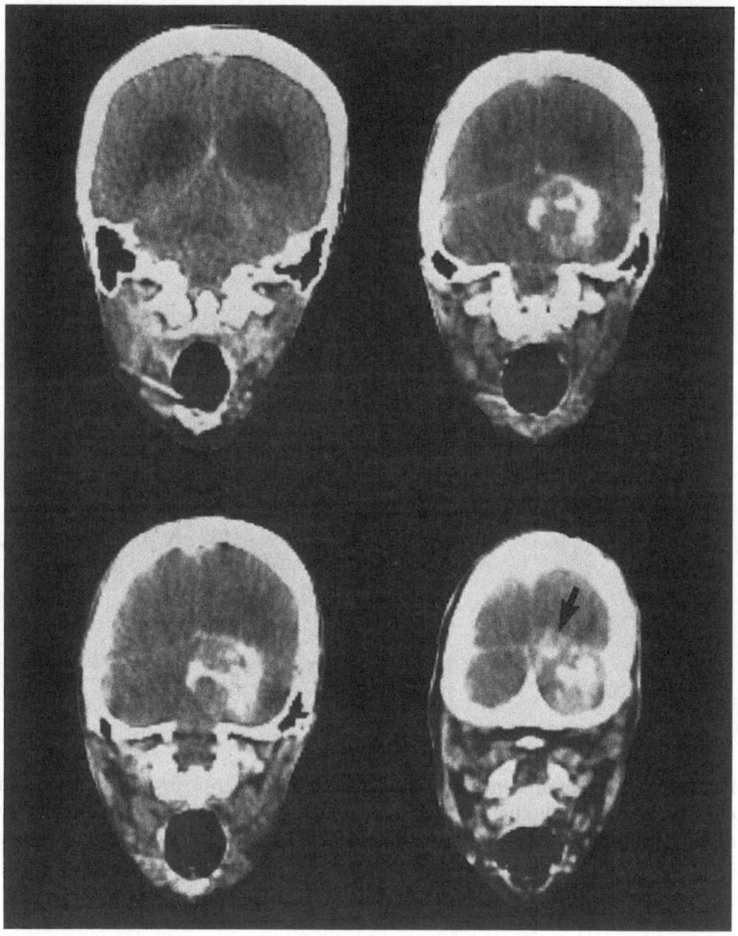

**Fig. D2.75.** Partially calcified subtentorial meningioma on the right in a 59-year-old patient. The most posterior coronary scan demonstrates the small supratentorial portion of the tumor (arrow). Extensive hydrocephalus. Postcontrast study

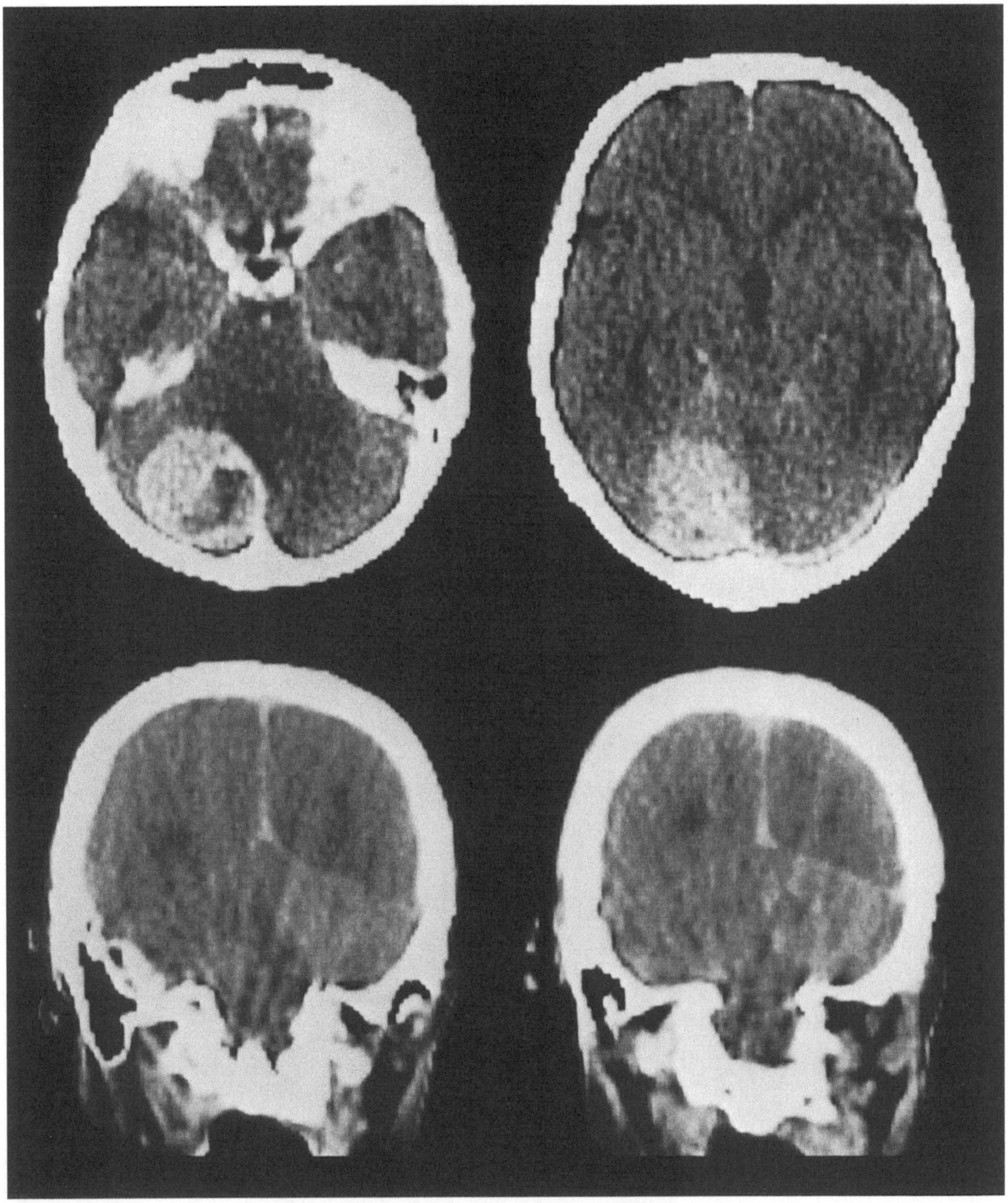

**Fig. D2.76.** Infratentorial meningioma on the left in 60-year-old female. Axial projections do not exclude the possibility of supratentorial extension of the tumor, which is suggested by sharp demarcation of the lesion at the midline (above right). Coronary projections demonstrate that the tumor is limited to an infratentorial location. Postcontrast study

**Fig. D2.77.** Meningioma above the right cerebellar hemisphere in a 46-year-old female. The tumor demonstrates isodense and hyperdense values in precontrast studies (above left). Significant inhomogeneous contrast enhancement (above right, below left). Slight displacement of the fourth ventricle to the left with moderate hydrocephalus. In addition, an angioma is demonstrated in the right parietal region near the ventricular system (below right) ►

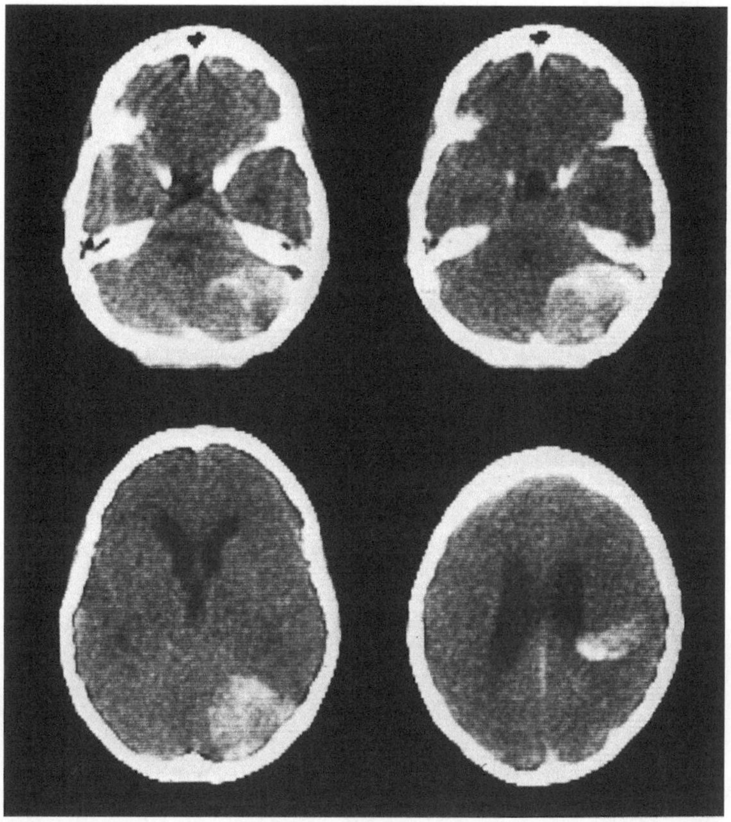

**Fig. D2.78.** Small meningioma at the right cerebellopontine angle in a 53-year-old female (precontrast studies on the left). Strong contrast enhancement (middle and right). Partial obliteration of the ambient cistern due to cephalad extension of the tumor. High density values in precontrast studies make a diagnosis of acoustic neurinoma less likely ▼

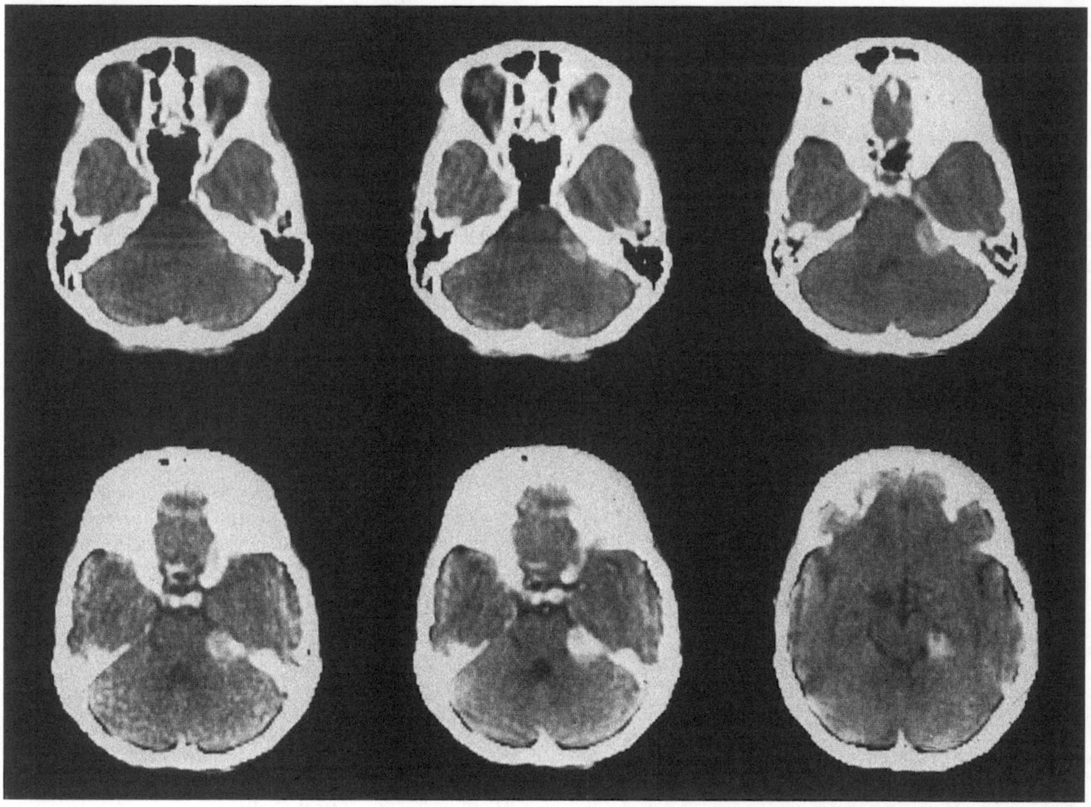

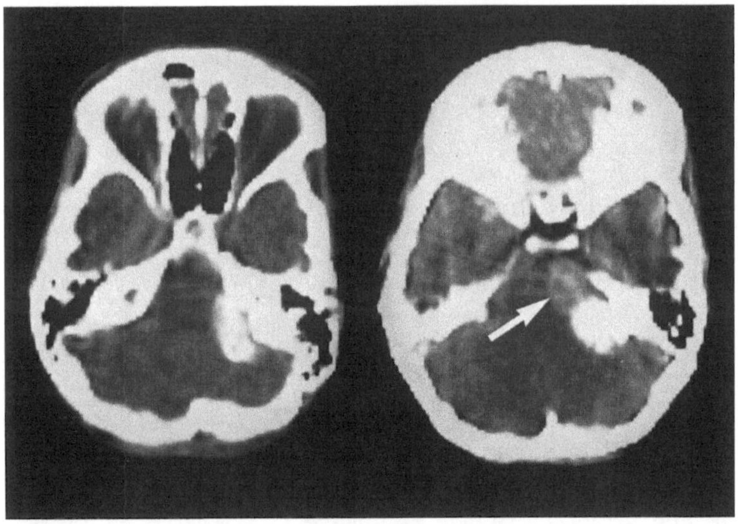

**Fig. D2.79.** Calcified meningioma on the petrous bone below the internal acoustic meatus in a 19-year-old patient with deficits of the basal cranial nerves on the right and signs of a lesion at the cerebellopontine angle. Contrast enhancement allows demonstration of an additional markedly less dense tumor at the right cerebellopontine angle (arrow), which proved to be an acoustic neurinoma at operation

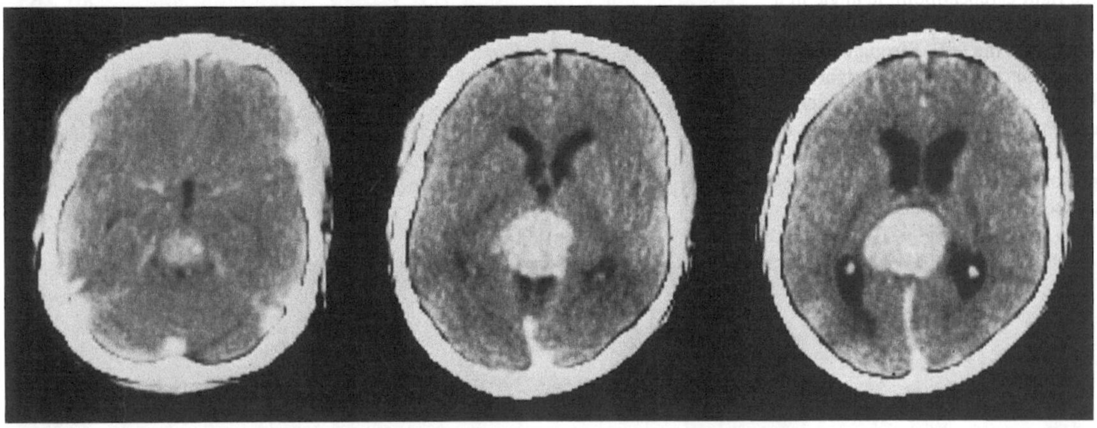

**Fig. D2.80.** Meningioma at the tentorial hiatus in a 44-year-old patient. The relations of the basal portions of the tumor to the margin of the tentorium suggests a diagnosis of meningioma rather than a tumor of the pineal body. Fine specks of calcification (left); homogeneous contrast enhancement. Dilatation of the ventricles due to blockage of the CSF passages at the aqueduct. Postcontrast study

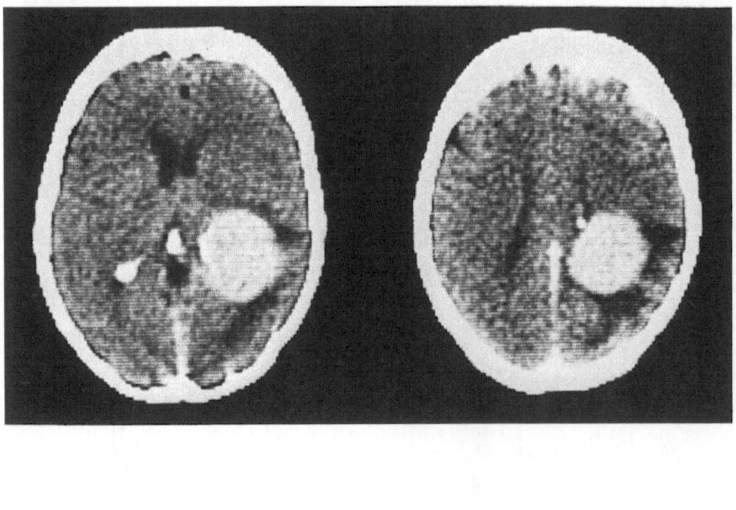

**Fig. D2.81.** Meningioma in the right lateral ventricle in a 73-year-old female. Sharp demarcation and very strong homogeneous contrast enhancement in the tumor located in the region of the trigonum. The calcified choroid plexus of the right lateral ventricle is displaced medially and appears on the medial border of the tumor (left). It is not possible to differentiate between perifocal edema and blocked CSF. Postcontrast study

## b) Malignant Meningiomas and Meningeal Sarcomas

As mentioned above meningiomas may demonstrate rapid growth. However, CT findings are characteristic of meningiomas if the growth rate is moderate.

If the tumor is rather undifferentiated, it is designated a malignant meningioma or meningeal sarcoma. The pattern characteristic of meningioma is absent in most of these tumors. *The surface of the lesion is usually blurred and sometimes irregular, while density values are inhomogeneous as a result of irregular contrast uptake due to regressive changes* (Figs. D2.82–85). VASSILOUTHIS and AMBROSE have reported similar findings (1979). Diagnosis of tumor type is not possible in these cases unless the CT scans demonstrate the origin of the tumor in the meninges (Fig. D2.83).

## c) Hemangiopericytomas

Hemangiopericytomas are tumors which may also be found in other parts of the body, although they have recently been classified with the meningiomas and designated as "hemangiopericytic meningiomas." CT findings in these tumors do in fact resemble those in meningiomas (Figs. D2.86, 87), and differentiation from meningioma is not possible on the basis of CT criteria alone. A few rare cases of congenital hemangiopericytomas have been discribed (Fig. D2.88).

## d) Primary Meningeal Melanomas and Leptomeningeal Melanosis

Circumscribed meningeal melanomas have the same CT appearance as metastases of melanoma (see p. 360, 363, 369).

Leptomeningeal melanosis is not detectable in the CT scan if mass effects or perifocal edema are not present, as one case in our series showed.

## e) Fibromas of the Dura Mater

In rare cases fibromas may originate in the dura mater; such tumors cannot be differentiated from meningiomas in the CT scan (Fig. D2.89).

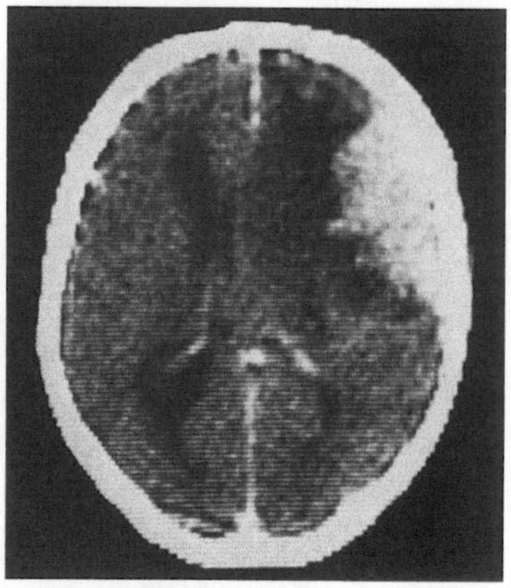

**Fig. D2.82.** Malignant meningioma in the right frontotemporal region in a 66-year-old female. Note the indistinct and irregular surface of the tumor as well as extensive perifocal edema. Major displacement of midline structures, especially near the septum pellucidum. Fairly homogeneous contrast enhancement within the tumor. Postcontrast study

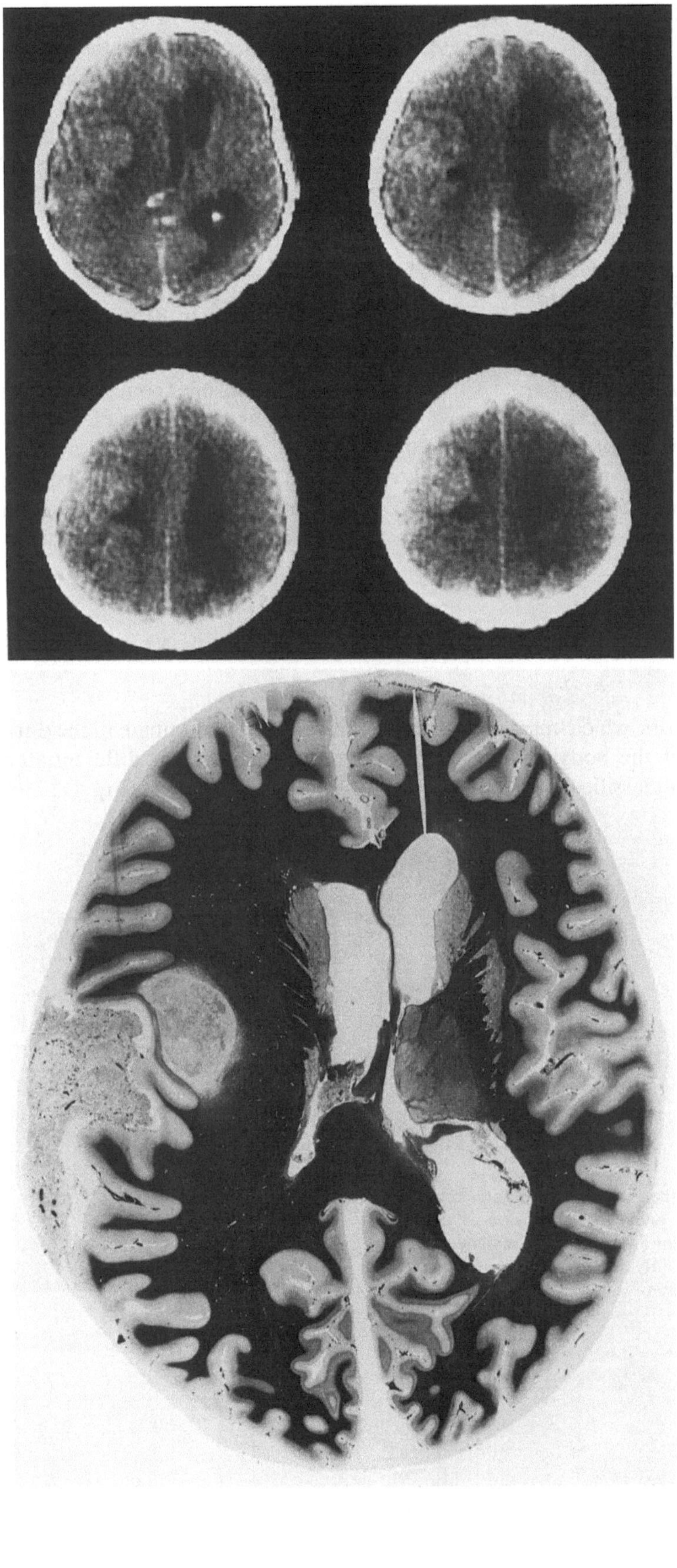

**Fig. D 2.83.** Malignant meningioma in the left temporoparietal region in a 59-year-old patient. The tumor is inhomogeneous and demonstrates irregular contrast enhancement. The knobby medial border of the tumor suggests a diagnosis of meningioma. Grade II–III perifocal edema. Major displacement of midline structures with dilatation of the contralateral ventricle (postcontrast study). Below: autopsy specimen in the same plane as the CT studies. The specimen shows tumor growth in the meninges with penetration of the white matter. (Courtesy of Dr. Gisela STOLTENBURG-DIDINGER, Institute of Neuropathology, Free University of Berlin)

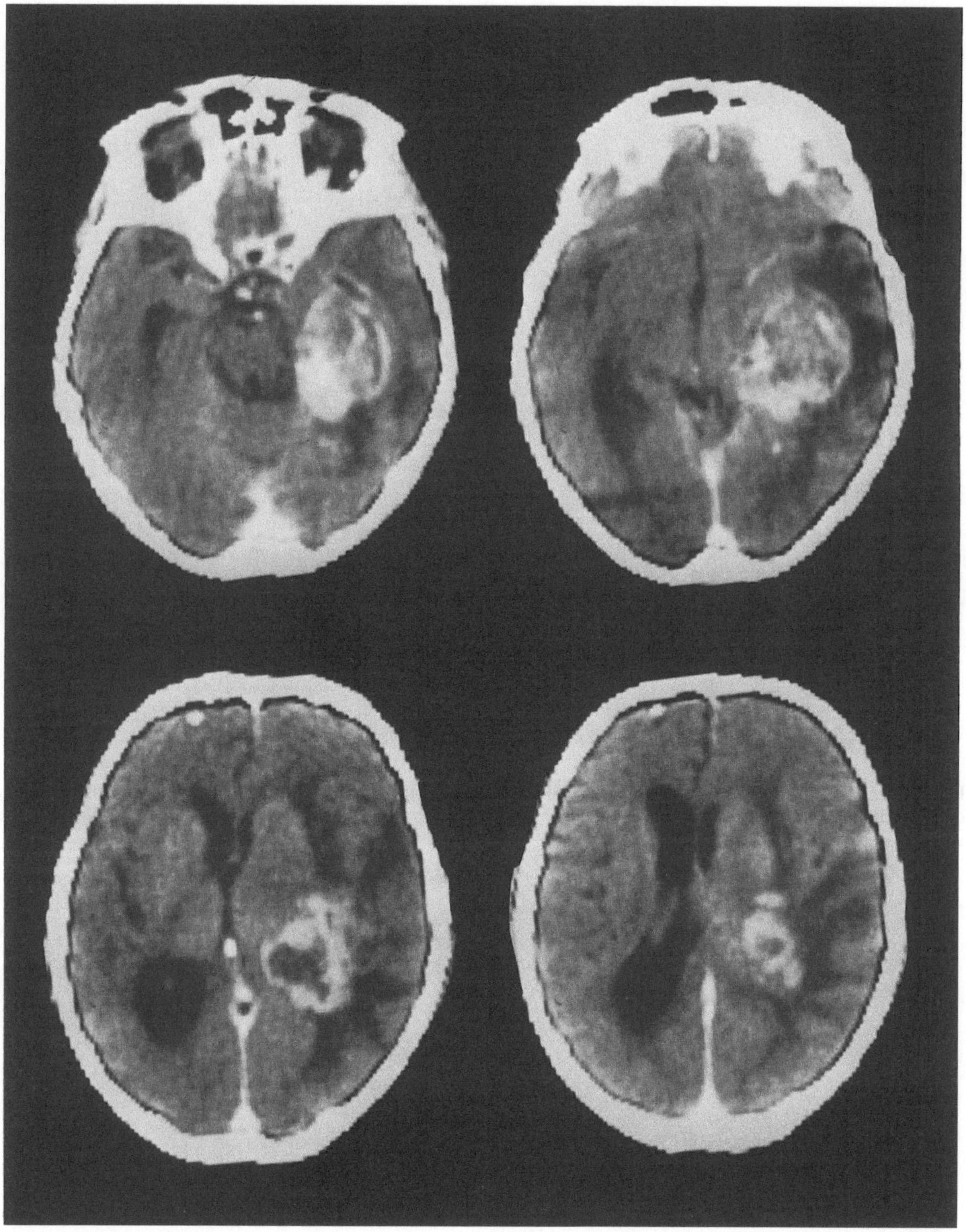

**Fig. D2.84.** Malignant meningioma in the right temporobasal region originating at the tentorium in a 60-year-old man. Atypical CT findings with many zones of low density representing regressive change within the tumor. Extensive perifocal edema with moderate displacement of midline structures. Compression of the brain stem at the tentorial hiatus with disruption of CSF circulation and contralateral dilatation of the ventricles. The CT findings do not allow a definite diagnosis of meningioma. Postcontrast study

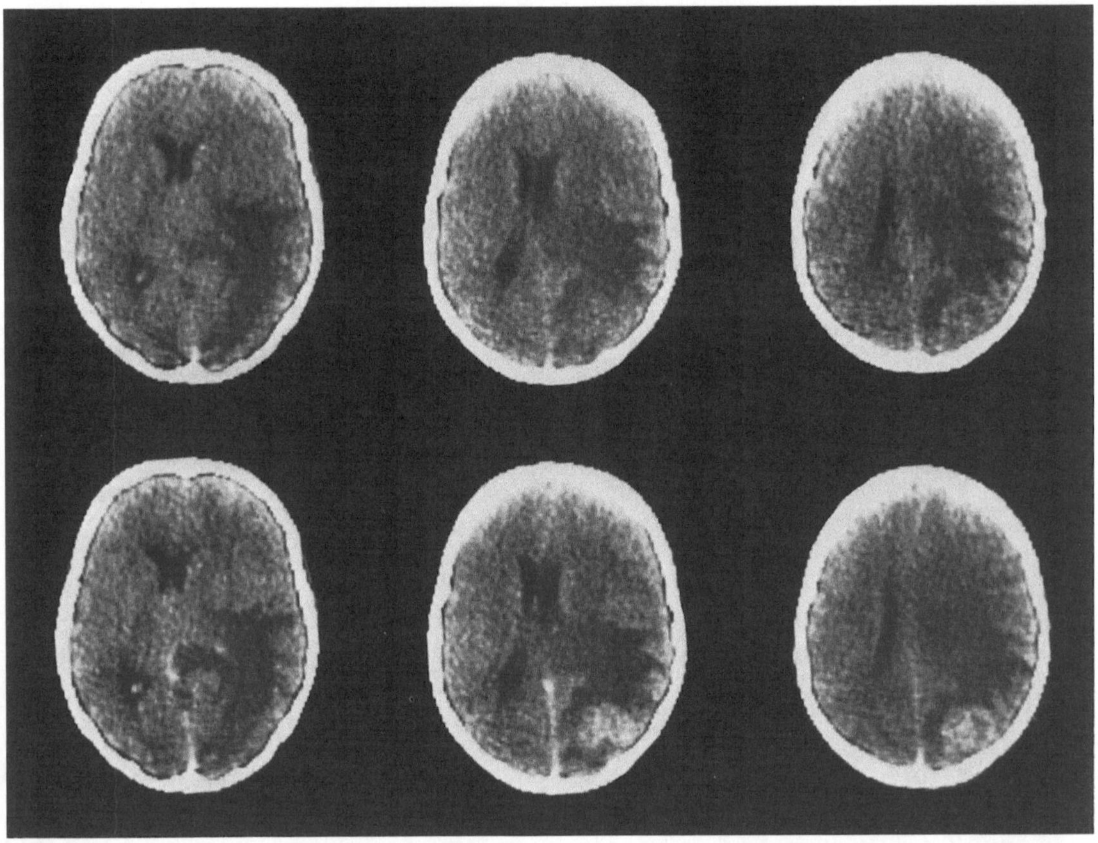

**Fig. D2.85.** Meningeal sarcoma in the right occipital region of a 38-year-old female. The tumor appears as an isodense and hypodense zone within an extensive area of edema near the vault. (Precontrast study, above). Moderate inhomogeneous increase in density values after contrast enhancement (below). Uncharacteristic CT findings

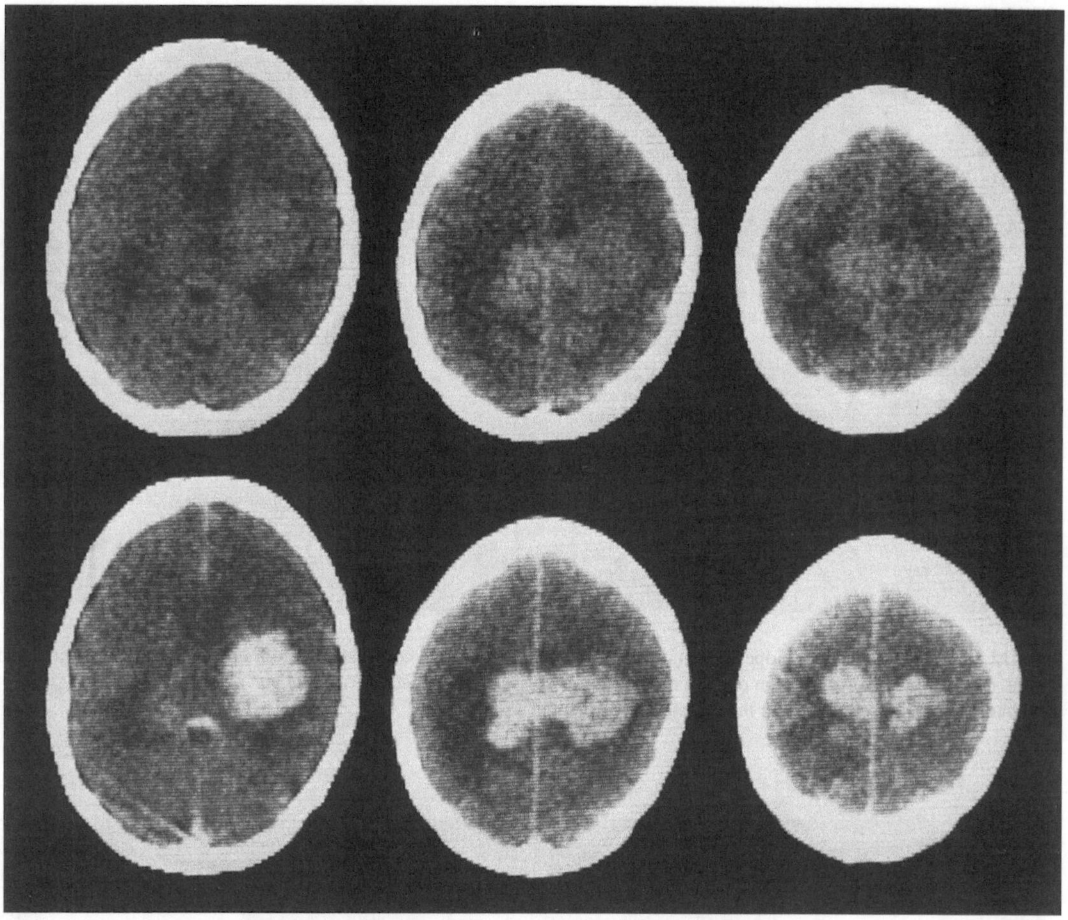

**Fig. D2.86.** Hemangiopericytic meningioma originating in the falx with bilateral extension in a 49-year-old female. Slightly hyperdense values in the precontrast study (above). Strong homogeneous contrast enhancement characteristic of meningioma (below)

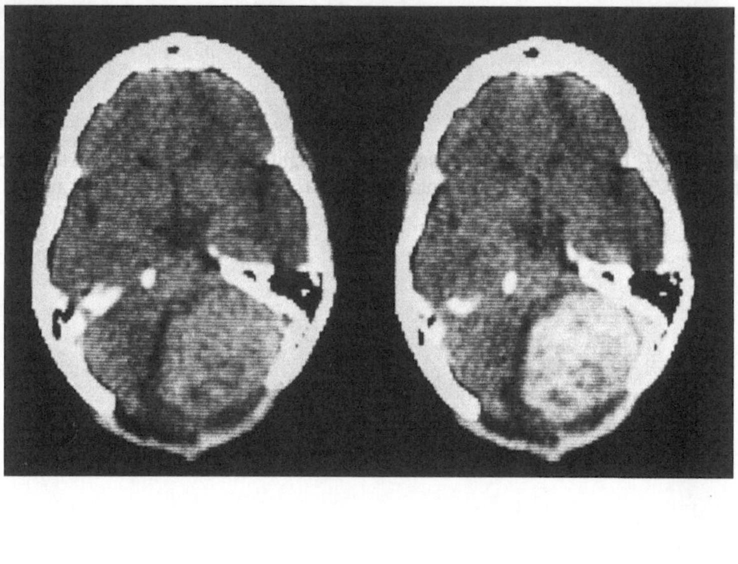

**Fig. D2.87.** Recurrence of hemangiopericytoma in the posterior fossa on the right. The tumor appears as a large hyperdense structure in the precontrast study (left). Generally homogeneous increase in density after contrast enhancement (right). CT findings characteristic of meningioma

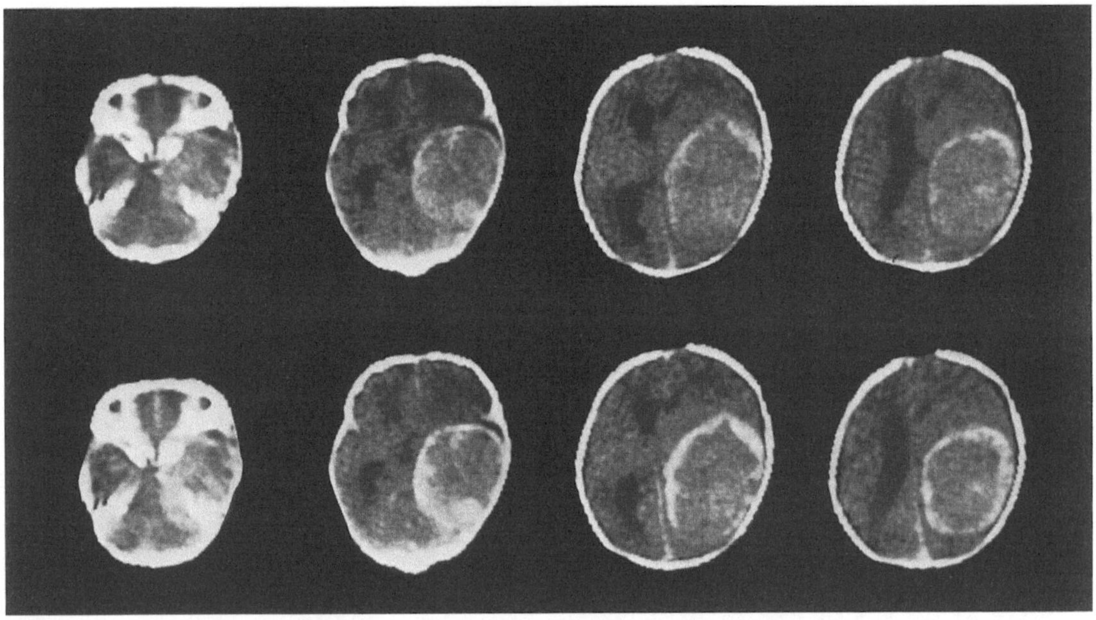

**Fig. D2.88.** Congenital hemangiopericytoma in a 13-day-old infant. The tumor involves a large portion of the right cerebral hemisphere. Rosette figure in the CT picture with slight marginal contrast enhancement. Above, precontrast studies; below, postcontrast studies

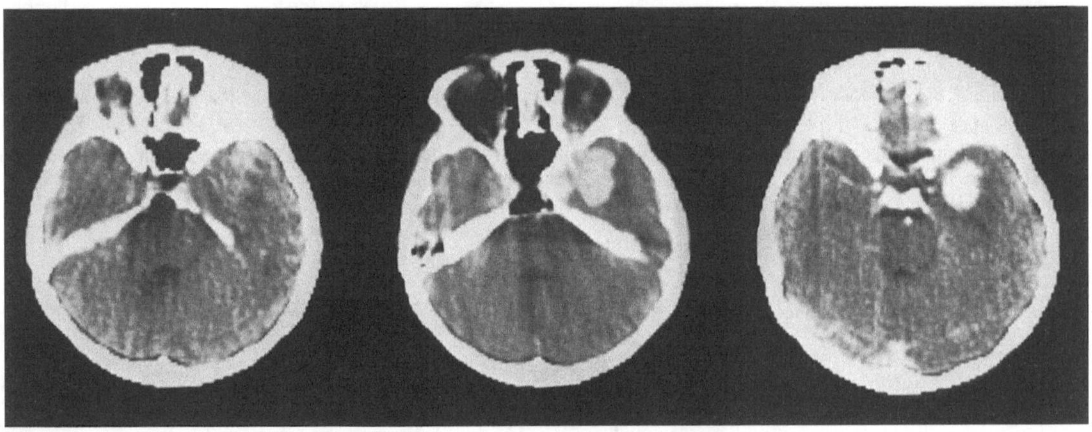

**Fig. D2.89.** Fibroma of the dura mater in the right parasellar region on the floor of the middle fossa in a 62-year-old female. CT findings characteristic of meningioma. Left, precontrast studies; middle and right, postcontrast studies

# 3. Neurinomas

| | |
|---|---|
| Incidence | 5–8% |
| Characteristic age at diagnosis | 35–60 years |
| Sex distribution | Females affected twice as often as males |
| Typical locations | 1. Originating in the eighth nerve at the cerebellopontine angle;<br>2. Originating in the fifth nerve at the base of the middle fossa |
| Characteristic clinical findings | ad 1. Deafness, vestibular disorders; hypesthesia in the distribution area of the trigeminal nerve and cerebellar symptoms in later stages of the disease;<br>ad 2. Pain and disorders of sensation in the distribution of the trigeminal nerve |
| Skull film | ad 1. Widening of the internal acoustic meatus<br>ad 2. Sharply delineated bone defect at the trigeminal impression of the petrous bone |
| EEG | Normal findings in most cases |
| Echoencephalography | Ventricular dilatation in large tumors |
| Serial brain scintigraphy | Strong radionuclide uptake common in tumors larger than 2 cm in diameter |
| Cerebral angiography | Displacement of normal vessels due to tumor, discrete staining of the tumor as a result of increased vascularization; slight tumor blush |
| Other contrast studies | Even small tumors may be demonstrated by cisternography (gas or positive contrast medium) |
| **Computed Tomography** | |
| Precontrast study | Tumors are often isodense and not demonstrable in plain scans; indirect tumor signs (displacement or obliteration of the fourth ventricle, dilatation or obliteration of the cerebellopontine cisterns) only in cases of large neurinomas |
| Contrast medium uptake | Significant, usually homogeneous contrast medium uptake in all cases |
| Appearance after contrast enhancement | Solid tumor nodule at the cerebellopontine angle or in the middle fossa attached to the midbrain or the pons; tumors smaller than 1.5 cm in diameter are rarely demonstrated with axial CT; perifocal edema common in large tumors |

Continuation

Continuation

**Differential Diagnosis**

ad 1. Meningioma
Metastasis
Ependymoma
Glomus tumor
Hemangioblastoma
Aneurysm
Basilar artery ectasia
Cerebellar sarcoma and abscess

ad 2. Meningioma
Pilocytic astrocytoma
Gangliocytoma and giant aneurysm

Reports in the literature indicate that neurinomas make up 3%–8% of all brain tumors. We found neurinoma in 196 cases (5.2%). Peak incidence occurs between the ages of 35 and 60 years, although some cases have been reported in patients younger than 20 years of age. Females are affected twice as often as males. Neurinomas are benign (grade I) tumors.

### Typical Locations

#### a) Acoustic Neurinomas

The majority of intracranial neurinomas are located in the cerebellopontine angle and originates in the eighth cranial nerve. Tumor growth starts in the auditory canal, usually on the vestibular nerve, and causes widening of the canal. The lesions vary greatly in size and do not show invasive growth, but expansion may lead to deformation and displacement of the brain stem and the adjacent cerebellar hemisphere with characteristic clinical findings.

Neurinomas vary in consistency from tough to soft, depending on the degree of regressive change. Cysts in the tumor are rare, but arachnoid cysts of various sizes may be found in the vicinity of acoustic neurinomas.

The facial nerve may be displaced and stretched as it crosses the capsule of the tumor. In some cases the nerve cannot be separated from the tumor itself.

Bilateral acoustic tumors are not uncommon and may represent a "forme fruste" of neurofibromatosis. Combination of acoustic neurinoma with an ipsilateral or contralateral meningioma is also possible (Fig. D2.79).

### Characteristic Clinical Findings

Unilateral hearing loss or deafness accompanied by a vestibular disorder is characteristic. Large tumors cause additional neurological deficits related to the fifth and seventh cranial nerves as well as signs of cerebellar dysfunction. Disruption of CSF circulation by large tumors may cause hydrocephalus, headache, or even papilledema.

#### b) Trigeminal Neurinomas

Neurinomas of the fifth cranial nerve are much less common than acoustic neurinomas. They originate in or near the Gasserian ganglion and cause continuous pain and paresthesia in the distribution of the trigeminal nerve.

Neurinomas originating in the other caudal cranial nerves are exceedingly rare and cause neurological deficits related to the affected nerve.

### Additional Diagnostic Procedures

Plain skull films and special projections demonstrate dilatation of the internal auditory canal in 40% to more than 80% of cases with acoustic neurinoma (Canigiani 1978). Destruction of the tip of the petrous bone may also occur, while secondary signs of increased intracranial pressure are found only in very large tumors.

Circumscribed bone defects at the trigeminal impression in the petrous bone are often found in cases of fifth nerve neurinoma.

The electroencephalogram is normal in the majority of cases with both types of neurinoma. Moderate ventricular dilatation is found at echoencephalography in all large acoustic neurinomas (SCHIEFER and KAZNER 1967).

BURROWS reported scintigraphic demonstration of acoustic neurinoma in 77% of cases (1978). Dynamic brain scans are capable of demonstrating large tumors, though small tumors almost certainly escape detection with this method.

Serial angiographic studies demonstrate displacement of the anterior inferior cerebellar artery as well as a slight tumor blush in acoustic neurinoma.

Pneumoencephalography and cisternography with positive contrast media are also capable of demonstrating neurinomas. The latter method is useful in demonstration of small tumors located in the internal auditory canal (WENDE and NAKAYAMA 1978).

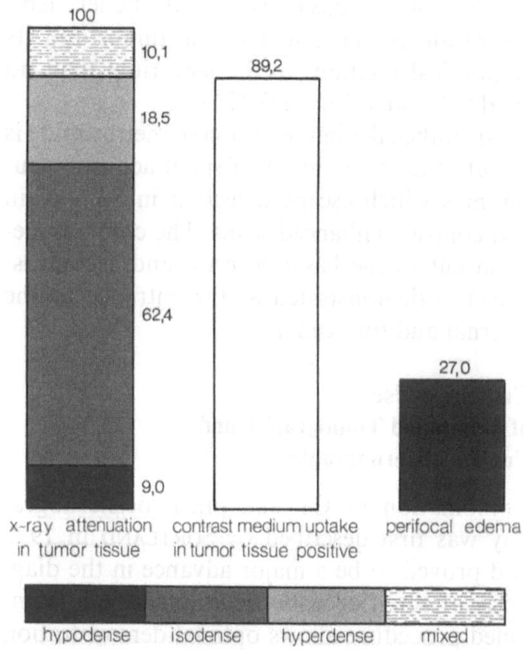


**Fig. D3.1.** X-ray attenuation, contrast medium uptake, and frequency of perifocal edema in neurinomas (percent)

## a) Acoustic Neurinomas

### Computed Tomography (Figs. D3.1–20)

#### Precontrast Study

*These tumors are usually isodense and not directly visible* in the precontrast scan (Figs. D3.2–5). In our series 61% of 190 acoustic neurinomas were isodense in the plain scan. Slight variations in density may be found. *Perifocal edema* may demarcate isodense tumors in some cases (Fig. D3.3). *Cystic formations* outside the tumor may also be identified (Fig. D3.8). *Displacement of the fourth ventricle* occurs in about 60% of cases and is a very important indirect sign of this tumor (Fig. D3.2), as is *failure to demonstrate the fourth ventricle* in technically adequate studies, which was the case in 17% of patients in our series. This is also true of *dilatation or unilateral obliteration of the cerebellopontine cistern* (Figs. D3.4, 5). Very large tumors may elevate and twist the ipsilateral temporal horn and compress the brain stem.

*Dilatation of the internal auditory canal* and other changes in the petrous bone may be found in CT scans evaluated with large window width (Fig. E18, p. 392).

#### Postcontrast Study

Neurinomas demonstrate rapid contrast uptake with maximum density values at 2 min after contrast administration in almost all cases. Subsequent decline is rather marked in the first hour following contrast application.

*Most neurinomas require contrast enhancement for demonstration in the CT scan.* Contrast uptake is intense and averaged 21 HU in our series. Of 194 neurinomas, 173 (89,2%) demonstrated contrast uptake, with a homogeneous pattern in most cases. Cysts and necrotic zones did not accept the contrast medium, with the result that ring structures appeared within the sharply delineated tumor in a few cases (Fig. D3.9). Very large acoustic neurinomas always demonstrate regressive changes which are easily recognizable in the CT scan (Figs. D3.10, 11, 13).

Size of the tumor is the decisive factor in CT demonstration. *Acoustic neurinomas smaller than 1.5 cm in diameter are demonstrated with axial projections only in exceptional cases* (Figs. D3.5, 6).

Coronary projections provide better demonstration of the extent of the tumor and its anatomical relations to the tentorium than do axial CT scans (Figs. D3.12, 13).

Intrathecal administration of metrizamide is useful in demonstration of small acoustic neurinomas which escape detection in both plain and contrast-enhanced scans. The contrast medium enters the basal cisterns, and a contrast defect is demonstrated at the entrance to the internal auditory canal.

**Combined Use of Computed Tomography and Pneumocisternography**

Combination of CT and pneumocisternography was first described by SORTLAND in 1978 and proved to be a major advance in the diagnosis of small acoustic neurinomas. The combined procedure allows optimal demonstration of the cerebellopontine cistern and the internal auditory canal with demonstration of very small tumors at these locations. KRICHEFF et al. (1979) and WENDE (1980) reported similar results.

*Procedure*

Following plain skull films and tomographic studies of the petrous bones, both pre- and postcontrast CT scans are made in order to demonstrate large space-occupying lesions in the cerebellopontine angle (see Table 4). If these studies are negative, lumbar puncture is performed with the patient in the sitting position, the head inclined toward the healthy ear, and 5–6 ml of air are injected rapidly. The air quickly rises to the cerebellopontine cistern and enters the internal auditory canal. CT studies with thin slices (5 mm or less) and a high resolution matrix (320 × 320, for example) are made with the patient lying on his side. The patient's head is rotated approximately 45° so that the air-filled cerebellopontine cistern and the internal auditory canal are uppermost. With the patient in this position the cerebellopontine angle is demonstrated in the CT scan. Rotation of the patient allows demonstration of the corresponding region on the opposite side (Fig. D3.15). Both intracanicular and extracanicular acoustic neurinomas can be demonstrated with a high degree of certainty using this technique (Figs. D3.16, 17).

**Table 4.** Order of neuroradiological studies in cases of suspected tumor at the cerebellopontine angle

1. Conventional skull films including special projections
2. Tomographic studies of the petrous bone
3. Precontrast and postcontrast CT studies
4. Combination of computed tomography and gas cisternography or cisternography with positive contrast media in cases with negative findings in 3

The procedure described above is both simple and diagnostically useful. It is also very safe, if the usual criteria for lumbar puncture are observed. Some patients report slight headache.

## b) Trigeminal Neurinomas

The trigeminal neurinomas observed in our series were characterized by strong, homogeneous contrast uptake. The tumors were located in the medial portion of the middle fossa in contact with the brain stem (Figs. D3.18, 19). Coronary projections may be useful in these tumors (Fig. D3.18).

**Differential Diagnosis**

Differential diagnosis of **acoustic neurinomas** must include *meningioma and metastasis as well as glomus tumor, angioblastoma, ependymoma, aneurysm, desmoplastic medulloblastoma, and brain abscess in rare cases.*

*Meningiomas* may be isodense in up to 14.4% of cases, though such a finding is rare in the cerebellopontine region. Contrast uptake is similar in neurinomas and meningiomas, but differentiation is usually possible on the basis of clinical findings. Otological examination is of prime importance in this regard. Calcification and extensive destruction of the petrous bones is more typical of meningioma, as is extensive growth and a sharply delineated tumor border at the tentorium, though very large acoustic neurinomas may have a similar appearance.

The history is decisive in the diagnosis of *metastasis*, since CT findings may be identical to those found in acoustic neurinoma. The same is true of *glomus tumors*, which may, however, cause extensive bone destruction. Otological examination is usually diagnostic in these cases, and coronary CT projections as well as conventional tomography demonstrate characteristic findings (Fig. D8.2, p. 344).

*Desmoplastic medulloblastomas* and solid *angioblastomas* may be found in the cerebellopontine angle with identical CT findings in both of these tumors.

*Plexus papilloma* may originate between the cerebellopontine angle and the lateral recess of the fourth ventricle. Differential diagnosis may be difficult if the tumor is uncalcified.

*Aneurysms of the basilar artery* protruding into the cerebellopontine angle can usually be diagnosed and differentiated from acoustic neurinomas as a result of the vessel's tortuous course and very intense contrast uptake in the vascular lesion (Figs. F71, 73–76, p. 449ff.).

*Epidermoid cysts of the cerebellopontine angle* have the same density as CSF and present no problems in differential diagnosis.

Differential diagnosis of **trigeminal neurinoma** include *meningiomas of Meckel's cave* and large *pilocytic astrocytomas* which may also demonstrate strong contrast uptake. Temporobasal *gangliocytomas* are similar in appearance, but usually contain calcification, which is never the case in trigeminal neurinoma. *Giant aneurysms of the carotid and posterior cerebral arteries* may have the same location as trigeminal neurinomas, but strong contrast uptake in these "tumors" makes the diagnosis easy. Thrombosed aneurysms show a ring of increased density representing the capsule of the vascular process (Fig. F67, p. 446).

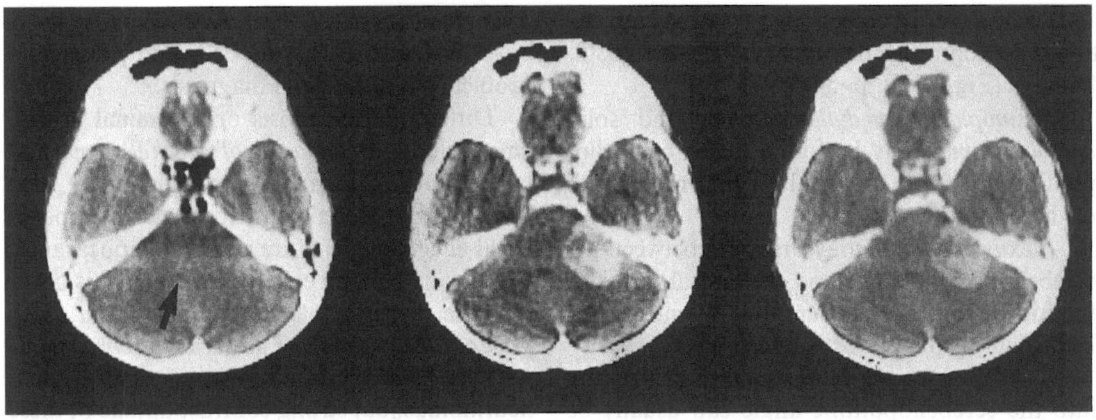

**Fig. D3.2.** Isodense acoustic neurinoma in a 55-year-old female with symptoms of a lesion at the cerebellopontine angle. Precontrast study (left): displacement of the fourth ventricle to the left (arrow) suggests the presence of a space-occupying lesion. Postcontrast study (right): inhomogeneous contrast uptake in the lesion (acoustic neurinoma), which has caused a large indentation of the caudal brain stem

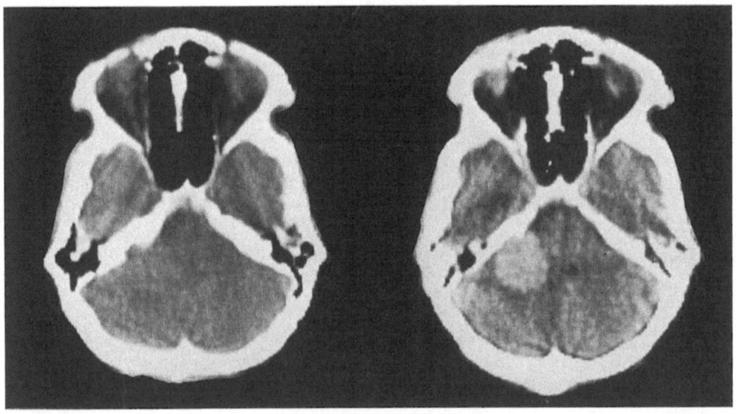

**Fig. D3.3.** Isodense acoustic neurinoma on the left in a 67-year-old patient. The precontrast study (left) demonstrates perifocal edema and widening of the internal acoustic pore, suggesting presence of a tumor. Strong contrast uptake within the tumor and major displacement of the fourth ventricle (right)

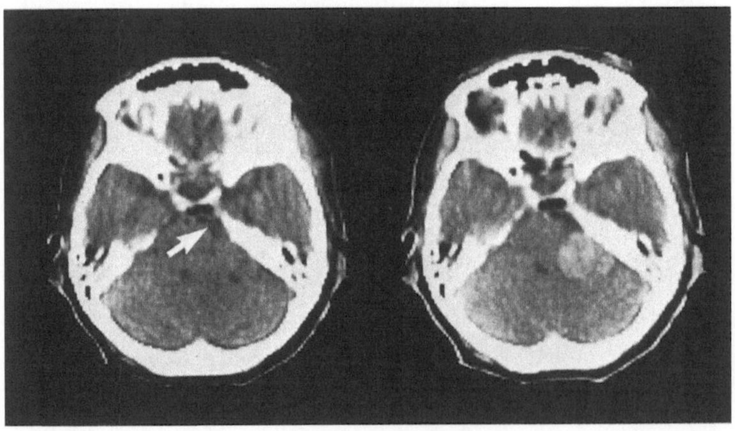

**Fig. D3.4.** Isodense acoustic neurinoma on the right in a 62-year-old female with displacement of the fourth ventricle and dilatation of the cerebellopontine cistern (arrow) suggesting the presence of a space-occupying lesion at the right cerebellopontine angle. Strong contrast uptake within the tumor (right)

---

**Fig. D3.7.** Large slightly hyperdense acoustic neurinoma on the left with considerable widening of the left internal acoustic pore and significant displacement of the fourth ventricle. Extensive perifocal edema (above, precontrast studies). The true extent of the tumor is evident in postcontrast studies (below). Forty-year-old female with symptoms of a lesion at the left cerebellopontine angle

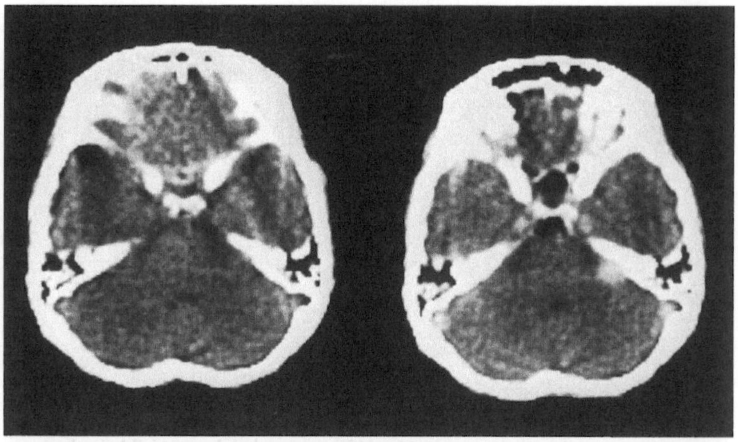

**Fig. D3.5.** Small isodense acoustic neurinoma on the right in a 46-year-old patient. Dilatation of the cerebellopontine cistern is demonstrated in the precontrast study and suggests the presence of a tumor (left). Strong contrast uptake within the tumor (right)

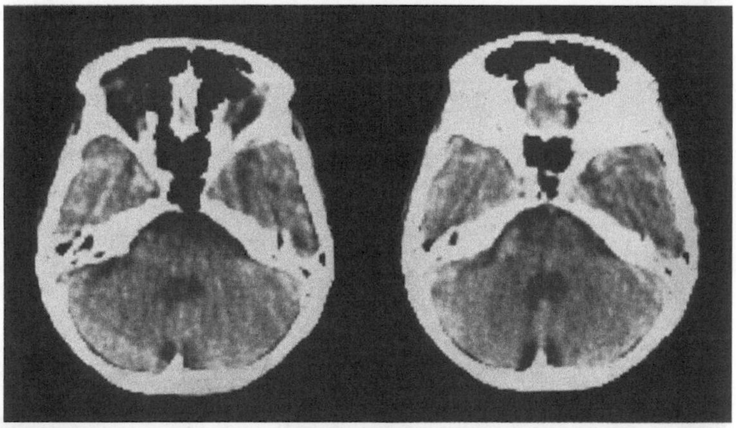

**Fig. D3.6.** Very small acoustic neurinoma on the left, barely visible in the precontrast study (left). Clear demonstration of the tumor at the posterior border of the pyramids in the postcontrast scan (right). The dark demarcation line between bone and tumor is an artifact. Fifty-three-year-old female with symptoms of a lesion at the left cerebellopontine angle

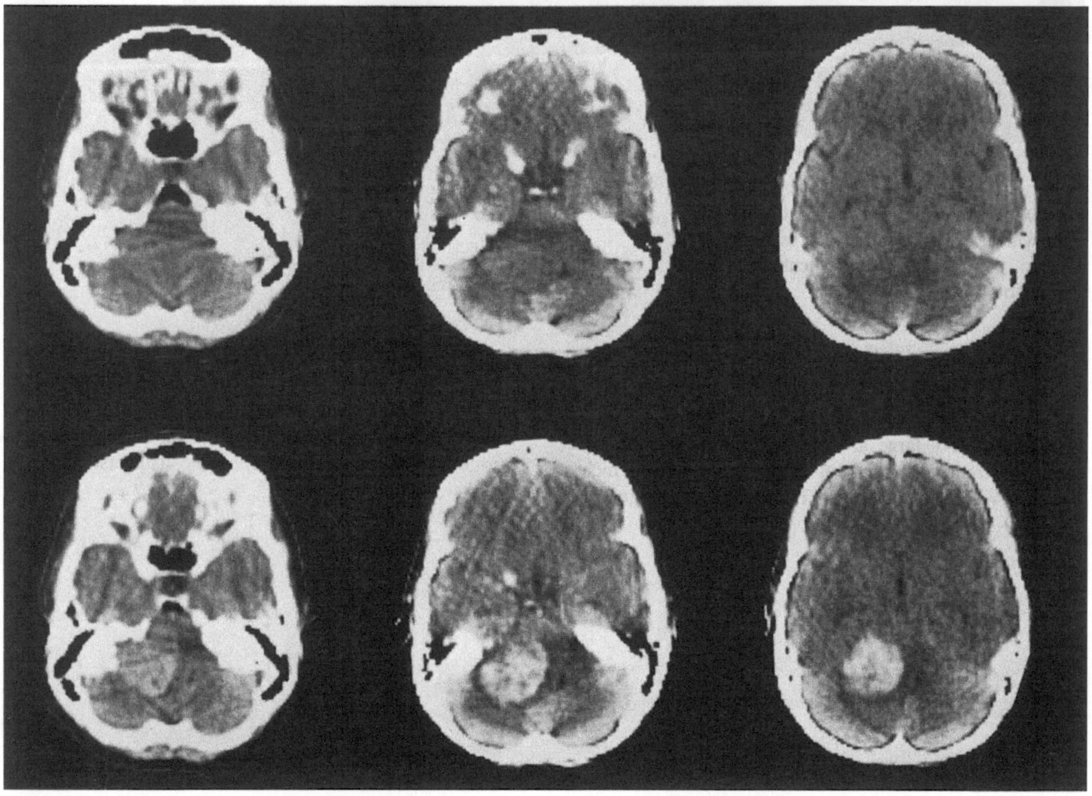

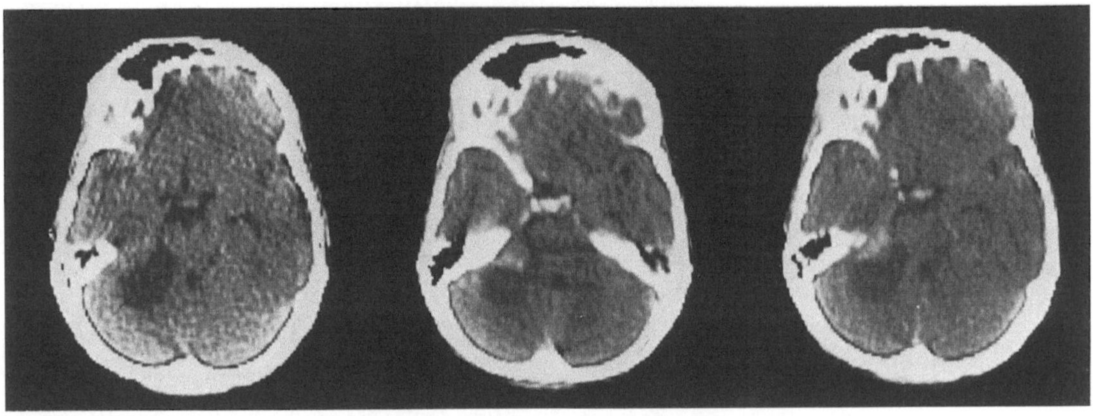

**Fig. D3.8.** Acoustic neurinoma on the left surrounded by a large cyst in a 47-year-old female. The tumor is clearly visible in the precontrast study (left). Clearer demonstration of solid tumor tissue after contrast enhancement (right)

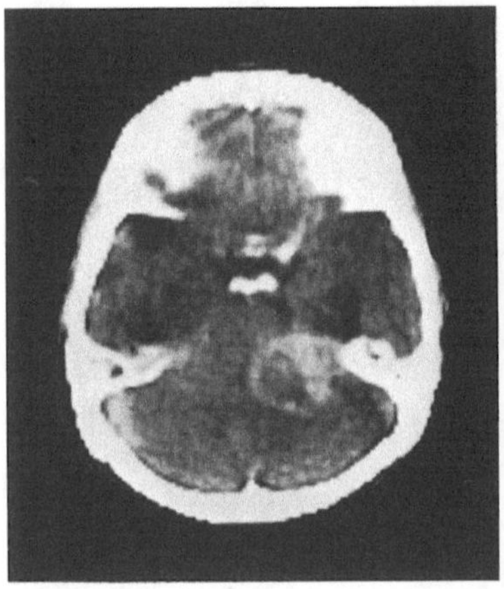

▲

**Fig. D3.9.** Acoustic neurinoma on the right with a central zone of necrosis and a ring of contrast enhancement in a 69-year-old male

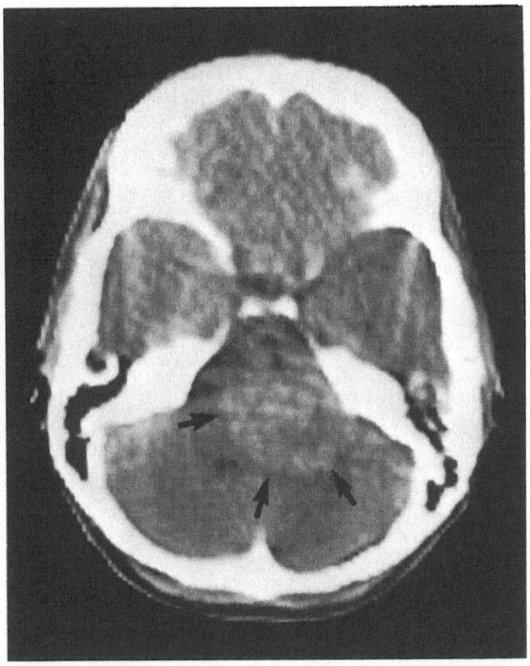

▲

**Fig. D3.10.** Very large acoustic neurinoma on the right, causing extreme displacement of the brain stem, which is not clearly delineated in the CT study. Initial diagnosis of brain stem tumor on the basis of CT findings. An acoustic neurinoma was found at operation. Postcontrast study

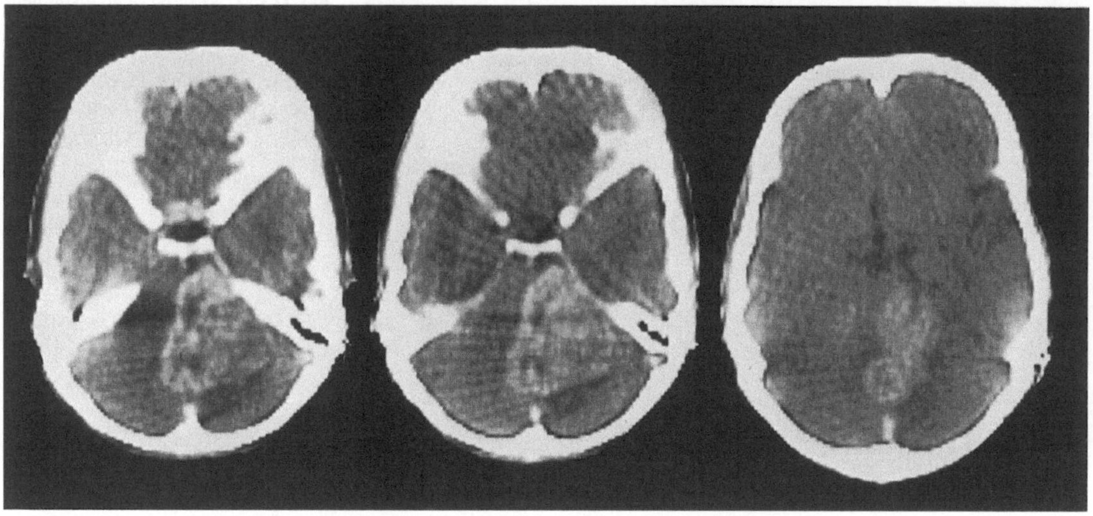

**Fig. D3.11.** Very large acoustic neurinoma with extensive regressive changes in a 37-year-old female. The tumor extends from the foramen magnum to the tentorium and the superior portion of the vermis cerebelli. Artifacts on the right due to a Holter valve. Postcontrast studies

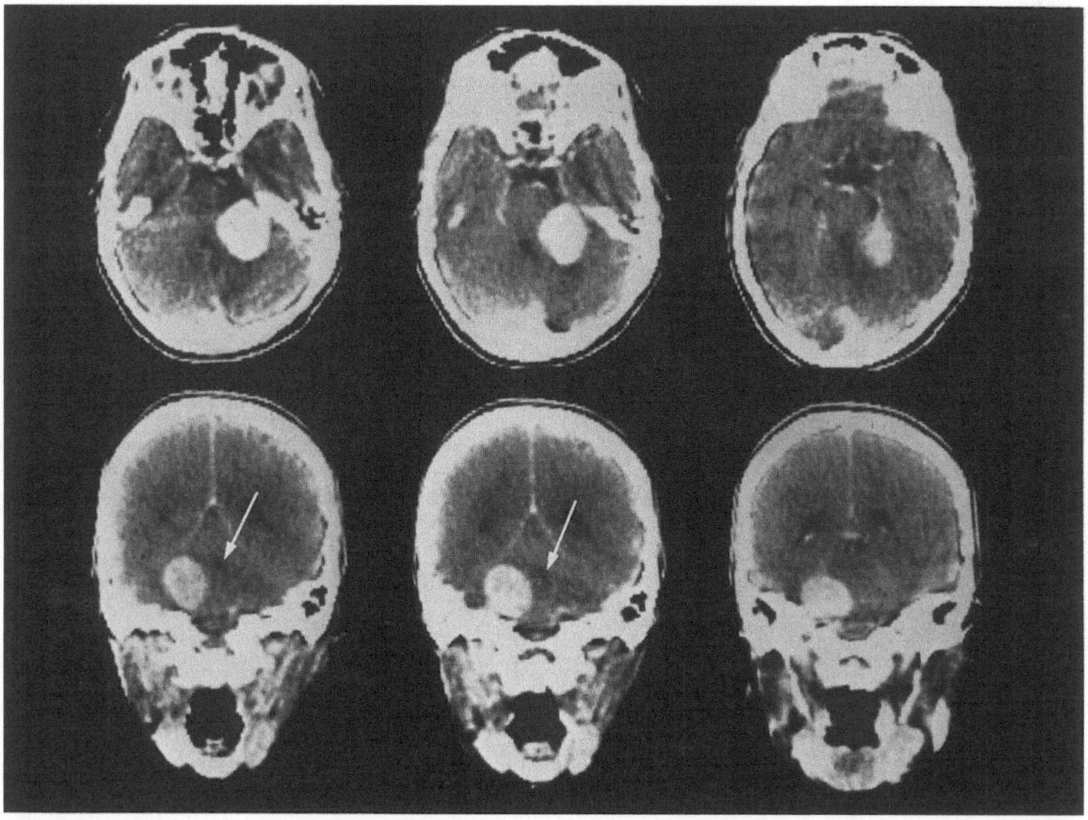

**Fig. D3.12.** Comparison of horizontal and coronary CT scans in an acoustic neurinoma on the right. Contrast enhancement with 30 g iodine. The coronary projection demonstrates displacement and comma-shaped deformation of the fourth ventricle (arrow). The tumor extends up to the tentorium (39-year-old patient)

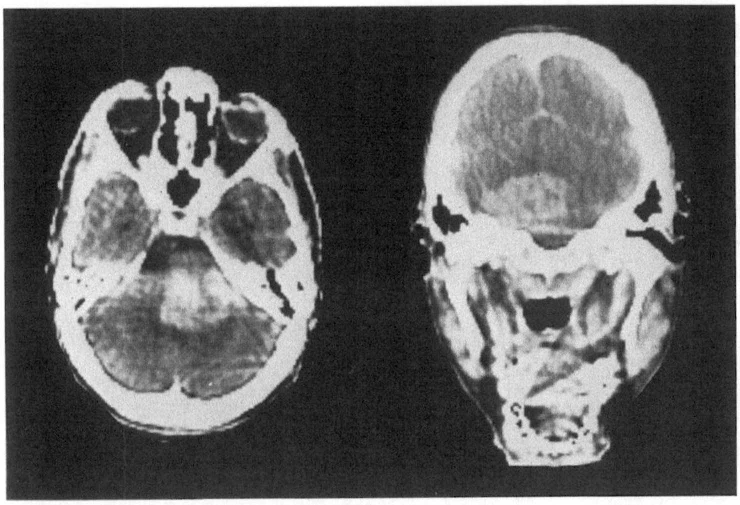

**Fig. D 3.13.** Very large acoustic neurinoma on the right with extension beyond the midline to the left in a 20-year-old patient. Horizontal and coronary projections. Postcontrast study

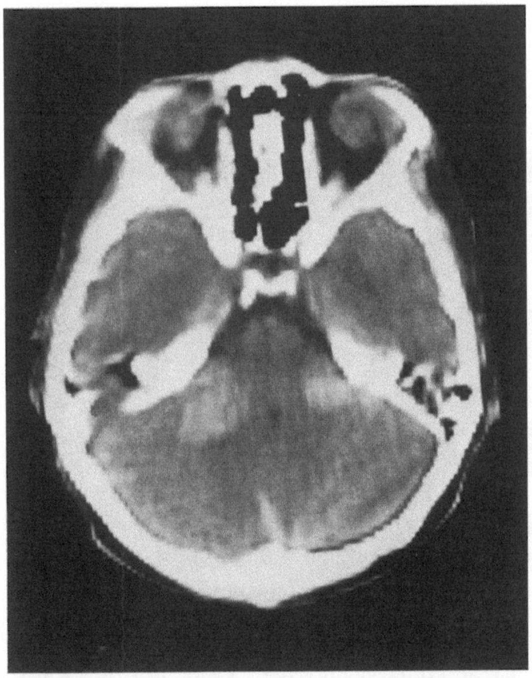

**Fig. D 3.14.** Bilateral acoustic neurinoma in a 55-year-old patient. Dilatation of the cerebellopontine cisterns bilaterally. Strong contrast enhancement within the tumor nodules

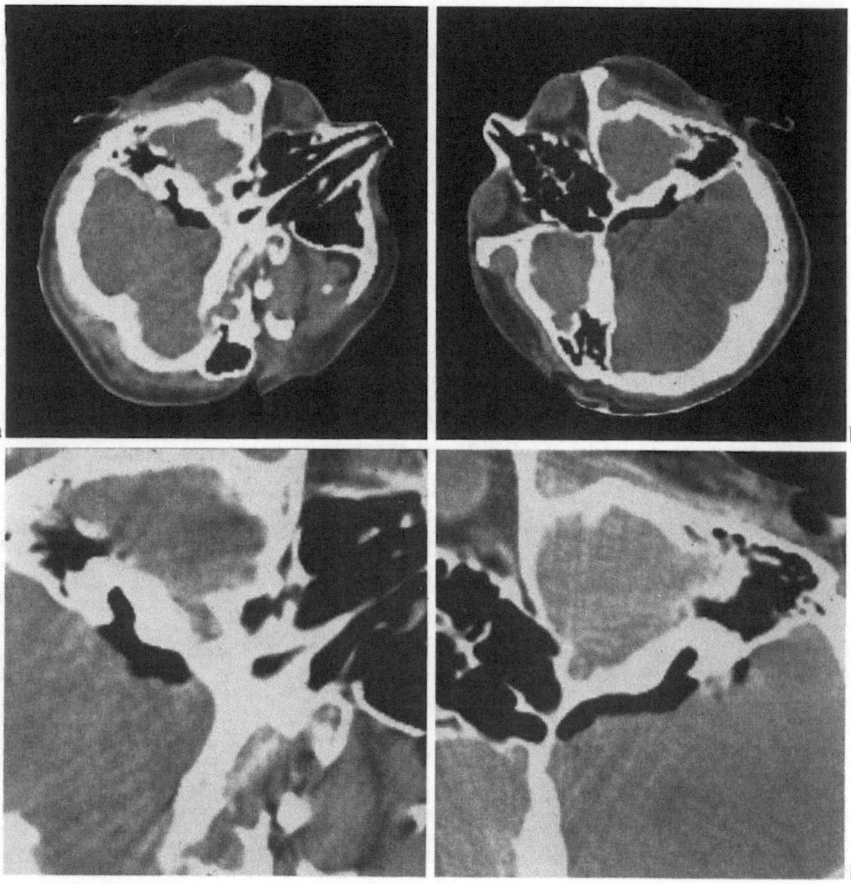

a b a' b'

**Fig. D3.15** a, b. Combined computed tomography and air cisternography with demonstration of the cerebellopontine cisterns and the internal acoustic meatus. Demonstration of the structures on the left (**a**, **a′**). After a change of head position air enters the internal acoustic meatus and the right cerebellopontine cistern (**b**, **b′**). Normal findings. **a′** and **b′** enlargements (5-mm slices)

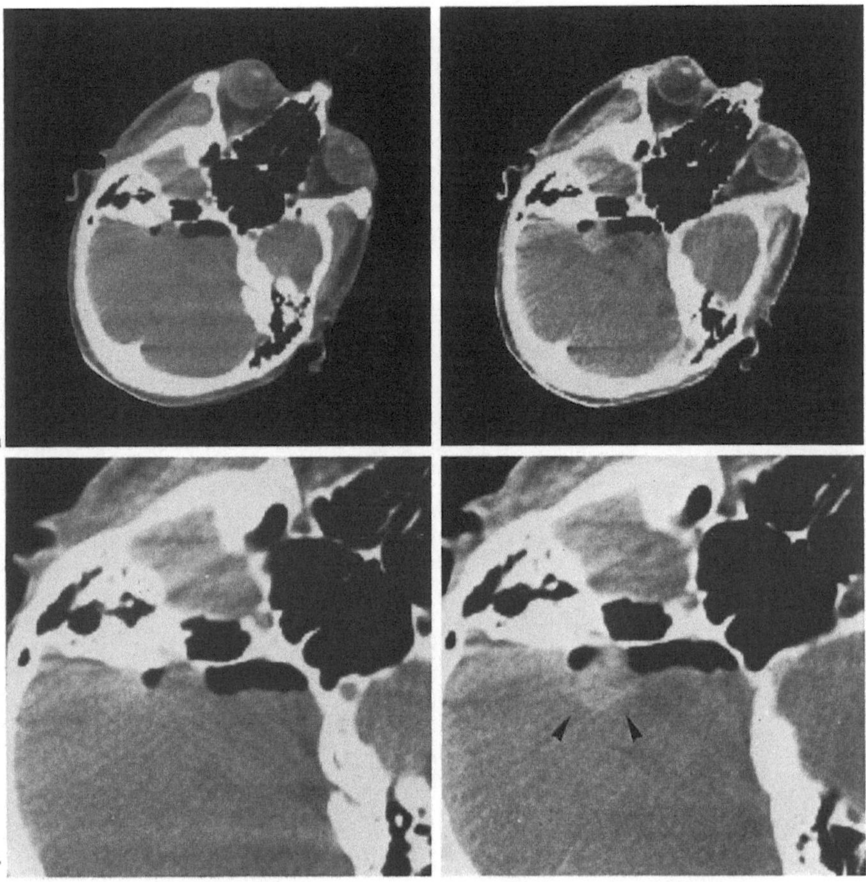

a b a′ b′

**Fig. D3.16** a, b. Combined computed tomography and air cisternography in a small acoustic neurinoma on the left. Air is present in the left cerebellopontine cistern; the acoustic neurinoma appears as a defect within the air-filled cistern (**a**, **a′**). Contrast enhancement allows clear delineation of the entire tumor (**b**, **b′**). **a′** and **b′** enlargements. (5-mm slices)

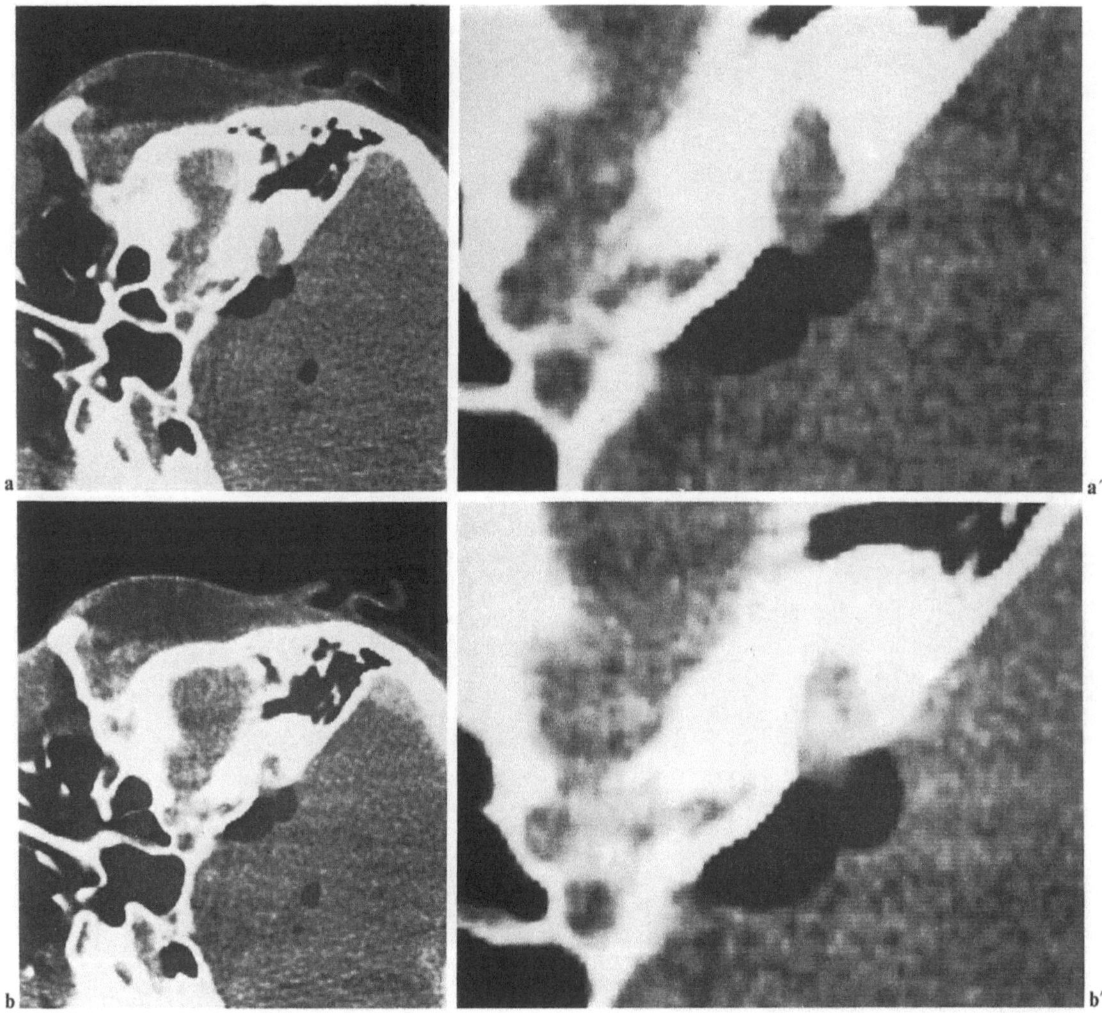


**Fig. D3.17** a, b. Combined computed tomography and air cisternography in a primarily intracanalicular acoustic neurinoma. The tumor fills the entire right internal meatus and demonstrates a small extracanalicular portion which is clearly delineated in the air-filled cerebellopontine cistern. **a′** and **b′** enlargements (5-mm slices). **b** and **b′** after contrast enhancement

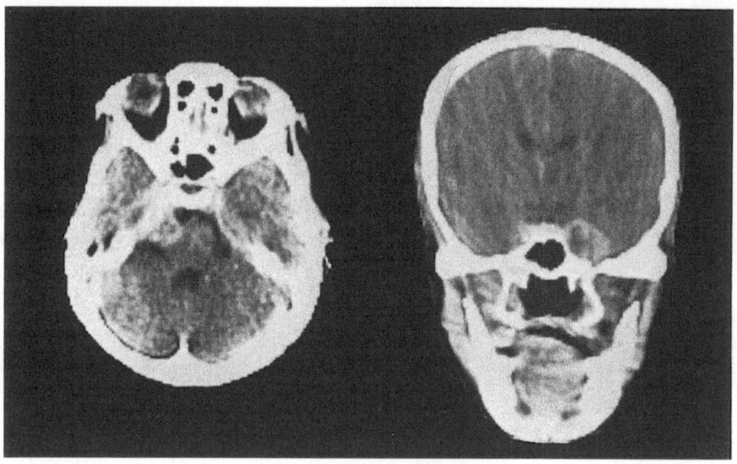

**Fig. D3.18.** Small trigeminal neurinoma on the left with inhomogeneous contrast uptake in both horizontal and coronary projections in a 58-year-old female. Typical site of this type of tumor. Postcontrast study

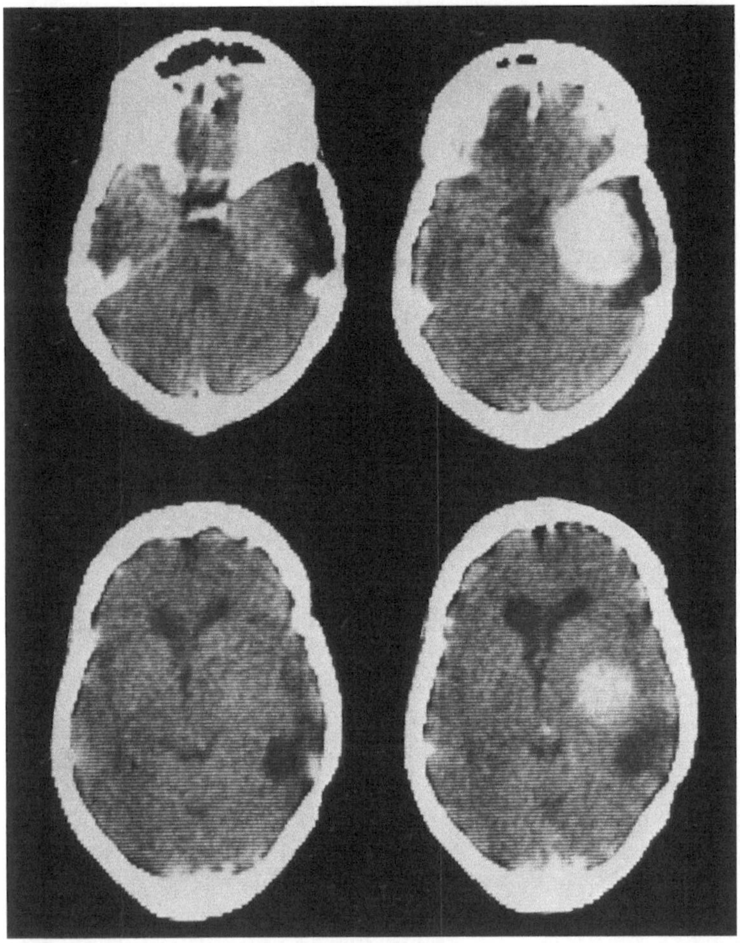

**Fig. D3.19.** Extensive recurrence of a trigeminal neurinoma on the right in a 65-year-old female. Solid tumor tissue appears isodense in precontrast studies (left) and demonstrates strong homogeneous contrast in the postcontrast study (right)

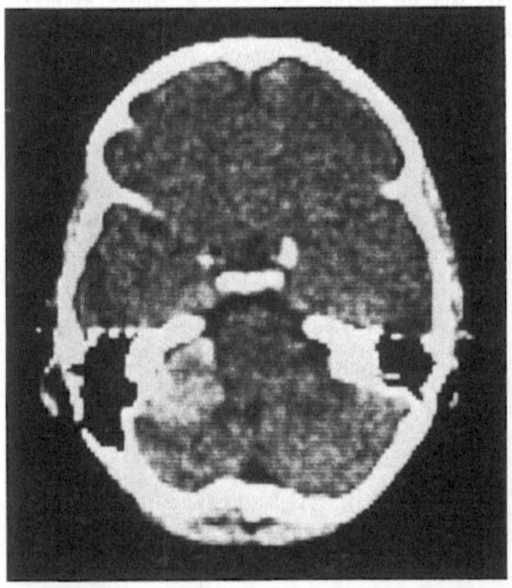

**Fig. D3.20.** Tenth nerve neurinoma on the left in a 14-year-old boy. The tumor is located slightly farther caudad than an acoustic neurinoma, but CT findings are similar in these tumors

# 4. Pituitary Adenomas

| | |
|---|---|
| Incidence | 8–12% |
| Characteristic age at diagnosis | 25–60 years |
| Sex distribution | Equal sex distribution |
| Typical locations | Sellar region |
| Characteristic clinical findings | Hormonal disorders (acromegaly, hyperprolactinemia, Cushing syndrome; pituitary insufficiency); visual disorders (chiasma syndrome) |
| Skull films | Primary changes of the sella |
| EEG | No findings |
| Echoencephalography | No findings |
| Serial brain scintigraphy | Tumors with large suprasellar portions demonstrate a perfusion pattern similar to that of meningioma with radionuclide uptake in static scans |
| Cerebral angiography | Elevation of the anterior cerebral artery in tumors with suprasellar extension; displacement and stretching of the carotid syphon in tumors with parasellar extension |
| Other contrast studies | Pneumocisternotomography demonstrates suprasellar extension of tumor |
| Special tests | Endocrinological studies |

**Computed Tomography**

| | |
|---|---|
| Precontrast study | Mostly hyperdense, rarely isodense zone filling the pentagon; inhomogeneous absorption pattern due to cyst formation in the tumor in some cases |
| Contrast medium uptake | Always positive in solid tumor portions |
| Appearance after contrast enhancement | Sharply delineated tumors in the suprasellar region and/or the entrance to the sella, with parasellar or retrosellar extension in some cases; cysts are clearly demonstrated; tumors limited to the sella (microadenomas) are usually not demonstrable with CT standard technique |

**Differential Diagnosis**

Suprasellar meningioma
Craniopharyngioma
Pilocytic astrocytoma
Aneurysm
"Empty sella"
Metastasis, chordoma, ectopic pinealoma, malignant lymphoma, tumors of the epipharynx, and histiocytosis X in rare cases

Pituitary adenomas are extracerebral tumors derived from the anterior pituitary lobe. ZÜLCH reported finding pituitary adenoma in 6.6% and OLIVECRONA in 8.6% of all intracranial tumors, while our collective demonstrated pituitary adenoma in 10% of cases (377 of 3,750 tumors). However, pituitary adenoma may comprise a larger proportion of all intracranial tumors, since endocrinological studies have allowed the diagnosis of microadenoma in an increasing number of cases in the recent past.

Pituitary adenomas are most common in middle-aged patients, but the peak incidence between the ages of 35 and 55 years (ZÜLCH) has shifted toward younger age groups with more frequent diagnosis of microadenomas.

Sex distribution is approximately equal, though microadenomas producing prolactin are more common in females.

## Location and Classification

Pituitary adenomas always originate in the sella and may extend to the suprasellar, parasellar, retrosellar, and/or subfrontal regions. Extension into the base of the skull may involve the cavernous sinus and the sphenoid sinus.

Large adenomas may extend in all directions simultaneously, and expansive growth is especially common in tumor recurrence after operation. Spread through the CSF pathways is a rare complication.

Very large pituitary adenomas with extension to the foramina of Monro may cause occlusive hydrocephalus.

Pituitary adenomas were previously classified according to histological criteria and described as eosinophilic, basophilic, chromophobic, or mixed types. The more *modern classification* derives from *endocrinological criteria,* and tumors are described as hormonally active or inactive (if immuncytochemical methods are available).

## Characteristic Clinical Findings

Purely intrasellar tumors may be characterized by *excessive hormone production* with corresponding clinical phenomena such as acromegaly, hyperprolactinemia (amenorrhea-galaktorrhea syndrome), or the Cushing syndrome as a result. These tumors and hormonally inactive lesions may exert pressure on the anterior pituitary lobe with consequent *pituitary insufficiency* and secondary hypogonadism, hypothyroidism, and adrenocortical insufficiency. When the pituitary adenoma extends beyond the sella and reaches the optic chiasma *bitemporal hemianopia,* observed in half of our cases, results. Irritation of the nerves serving the external ocular muscles – especially the third cranial nerve – occurs in rare cases of parasellar extension of the tumor and may cause double vision.

Headache occurs as a result of blockage of the foramen of Monro, after hemorrhage in the tumor and as the typical frontal headache found in acromegaly.

## Additional Diagnostic Procedures

*Conventional radiology* continues to play the decisive role in diagnosis of pituitary adenoma. The overwhelming majority of microadenomas may be detected on the basis of double contours or unilateral excavation of the sella on plain skull films or tomographic studies. However, a normally configured sella without enlargement or deformation does not exclude the diagnosis of microadenoma. Special endocrinological studies are necesssary for diagnosis in many of these cases, especially with Cushing's disease.

Tumor growth beyond a diameter of 8 mm results in enlargement of the cavum sellae, thinning of the floor of the sella, and increased radiolucency of the dorsum sellae, which may be further deformed with enlargement of the sellar aperture. *Serial brain scintigraphy* demonstrates only large suprasellar adenomas. Perfusion patterns and radionuclide uptake are comparable to those found in meningiomas.

*Angiographic findings* in large adenomas with suprasellar expansion reveal elevation of the horizontal segment of the anterior cerebral artery, stretching or lateral displacement of the carotid siphon, especially in parasellar growth of the tumor.

Normal vascular findings do not exclude the possibility of suprasellar or parasellar tumor growth, since the adenoma may lack a capsule and fail to displace vessels as it grows. Suspicion of parasellar tumor growth is an indication for angiography.

*Pneumoencephalography and cisternography* were the decisive procedures in diagnosis of suprasellar adenomas before the introduction of computed tomography, but these two procedures have largely been supplanted by the newer technique. Pneumocisternography is no longer justified even in cases with unclear CT findings or when an empty sella is suspected, since CT scanning after intrathecal injection of metrizamide will solve these diagnostic problems with a higher degree of reliability.

## Computed Tomography (Figs. D4.1–30) (see also pp. 382f., 392).

### Precontrast Study

Pituitary adenomas appear as sharply delineated, round, or oval hyperdense (65.8%) or isodense (17.5%) lesions which partially or totaly fill the chiasmatic cistern (Fig. D4.2). 12.5% of adenomas demonstrate mixed density due to cysts or residues of hemorrhage in the tumor (Figs. D4.13, 15). Cysts may be found outside the actual tumor in some cases (Figs. D4.19, 20).

Calcification is extremely rare, occurring in less than 1% of all adenomas (Fig. D4.11). Only a few adenomas are uniformly hypodense, the result of cystic change (4.2%). Attenuation values in solid tumor tissue average 35–50 HU. Higher density values within an adenoma suggest hemorrhage in the tumor, especially if the patients complain of sudden onset of headache and visual disorders (Figs. D4.16, 17). This development is extremely rare, occurring in 1% of cases in our series, and may entail paralysis of the extraocular muscles and severe endocrine disorders. CT is also useful in demonstration of postoperative hemorrhage (Fig. D4.18).

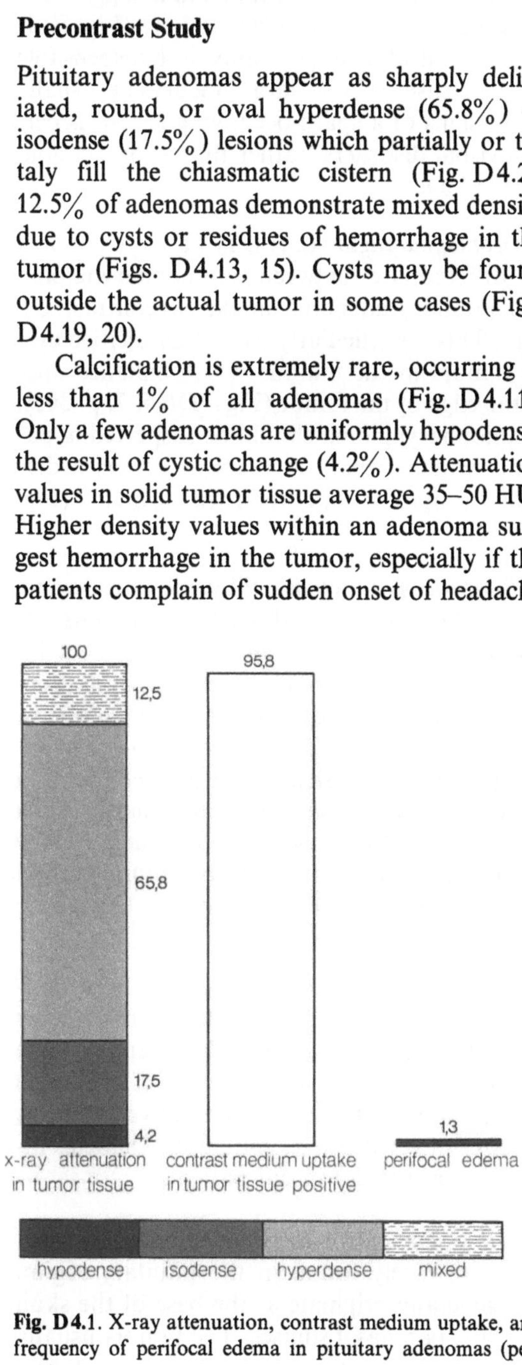


**Fig. D4.1.** X-ray attenuation, contrast medium uptake, and frequency of perifocal edema in pituitary adenomas (percent)

### Postcontrast Study

There is a significant increase in absorption values in solid tumor after contrast enhancement in more than 95% of cases. The increase in density is homogeneous and averages 16 HU (range 12–34 HU), depending mainly on the amount of contrast medium employed. The maximum is attained shortly after injection and the decrease in density values is correspondingly rapid.

The pituitary adenoma with suprasellar expansion usually appears as a sharply delineated hyperdense zone within the chiasmatic cistern (Figs. D4.3, 4, 6, 7). Contrast enhancement may be necessary for determination of the exact configuration of the tumor. Parasellar, retrosellar, and subfrontal portions of the adenoma are much more clearly demonstrated after contrast enhancement and may indeed require contrast enhancement for demonstration (Figs. D4.8–10). These findings are especially important in the choice of the operative approach to the tumor. Cysts and areas with past hemorrhage or regressive changes do not accept contrast media and appear as sharply delineated zones of relatively low density in the contrast-enhanced scan (Figs. D4.12–15). Large vessels such as the internal carotid and basilar arteries appear as round circumscribed structures at the edge of the tumor on horizontal slices and demonstrate very high density values after contrast enhancement (Figs. D4.9, 14). Coronary projections may show longer segments of these two vessels; in some cases the carotid bifurcation into the anterior cerebral and middle cerebral arteries is visible. Contrast uptake in the cavernous sinus may simulate parasellar extension of the tumor.

*Coronary projections define the suprasellar extent of the adenoma and its relations to adjacent brain structures* (Figs. D4.4, 5). *Intrathecal administration of metrizamide* allows better demonstration of pituitary adenomas in the CT scan, since the tumor appears as a defect within the hyperdense basal cisterns (Fig. D4.21).

Invasion of the sphenoid sinuses by the tumor is evident when the sphenoid cells, which usually contain air, are filled with hyperdense tissue after contrast enhancement (Fig. E7, p. 382). Lateral extension is evident in horizontal slices when the tumor has penetrated the cavernous sinus and invades the middle fossa (Fig. D4.8).

*Pituitary adenomas confined to the sella* must reach the sellar aperture before they can be demonstrated in the CT scan (Figs. D4.22–24). This is true especially for CT scanners of the first and second generations.

Endocrinological studies reveal *microadenomas* which escape detection with standard CT technique when the tumors are smaller than 5 mm in diameter. However, most microadenomas can be demonstrated when reformated images from extremely thin slices (1.5 to 2 mm) are used (TURSKI et al. 1981) (Fig. D4.29).

**Empty sella** is defined as radiological evidence of sellar enlargement with herniation of the opticochiasmatic cistern into the sella. CT studies show a zone with CSF density at the entrance to the sella (Figs. D4.25–27). This is a common finding in 30% of all patients over 40 as a result of involution of the pituitary gland with descent of the diaphragma sellae. The *pituitary stalk* may occasionally appear in the posterior segment of the sellar aperture (Fig. D4.28).

Approximately 20% of patients with microadenoma also demonstrate herniation of the opticochiasmatic cistern into the pituitary fossa. A diagnosis of "empty sella" may be made in these cases and can be confirmed by intrathecal administration of metrizamide with subsequent CT studies. The intrasellar cistern, which is opacified by the contrast medium, can be visualized within the sella, especially in coronary projections.

## Differential Diagnosis

*1. Suprasellar Meningioma.* Suprasellar meningeomas and pituitary adenomas have similar density, contrast uptake, and locations, and cannot be differentiated in the precontrast CT scan (Figs. D2.12). Differentiation may be possible as a result of typical changes in bony structures associated with meningioma visible in the plain skull film. Sellar enlargement and endocrine disorders are not found with this tumor (see Fig. D4.30).

*2. Aneurysms.* Large aneurysms of the carotid artery and the circle of Willis may simulate pituitary adenoma, though contrast uptake in these cases is extremely high (Fig. F60). Crescent-shaped and ring-shaped calcifications are often found in the wall of the aneurysms, both in CT studies and plain films, and suggest the possibility of a vascular lesion (Fig. F61, p. 444). Carotid angiography is indispensable in such cases. These large aneurysms usually cause signs of a space-occupying lesion, generally visual disorders, rather than subarachnoid hemorrhage.

*3. Craniopharyngioma.* It is not always possible to differentiate between craniopharyngioma and pituitary adenoma in the precontrast CT scan. This is particularly true of uncalcified cystic tumors in the midline which enhance only at the edge of the tumor (Figs. D6.6, 7, p. 303). Craniopharyngioma should be suspected in patients younger than 25 years of age with diabetes insipidus and retarded growth (Fig. D4.30).

*4. Pilocytic Astrocytoma.* Pilocytic astrocytoma of the optic chiasma and the hypothalamus was formerly designated as optic glioma, spongioblastoma of the hypothalamus, or infundibuloma. It is often irregular, may involve one or both optic nerves and may extend to the hypothalamic region. Calcification is as common in pilocytic astrocytoma as in craniopharyngioma but is not characteristic of adenoma. Density values before and after contrast administration may resemble those in adenoma (Fig. G12, p. 471).

*5. Ectopic Pinealoma or Germinoma.* CT findings may be quite similar to those in pituitary adenoma (Fig. D1.245). The patients are usually children and adolescents. As in all rare tumors found in this region, definitive diagnosis requires direct tissue examination. Diabetes insipidus was present in our patients.

*6. Other Tumors in the Sellar Region. Metastases* are rarely found in the pituitary region and generally originate at the base of the skull or in the paranasal sinuses. The tumors usually are associated with radiological and CT evidence of bone destruction, as is also the case in other malignant tumors of this region such as epipharynx carcinoma or sarcoma and aesthesioneuroblastoma (see Chap. E, p. 378).

Our series includes a number of *chordomas* of this region. The tumors demonstrate numerous small calcifications and take up contrast media readily (Figs. D7.6, 7, p. 339 f.). CT findings are quite different from those in adenoma.

We were not able to differentiate between a *malignant lymphoma* of the sellar region and pituitary adenoma (Fig. D1.212, p. 167). The same is true of *histiocytosis X*, which may originate at any point in the hypothalamo-pituitary axis (Figs. D1.229–231, p. 178).

A **choristoma** was found in a 50-year-old male. The tumor is a malformation of the posterior pituitary lobe. It appeared as a large sharply delineated mass lesion in the suprasellar region which differed from the usual presentation of pituitary adenoma in its enormous suprasellar extension (Fig. D4.31). ZÜLCH also reports *gangliocytomas* of the sellar region, but we did not observe this tumor in our series.

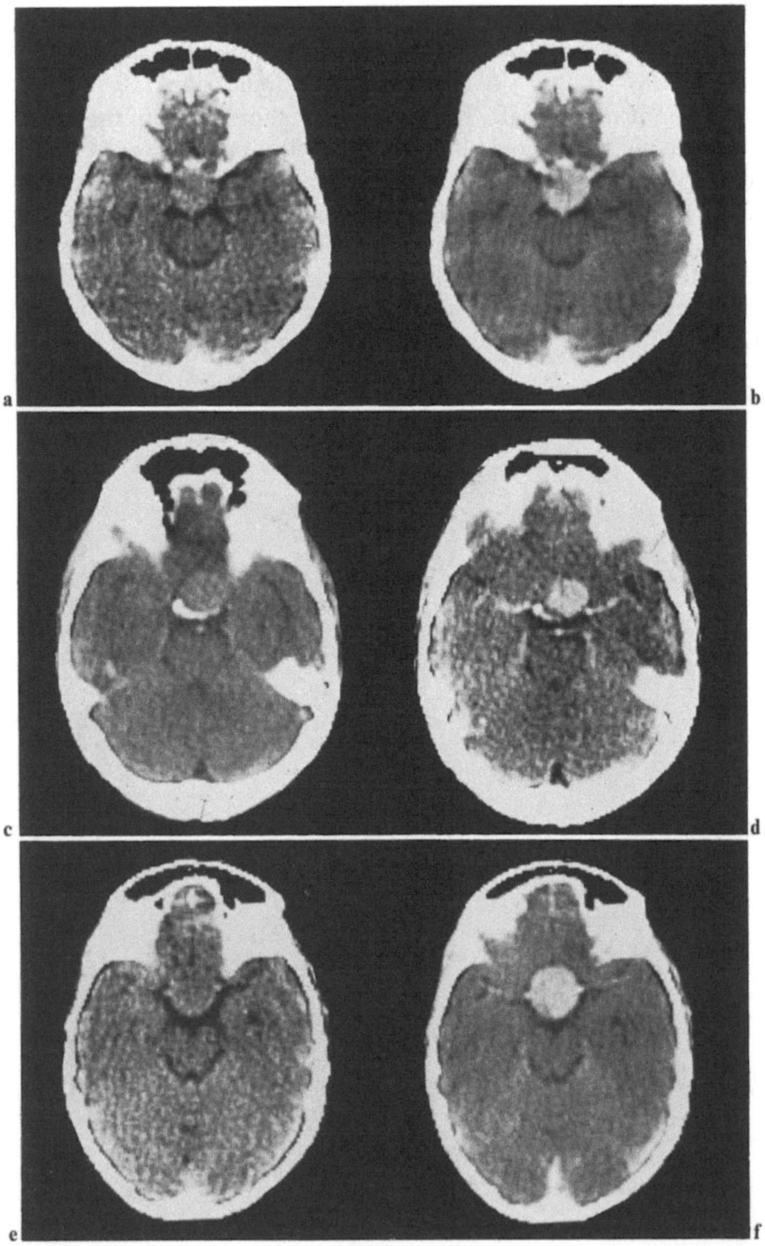


**Fig. D4.2** a–f. Typical CT findings in pituitary adenomas. (**a, b**) Suprasellar adenoma in a 64-year-old female. The tumor appears hyperdense in the precontrast study (**a**) and completely fills the chiasmatic cistern; strong contrast uptake (**b**). (**c, d**) Asymmetrical adenoma with slightly hyperdense absorption values in the precontrast study (**c**) and strong contrast uptake (**d**) in a 24-year-old patient. Note the unilateral atrophy of the dorsum sellae. (**e, f**) Large symmetrical pituitary adenoma in a 40-year-old patient. The tumor appears isodense in precontrast studies (**e**), but it is clearly delineated within the chiasmatic cistern. Strong contrast uptake (**f**)

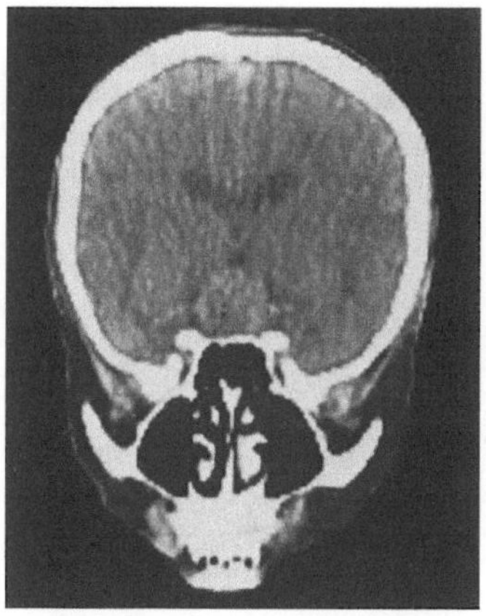

Fig. D4.4. Large suprasellar pituitary adenoma in a 50-year-old female. Coronary projections demonstrate partial obliteration of the third ventricle by the tumor

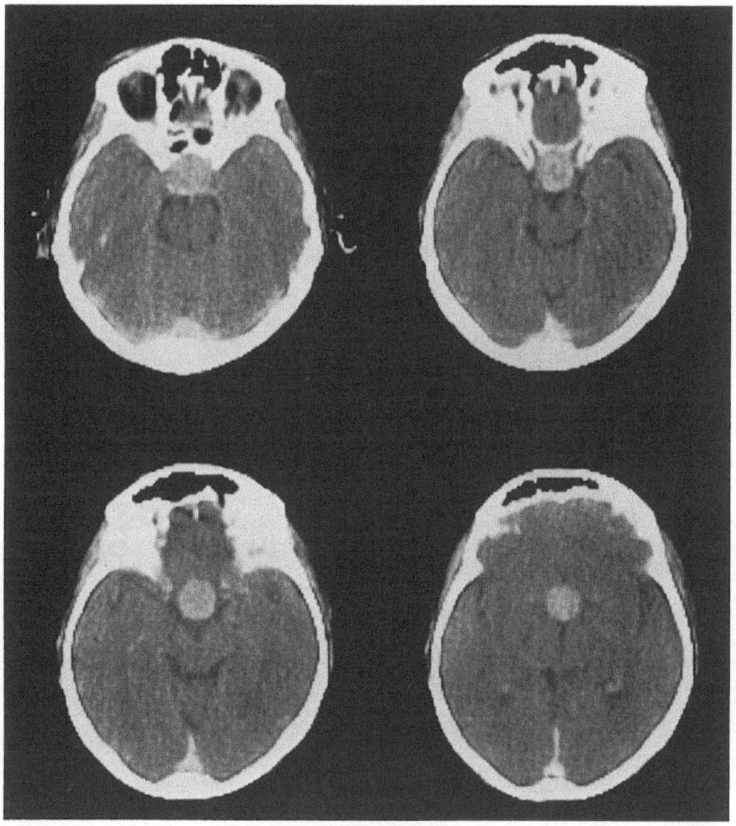

Fig. D4.3. Symmetrical pituitary adenoma with intrasellar and suprasellar extension in a 50-year-old patient with bitemporal hemianopsia. Postcontrast study

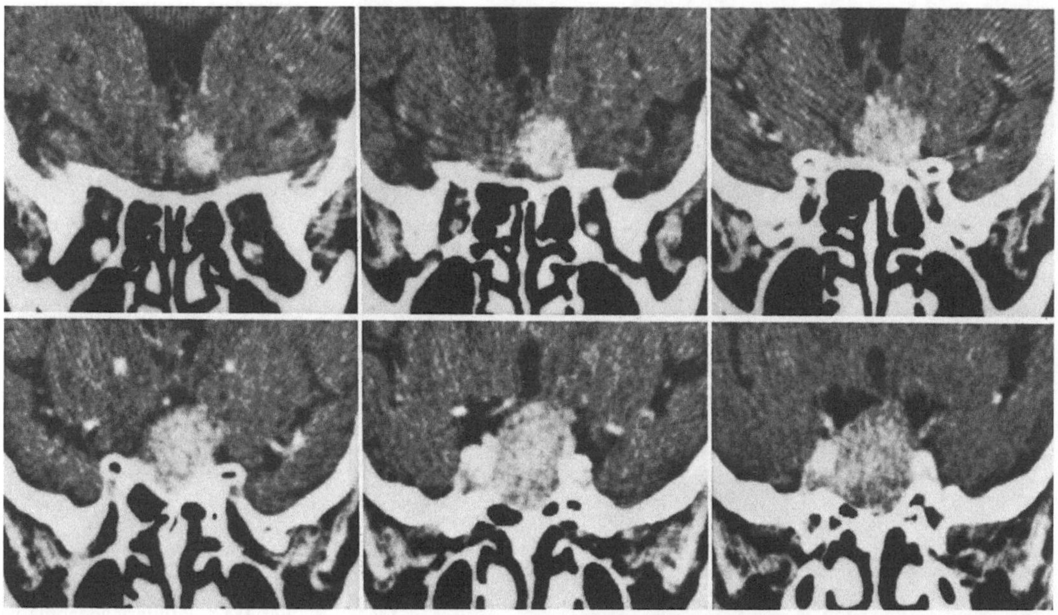

Fig. D4.5. Asymmetrical pituitary adenoma with intrasellar and suprasellar growth in a 72-year-old female. Extent of tumor growth is demonstrated well in the coronary projection. Postcontrast study. (Courtesy of Prof. FELIX, Dept. of Radiology, Klinikum Charlottenburg, FU Berlin)

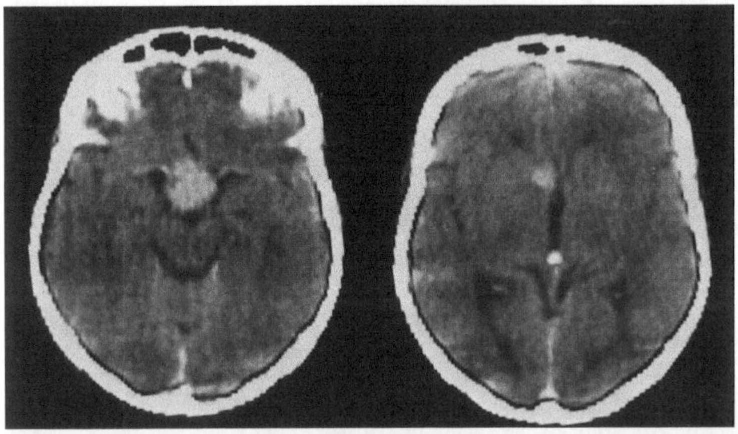

**Fig. D4.6.** Pituitary adenoma with suprasellar extension as far as the foramen of Monro on the left. The tumor has not caused blockage of the foramen. Postcontrast study ◄

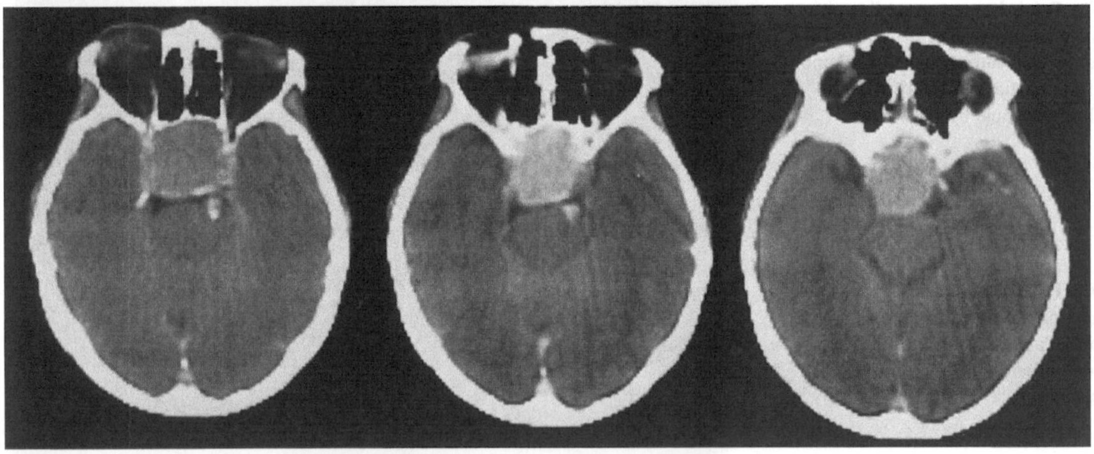

▲

**Fig. D4.7.** Large pituitary adenoma extending into the sphenoid sinus. Total destruction of the dorsum sellae. Postcontrast study

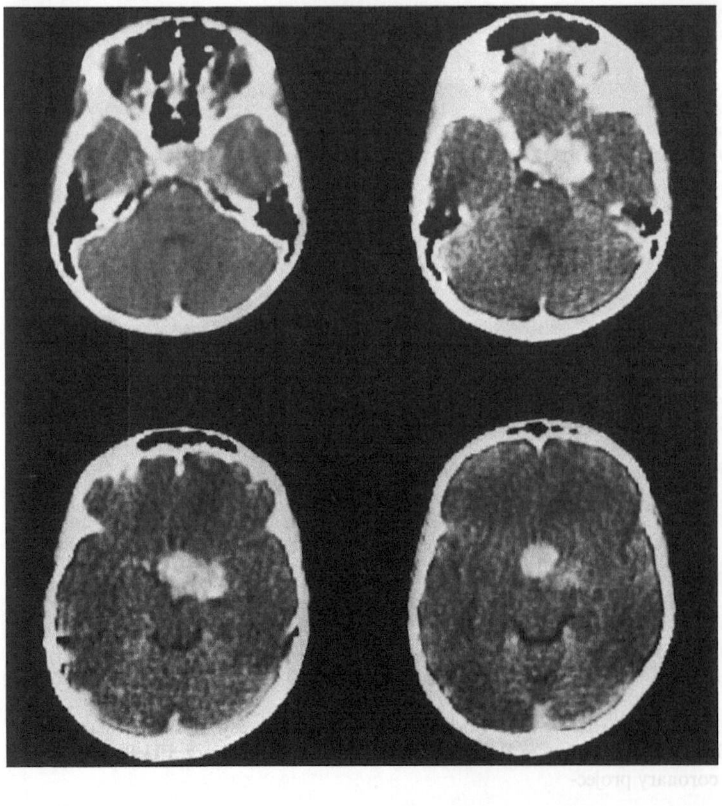

◄

**Fig. D4.8.** Pituitary adenoma with intrasellar, suprasellar, and parasellar growth on the right in a 43-year-old female. Postcontrast study

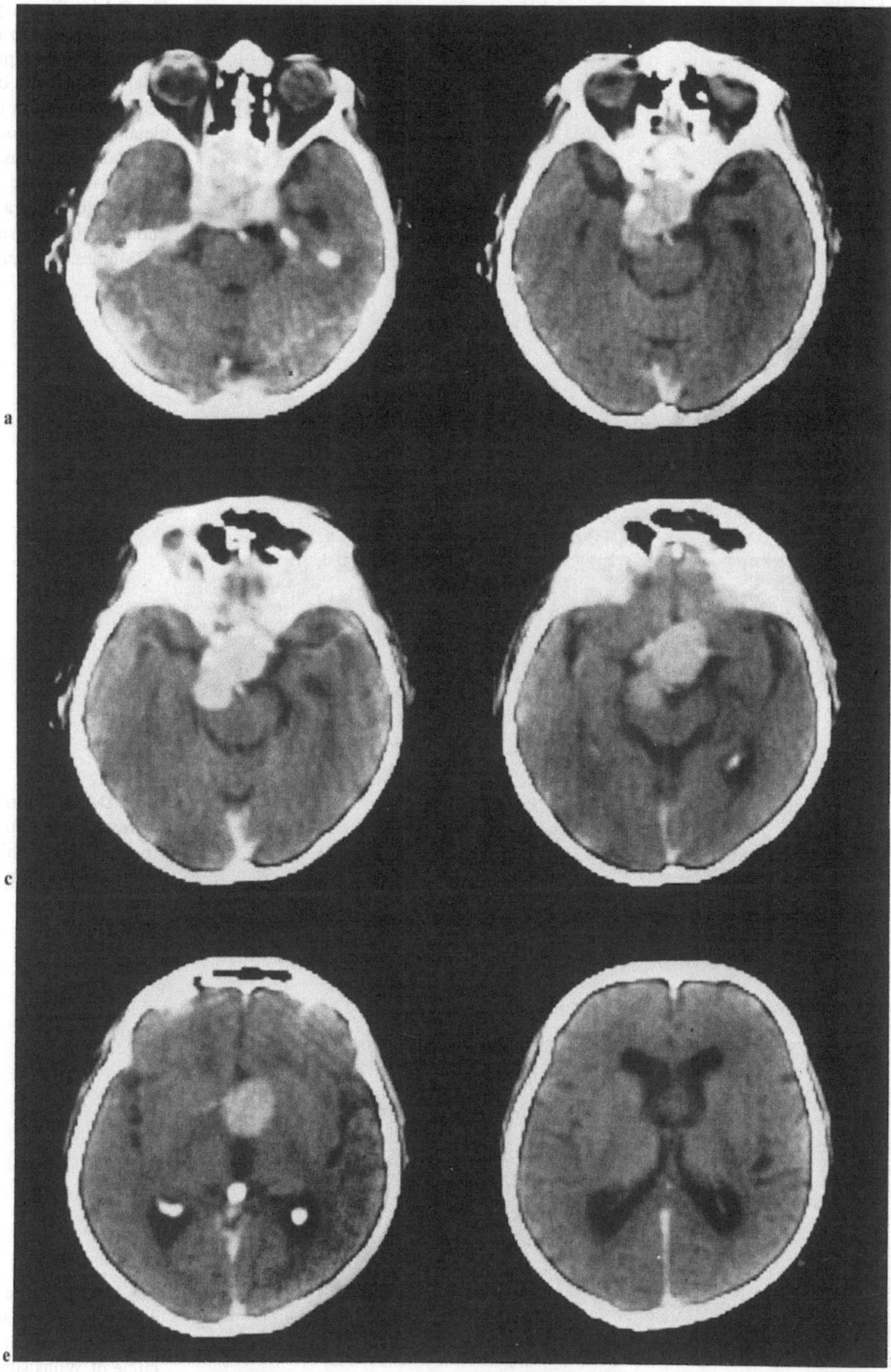

a b c d e f

**Fig. D4.9** a–f. Large pituitary adenoma in a 71-year-old patient. The tumor has penetrated the sphenoid sinus (**a**). A retrosellar offshoot of the tumor extends toward the left cerebral peduncle (**b**, **c**, **d**). Significant suprasellar growth with incipient blockage of the foramina of Monro (**e**, **f**). Postcontrast study

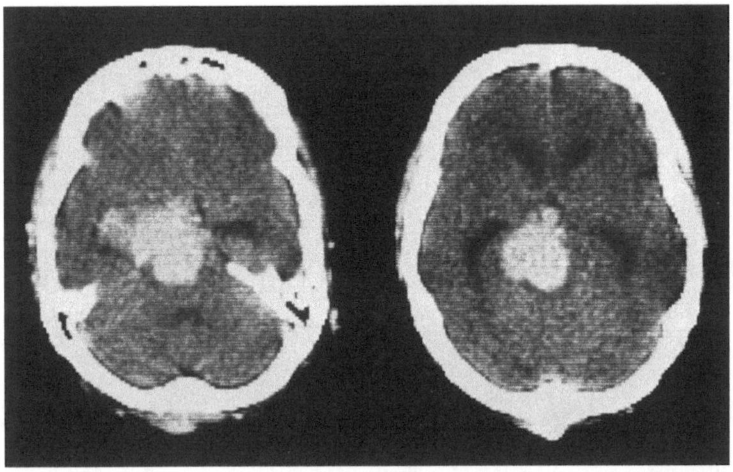

**Fig. D4.10.** Pituitary adenoma with an atypical growth pattern in the parasellar, subtemporal, and retrosellar regions with disruption of CSF circulation in the third ventricle and the aqueduct in a 36-year-old male with signs of increased intracranial pressure. The tumor was not recognized as a pituitary adenoma at initial evaluation of the CT studies. Postcontrast study

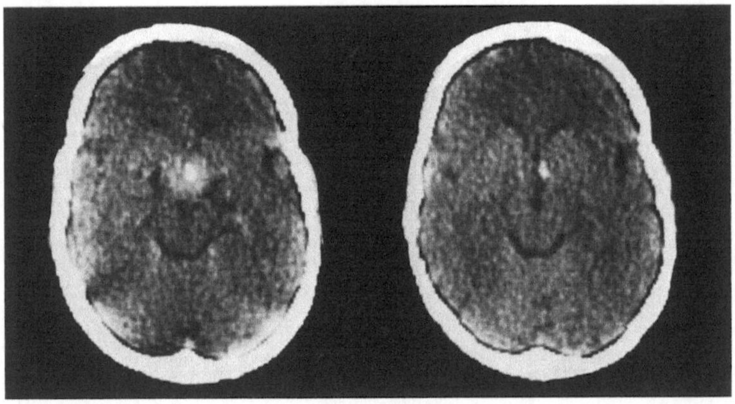

**Fig. D4.11.** Suprasellar growth of a pituitary adenoma in a 49-year-old patient with a chiasma syndrome. Fine calcification in the upper portions of the tumor. Postcontrast study

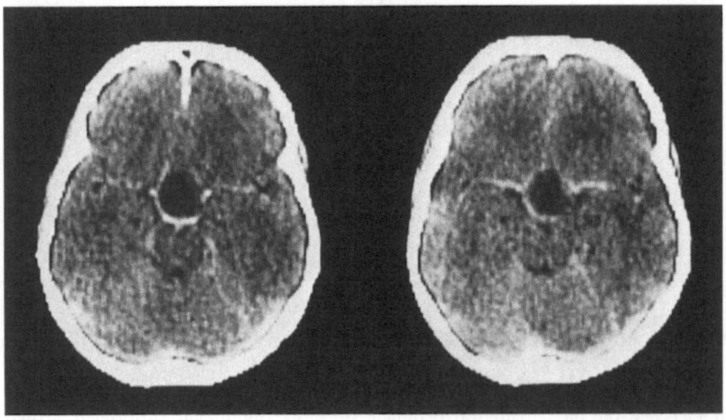

**Fig. D4.12.** Cystic pituitary adenoma in a 48-year-old female. Contrast enhancement demonstrates the circle of Willis surrounding a hypodense zone. No evidence of contrast uptake within the tumor capsule

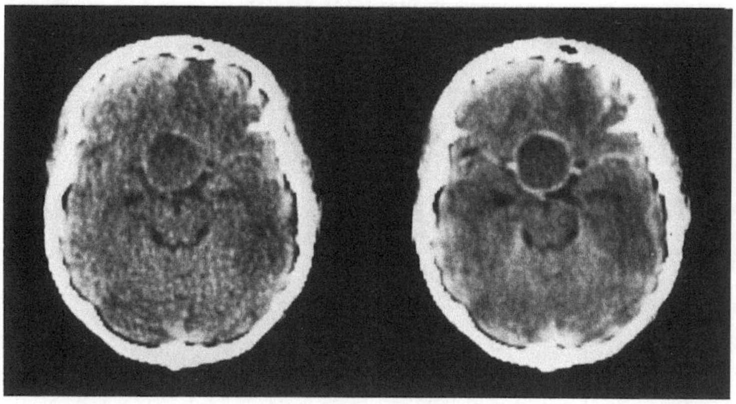

**Fig. D4.13.** Large cystic pituitary adenoma in a 24-year-old female with a chiasma syndrome and secondary amenorrhea (left, precontrast study). There is strong contrast enhancement within the capsule in the postcontrast study (right). Density values within the cyst remain unchanged at 27–28 HU. Xanthochromic fluid was found in the cyst at operation

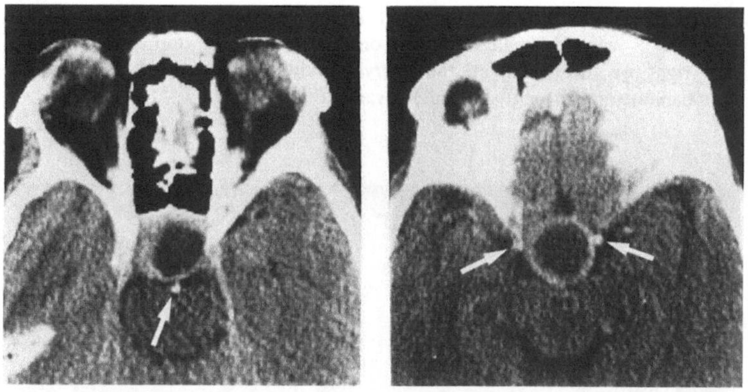

**Fig. D4.14.** Cystic pituitary adenoma in a 70-year-old female with a chiasma syndrome. Ring enhancement of the solid portions of the tumor. Strong contrast uptake in the large arteries [right and left internal carotid and basilar arteries (arrows)] adjacent to the tumor capsule. Demonstration of old liquefied hematoma within the adenoma at operation

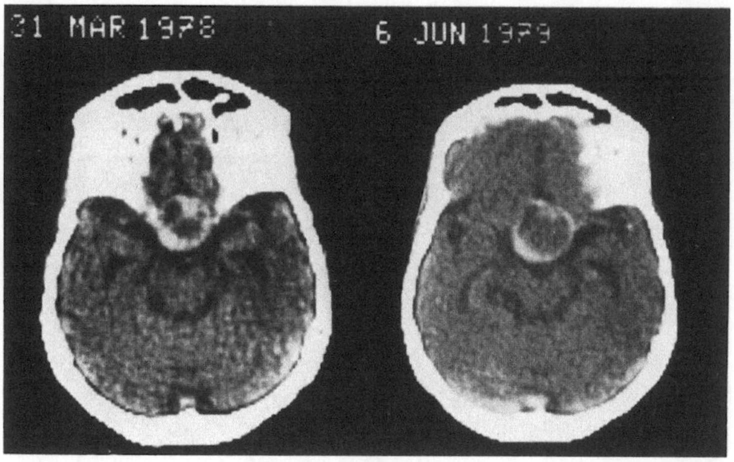


**Fig. D4.15.** Follow-up studies of a cystic pituitary adenoma. Initial CT on March 13, 1978: Large polycystic adenoma in a 74-year-old patient. Follow-up studies on June 6, 1979, 15 months after transsphenoidal resection of the tumor: demonstration of a large recurrent tumor, again with a cyst

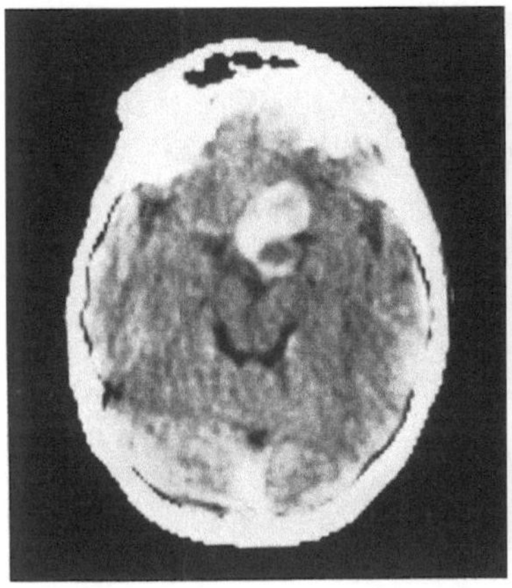

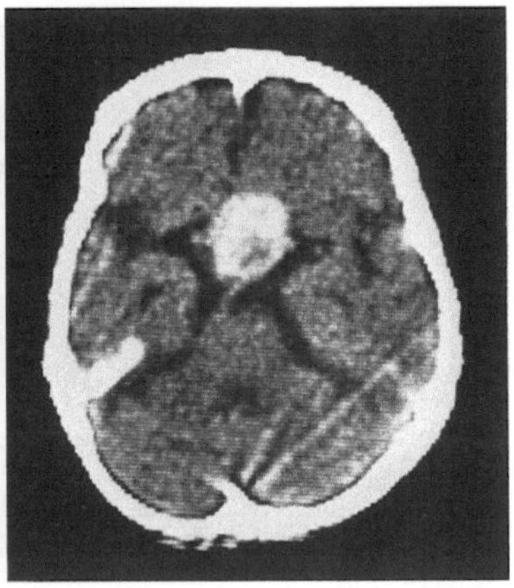

**Fig. D4.17.** Massive hemorrhage in a pituitary adenoma in a 69-year-old man with sudden onset of total blindness. Density values within the tumor are those found in freshly coagulated blood (80–85 HU)

▲

**Fig. D4.16.** Pituitary adenoma with extension to the right subfrontal region with evidence of recent and past hemorrhage in a 38-year-old female with acute onset of blindness in the right eye and incomplete third nerve paralysis. The tumor demonstrates strongly hyperdense values (70–80 HU) in the precontrast study. At operation these regions were found to contain recent hemorrhage. Past hemorrhage posterior to the recent bleeding has the same appearance as a cyst. Postcontrast study

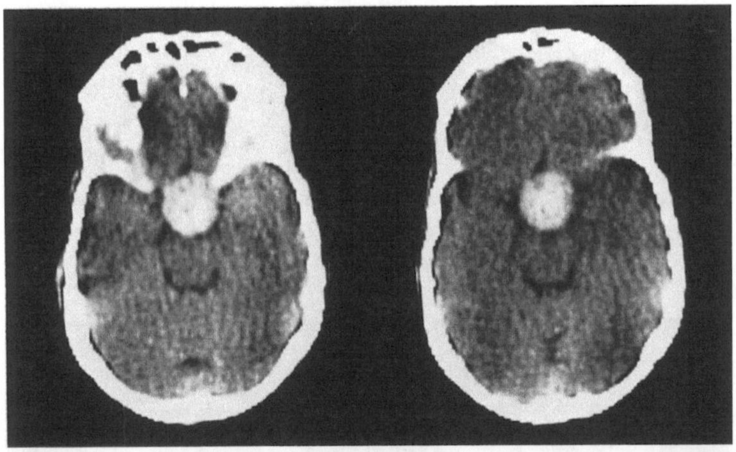

**Fig. D4.18.** CT findings 6 days after transsphenoidal removal of a pituitary adenoma in a 46-year-old patient. Hemorrhage in the area of the former tumor. High attenuation values in precontrast studies pointing to freshly coagulated blood

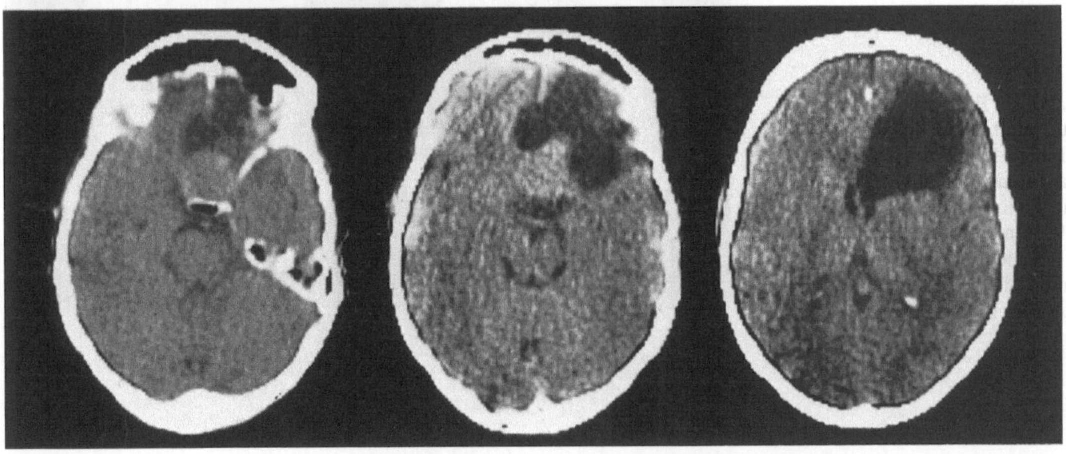

**Fig. D4.19.** Large suprasellar pituitary adenoma in a 37-year-old male with impotence, visual disorders, and an organic brain syndrome. The precontrast study shows a slightly hyperdense suprasellar tumor with a large marginal cyst occupying almost the entire right frontal lobe

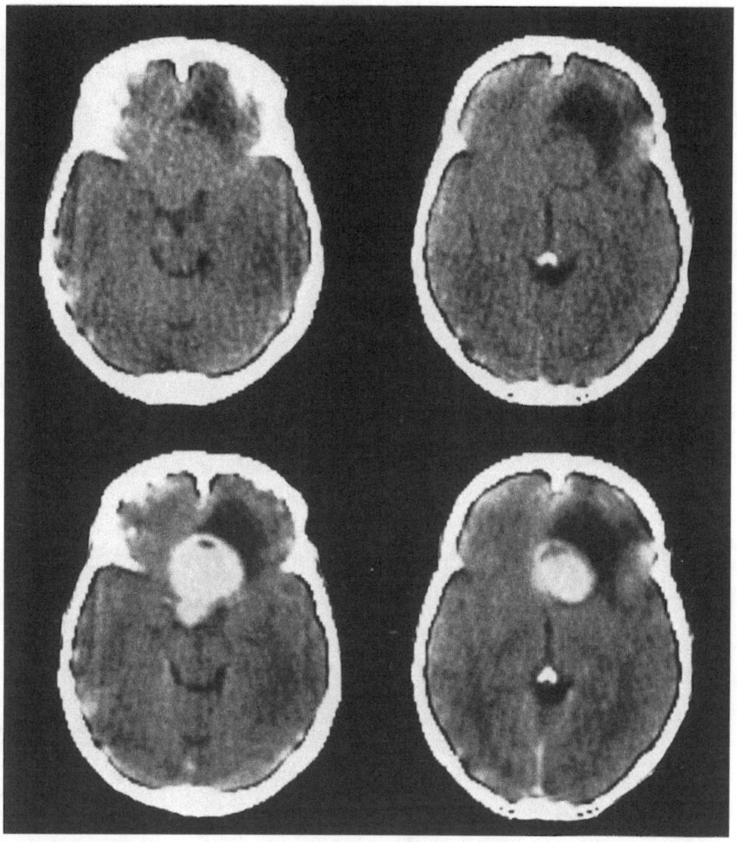

**Fig. D4.20.** Extensive suprasellar and retrosellar recurrence of a pituitary adenoma with a marginal cyst in the right frontal lobe of a 35-year-old female. The tumor appears isodense in the precontrast study (above). There is strong almost homogeneous contrast uptake in the solid portion of the tumor (below)

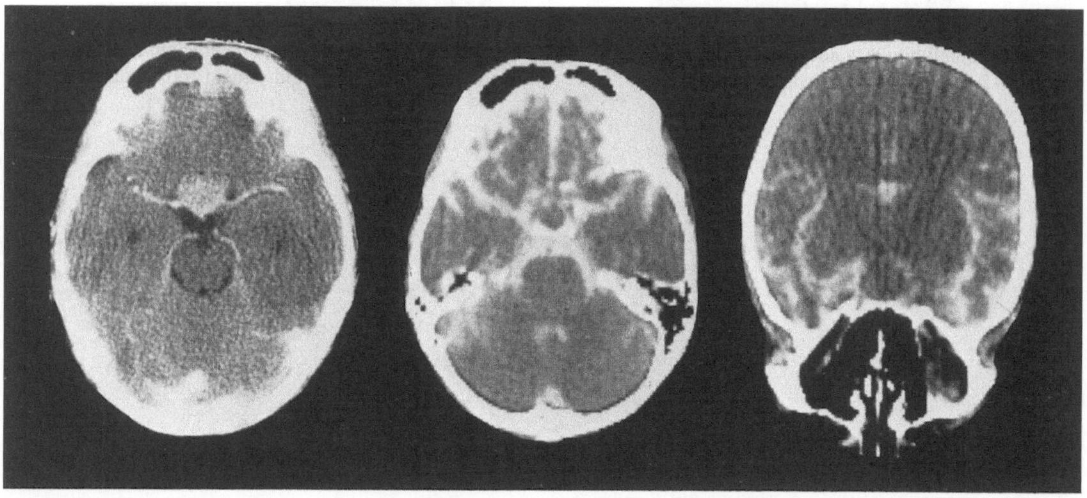

**Fig. D4.21.** Demonstration of a suprasellar pituitary adenoma in both horizontal and coronary projections after intrathecal administration of metrizamide in comparison to postcontrast studies in horizontal projection. The tumor appears as a contrast defect within the hyperdense basal cisterns. Twenty-six-year-old man with chiasma syndrome

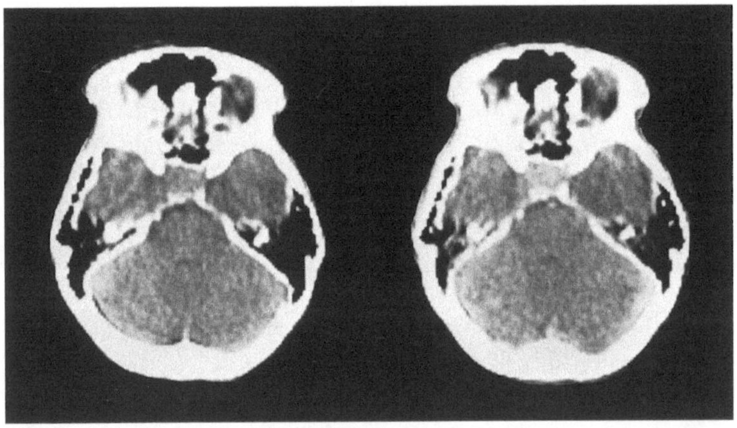

**Fig. D4.22.** Intrasellar pituitary adenoma with asymmetrical growth before (left) and after contrast enhancement (right) in a 39-year-old female with secondary amenorrhea

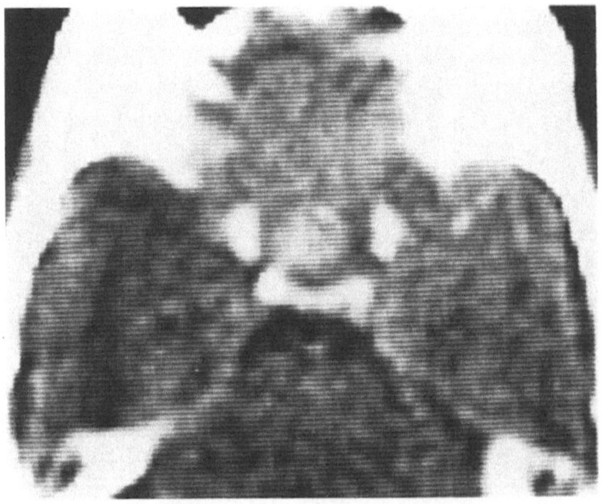

**Fig. D4.23.** Small pituitary adenoma at the entrance to the sella in a 15-year-old boy (postcontrast study)

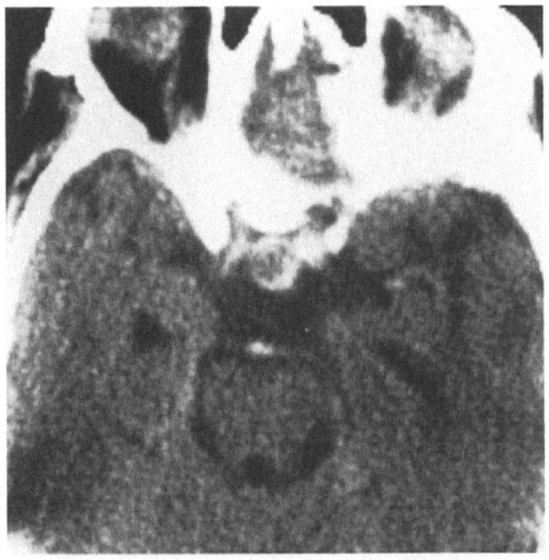

**Fig. D4.24.** Very small pituitary adenoma at the entrance to the sella in a 73-year-old patient (postcontrast study)

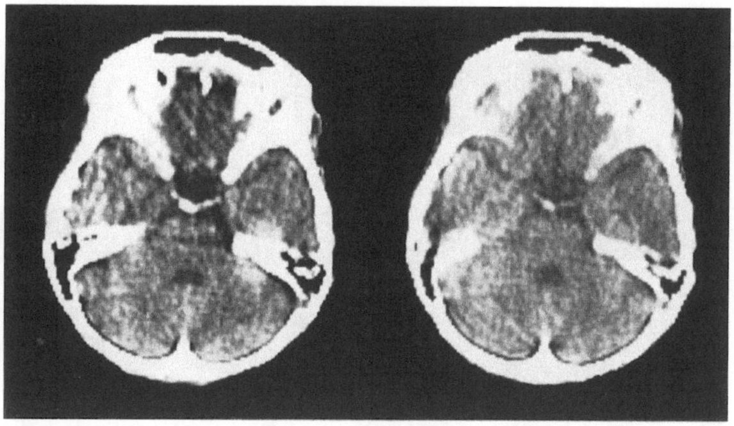

**Fig. D4.25.** Empty sella in a 36-year-old female with a radiological diagnosis of an enlarged sella. A large zone with CSF density is demonstrated at the entrance to the sella in both precontrast and postcontrast studies

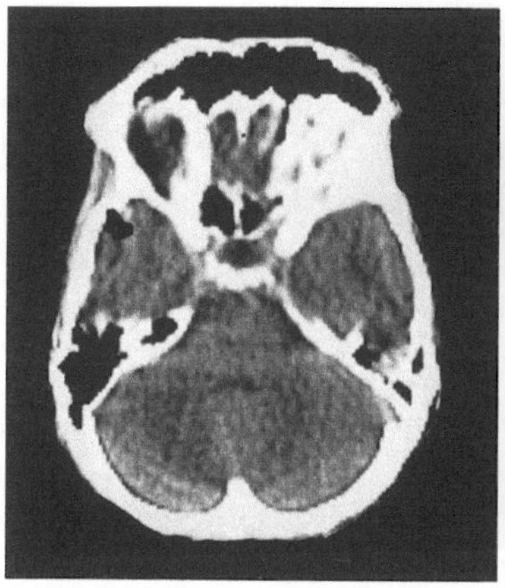

**Fig. D4.26.** Small empty sella in a 40-year-old man with radiological diagnosis of sellar enlargement. Hypodense zone at the entrance to the sella

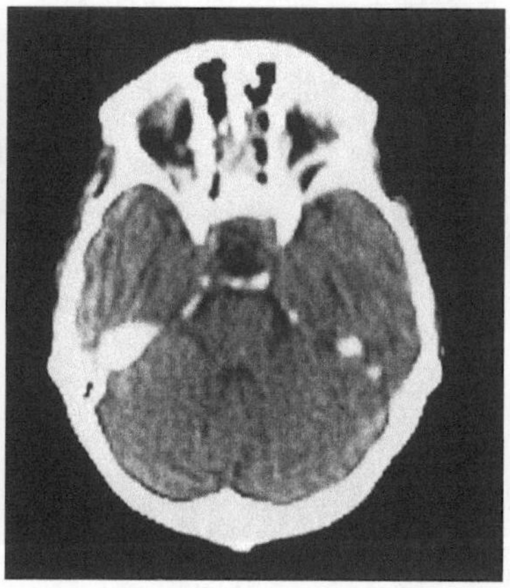

**Fig. D4.27.** Empty sella in a 57-year-old patient after transsphenoidal resection of a pituitary adenoma

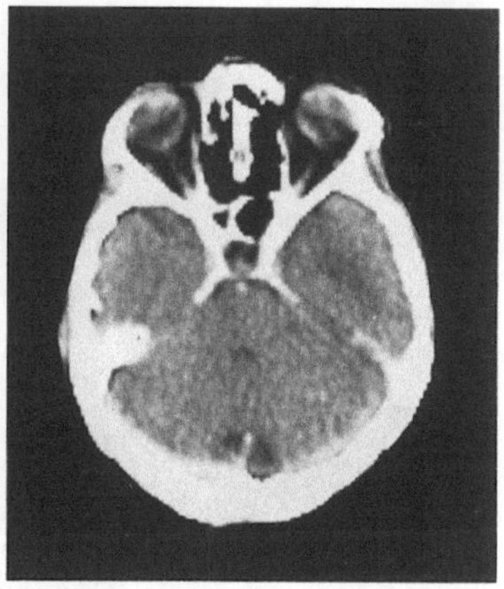

**Fig. D4.28.** Demonstration of the pituitary stalk at the entrance to the sella in a 66-year-old female

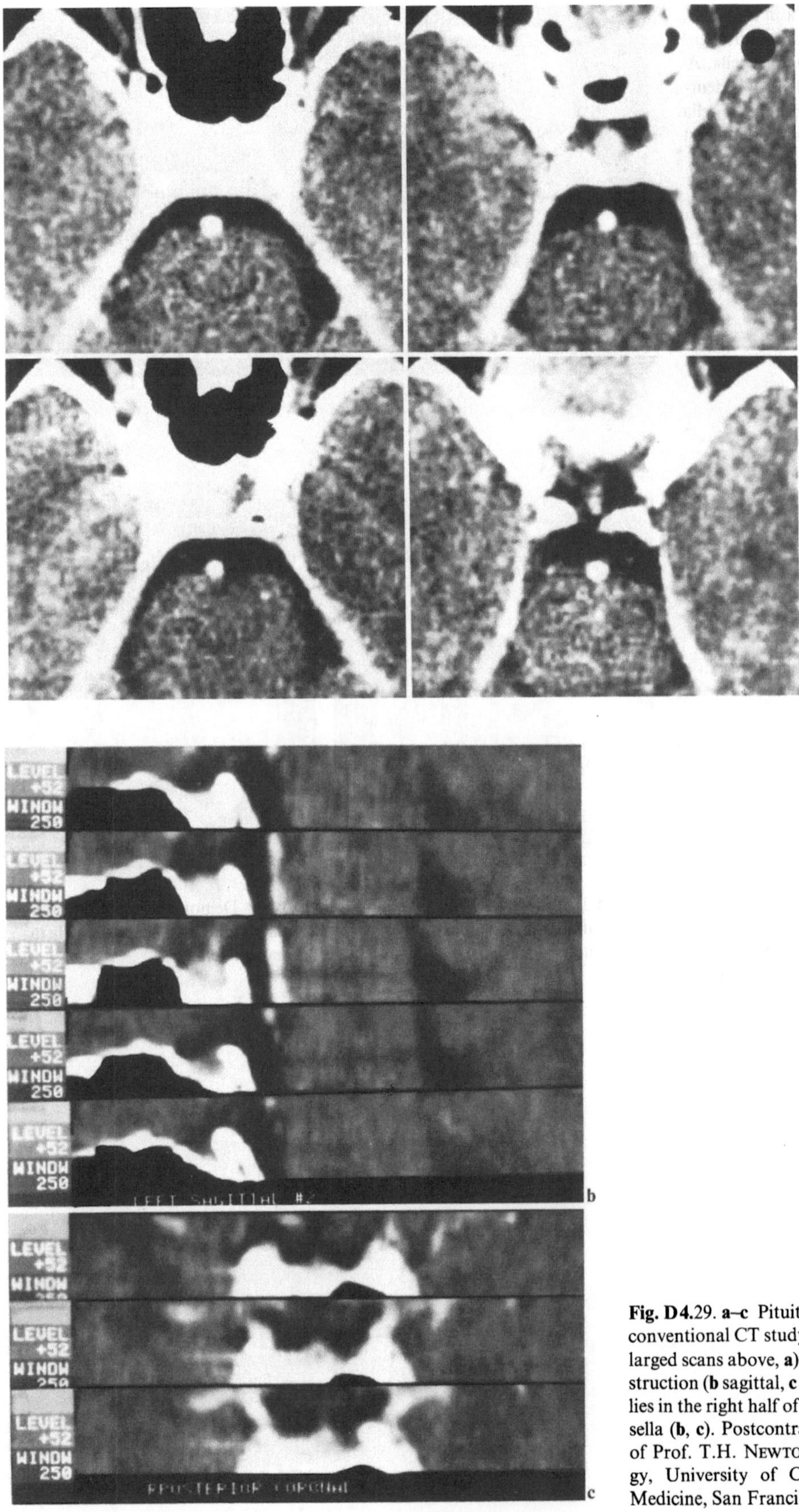


a

b

c

**Fig. D4.29. a–c** Pituitary microadenoma in conventional CT study (group of four enlarged scans above, **a**) and vertical reconstruction (**b** sagittal, **c** coronal). The tumor lies in the right half of the slightly enlarged sella (**b**, **c**). Postcontrast studies. (Courtesy of Prof. T.H. NEWTON, Dept. of Radiology, University of California, School of Medicine, San Francisco, California, USA)

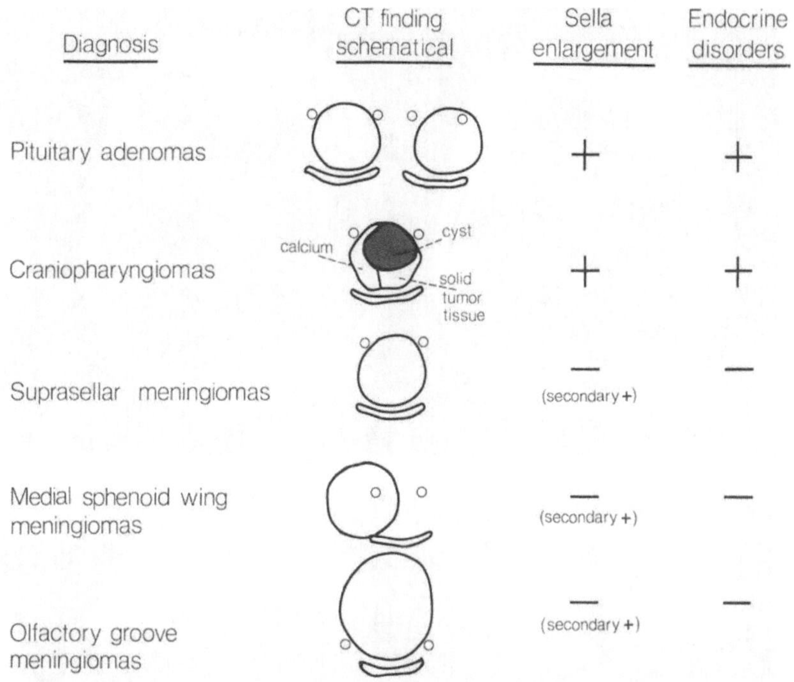


**Fig. D4.30.** Differential diagnosis of the most common suprasellar and parasellar tumors on the basis of CT findings, sellar changes, and endocrine disorders

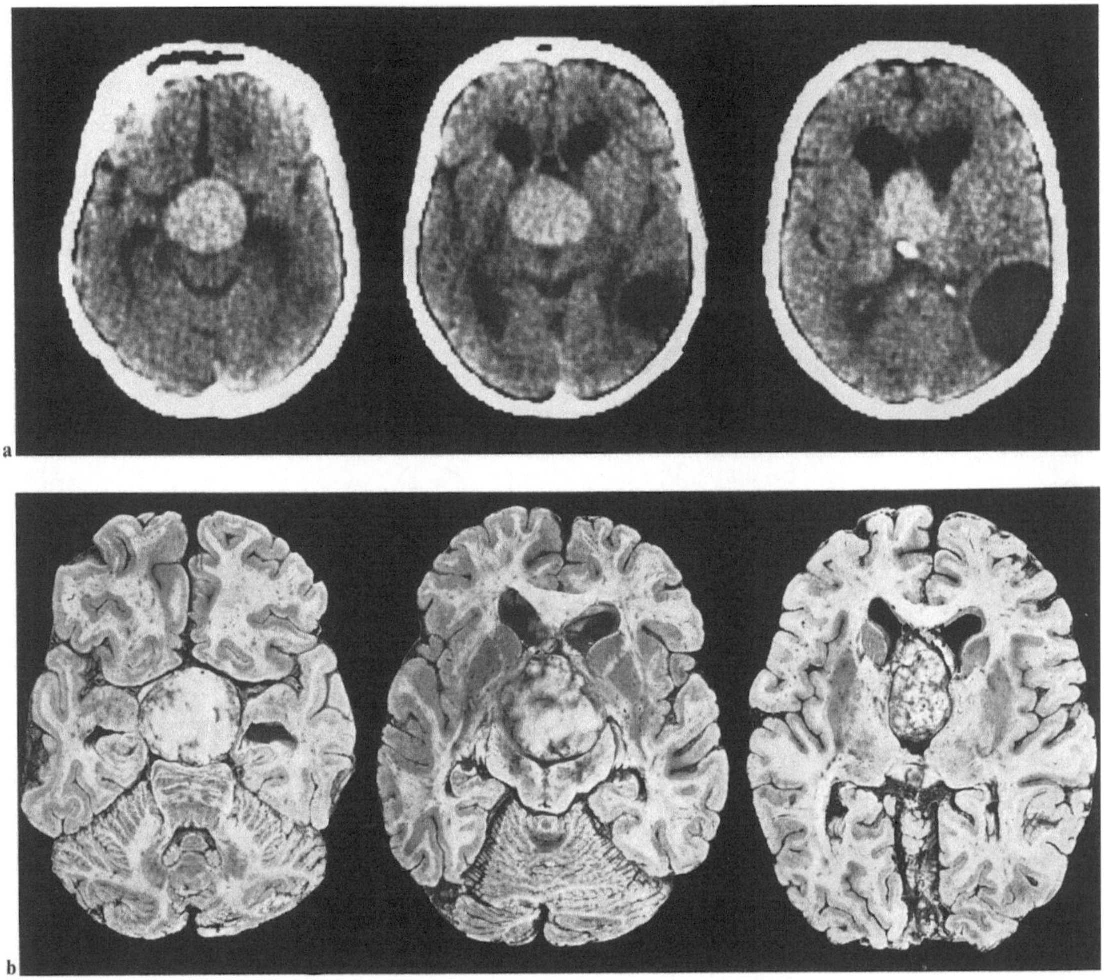

**Fig. D4.**31 a, b. Choristoma of the posterior pituitary in a 58-year-old man. Large suprasellar tumor with hyperdense values in the precontrast scan, bilateral blockage of the foramina of Monro by the tumor. Demonstration of an arachnoid cyst in the right posterior temporal region as incidental finding. Postcontrast study (**a**). (**b**) Autopsy specimens in the same planes as the CT studies demonstrate identical anatomical relations. (Courtesy of Priv. Doz. Dr. G. EBHARDT, Neuropathological Institute, Free University of Berlin)

# 5. Tumors of the Blood Vessels

## Hemangioblastomas

| | |
|---|---|
| Incidence | 1–2% (most common cerebellar tumor in adults) |
| Characteristic age at diagnosis | 30–60 years |
| Sex distribution | Preponderance of males |
| Typical locations | Cerebellum |
| Characteristic clinical findings | Signs of cerebellar dysfunction |
| Skull film | Secondary changes of the sella |
| EEG | Uncharacteristic changes |
| Echoencephalography | Ventricular dilatation |
| Serial brain scintigraphy | Perfusion pattern similar to that of arteriovenous malformation in large solid tumors; radionuclide uptake in this tumor tissue |
| Cerebral angiography | Strong contrast uptake in the tumor nodule, often in combination with an avascular space (cyst) |

**Computed Tomography**

| | |
|---|---|
| Precontrast studies | Hypodense area in most cases |
| Contrast medium uptake | Marked in solid tumor nodules |
| Appearance after contrast enhancement | Large cyst with or without marginal tumor nodule, occasionally with rim enhancement; solid tumor without cystic portions in rare cases |

**Differential Diagnosis**

*Lesion with Large Cyst*

Pilocytic astrocytoma
Arachnoid cyst
So-called simple cyst
Occlusion of the foramina of Magendie and Luschka with large fourth ventricle
Epidermoid of the fourth ventricle
Large cerebellomedullar cistern

*Tumor with Ring Structures and Centrally Located Cyst*

Pilocytic astrocytoma
Metastasis
Abscess and monstrocellular sarcoma

*Solid Tumor Nodule*

Metastasis
Meningioma
Acoustic neurinoma
Aneurysm/angioma
Malignant lymphoma

Synonyms: *angioblastoma, hemangioendothelioma, Lindau tumor*. These are grade I tumors which originate in the cerebral vessels. ZÜLCH reported finding these lesions in 1.3% of all intracranial tumors, while CUSHING found 1.2% and OLIVECRONA 2.3%. Hemangioblastomas comprised 1.1% of tumors in our series.

Peak incidence lies between the ages of 30 and 60 years; this tumor is very rare in children. Males are affected twice as often as females. Somewhat higher familial incidence has been reported.

### Typical Location – Characteristic Clinical Findings

Almost all hemangioblastomas originate in the cerebellum, often in association with a large cyst, rarely in the spinal cord, and very rarely in the cerebral hemispheres. It is the most common cerebellar tumor in adults, and signs of cerebellar dysfunction predominate.

### Additional Diagnostic Procedures

Plain skull films, electroencephalography, and echoencephalography provide nonspecific changes suggestive of an intracranial space-occupying lesion.

Serial brain scintigraphy is positive with perfusion patterns typical of a-v malformation as well as early radionuclide uptake in cases of large solid tumor.

A typical vascular blush in the solid portions of the tumor is found in the angiogram. An avascular space may be demonstrated in the presence of a large cyst.

## Computed Tomography (Figs. D 5.1–10)

### Precontrast Study

In a large majority of cases (73%) the lesion appears as a *sharply delineated hypodense zone in the posterior fossa* (Figs. D 5.2–5). This figure represents the cystic portion of the tumor, which has a mean density of 20–22 HU. In one case we measured only 12 HU (see Fig. D 5.2).

The solid tumor differs only slightly in absorption from surrounding normal cerebellar tissue if the lesion is not isodense.

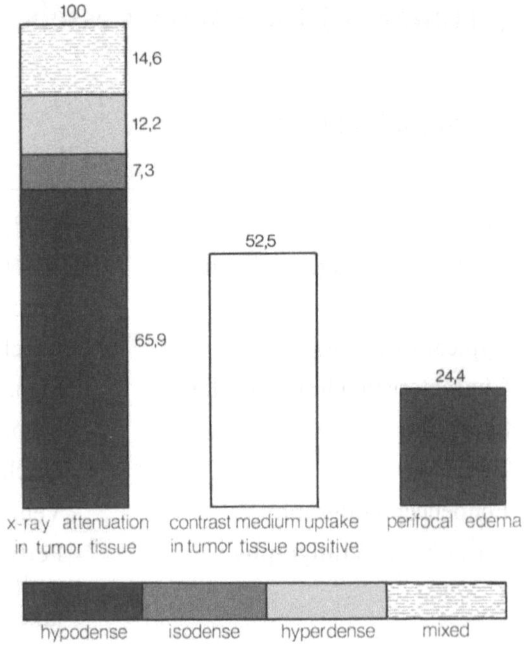


**Fig. D 5.1.** X-ray attenuation, contrast medium uptake, and frequency of perifocal edema in hemangioblastomas (percent)

### Postcontrast Study

Contrast uptake occurs only in the solid portions of the tumor and results in average increases in density of 15–20 HU. The vascular nature of the tumor causes a rapid increase in attenuation immediately after contrast administration with an equally rapid decrease.

Contrast enhancement demonstrated the solid portion of the tumor in approximately half of our cases. Contrast uptake may result in a variety of structures including a small marginal tumor nodule with a large cyst (Figs. D 5.5, 6), ring blush of the tumor (Figs. D 5.7–9), and large solid tumors with rather homogeneous contrast enhancement (Fig. D 5.10).

Slight or moderate perifocal edema is found in a small number of patients with hemangioblastomas containing large portions of solid tumor.

### Differential Diagnosis

Tumors with a **large cyst** also suggest a diagnosis of *pilocytic astrocytoma*, although this tumor occurs most often in children. Calcification is typical of pilocytic astrocytoma, and slight contrast uptake in the entire wall of the cyst is only found in this tumor.

Measurement of attenuation values within the cyst allows differentiation between an *arachnoid cyst* and a cyst accompanying angioblastoma or other cerebellar tumor. The contents of an arachnoid cyst have the same density as CSF, while the absorption values in the cyst in angioblastoma are considerably higher (see above). It is not possible to differentiate between a so-called *simple cyst* (Fig. F 40, 41) and a cyst accompanying angioblastoma, since the xanthochromic fluid in a simple cyst may have somewhat higher density values than CSF. Extreme dilatation of the fourth ventricle due to *obstruction of the foramina of Magendie and Luschka* with simultaneous stenosis of the aqueduct ("entrapped fourth ventricle") may resemble a midline cyst in angioblastoma. The same is true of *epidermoid of the fourth ventricle*. Density values in both entities are close to those of CSF, which is of considerable help in diagnosis.

A **circular tumor** with a cyst at its center also suggests *pilocytic astrocytoma* of the cerebellum. However, in some cases CT findings may not allow certain differentiation.

*Cerebellar metastases and abscesses* may occasionally produce similar CT findings. In these cases the history and other clinical findings usually suggest the diagnosis.

It is not possible to differentiate between cerebellar angioblastoma and *monstrocellular sarcoma* with the CT scan alone.

**Solid tumor nodules** may be found in a number of tumors and vascular disorders including *metastasis, meningioma, acoustic neurinoma, giant aneurysm, cerebellar a.v. malformation, ectasia of the basilar artery, and malignant lymphoma*. The history, physical examination, vestibular function studies, plain skull films, and angiographic studies often help in differentiation of these solid tumors.

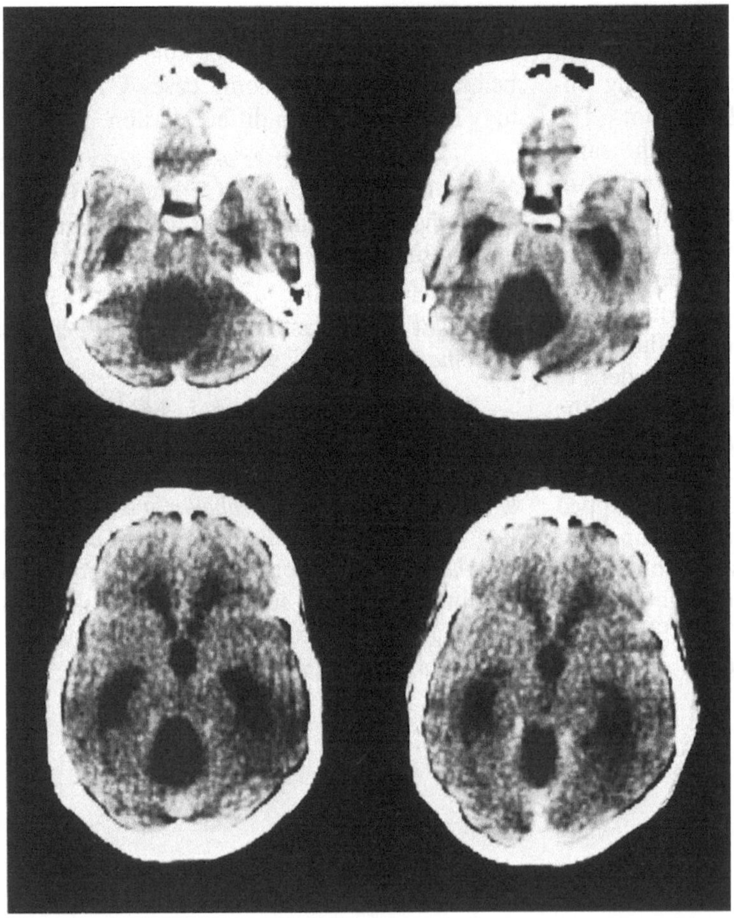

**Fig. D5.2.** Large cystic hemangioblastoma in the cerebellar vermis with extreme hydrocephalus in an 18-year-old patient. Density values within the cyst (12 HU) are slightly higher than those of CSF. Contrast enhancement fails to demonstrate a solid tumor nodule. (left, precontrast study; right, postcontrast study)

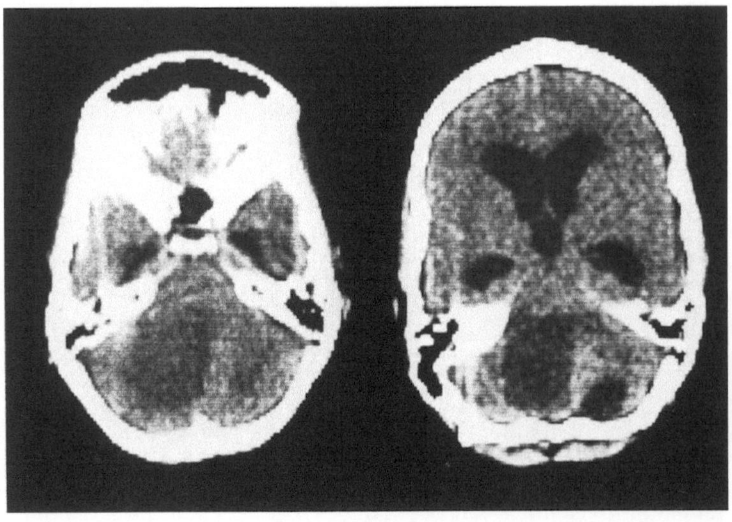

**Fig. D5.3.** Multichambered hemangioblastoma in the posterior fossa of a 12-year-old child. The cyst contents have significantly higher density values than CSF. No demonstration of solid tumor tissue. Marked hydrocephalus. Postcontrast study

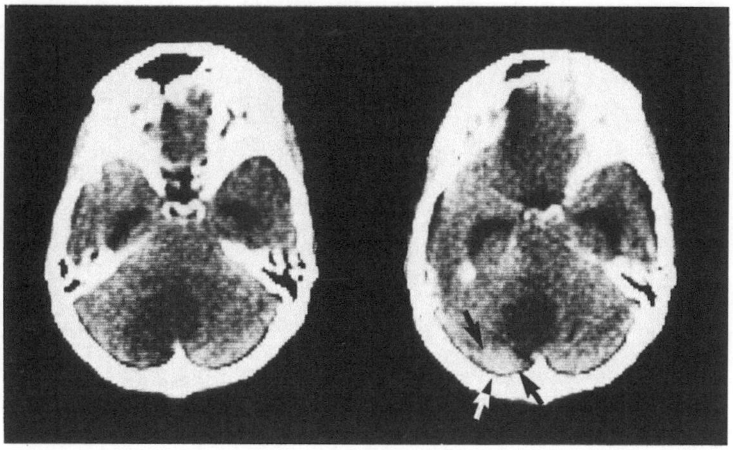

**Fig. D5.4.** Cystic hemangioblastoma of the cerebellar vermis and the left cerebellar hemisphere in a 34-year-old patient. Contrast enhancement reveals a small hyperdense region (arrows) in the left cerebellar hemisphere, representing a solid hemangioblastoma

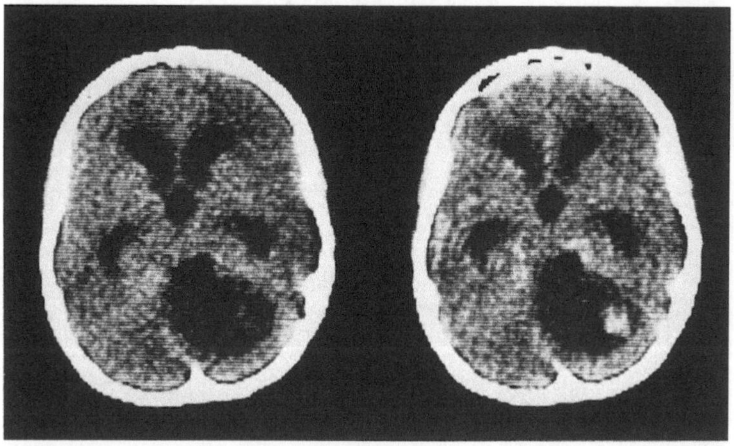

**Fig. D5.5.** Large cystic hemangioblastoma in the right cerebellar hemisphere in a 19-year-old female. There is a small hypodense nodule of solid tissue on the right lateral wall of the cyst (left); strong contrast uptake within the tumor nodule, which supports a diagnosis of hemangioblastoma (right)

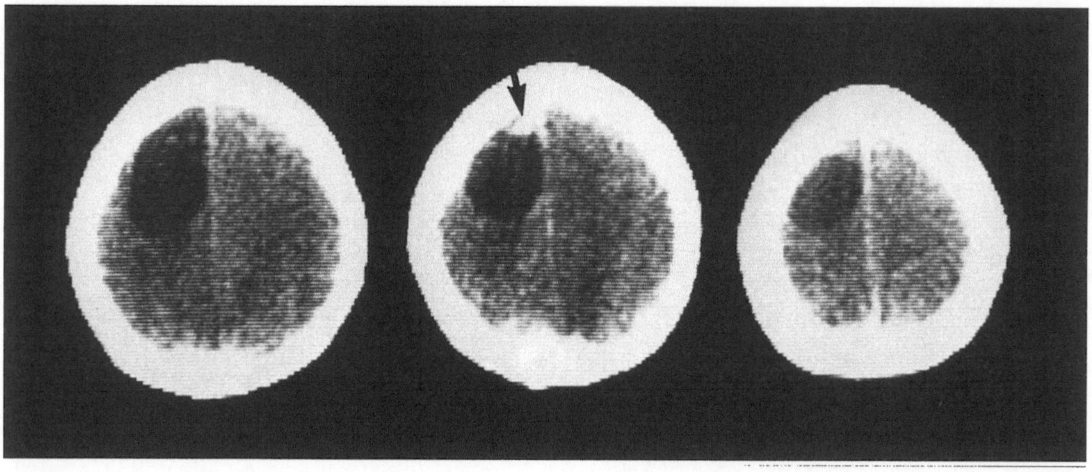

**Fig. D5.6.** Cerebral hemangioblastoma in a 17-year-old man with focal seizures. Demonstration of a large hypodense lesion with a circumscribed marginal zone of solid tissue with contrast uptake (arrow) representing a hemangioblastoma nodule. Rare location for hemangioblastoma. Postcontrast study

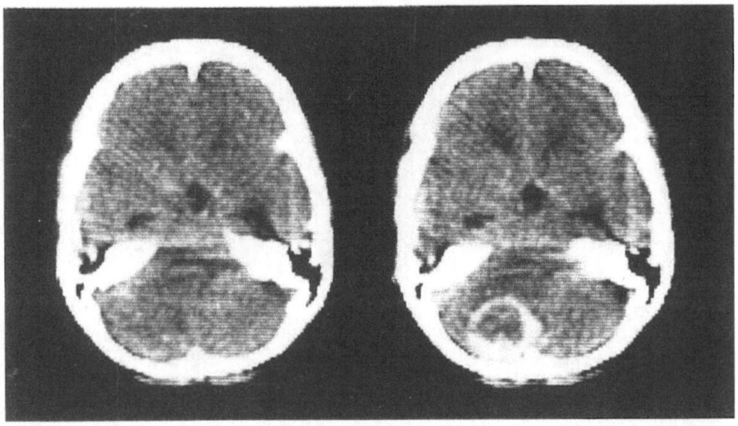

**Fig. D5.7.** Isodense hemangioblastoma in the left cerebellar hemisphere without evidence of a cyst in the precontrast study (left) in a 38-year-old female with cerebellar symptoms. Demonstration of a strongly hyperdense ring structure after contrast enhancement (right), which suggests the presence of a highly vascularized lesion

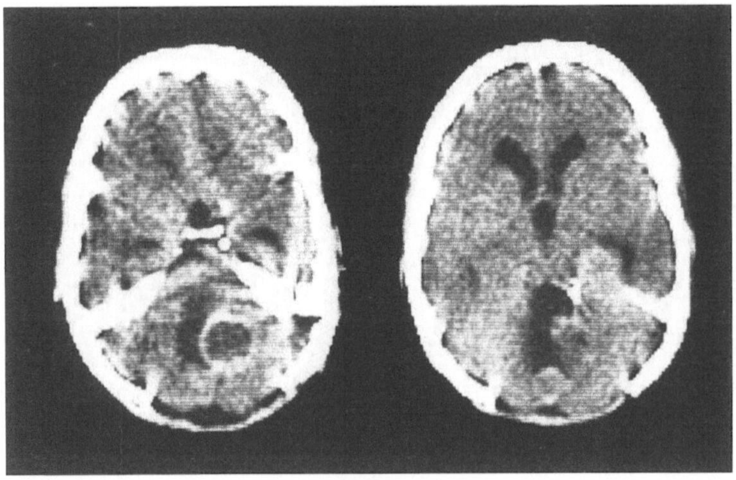

**Fig. D5.8.** Recurrent hemangioblastoma in the right cerebellar hemisphere of a 33-year-old female with additional hemangioblastomas in the choroid and the spinal cord. Ring enhancement of the tumor nodule. Postcontrast study

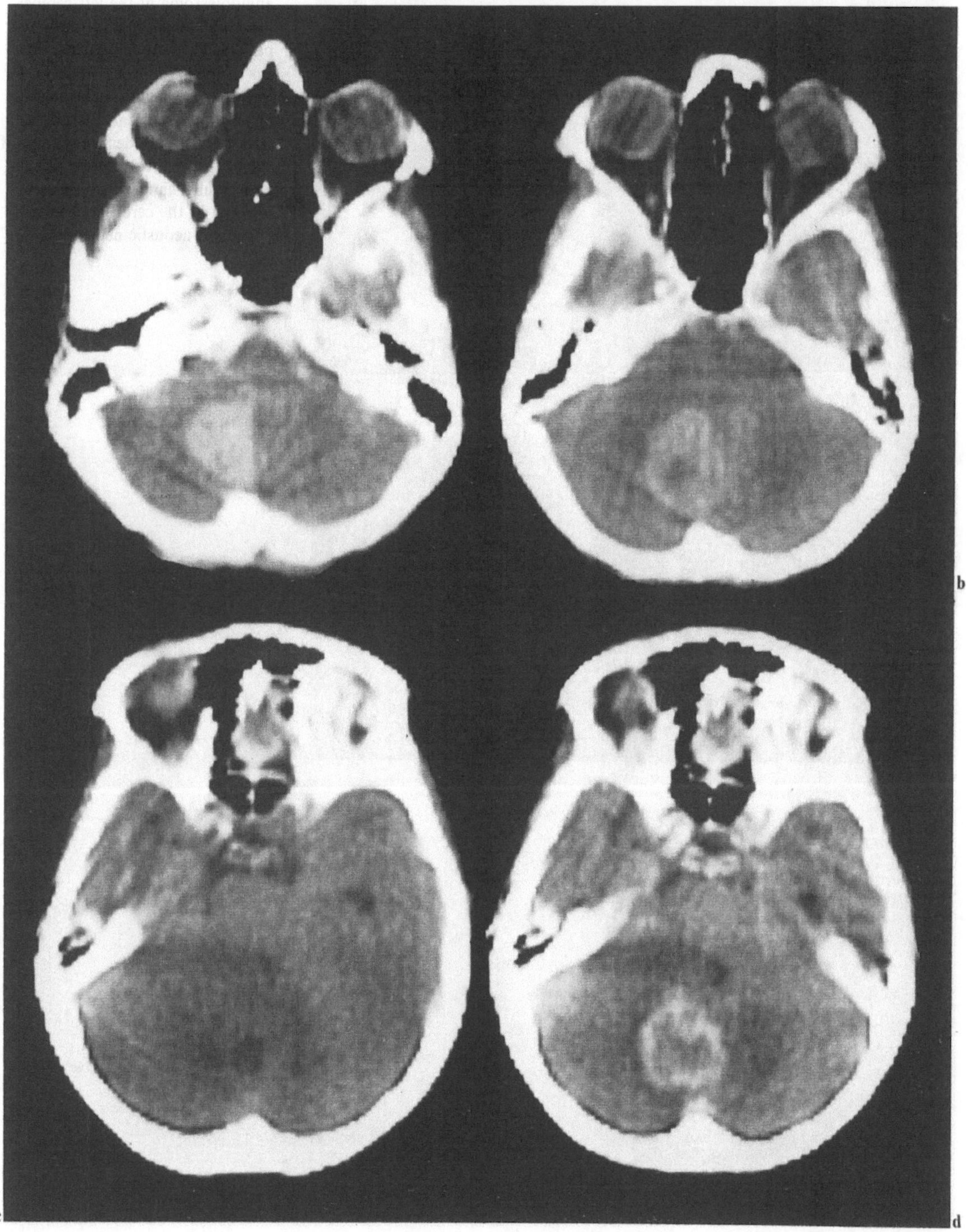

**Fig. D5.9** a–d. Large solid hemangioblastoma in the cerebellar vermis in a 60-year-old female. Isodense and slightly hypodense values in the precontrast CT scan (**c**). Contrast enhancement (**a, b, d**) produces an increase in density values within the tumor and demonstrates central zones of necrosis. The intensity of contrast uptake is apparently attenuated by use of a large window width. Perifocal edema in both cerebellar hemispheres (slight contrast due to window width of 200 HU)

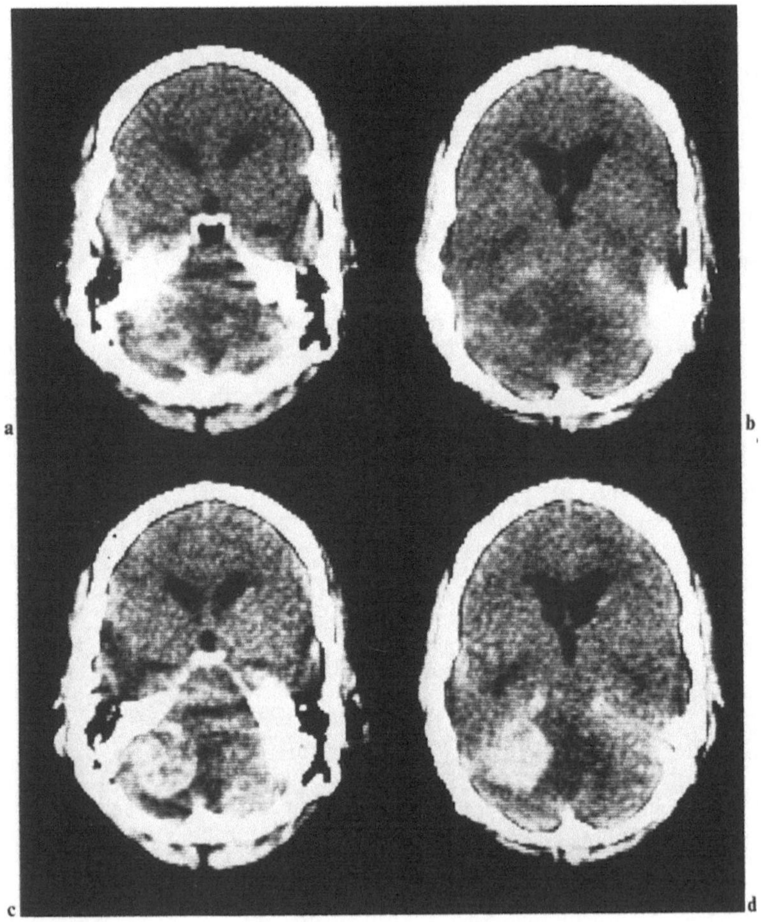

**Fig. D5.10** a–d. Large solid hemangioblastoma at the left cerebellopontine angle in a 34-year-old patient. Partially hyperdense values in the precontrast study (**a**, **b**). Very strong, slightly inhomogeneous contrast uptake within the tumor (**c**, **d**) with demonstration of extensive perifocal edema. Diagnostic alternatives include meningioma at the cerebellopontine angle and acoustic neurinoma

# 6. Dysontogenetic Tumors

## a) Hamartomas

Hamartomas are very rare gliomatous lesions without evident proliferative tendencies. They demonstrate little or no mass effect and are most often found in the temporal lobe. Histological studies may reveal all types of slow-growing gliomas arrested at an early developemental stage. Patients with these malformations often present with convulsions – usually psychomotor seizures – in childhood and adolescence. Neurological examination is generally normal while the EEG demonstrates focal activity in the temporal lobe corresponding to the psychomotor character of the seizures.

### Computed Tomography (Figs. D 6.1–3).

Hamartomas are almost always visible in the precontrast scan, since calcification and cysts are very common (Figs. D 6.1–3). A significant increase in density following contrast administration is observed in some cases (Fig. D 6.3).

Hamartoma must always be considered in the differential diagnosis of a temporal lobe lesion in a young epileptic patient. However, this is only one of a number of possibilities, since other lesions may produce the same or similar CT findings. The most common *alternative diagnoses* are *pilocytic astrocytoma* with a cyst and calcification or calcified *oligodendroglioma* and *gangliocytoma*. Transitional forms may also occur (Fig. D 6.3). Hemorrhage in a hamartoma occurred in one case in our series, which emphasizes the malformative character of the lesion, though this finding is rather exceptional.

## b) Cavernous Hemangiomas

Cavernous hemangiomas (synonym: cavernoma) are very rare intracranial malformative tumors which may occur in all regions of the brain but most often develop in the cerebral hemispheres. The tumors have also been found in the lateral ventricles, in the basal ganglia, the brain stem, and the cerebellar hemispheres. Cavernomas may also originate in the dura mater (Fig. D 6.5), most often on the floor of the middle fossa (Mori et al. 1980). Presenting signs are a function of location, with seizures predominating in tumors of the cerebral hemispheres and cranial nerve deficits – especially of the second and third cranial nerves – when the cavernoma is located at the base of the skull. Incidence is highest in adolescents and young adults, but the tumor has also been found in infants as a congenital lesion.

### Computed Tomography (Figs. D 6.4, 5)

Cavernous hemangiomas usually demonstrate high density values in the precontrast scan, and calcification is a common finding (Figs. D 6.4a and b, 5). Contrast enhancement generally results in a significant increase in density values with an appearance resembling meningioma. This is especially true of cavernomas in the middle cranial fossa. The tumors are usually spherical or nodular and sharply delineated against surrounding brain tissue. An accurate prediction of histological diagnosis on the basis of CT studies is virtually impossible. Very strong contrast uptake suggests a highly vascularized lesion, though a meningioma cannot be excluded on the basis of such findings.

A cavernoma may be suspected when the tumor is confined to the cerebral parenchyma, since other tumors of similar appearance were not demonstrated in the brain tissue in our series (Fig. D 6.4a).

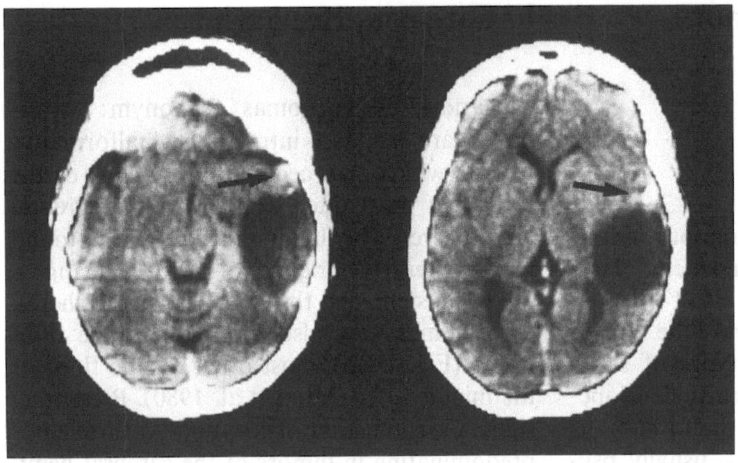

**Fig. D6.1.** Hamartoma in the right temporal lobe of a 25-year-old female with psychomotor seizures. CT studies demonstrate a large cyst in the right temporal lobe with adjacent small areas of very high density (arrows), which were found to be partially calcified at operation. Postcontrast study. (Studies courtesy of Dr. BACKMUND, Neurology Department of the Max-Planck-Institute of Psychiatry, Munich)

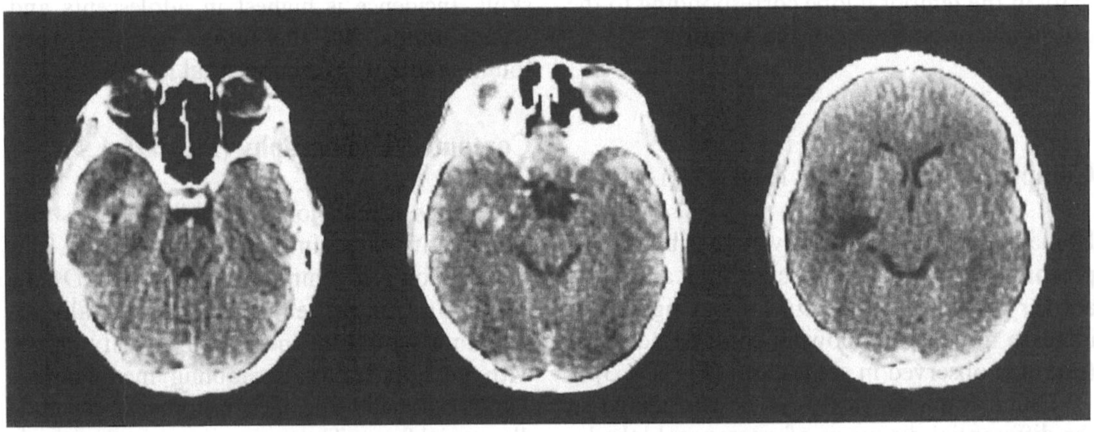

**Fig. D6.2.** Hamartoma in the left temporal lobe of a 15-year-old boy with psychomotor seizures. The tumor demonstrates inhomogeneous density values, with many calcified specks as well as larger areas of calcification. Demonstration of a small cyst in the posterior portion of the tumor (right). Slight increase in density after contrast enhancement. Postcontrast study

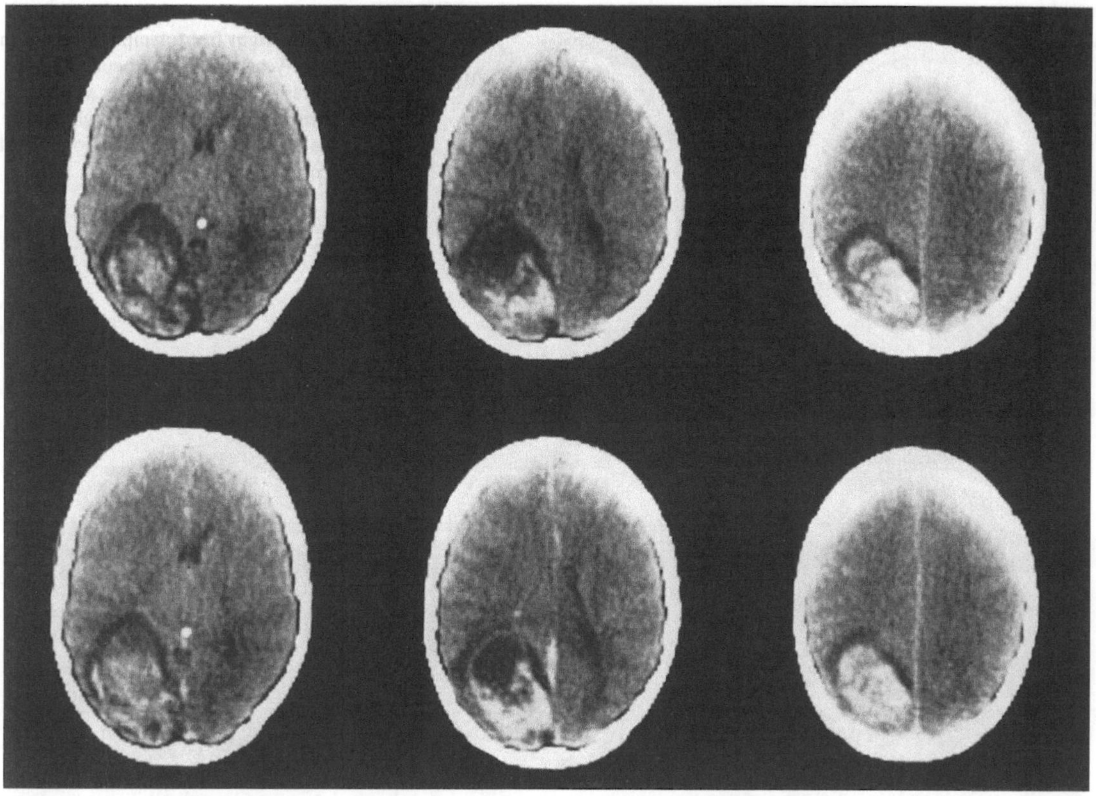

**Fig. D6.3.** Combination of hamartoma and oligodendroglioma with hemorrhage in the left occipital lobe of a 17-year-old female with a history of seizures for several years. Precontrast studies (above) reveal a sharply delineated lesion with inhomogeneous density values. The strongly hyperdense portions represent coagulated blood. Postcontrast studies demonstrate a significant increase in density within the previously isodense portions of the tumor (below, left) as well as delicate contrast uptake within the capsule (below, middle). CT studies suggested the presence of a tumor with cystic and solid elements as well as recent hemorrhage, findings which were confirmed at operation

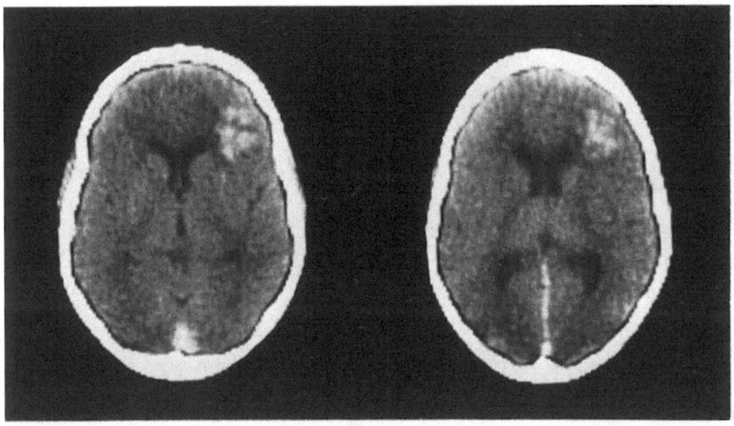

a

**Fig. D6.4**a. Cavernous hemangioma in the right frontotemporal region in a 14-year-old girl with epileptic seizures. The lesion appears as an irregular area with very high density values suggesting calcification. Slight contrast uptake

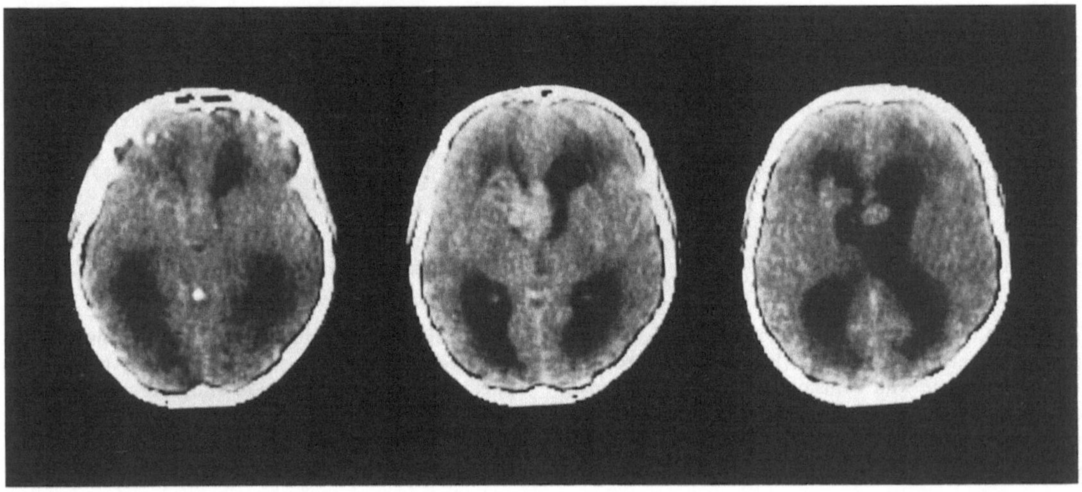

b

**Fig. D6.4**b. Cavernoma at the left foramen of Monro with extension into the left anterior horn, obstructive hydrocephalus and periventricular lucency. Irregular configuration and hyperdense values in the precontrast study. Little change in the postcontrast study. A cavernoma with numerous remnants of past hemorrhage was found at operation (17-year-old girl with headache and papilledema)

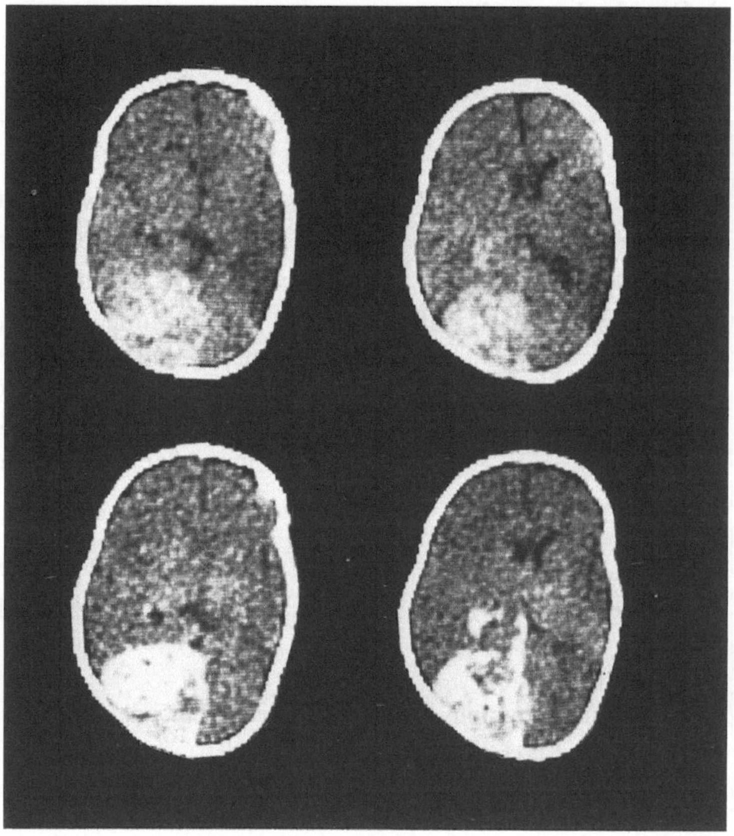

**Fig. D6.5.** Congenital cavernous hemangioma in the left occipital lobe of a 3-month-old infant. The tumor demonstrates high density values in the precontrast study (above), and there is a further increase in radiation attenuation after contrast enhancement (below). The extent of contrast uptake suggests the presence of a vascular lesion

## c) Craniopharyngiomas

| | |
|---|---|
| Incidence | 2–4% |
| Characteristic age at diagnosis | All age groups with peak incidence at 10 years |
| Sex distribution | Preponderance of males |
| Typical location | Suprasellar region |
| Characteristic clinical findings | Visual disorders; signs of increased intracranial pressure; pituitary insufficiency, dwarfism, and delayed puberty in children; Fröhlich's disease in rare cases; diabetes insipidus not uncommon |
| Skull film | Suprasellar calcifications, primary changes of the sella, signs of increased intracranial pressure in children |
| EEG | Uncharacteristic changes |
| Echoencephalography | Tumor echo in the midline, dilatation of the lateral ventricle subsequent to blockade of the foramen of Monro |
| Serial brain scintigraphy | Radionuclide uptake in large solid portions of the tumor |
| Cerebral angiography | Elevation of the horizontal portion of the anterior cerebral artery in some cases |
| Other contrast studies | Pneumoencephalography demonstrates suprasellar extent of the tumor |
| Special tests | Endocrinological studies |
| **Computed Tomography** | |
| Precontrast study | Not uniform; hyperdense zones caused by calcifications; hypodense zones due to cystic portions; solid uncalcified portions of the tumor often isodense |
| Contrast medium uptake | Restricted to solid uncalcified portions of the tumor |
| Appearance after contrast enhancement | Suprasellar tumor nodule with calcification and cysts in many cases |

**Differential Diagnosis**

Pituitary adenoma
Pilocytic astrocytoma
Gangliocytoma
Meningioma
Chordoma
Aneurysm of the carotid artery
Carcinoma of the epipharynx

Craniopharyngioma develops from the craniopharyngic duct and may occur at both intrasellar and suprasellar locations. It is the second most common tumor of the sellar region after pituitary adenoma. Incidence is reported as ranging from 2%–4% in the literature and accounted for 2.2% of all tumors in our series. It is a grade I lesion.

### Characteristic Clinical Findings

Deficient production of growth hormone results in *pituitary dwarfism* with delayed puberty, and – very rarely – Fröhlich's syndrome.

*Diabetes insipidus* is observed in many cases and may terminate in antidiabetes.

*Suprasellar extension of the tumor results in visual disorders* while *blockage of the foramina of Monro* causes increased intracranial pressure.

### Additional Diagnostic Procedures

Fine calcification is a common finding on plain skull films, though massive calcification may occur. Bone destruction of the sella is unusual, in contrast to the typical findings in pituitary adenoma. Separation of the cranial sutures and pronounced digital impressions may be observed as signs of increased intracranial pressure in children. EEG shows nonspecific changes in large tumors, while echoencephalography demonstrates a tumor echo complex near the midline. Dilatation of the lateral ventricles is detectable in cases of blockage of the foramina of Monro. Serial brain scintigraphy reveals the solid uncalcified portion of the tumor and demonstrates perfusion defects in large cysts. Cerebral angiography may reveal elevation of the horizontal part of the anterior cerebral artery without demonstration of a tumor blush or pathological vessels.

Pneumoencephalography can show the suprasellar extent of the tumor.

Endocrinological function studies reveal characteristic hormonal deficits.

## Computed Tomography (Figs. D6.6–16)

### Precontrast Study

Craniopharyngioma presents with a wide variety of findings in the CT scan, since the tumor may contain calcified, cystic, and solid elements (Figs. D6.8–14). Approximately 80% of tumors are hyperdense or mixed density lesions. Purely hypodense zones represent large *cystic structures* (Figs. D6.9, 16), with Hounsfield values approaching those of CSF. Some craniopharyngioma cysts demonstrate X-ray absorption slightly lower than that found in normal brain tissue (Fig. D6.11). AMBROSE (1974) reported a case of a chambered cyst in a craniopharyngioma with negative EMI numbers, but we did not observe a similar phenomenon in our series of 81 patients with this type of tumor.

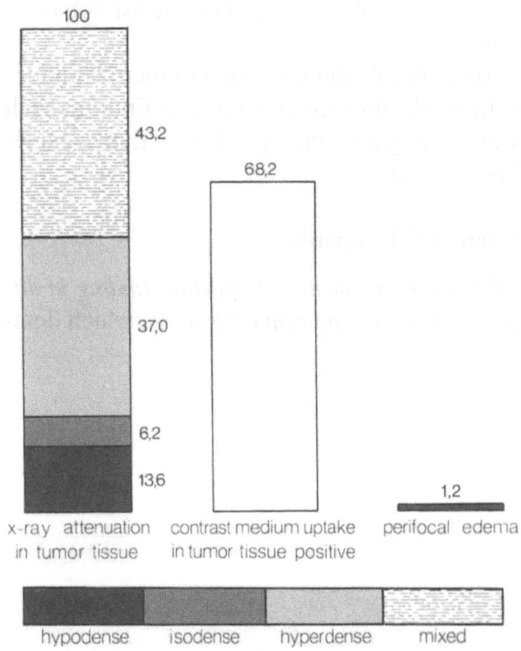


**Fig. D6.6.** X-ray attenuation, contrast medium uptake, and frequency of perifocal edema in craniopharyngiomas (percent)

*Calcification* may vary in form and extent, ranging from fine flecks to conglomerates the size of a chestnut, which appear as sharply delineated high density zones (Figs. D6.11–15). The *solid portions of the tumor* are usually isodense or slightly hypodense (Fig. D6.12), so that solid tumors can only be detected on the basis of indirect signs in the plain scan.

### Postcontrast Study

Contrast administration is followed by an average increase in density of 12–14 HU in about two-thirds of cases.

Contrast uptake is limited to the solid uncalcified portions of the tumor. A combination of solid, calcified, and cystic elements may produce bizarre figures, especially in cases of recurrent tumor (Figs. D6.10, 14, 15). Ring enhancement is occasionally seen in cystic tumors (Figs. D6.7, 8, 11) and delineation of slightly hypodense cysts is improved after contrast enhancement.

Intrathecal administration of metrizamide is useful in clarification of equivocal findings such as those in cystic tumors with very thin capsules (Fig. D6.16).

### Differential Diagnosis

*Calcification is the most important finding in differentiation from pituitary adenoma,* which demonstrates calcification in only 1% of cases. However, *CT findings may be identical in some cases of craniopharyngioma and pituitary adenoma* (Figs. D4.13, D6.8). A detailed discussion of the differential diagnosis of suprasellar space-occupying lesions is found in Chap. D4 on pituitary adenomas (see p. 272f.).

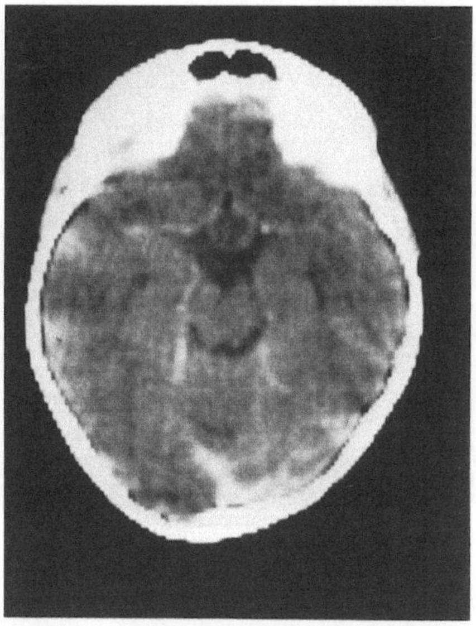

**Fig. D6.7.** Small cystic craniopharyngioma in an 11-year-old boy with dwarfism and hormonal disorders. The postcontrast study shows a spherical space-occupying lesion with slight marginal contrast uptake in the region of the pentagon. Density values within the cyst are significantly higher than those of CSF

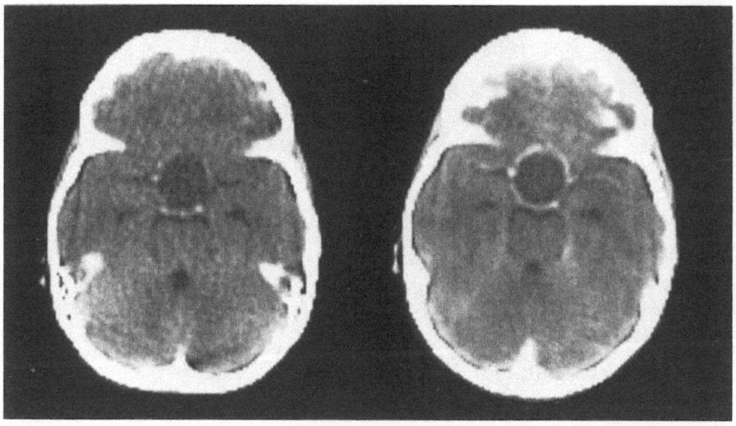

**Fig. D6.8.** Large cystic craniopharyngioma filling the entire chiasmatic cistern in a 12-year-old girl with rapidly progredient loss of sight (precontrast study: left). Demonstration of a ring structure representing the solid portion of the tumor after contrast enhancement (right). Similar findings may be found in pituitary adenoma with cysts or past hemorrhage. The patient's age is the most important factor in differentiating between the two lesions

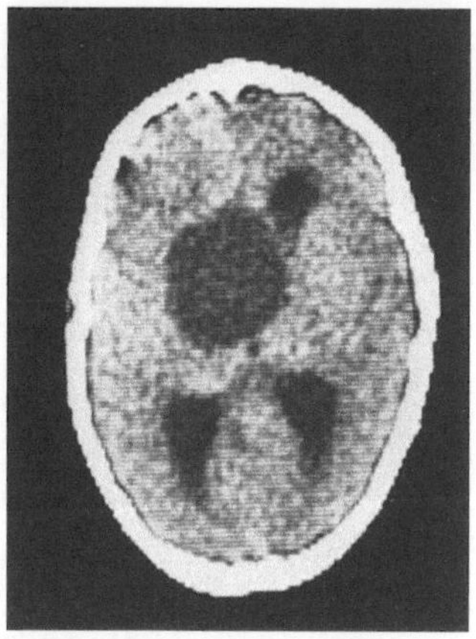

**Fig. D6.9.** Craniopharyngioma with a very large cyst in a 8-year-old boy 2 years after partial resection of the tumor. Density values within the cyst are significantly higher than those of CSF

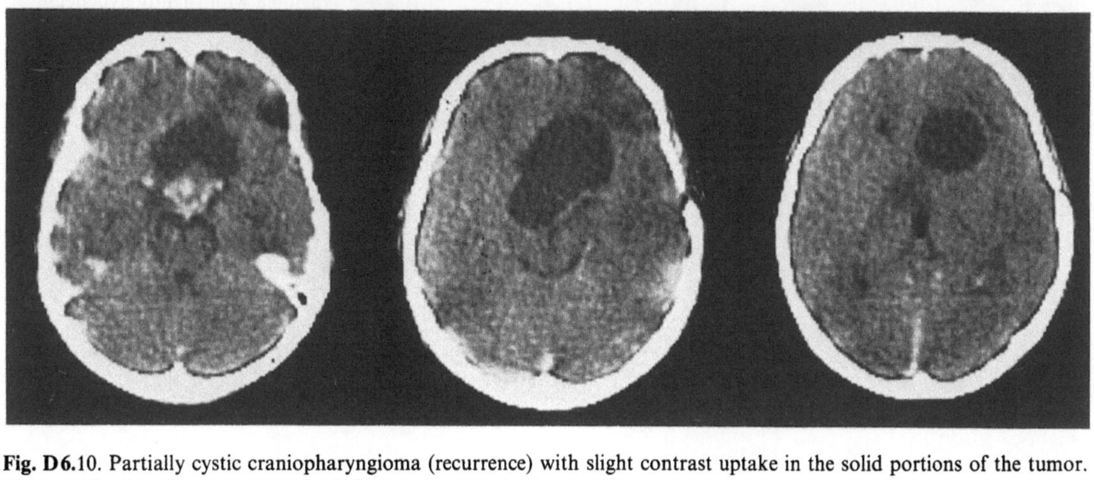

**Fig. D6.10.** Partially cystic craniopharyngioma (recurrence) with slight contrast uptake in the solid portions of the tumor. Fine calcification (21-year-old patient). Postcontrast study

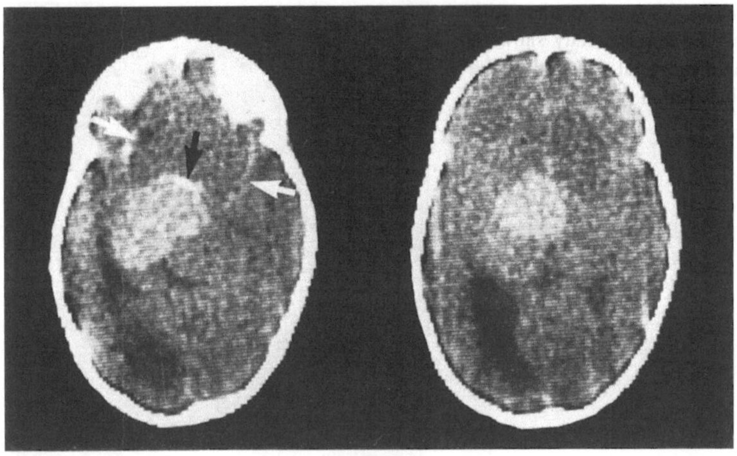

**Fig. D6.**11. Giant craniopharyngioma in a 4-year-old boy with dwarfism, visual disorders, and signs of increased intracranial pressure. Postcontrast studies demonstrate a large solid tumor with extension to the left temporal lobe and blockage of the foramen of Monro on the left. Large isodense cyst within the tumor in the anterior fossa with slight marginal contrast uptake (white arrow). Calcification at the anterior margin of the tumor (black arrow). Postcontrast study

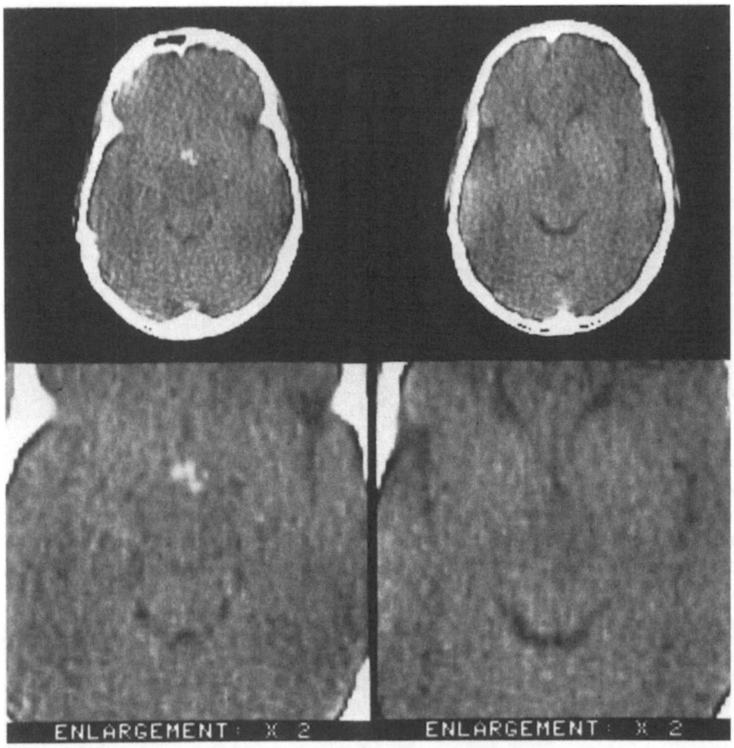


**Fig. D6.**12. Large solid craniopharyngioma with slightly hypodense values and a small marginal calcification in a 50-year-old man. The chiasmatic and prepontine cisterns are entirely filled by tumor. (Precontrast CT)

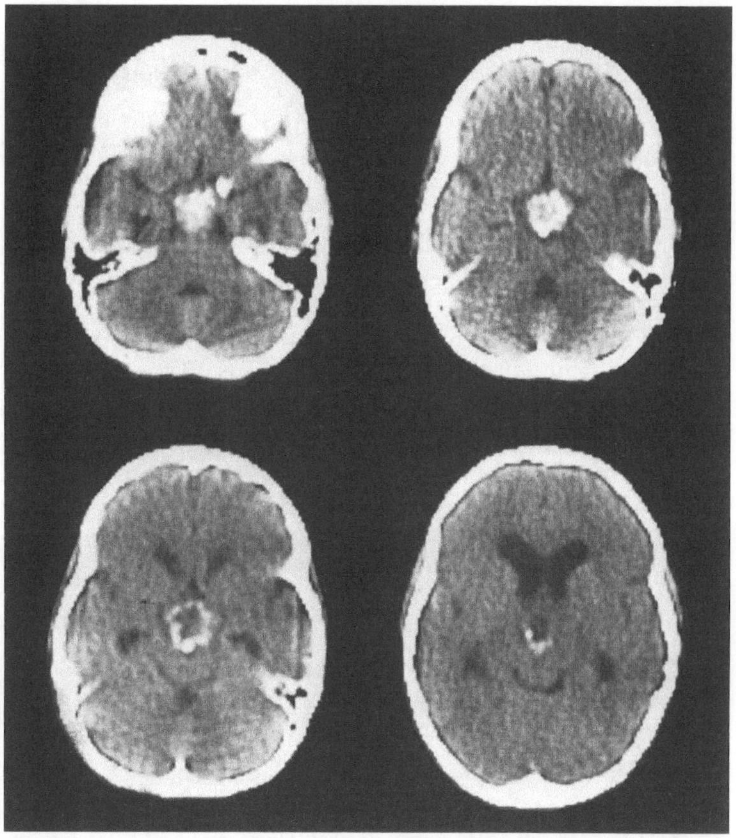

**Fig. D6.13.** Highly calcified craniopharyngioma in a 23-year-old female with headache and secondary amenorrhea. CT studies were made after calcification was demonstrated in plain skull films. Precontrast study

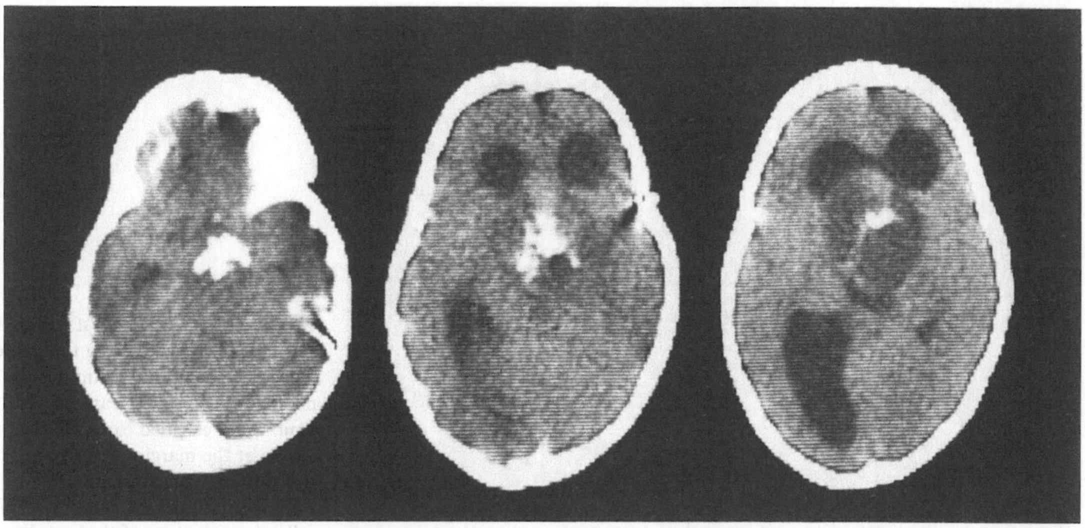

**Fig. D6.14.** Recurrence of craniopharyngioma in a 12-year-old girl. The tumor is composed of a solid highly calcified tumor mass and a large cyst with suprasellar extension which has led to blockage of both foramina of Monro. The right occipital horn does not appear in the CT scan due to oblique head position

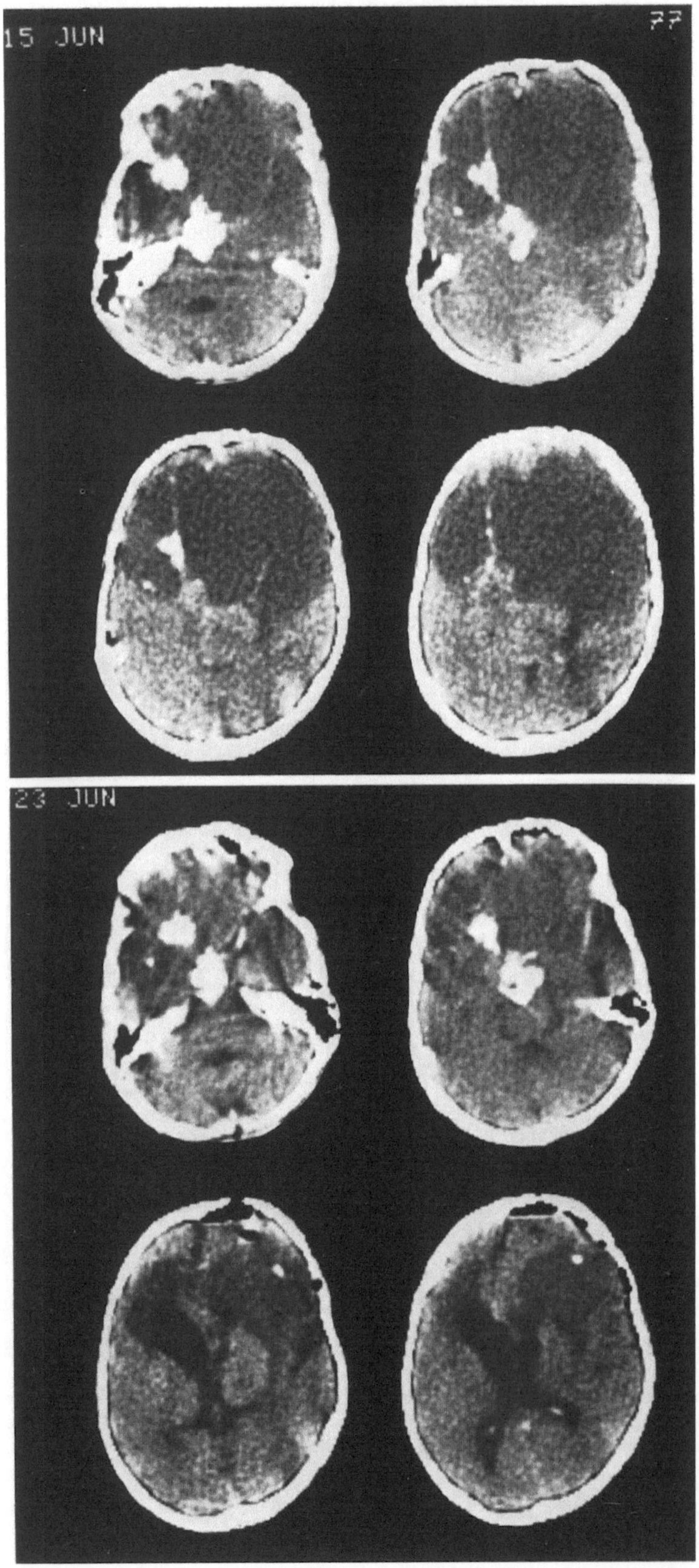


**Fig. D6.**15. Very large cyst within a craniopharyngioma filling the entire anterior fossa and a portion of the middle fossa in a 33-year-old patient. Solid calcified elements are visible at the margin of the tumor (CT studies from June 15, 1977). Follow-up studies on June 23, 1977 following puncture of the cyst demonstrate a significant reduction in size of the cyst and considerable normalization of the ventricular system. Dilatation of the left anterior horn. Tumor recurrence 18 months after initial resection. The patient was somnolent on admission to hospital

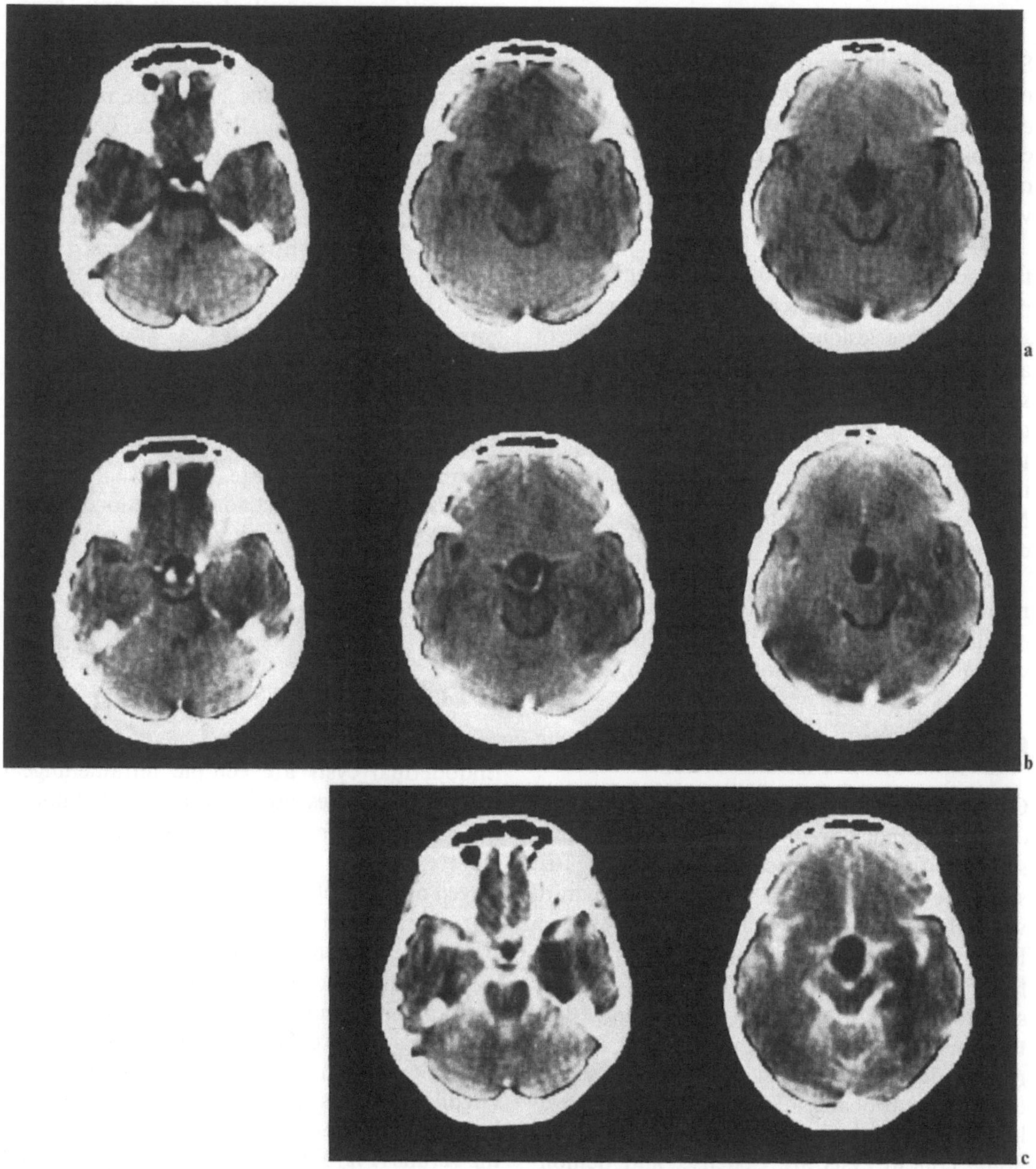


**Fig. D6.16** a–c. Cystic craniopharyngioma in a 45-year-old female with visual disorders (enlargement of the physiological blind spot bilaterally). (**a**) Large hypodense zone (18–25 HU) within the chiasmatic cistern. (**b**) Narrow marginal zone of increased density after contrast enhancement. (**c**) Combined cisternography with metrizamide and computed tomography demonstrates that there is no communication between the cystic lesion and the CSF spaces

## d) Colloid Cysts

Synonyms include *cyst of the foramen of Monro, ependymal cyst, paraphyseal cyst, and neuroepithelial cyst*. These lesions originate in the tela choroidea of the choroid plexus at the junction of the lateral ventricle and the roof of the third ventricle.

The "tumors" are in fact rare malformations containing a mucous membrane which produces a yellow-greenish gelatinous substance. These lesions accounted for 0.25% of all cases in our series. Colloid cysts range in size from a few millimeters to the size of a cherry with clinical findings related to size of the tumor. Some cysts may act as a valve with intermittent occlusion of the foramina of Monro and hydrocephalus confined to the lateral ventricles.

Patients with this malformation suffer intermittent headache and signs of increased intracranial pressure. Sudden loss of consciousness without convulsions is not uncommon.

### Computed Tomography (Figs. D 6.17, 18)

CT findings are characteristic and allow unequivocal prediction of the histological diagnosis. One finds a spherical, sharply delineated structure in the anterior portion of the third ventricle between the two foramina of Monro. Hyperdense values in the precontrast scan are found in approximately 80% of cases, with absorption values approaching 60 HU, suggesting the presence of calcification or recent hemorrhage (Fig. D 6.17). The high density of the colloid is most probably related to its high electrolyte concentration (ISHERWOOD et al. 1977). Some colloid cysts are isodense, and demonstration with CT is very difficult (Fig. D 6.18). *Dilatation of both lateral ventricles with a normal third ventricle suggests the presence of an isodense colloid cyst*. Additional slices may be necessary for demonstration in some cases, since the colloid cyst may escape detection in standard 1-cm slices. Experience shows that colloid cysts do not enhance, with the result that density values are virtually identical before and after contrast administration. Superposition of the adjacent choroid plexus may simulate an increase in density, as is also the case when precontrast and postcontrast sections are not absolutely identical.

#### Differential Diagnosis

Tumors in the same location in the anterior portion of the third ventricle may be plexus papillomas or meningiomas in very rare cases. Both tumors demonstrate a significant increase in density after contrast administration. The exact spherical configuration of the colloid cyst is hardly ever found in these two tumors.

## e) Endodermal Cysts

Endodermal cysts are ectopic intrameningeal nests of tissue resembling the endothelium of the gastrointestinal tract. They are found almost exclusively in the spinal canal. We observed one case of endodermal cyst in the posterior fossa, where the lesion appeared as a sharply delineated hyperdense midline structure located near the vault (Fig. D 6.19 a). A diagnosis of meningioma was considered but rejected since the structure did not take up contrast media. At operation a large cyst containing a dark viscous fluid was found between the cerebellar hemispheres extending over the entire length of the vermis (Fig. D 6.19 b). We recently observed a low density endodermal cyst in the fourth ventricle. Similar observations are reported in the literature.

**Fig. D6.17.** Colloid cyst of the third ventricle with occlusive hydrocephalus secondary to blockage of both foramina of Monro in a 17-year-old patient with intermittent headache. The colloid cyst appears spherical and lies typically in the anterior portion of the third ventricle where it acts as a valve and blocks both lateral ventricles. Hyperdense values (64 HU) in the precontrast study. No increase in density values after contrast enhancement

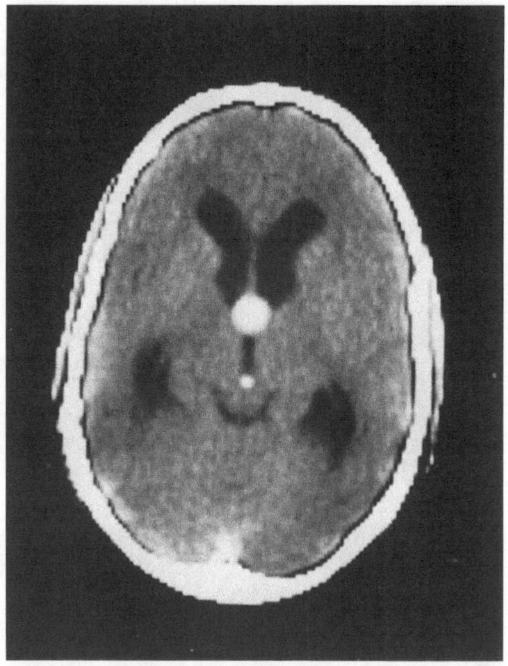

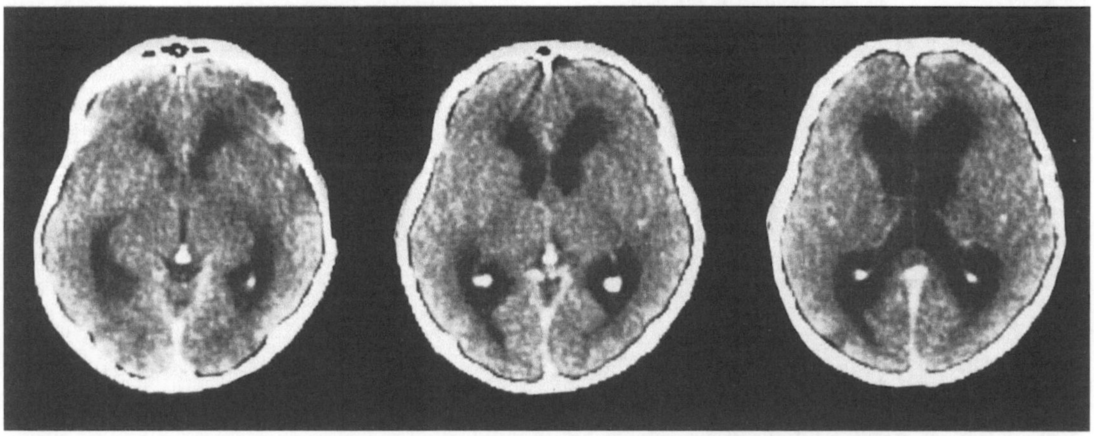

**Fig. D6.18.** Isodense colloid cyst at a typical location in a 43-year-old patient with signs of increased intracranial pressure. Presence of a hemispherical defect between the anterior horns suggests the presence of the cyst (middle). Normal width of the third ventricle posterior to the cyst indicates the location of the lesion (left). Extreme hydrocephalus secondary to a blockage of both foramina of Monro

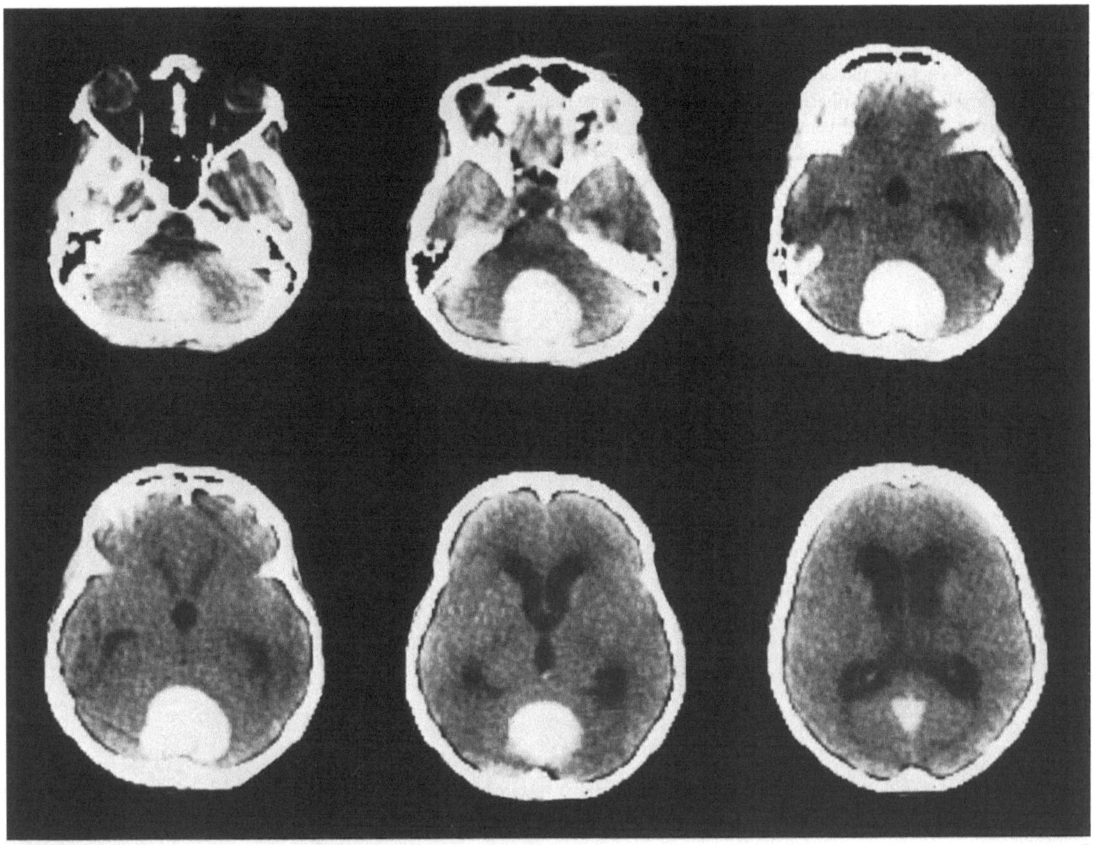

a

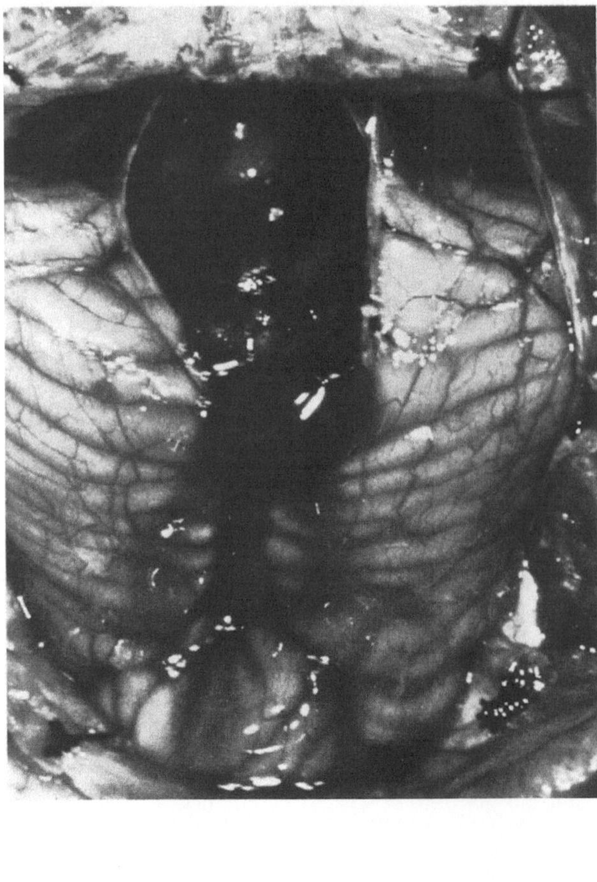

b

**Fig. D6.**19 a, b. Endodermal cyst in the midline of the posterior fossa in a 29-year-old female with signs of cerebellar dysfunction. (**a**) The lesion appears as a sharply delineated zone with extremely high density values (96 HU). No change after contrast enhancement. The fact that a dermal sinus in the midline had been resected several years before suggested the presence of a malformation. An alternative diagnosis of meningioma was rejected, since the standard deviation of the density values was only 5 HU. This degree of homogeneity is not found within calcified meningiomas. (**b**) A large cyst containing an oily dark brown fluid was found in the midline at operation. Patient in a sitting position. An identical CT finding in a 44-year-old woman was diagnosed as an atypical dermoid cyst at histological examination

## f) Lipomas

Lipomas are rare intracranial lesions discovered as incidental findings at autopsy in the majority of cases in the literature. VONDERAHE and NIEMER (1944) found four intracranial lipomas in 5,000 autopsies while BUDKA (1974) reported nine lipomas in 1956 selected neuropathological autopsy cases (0.46%). Our series includes 14 cases among 3,750 intracranial tumors (0.37%). Histological studies reveal fully differentiated fat cells, often with other structures such as blood vessels, reticular tissue, and muscle fibres. Fibrosis, calcification, and even ossification may be found, especially in the marginal portions of the tumor.

Intracranial lipomas are ectopic malformative lesions and not tumors in the strictest sense. WILLIS (1948) describes them as superfluous tumor-like structures composed of an incongruous mixture of tissues. They are related to teratoid lesions and grow at the same rate as normal tissue, in contrast to the disorderly growth pattern of ventricular tumors in tuberous sclerosis and neurofibromatosis. As a result, clinical manifestations are not due to growth of intracranial lipomas but rather to the effects of regressive alterations within the lipoma on the surrounding tissues.

Of these lesions, 28%–50% are located in the corpus callosum, while others are found in the tuber cinereum and the quadrigeminal region. KREINER (1935) reviewed the literature and used his own observations to develop a grouping of intracranial lipomas on the basis of location.

1. Ambient cistern, quadrigeminal region
2. Chiasmatic cistern and infundibulum
3. Interpeduncular cistern
4. Cistern of the Sylvian fissure
5. Lateral pontine cistern (cerebellopontine angle)
6. Cerebellomedullar cistern
7. Tela choroidea of the lateral ventricle and the third ventricle, choroid plexus, and velum triangulare
8. Cistern of the corpus callosum

KREINER's study includes five cases of lipoma in the corpus callosum combined with small tumors in the choroid plexus of the lateral ventricle (see Figs. D 6.25, 26).

The literature gives the impression that lipomas rarely cause neurological symptoms and signs. Lipomas of the corpus callosum usually cause epileptic seizures, and hemiparesis and other neurological disorders are rare. Ten of our 14 patients with intracranial lipomas had neurological symptoms related to the tumor.

### Computed Tomography (Figs. D 6.20–30)

CT diagnosis of lipoma is based on typical location and characteristic density values. Fatty tissue has attenuation values near −100 HU on the Hounsfield scale, and these values are typical of lipoma. *Small tumor nodules which occupy less than a whole slice may show higher attenuation values due to the partial volume effect.* Intravenous contrast administration does not result in a significant increase in attenuation values.

A *calcified layer at the margin of a large lipoma* in the corpus callosum is a characteristic finding that may also be visible on plain skull films and allows prediction of the histological diagnosis. The calcified layer is especially well demonstrated in coronary projections (Fig. D 6.27b). We did not observe calcification in lipomas at other locations. Lipoma is often accompanied by partial or total aplasia of the corpus callosum, which results in divergence of the lateral ventricles (Figs. D 6.26–28). Multiple lipomas may occur, especially near the choroid plexus of the lateral ventricles (Figs. D 6.25, 26). Figures D 6.20–30 provide examples of intracranial lipomas at typical locations.

#### Differential Diagnosis

*Dermoid cysts* and *teratomas* may demonstrate density values similar to those in lipomas. They are also very rare, in contrast to epidermoid cysts, which have the same density as CSF and present few problems in differential diagnosis. Since dermoid cysts and teratomas are rare, experience is limited, but four locations would seem to be predisposed: the third ventricle, with the tumor originating in the pineal body; the ambient cistern; the fourth ventricle; and the sphenoid bone with extension into the frontal or temporal lobe. We have not found a single verified report of lipoma at the last two locations. The *inhomogeneity of the cyst contents in dermoids and teratomas is an additional parameter in the diagnosis* of these hypodense lesions. Histograms demonstrate homogeneous distribution of density values in lipoma only if the tumor measures at least 25–30 mm in diameter. Variation is greater in small lipomas as a result of the partial volume effect, and standard deviation of attenuation values in these tumors may be similar to that in dermoid cysts.

Lipomas in the ambient cistern are generally much smaller than dermoid cysts found in this region. The characteristic calcified layer in lipoma allows easy differentiation between dermoid cyst of the third ventricle and lipoma of the corpus callosum.

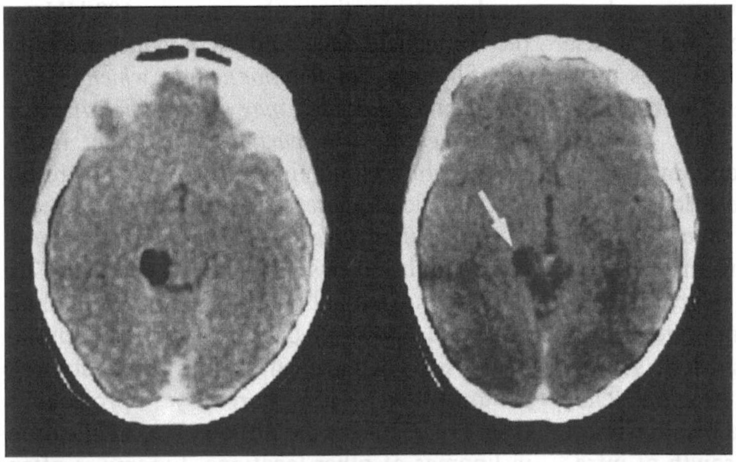

**Fig. D6.20.** Lipoma in the left ambient cistern of a 9-year-old boy with brain stem seizures. Extremely hypodense lesion (−48 to −52 HU) of the size of a hazelnut

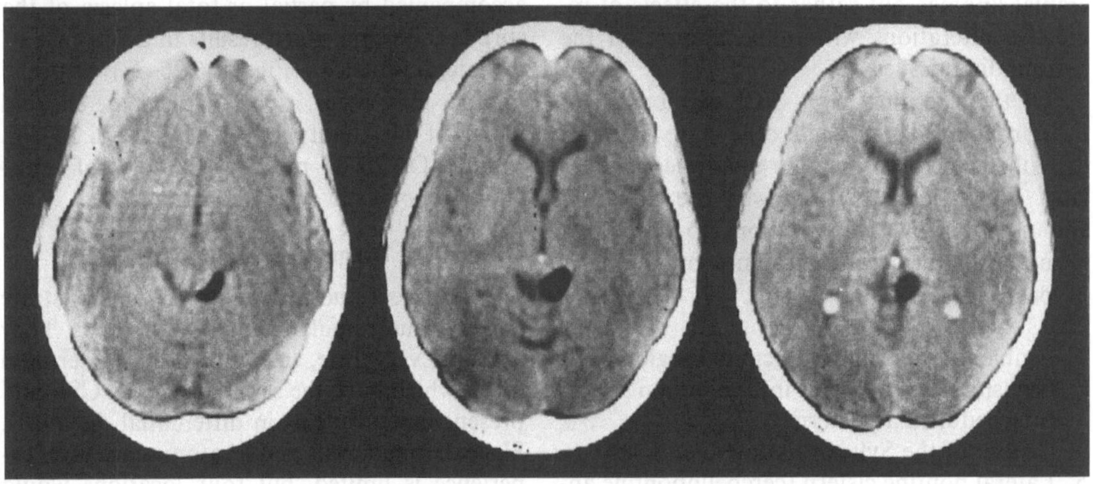

**Fig. D6.21.** Lipoma in the right ambient cistern and the lamina tecti of a 36-year-old female with a 2-year history of headache and a single epileptic seizure. Mean density −72 to −88 HU. Diagnosis confirmed at operation

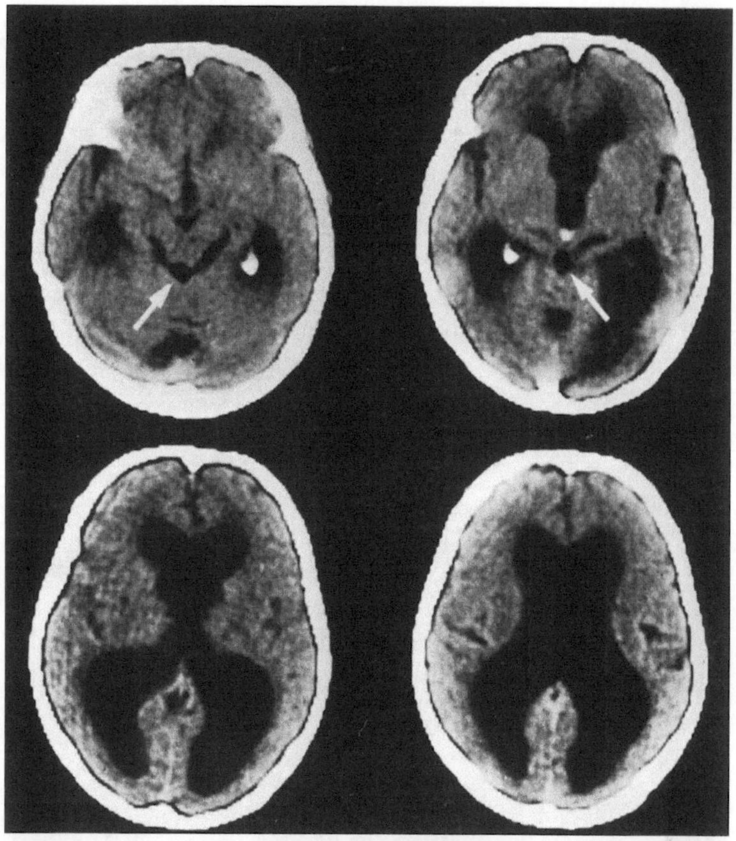

**Fig. D6.22.** Lipoma in the lamina tecti of a 67-year-old man with pronounced hydrocephalus secondary to disruption of the CSF circulation at the aqueduct. Mean density −70 HU

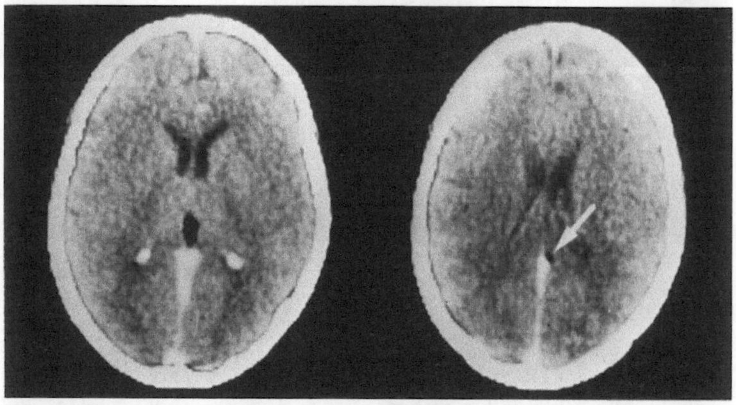

**Fig. D6.23.** Lipoma in the region of the velum interpositum in a 43-year-old female. Mean density −40 HU. Incidental finding

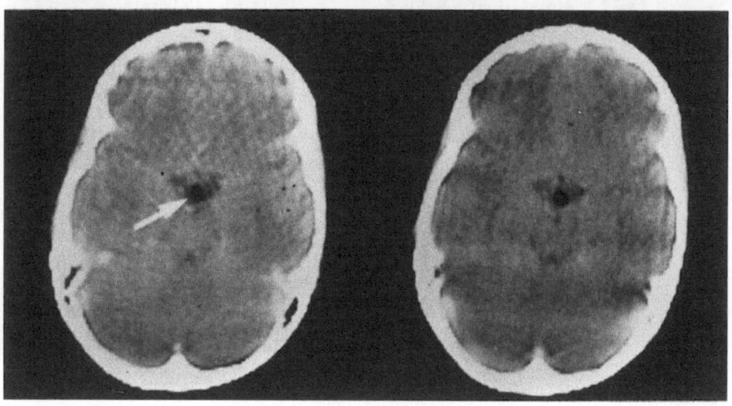

**Fig. D6.24.** Lipoma in the chiasmatic cistern, probably at the infundibulum in a 12-year-old boy with conspicuously aggressive behavior. Density −42 HU

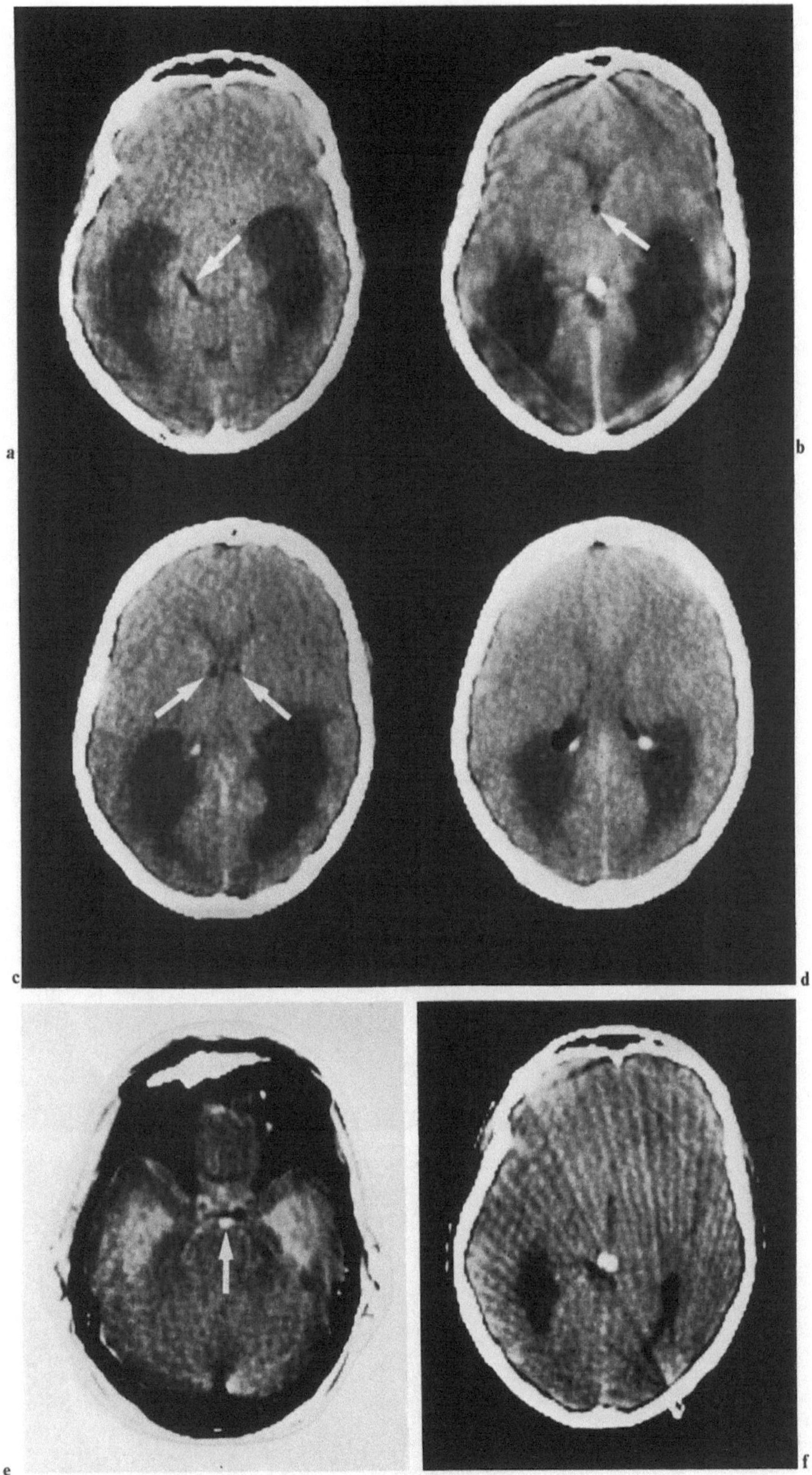
a b c d e f

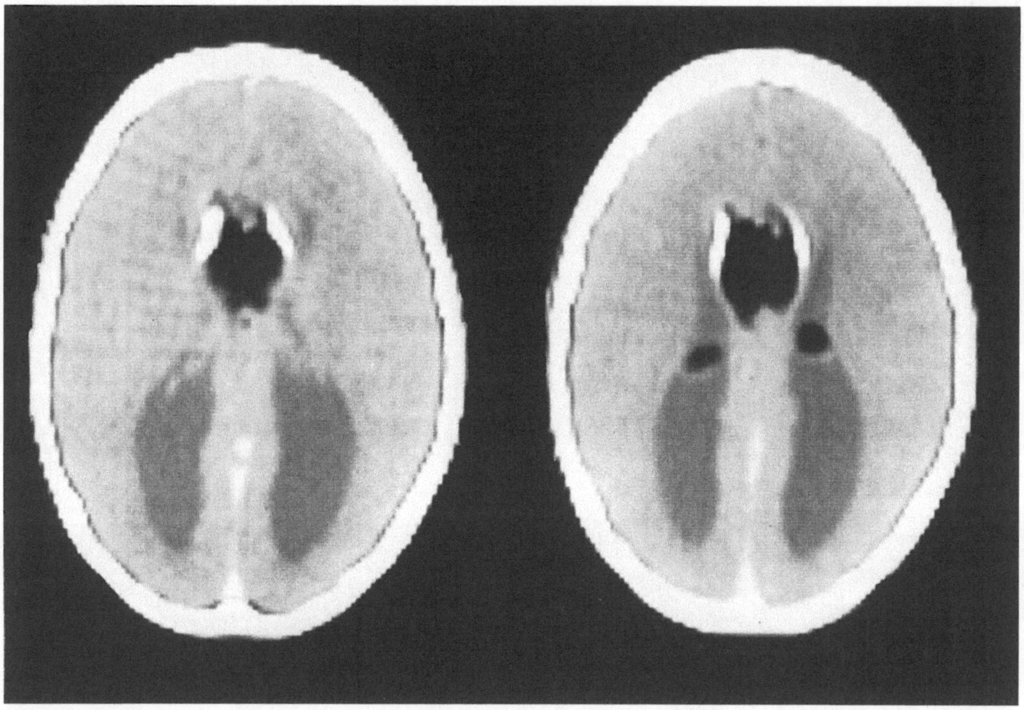

**Fig. D6.26.** Lipomas in the choroid plexus of both lateral ventricles combined with a lipoma in the corpus callosum with a typical calcified shell at the interface with normal brain tissue. Twenty-one-year-old female with a 2-year history of psychomotor seizures and intermittent headache for 3 months. The headaches are probably due to dilatation of the occipital horns. Density values in the lipomas range from −33 HU (left choroid plexus) to −67 HU (right choroid plexus) and −106 HU (corpus callosum)

◄

**Fig. D6.25** a–f. Multiple intracranial lipomas in a 60-year-old man with a severe organic brain syndrome, loss of vision, dizziness, and a disorder of bladder function. (**a**) Small lipoma on the left side of the ambient cistern (arrow). (**b**) Small lipoma in the anterior portion of the third ventricle (arrow). (**c**) Small lipomas in the choroid plexus of both lateral ventricles near the foramina of Monro (arrows). (**d**) Lipomas in the glomus of the choroid plexus in both lateral ventricles with occlusion of both occipital horns and resultant extreme hydrocephalus with periventricular lucency. (**e**) Small lipoma in the interpeduncular fossa (arrow). The reversed CT scan allows better demonstration of the lipoma. (**f**) Significant reduction of ventricular dilatation 6 weeks after a drainage operation. Artifacts due to metallic portions of the valve.

Density values range between −15 and −52 HU in the various lipomas

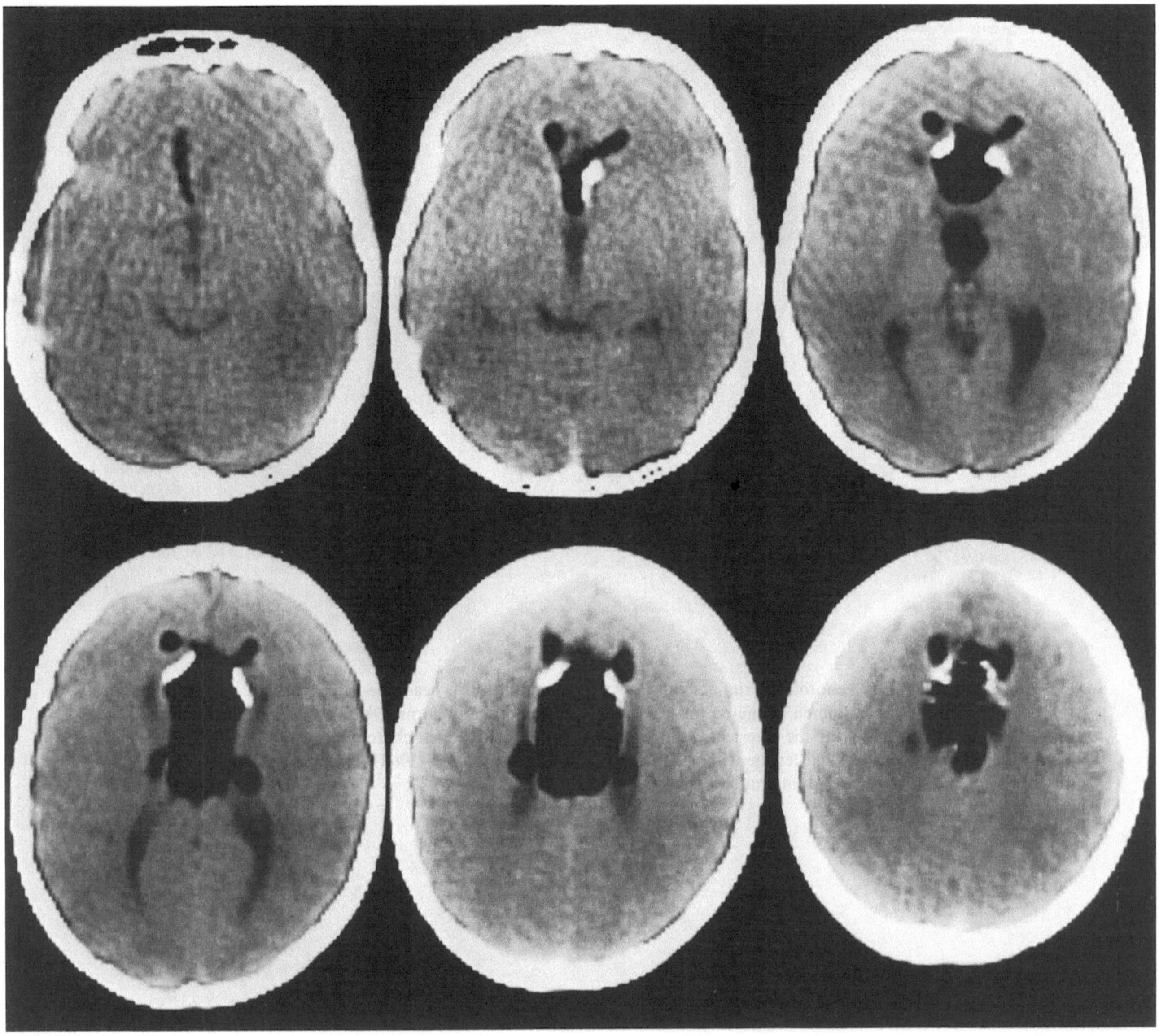

a

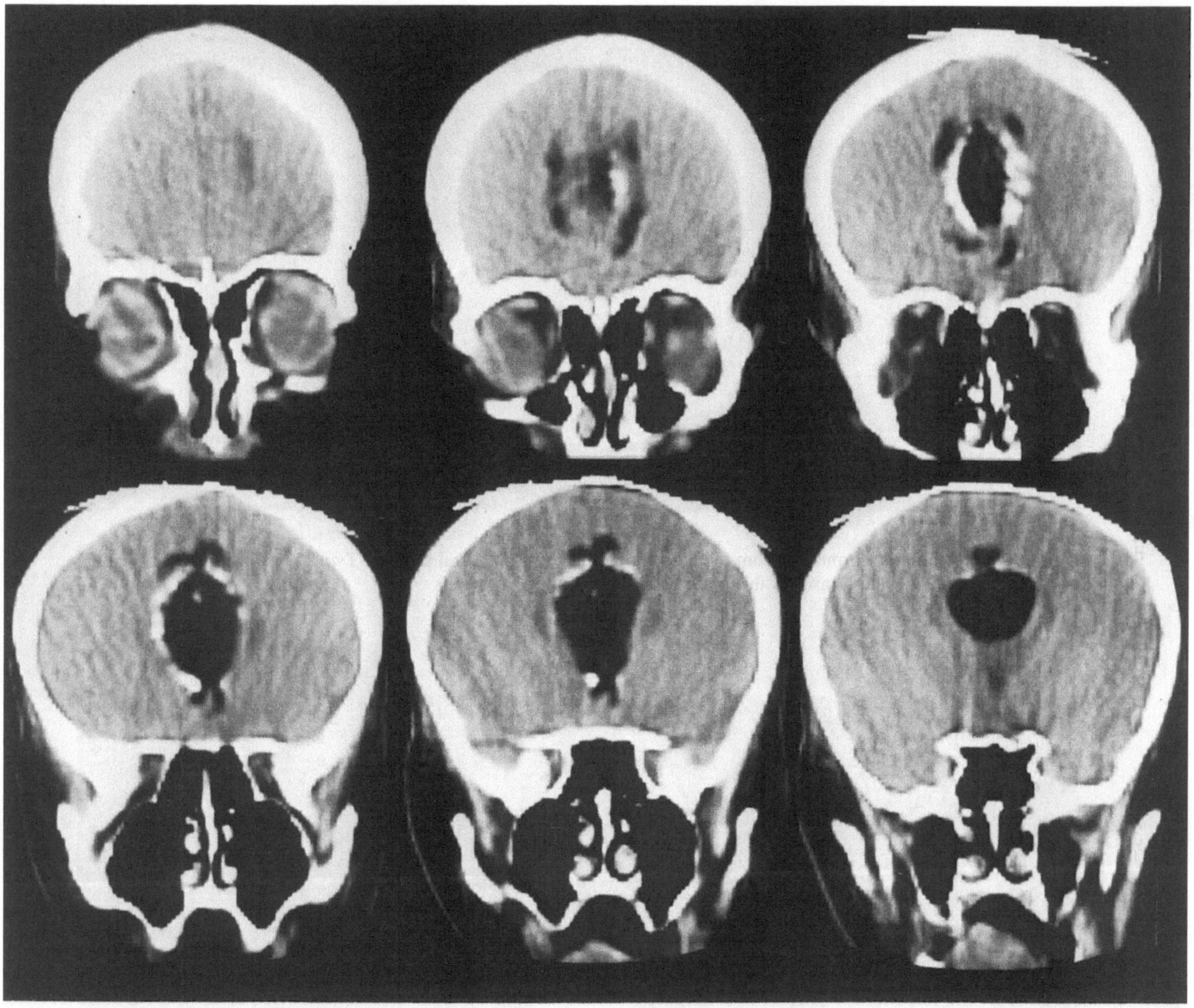

b

**Fig. D6.27** a, b. Atypical lipoma in the corpus callosum of a 22-year-old female with cerebral seizures. (**a**) Horizontal projections: large lipoma involving almost the entire corpus callosum (aplasia of the corpus callosum) with narrow zone of calcification at the margin of the tumor and multiple small lipomas in the lateral ventricle adjacent to the main tumor. (**b**) Coronary projection: better demonstration of the bowl-shaped calcification. Plain skull films usually reveal typical calcification in these patients

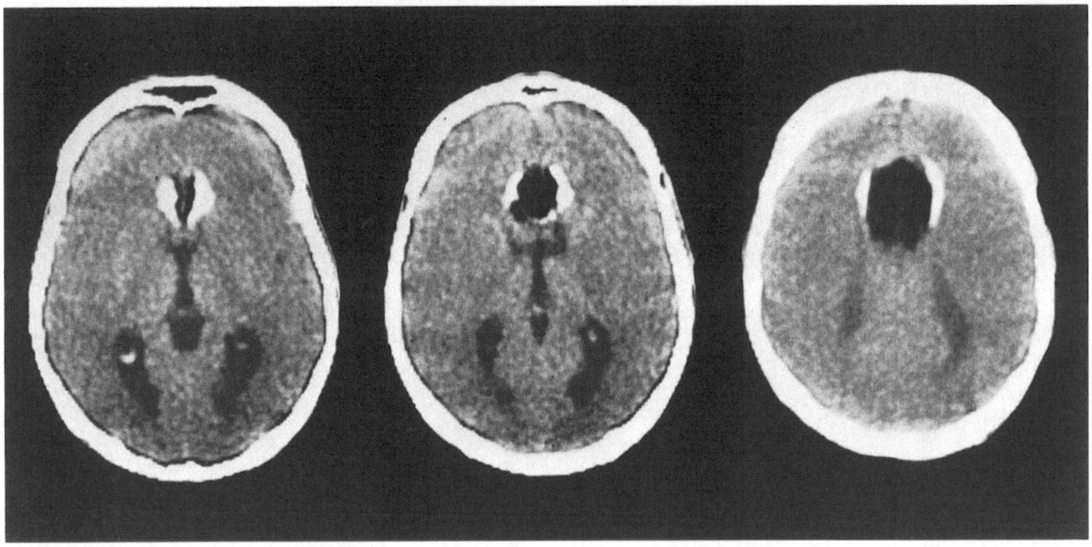

**Fig. D6.28.** Lipoma in the corpus callosum of a 20-year-old male with cerebral seizures. Typical bowl-shaped calcification at the margin of the lipoma. Density at the center of the lipoma −55 EMI units

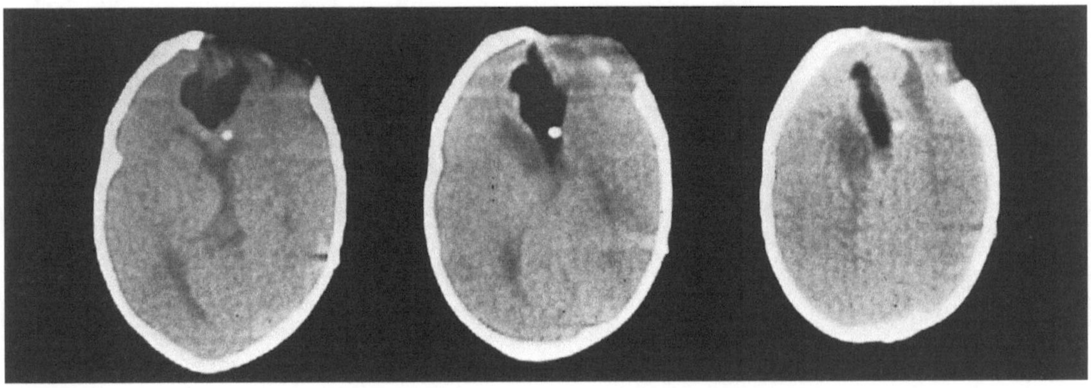

**Fig. D6.29.** Large lobulated lipoma between the frontal lobes (origin in the anterior corpus callosum?) in a child who had undergone resection of a right frontal encephalocele. Mean density −117 to −125 HU

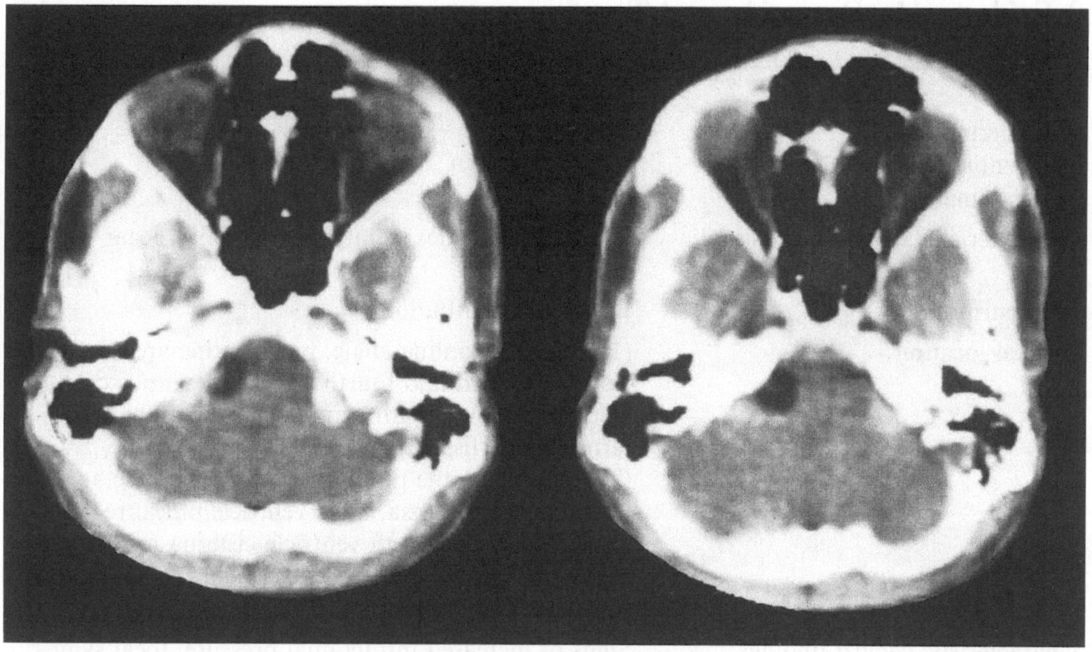

**Fig. D6.30.** Small lipoma at the tip of the left pyramid in an 18-year-old patient with signs of a lesion at the cerebellopontine angle. Mean density −55 HU

## g) Epidermoids, Dermoids, and Teratomas

| | |
|---|---|
| Incidence | |
| Epidermoids (1) | 0.6–1.5% |
| Dermoids (2) | 0.1% |
| Teratomas (3) | 0.3% |
| Characteristic age at diagnosis | 2nd to 4th decades; teratomas may also occur in young children |
| Sex distribution | Equal sex distribution |
| Typical location | (1) Cerebellopontine angle, parapontine area, lateral ventricles, third and fourth ventricles, corpus callosum, chiasma, quadrigeminal region, ambient cistern, Sylvian fissure, and skull vault<br>(2) Adjacent to the pituitary, cleft lines in the anterior and middle fossa, third ventricle/pineal region, ambient cistern, fourth ventricle cisterna magna<br>(3) Pineal region, third ventricle, sella region, lateral ventricle |
| Characteristic clinical findings | Signs of increased intracranial pressure, focal symptoms, "aseptic meningitis" |
| Skull film | Bone destruction |
| EEG | Uncharacteristic findings |
| Echoencephalography | Ventricular dilatation common |
| Serial brain scintigraphy | Perfusion defect in many cases; no radionuclide uptake |
| Cerebral angiography | Displacement of normal vessels |
| Pneumoencephalography | Epidermoids cause a characteristic pattern of irregularly distributed air around the tumor |

**Computed Tomography**

| | |
|---|---|
| Precontrast study | ad 1. Hypodense zone with CSF density; marginal calcification in some cases<br>ad 2. Very low density zone (density of fatty tissue); marginal calcification in many cases; rarely hyperdense area mimicking meningioma<br>ad 3. Similar to 2, otherwise inhomogeneously distributed density values due to mixture of various tissues |
| Contrast medium uptake | Positive in malignant teratomas, also positive in exceptional cases of hyperdense epidermoids |
| Appearance after contrast enhancement | No change in 1 and 2; variegated picture in malignant teratomas |

**Differential Diagnosis**

ad 1. Arachnoid cyst
- Other cysts
- Cysticercosis
- Cavities secondary to hemorrhage
- Gumma

ad 2. and 3. Lipoma

Epidermoids, dermoids, and teratomas are rare malformations. ZÜLCH found them in 1.8% of cases in a series of 9,000 tumors, with equal distribution between the two sexes. These tumors accounted for approximately 1% of cases in our series.

Epidermoid cysts, also known as pearl tumors or cholesteatomas, are the most common tumors in this group, accounting for approximately three-quarters of the total. Epidermoids and dermoids are most often diagnosed in the middle aged, while teratomas are usually found in children.

Epidermoids consist of keratin derived from the epidermis as well as connective tissue arranged in layers and surrounded by a thin membrane, which is responsible for the transparency and mother of pearl sheen of the tumors (Fig. D 6.36 b). Dermoids may contain partially saponified fatty tissue as well as cutaneous accessory organs with hair follicles, hair, sebaceous glands, and sweat glands.

Teratomas contain epidermal material and accessory organs as well as bone, cartilage, endodermal tissue, and other histological structures.

*Typical locations* are listed on p. 320.

Clinical symptoms and signs include increased intracranial pressure and focal neurological signs as well as *"aseptic meningitis,"* which is caused by the presence of epidermal tissue or fat in the CSF spaces.

### Additional Diagnostic Procedures

Plain skull films are useful only in epidermoids originating in the diploe of the cranial vault. Dermoid cysts of the anterior fossa cause bony destruction. Teratomas may show extensive intracranial calcifications or teeth. In the pneumoencephalogram epidermoid cysts may demonstrate a mottled distribution of air at the margin of the tumor as a result of penetration of the air into the arachnoid membranes encapsulating the epidermal tissue.

## **Computed Tomography** (Figs. D 6.31–52)

### Precontrast Study

All three types of malformative tumors demonstrate low density values and suggest the diagnosis of cyst. Calcification may be seen at the margin of the tumor (Figs. D 6.48, 51). Density measurements are decisive in the differentiation of these tumors. *Epidermoids have attenuation values similar to those of CSF,* ranging from +2 to +10 HU, and demonstrate the same shades of gray as CSF in the analog picture (Figs. D 6.31–40, 44). Our experience with 27 epidermoids corroborates the results reported by FAWCITT and ISHERWOOD (1977) as well as NEW and SCOTT (1975). However, GYLDENSTED and KARLE (1977) reported three suprasellar tumors, and BRAUN et al. (1977) found three epidermoids in the posterior fossa with isodense or hyperdense appearance. Some of these tumors took up contrast media, so that a diagnosis of meningioma was considered. It is not possible to ascertain whether the tumors reported in these articles are in fact the same epidermoid tumors defined above. One lesion was described as a "black mass" (compare Fig. D 6.19).

HASEGAWA et al. (1981) reported a case of intracranial epidermoid with homogeneous high density, while KIM et al. (1981) observed a dermoid tumor presenting as a high-density lesion in the noncontrast CT, both tumors mimicking meningioma. A recent case of suprasellar epidermoid with hyperdense attenuation values was found to contain old hemorrhage and keratin (KAZNER et al., unpublished)

*Mean density values in dermoid cysts lie in the negative range of the Hounsfield scale* as a result of the high fat content of these lesions. Mean density values as low as −100 HU may be found, depending on the degree of saponification. Dermoids have a somewhat darker shade of gray than CSF in the analog picture (Figs. D 6.44–49). Standard deviation may be very high, sometimes more than 20 HU, as a result of the great range in density values of the individual components of the dermoid cyst.

Recently we observed a *hyperdense dermoid cysts* in a 44-year-old female with occipital headache. The CT scan showed a sharply delineated mass in the posterior fossa extending from the upper cerebellar vermis to the spinal canal ending at C3. Mean density values of +84 to +88 HU were measured in the precontrast CT without further increase after contrast-enhancement. The CT picture was identical to the case in Fig. D 6.19. At operation a dermal sinus was found ending in an encapsulated dark-brown, predominantly fluid malformative tumor with keratinic masses, hair and calcified elements. The highly viscous brownish fluid contained 32.8 g/dl of protein, which probably explains the high attenuation values.

CT findings in teratoma are not uniform. Fatty components with negative density values predominate, and differentiation from dermoid cysts may be impossible in individual cases (Fig. D6.51). The other elements of the teratoma may have very *high density values,* with the result that measurements at various locations within the tumor produce even greater variation. Analysis of the CT picture with different window levels demonstrates the individual components of the tumor (Fig. D6.50).

## Postcontrast Study

*We never observed a measurable increase in density in cases of epidermoid and dermoid.* Positive contrast enhancement was only found in malignant teratomas with bizarre tumor structures (Fig. D6.52).

*Intrathecal administration of metrizamide* may be helpful in differentiation of other cystic lesions, especially in epidermoids of the ambient cistern (Fig. D6.37).

## Differential Diagnosis

*1. Epidermoid Cysts. Arachnoid cysts* near the vault cause characteristic thinning and bulging of the vault. Arachnoid cysts in the quadrigeminal region have the same absorption values as epidermoids and demonstrate no other characteristics which might allow certain differentiation. The same is true of arachnoid cyst in the cisterna magna. Arachnoid cysts are always spherical or oval in shape, while an irregular configuration suggests a diagnosis of epidermoid.

A *solitary cysticercus,* an *old hemorrhagic cavity,* and a *gumma* may all demonstrate hypodense zones with the same density as CSF as well as marginal calcification, so that differentiation from epidermoid cyst may be difficult, if not impossible. A lesion confined to the brain parenchyma without contact with the CSF space is probably not an epidermoid.

*2. Dermoid Cysts and Teratomas.* Since density values are extremely low in these cases, *lipoma* is the only alternative in differential diagnosis, and problems arise only in lesions of the ambient cistern, where both lipomas and dermoids are found (Figs. D6.21, 39).

Malignant teratomas in young children fail to demonstrate the low density zones found in benign teratomas. Other malignant tumors occurring in childhood must be considered in the differential diagnosis of such lesions. Hyperdense epidermoids and dermoids may simulate calcified meningiomas. Contrast enhancement is usually negative in such cases.

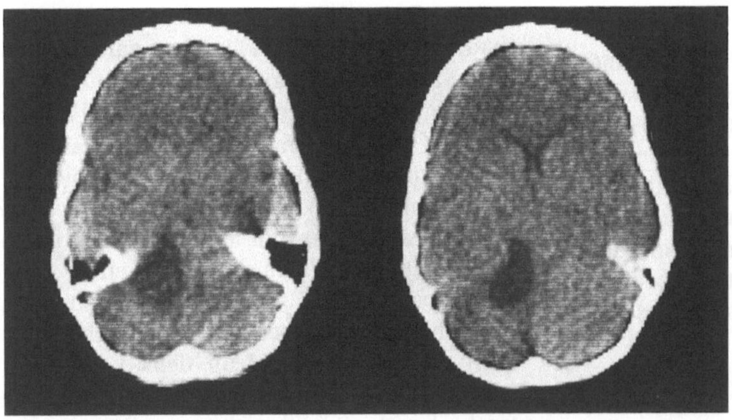

**Fig. D6.31.** Epidermoid cyst in the left cerebellopontine angle with extension to the ambient cistern in a 25-year-old female with signs of cerebellar dysfunction on the left. Density values within the tumor similar to those of CSF

**Fig. D6.32.** Parapontine epidermoid cyst on the left with extension to the left cerebellopontine angle in a 40-year-old male with deficits of the caudal cranial nerves on the left. Density values slightly higher than those of CSF (+8 HU)

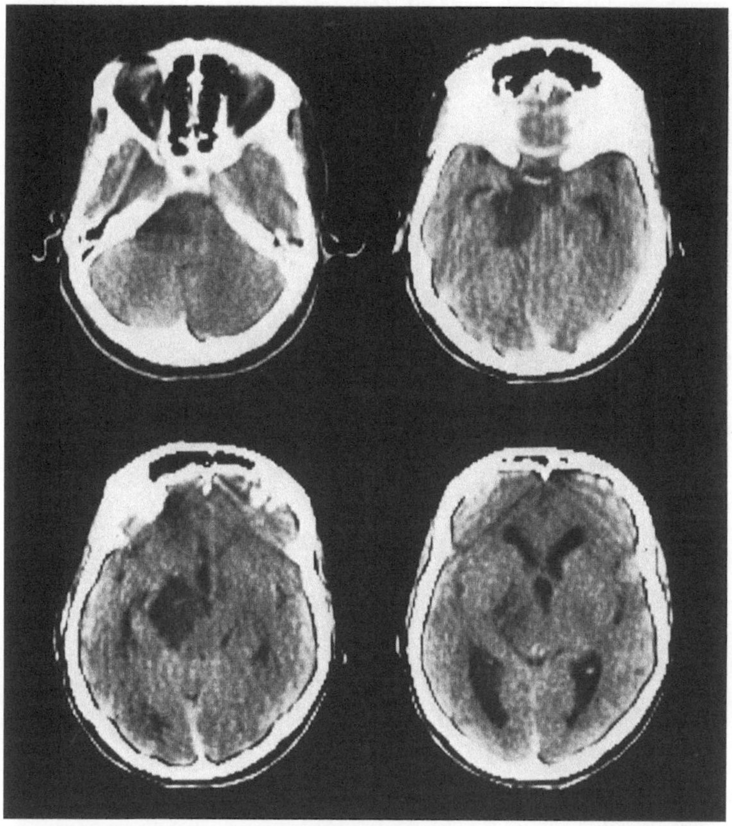

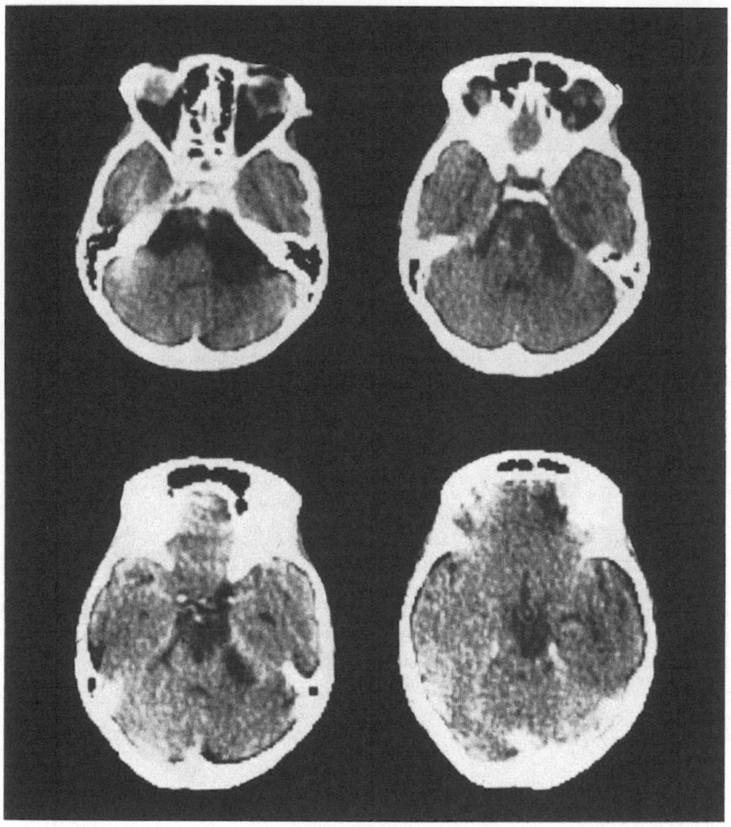

**Fig. D6.33.** Epidermoid cyst anterior to the pons with extension to both cerebellopontine angles, more pronounced on the right. Density values similar to those of CSF. Fifty-eight-year-old female with facial nerve paralysis on the right and spasticity on the left

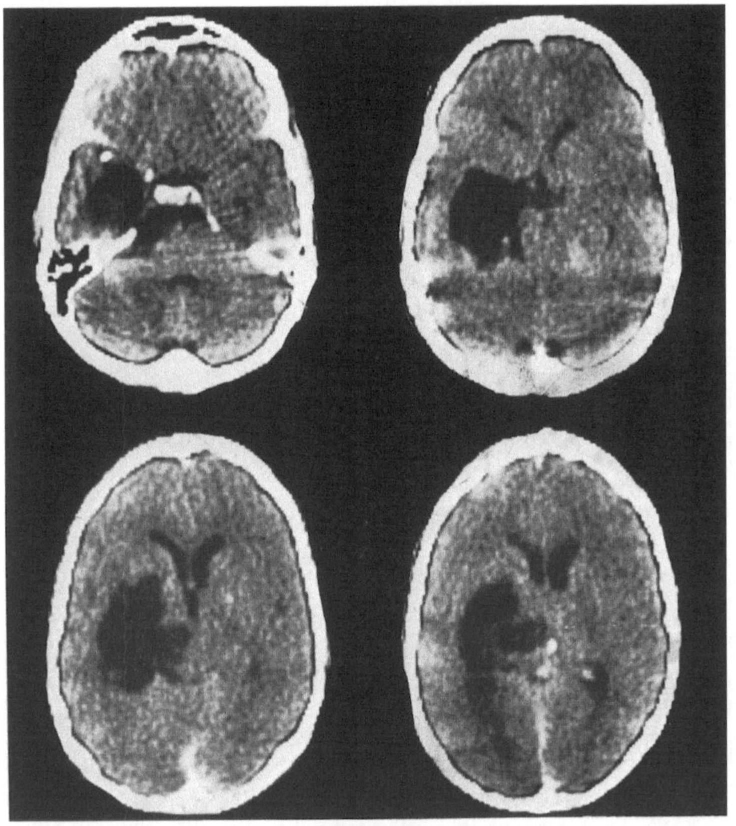

**Fig. D6.34.** Para- and prepontine epidermoid cyst on the left with extension to the subtemporal region and the ambient cistern in a 42-year-old patient. Mean density +9.7 to +13.5 HU

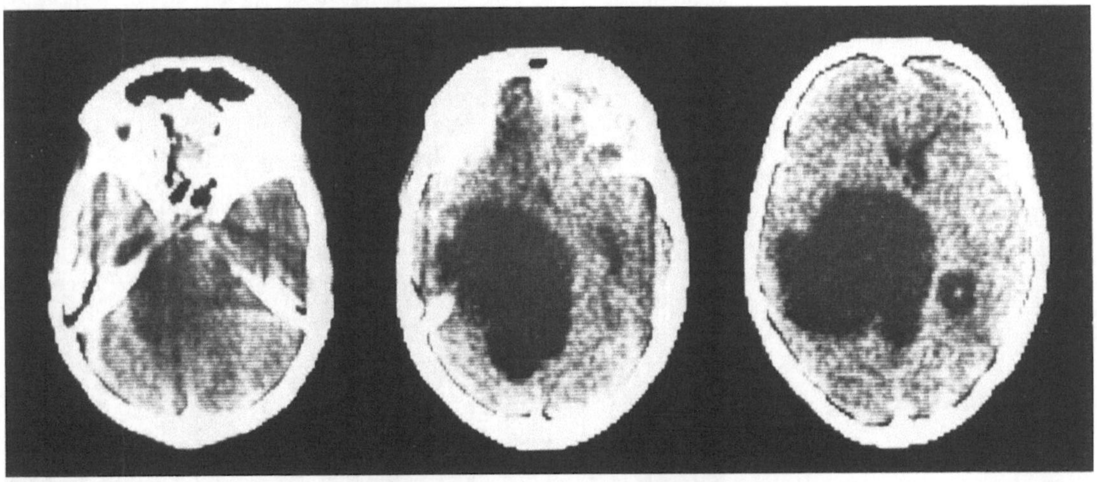

**Fig. D6.35.** Epidermoid cyst originating in the left cerebellopontine angle with extension through the tentorium into the left cerebral hemisphere in a 26-year-old female with signs of brain stem dysfunction. Density values range between 0 and +5 EMI units. Some pixels demonstrate values as low as −15 EMI units

**Fig. D6.36.** (**a**) Epidermoid cyst in the fourth ventricle of a 29-year-old female with signs of cerebellar dysfunction. Density values similar to those of CSF. Differential diagnosis includes arachnoid cyst and so-called simple cerebellar cyst. (**b**) The characteristic mother-of-pearl surface of the tumor is visible at operation

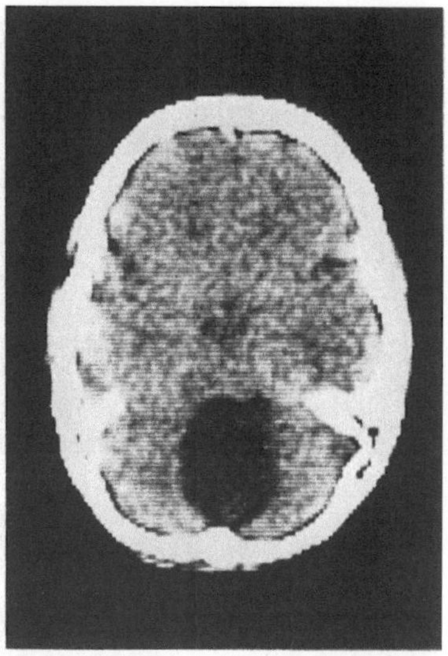

a

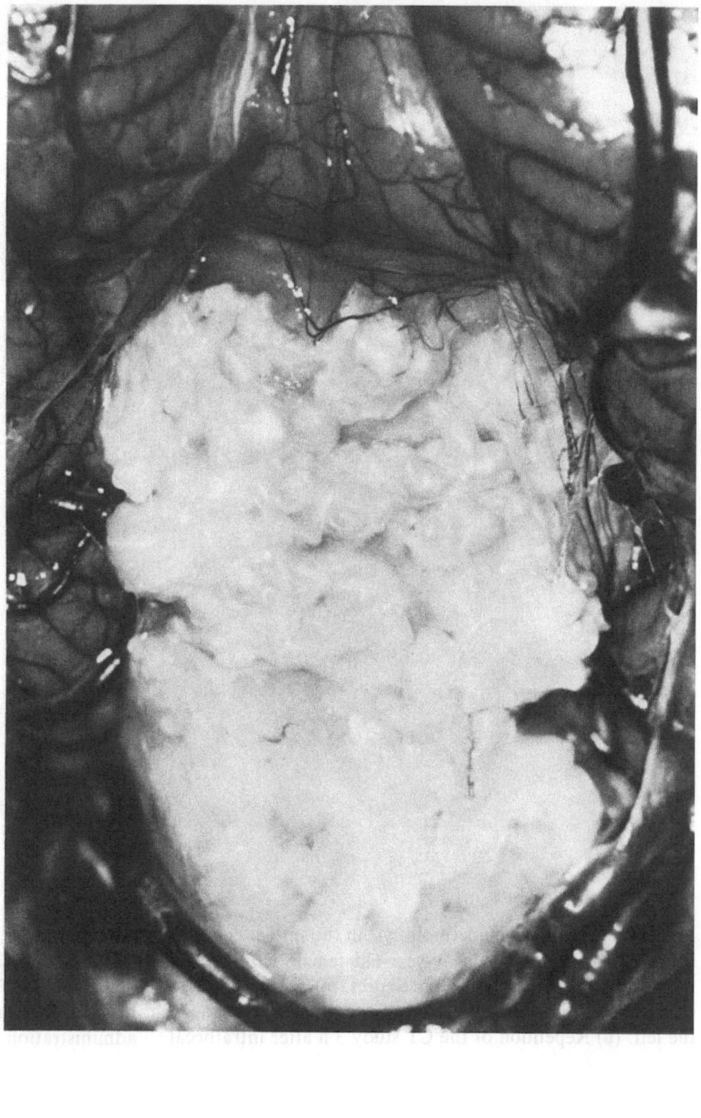

b

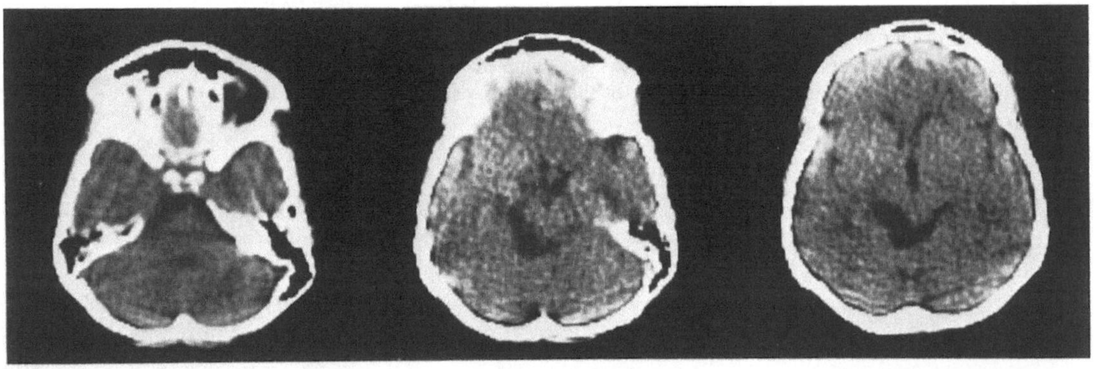

a

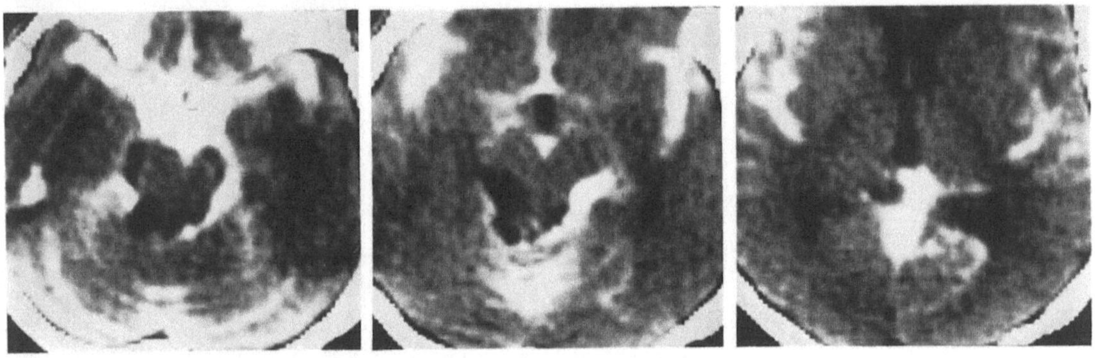

b

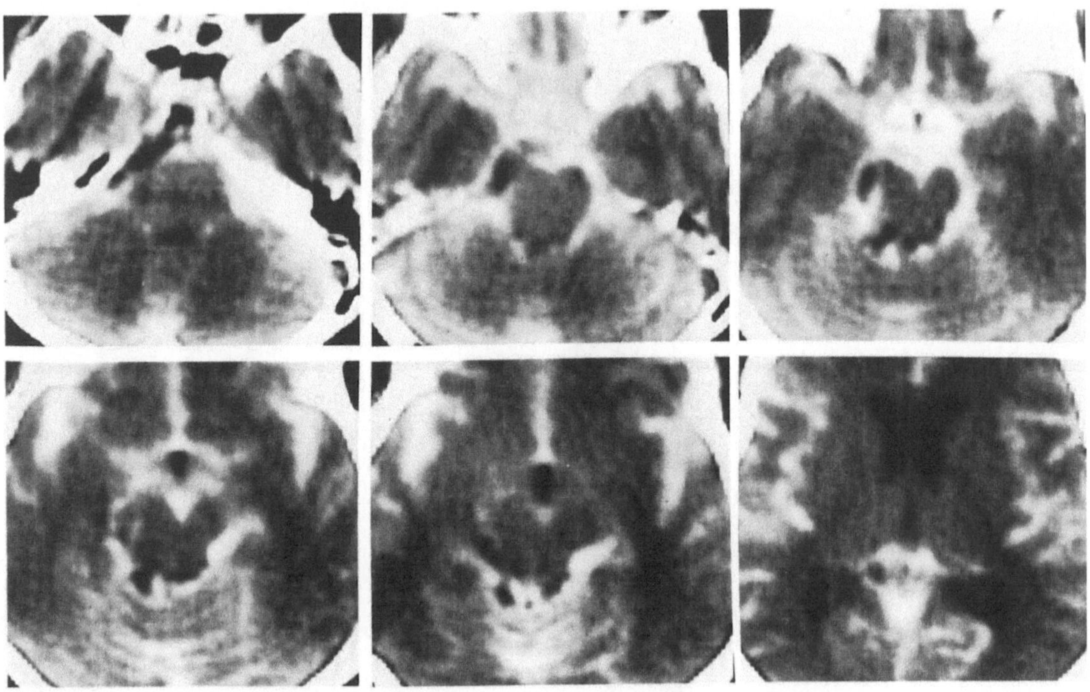

c

**Fig. D6.**37a–c. Small epidermoid cyst in the ambient cistern, primarily on the left in a 49-year-old female with cranial nerve deficits and psychomotor seizures. (**a**) The precontrast study shows apparent dilatation of the ambient cistern on the left. (**b**) Repetition of the CT study 3 h after intrathecal administration of metrizamide reveals that the apparent dilatation is in fact a space-occupying lesion with the same density as CSF. Diagnosis of an epidermoid cyst. (**c**) Contrast medium has penetrated the epidermoid cyst 6 h after administration

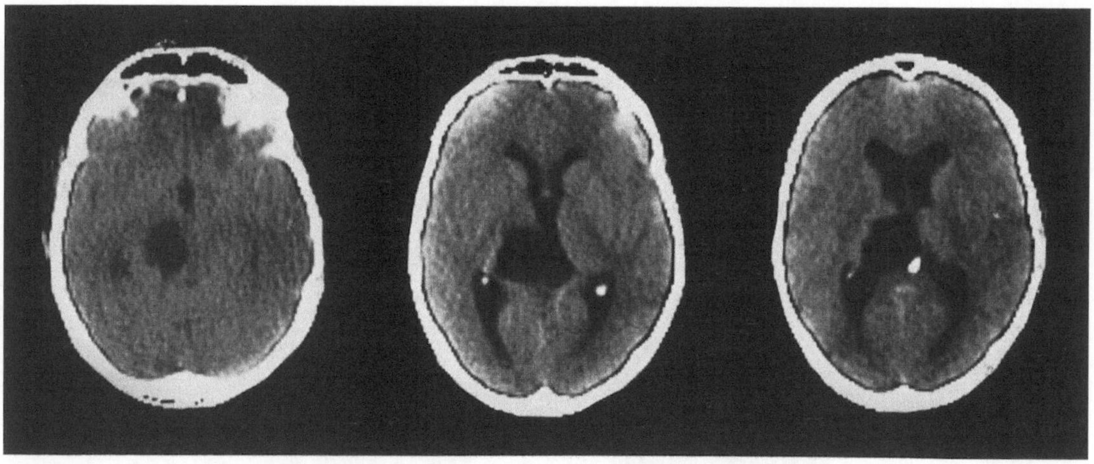

**Fig. D6.38.** Large epidermoid cyst with similar density as CSF (9.8 HU) in the lamina tecti, the left thalamus, and the left cerebral peduncle in a 47-year-old man with slowly progredient right hemiparesis. The picture on the right demonstrates a delicate membranous structure between the left occipital horn and the epidermoid cyst. This finding was decisive in making the diagnosis. Incipient hydrocephalus

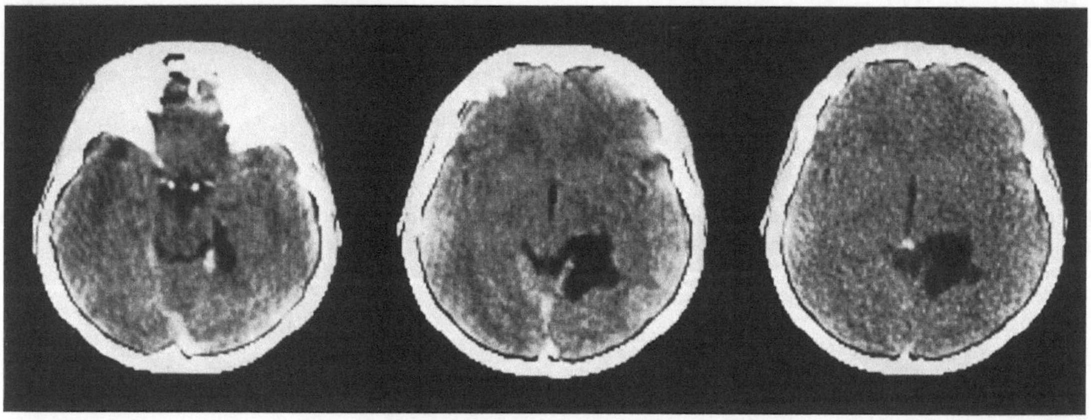

**Fig. D6.39.** Epidermoid cyst in the right ambient cistern with extension to the right occipital lobe and the right cerebral peduncle in a 34-year-old female with intermittent left hemiparesis. False diagnosis of multiple sclerosis several years previously. The lesion has the same density as CSF

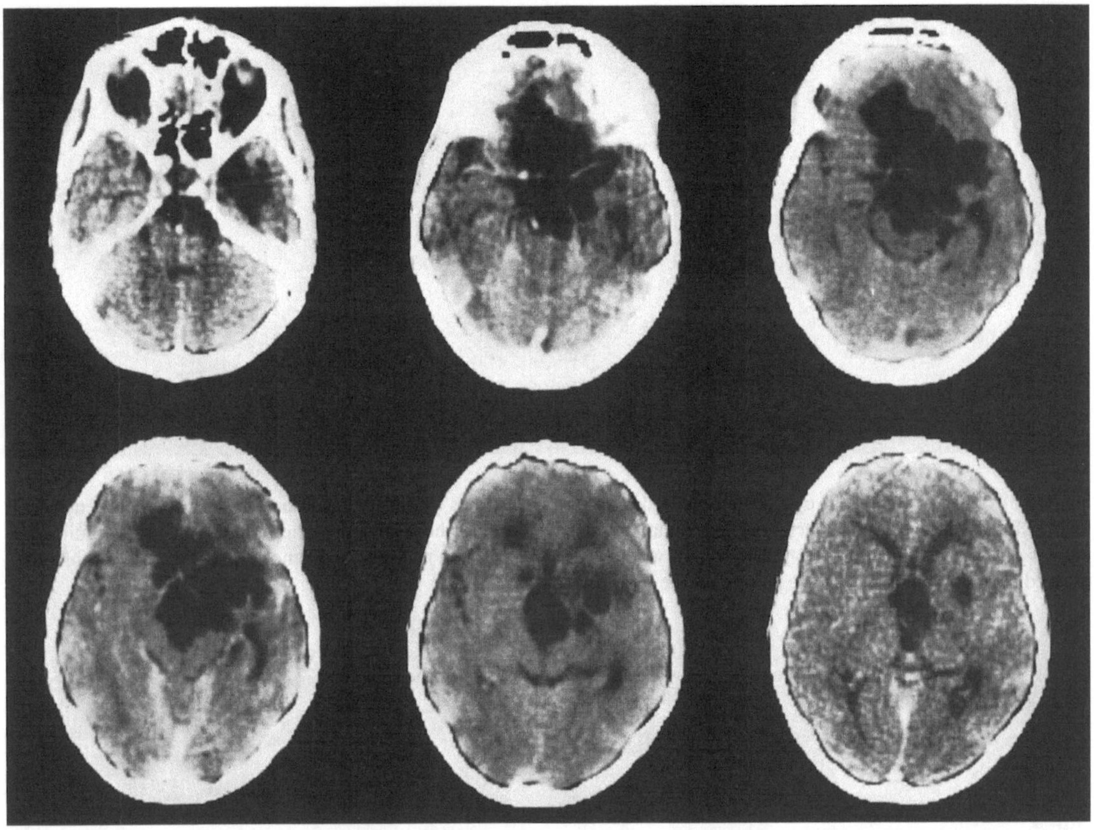

**Fig. D6.40.** Very large irregularly shaped epidermoid cyst at the base of the middle fossa with extension to the interpeduncular cistern and the prepontine region as well as to the subtemporal and subfrontal regions with penetration of the third ventricle in a 35-year-old patient

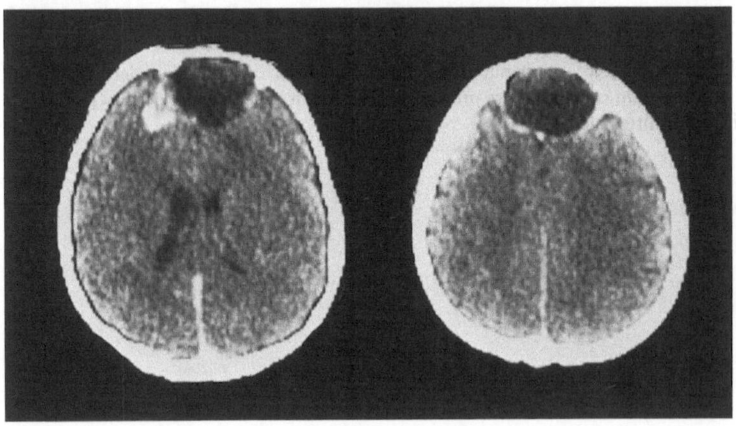

**Fig. D6.41.** Epidermoid in the diploe of frontal bone of a 53-year-old patient. The tumor is predominantly hypodense and delineated against normal brain tissue by a calcified membrane. A hyperdense zone adjacent to the epidermoid on the left demonstrated increased density values after contrast enhancement. This structure proved to be granulation tissue

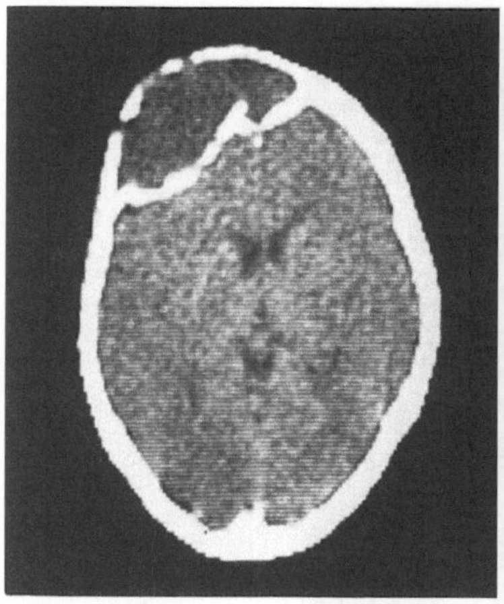

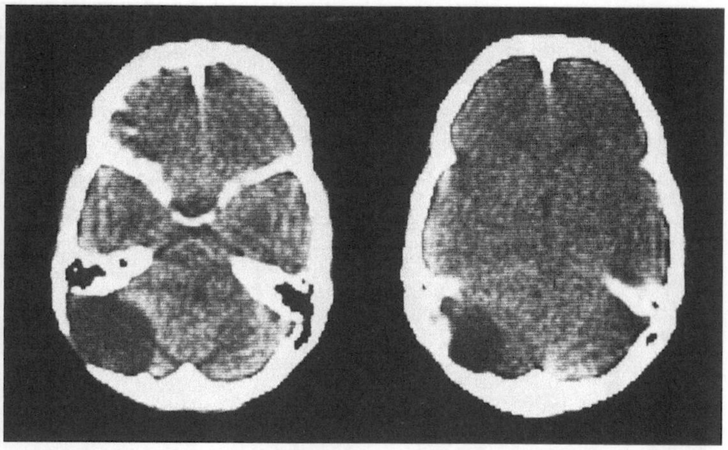

**Fig. D6.42.** Large epidermoid in the vault of a 68-year-old female admitted with protrusion of the left frontal bone and a tentative diagnosis of osteomyelitis. Solid bone delineates the malformative tumor against the cranial cavity. Density values within the epidermoid cyst are slightly higher than those in CSF

**Fig. D6.43.** Extradural epidermoid cyst in the posterior fossa on the left with destruction of the skull bone in 41-year-old female. Typical bone changes associated with a space-occupying lesion with CSF density allowed the correct diagnosis

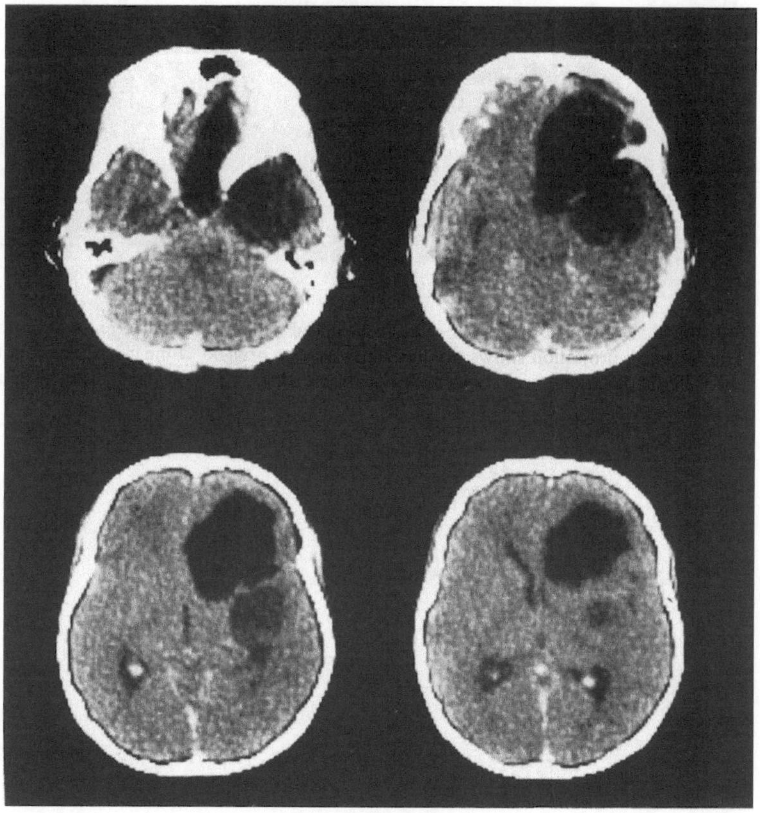

**Fig. D6.44.** Combination of a dermoid cyst originating in the sella with extension to the right frontal region and an epidermoid located in the right temporal region. The tumors are separated by the Sylvian fissure and the blood vessels located there. Mean density values in the dermoid −3 HU, in the epidermoid +6 HU. Twenty-year-old patient with extreme headache and papilledema

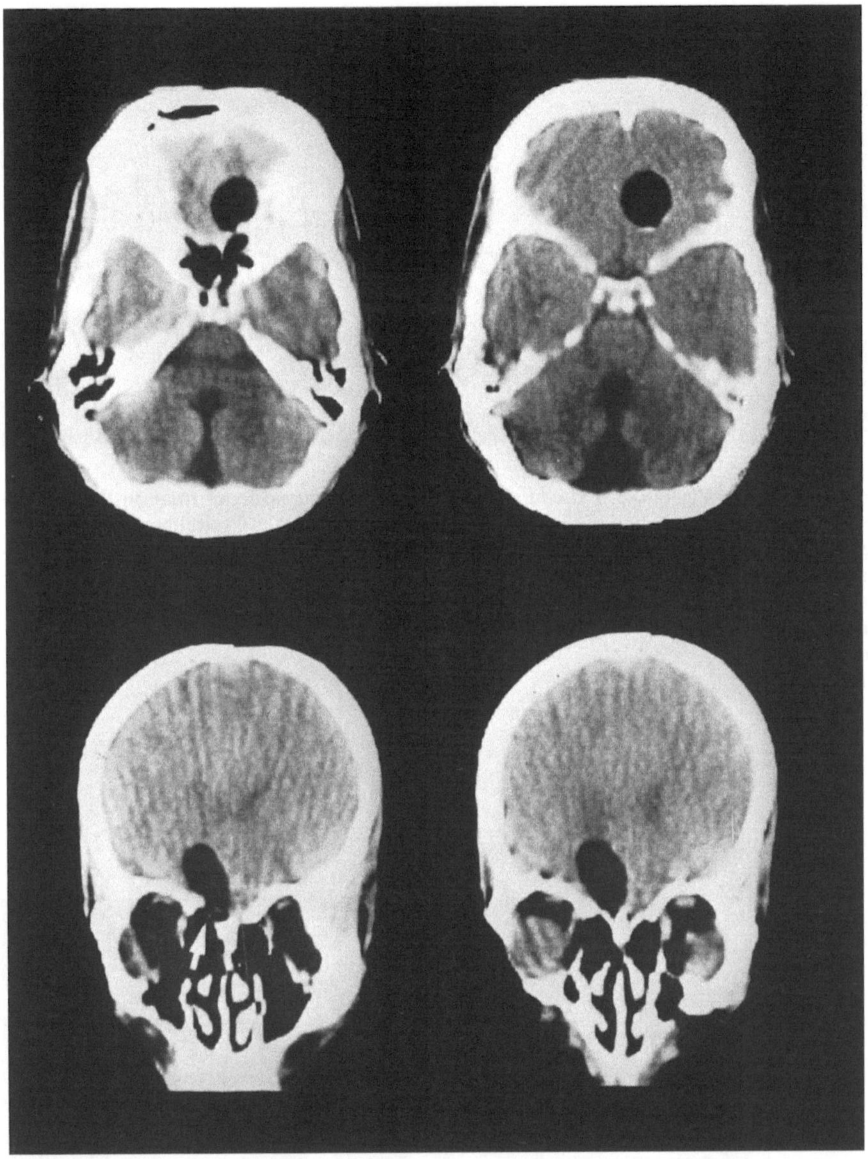

**Fig. D6.45.** Dermoid cyst in the right frontobasal region. The coronary projection shows that the dermoid cyst originates in the ethmoid bone, which demonstrates thinning and an excavation (arrow). Mean density values −68 HU. Fine calcification in the walls of the cyst (above right). Incidental finding of aplasia of the cerebellar vermis

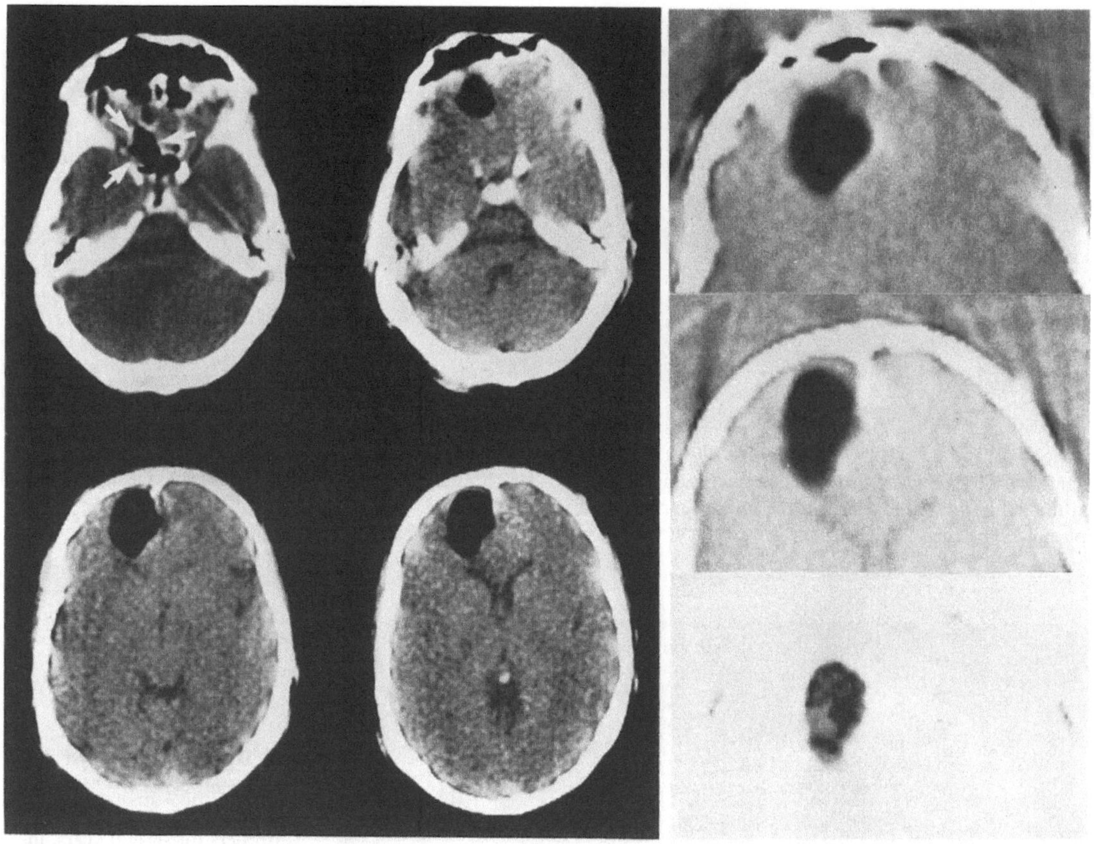

a b

**Fig. D6.46** a, b. Dermoid cyst in the left frontal region of a 40-year-old patient with occasional epileptic seizures. (**a**) Extremely hypodense zone (−61 EMI units) in the left frontal lobe. The tumor originates in the ethmoid bone, which shows a sharply delineated bone defect (arrows). (**b**) Wide range of density values within the tumor demonstrated by changing the window level and window width. A cyst containing saponified material and hair, surrounded by highly refractive oily liquid, was found at operation

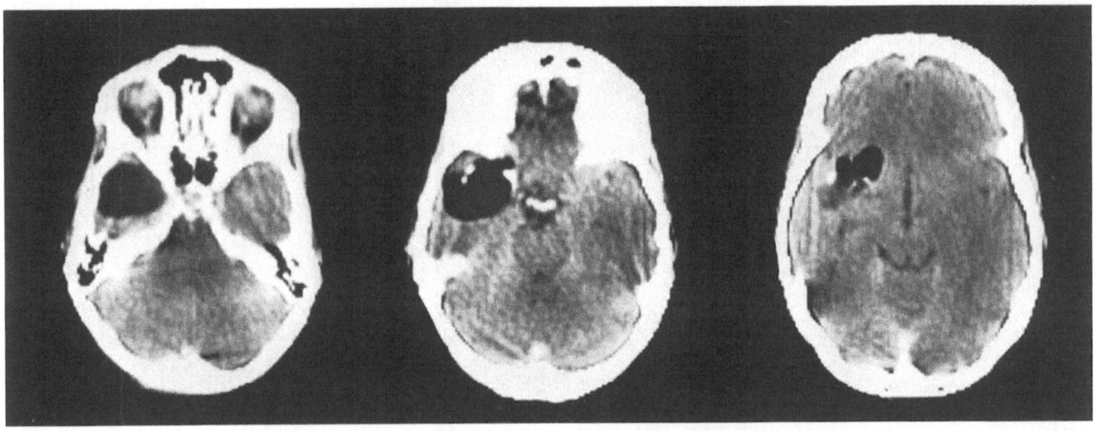

Fig. D6.47. Dermoid cyst at the base of the middle fossa on the left with a bone defect in the medial portion of the sphenoid wing (middle). Delicate calcification at the margin of the dermoid cyst, which has mean density values of −66 HU (33-year-old patient)

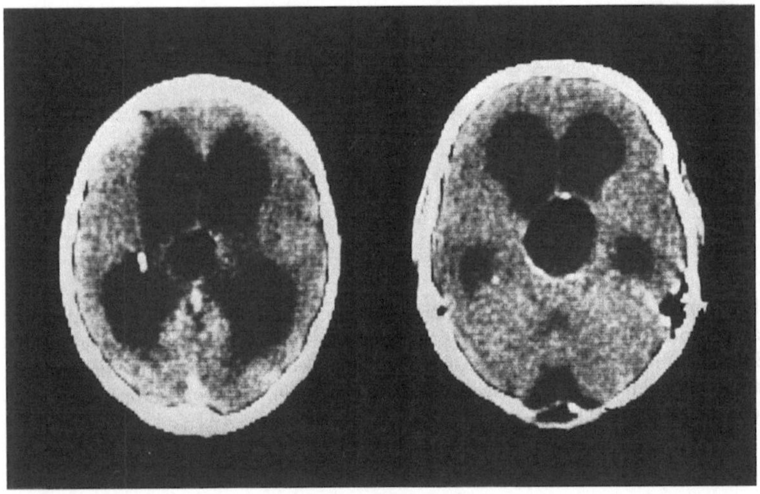

Fig. D6.48. Dermoid cyst in the third ventricle of a 32-year-old patient with a history of visual disorders for several years, incorrectly diagnosed as multiple sclerosis. Mean density values in the dermoid cyst −35 EMI units. Fine calcification in the capsule of the tumor. Extreme hydrocephalus. The bright speck in the left lateral ventricle represents the tip of a ventricular catheter after Torkildsen drainage

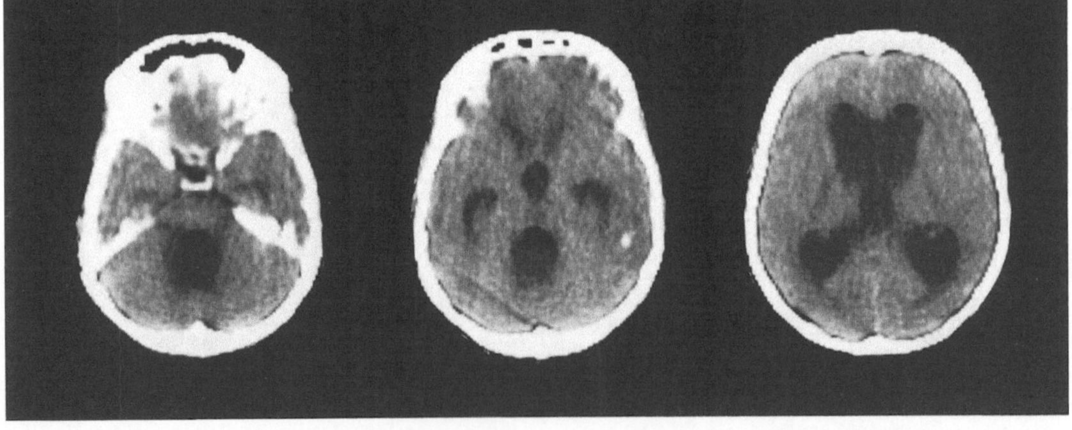

Fig. D6.49. Dermoid cyst in the fourth ventricle of a 31-year-old female with headache, vomiting and unsteady gait. Extremely hypodense zone (−50 HU) in the anterior segment of the fourth ventricle. Fatty tissue in both anterior horns. Significant dilatation of the ventricles

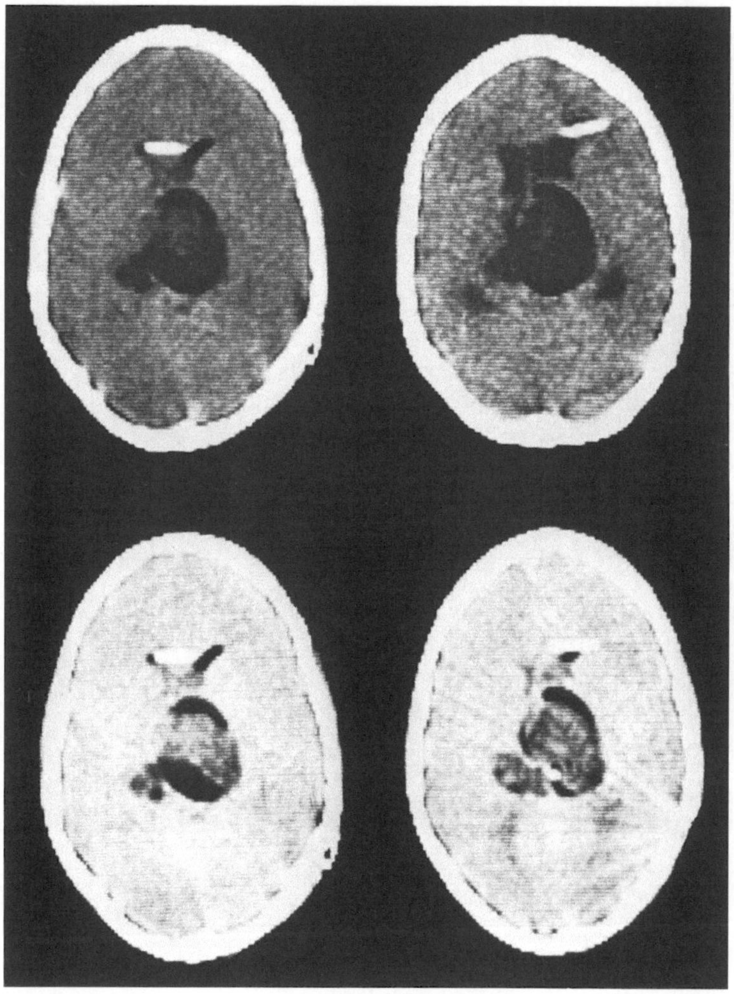

**Fig. D6.50.** Teratoma in the third ventricle of a 12-year-old boy in whom an "inoperable" midline tumor was diagnosed at the age of 8 years. Ventriculoatrial shunt in the lateral ventricle. CT studies demonstrate a very hypodense, conspicuously inhomogeneous lesion, especially in studies with lower window level (below). Free fatty tissue in both anterior horns, visible as small hypodense figures adjacent to the tip of the ventricular catheter. Mean density values −25 EMI units with lowest values at −54 units

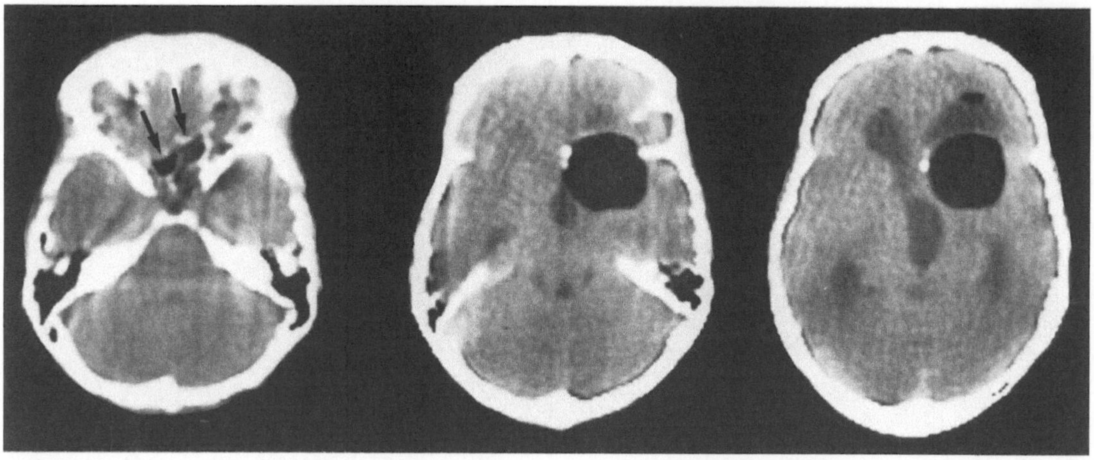

**Fig. D6.51.** Dermoid cyst/teratoma in a 34-year-old female with intermittent left hemiparesis. Tentative diagnosis of multiple sclerosis. CT: Cystic lesion with extremely low density values (−71 to −77 HU). Calcification in the medial wall. The basal slice demonstrates bone excavation near the planum sphenoidale (arrows), the origin of the tumor. Fatty tissue in both anterior horns, more pronounced on the right. A large dermoid cyst was found at operation. The medial wall of the tumor contained dense solid material, which proved to be a teratoma

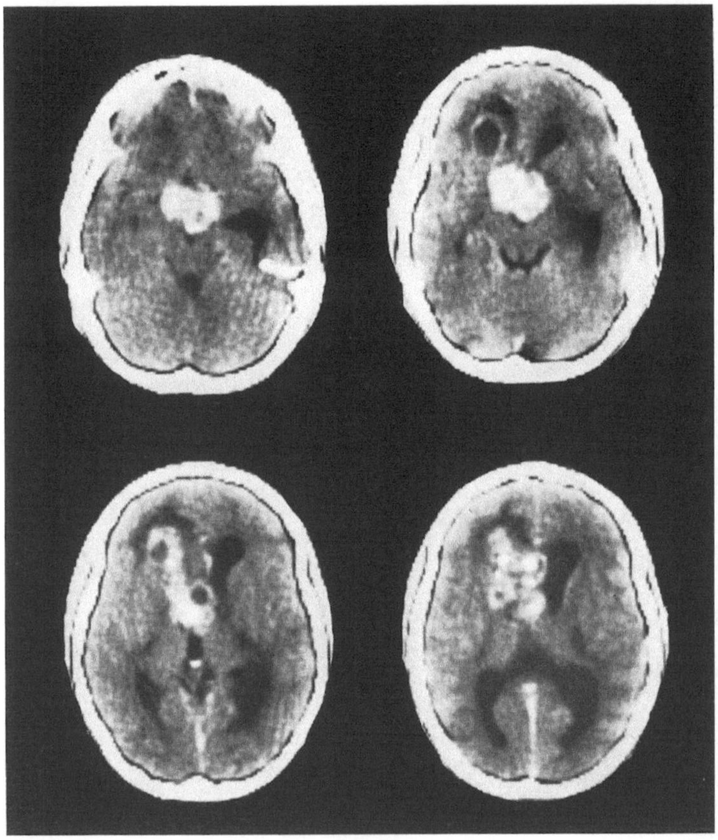

**Fig. D6.**52. Malignant teratoma in a 9-year-old boy. The tumor originates in the sella and has extended through the hypothalamus to the left lateral ventricle and the basal ganglia on the left. Significant contrast uptake within the inhomogeneous tumor. Slight perifocal edema. Ventricular dilatation secondary to blockage of both foramina of Monro. Histological type cannot be predicted on the basis of CT findings

# 7. Intracranial Tumors of Skeletal Origin

Osteomas, chondromas, and chordomas are the intracranial tumors derived from skeletal elements.

**Osteomas** may occur in all parts of the skull and present with attenuation values similar to those of bone. They appear as sharply delineated hyperdense zones in close relation to the vault or the base of the skull (Fig. D 7.1). The cerebellopontine angle is a common location for these tumors (Fig. D 7.2). Osteomas are easily identified with the help of plain skull films (see p. 397 f.).

Osteosarcomas and osteochondrosarcomas are the malignant forms of these tumors and demonstrate no characteristic differences from the benign forms in the CT scan (Fig. D 7.3).

Intracranial **chondromas** are very rare. They are high density lesions with numerous calcified elements irregularly distributed throughout the tumor (Figs. D 7.4, 5). Solid uncalcified tissue enhances significantly. Chondromas originate in the dura mater, especially in the region of the falx cerebri and at the base of the skull, where they are most often encountered at the foramen lacerum and the tip of the petrous bone (ZÜLCH 1958, 1975).

**Chordomas** are only found at the base of the skull, at the clivus, or in the subsellar region. They may demonstrate destructive growth toward the nasopharynx, optic chiasm, or foramen magnum.

Chordomas demonstrate high density values and mottled calcification in the CT scan (Figs. D 7.6, 7). There is strong contrast uptake in the solid uncalcified portions of the tumor. Horizontal projections do not always reveal the relations of a clivus chordoma to the base of the skull (Fig. D 7.8), and additional coronary projections are useful in this regard.

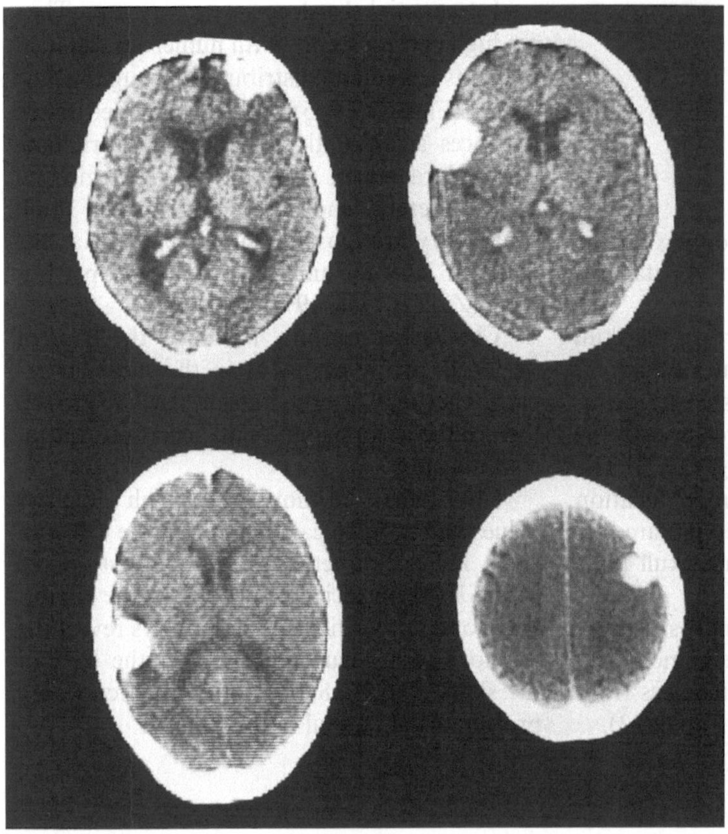

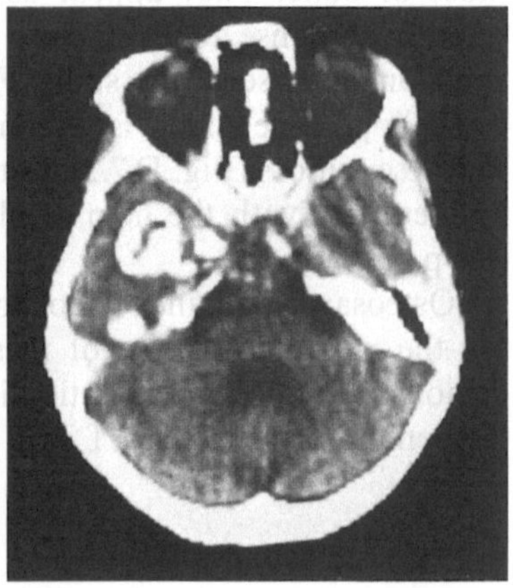

**Fig. D7.1.** Four examples of intracranial osteomas adjacent to the skull vault at different locations. The tumors have the same density as bone and are closely related to the vault. Space-occupying effects are rare, and there is no evidence of perifocal edema

**Fig. D7.3.** Osteochondrosarcoma at the base of the middle cranial fossa on the left in a 51-year-old patient. Spherical lesion with bone density and a central uncalcified zone

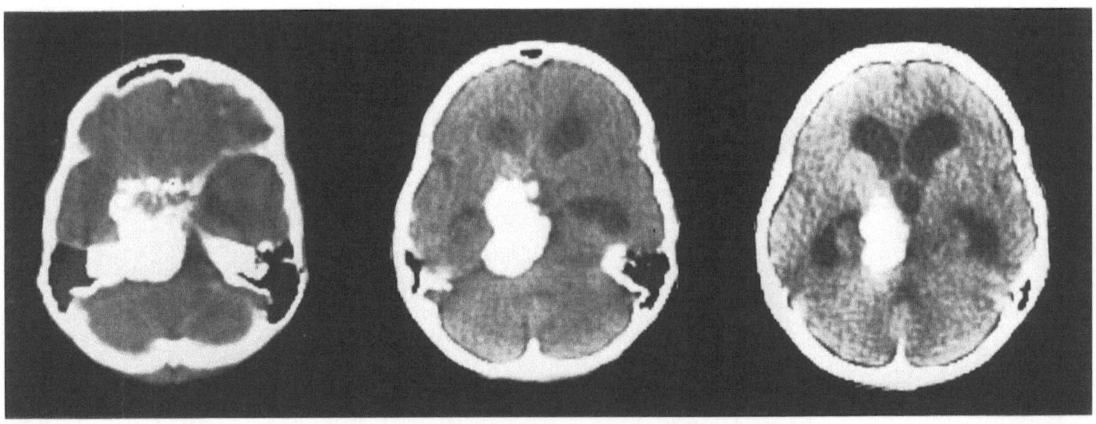

**Fig. D7.2.** Very large osteoma at the base of the middle fossa with extension into the cranial cavity and occlusive hydrocephalus secondary to blockage of the aqueduct in a 74-year-old female

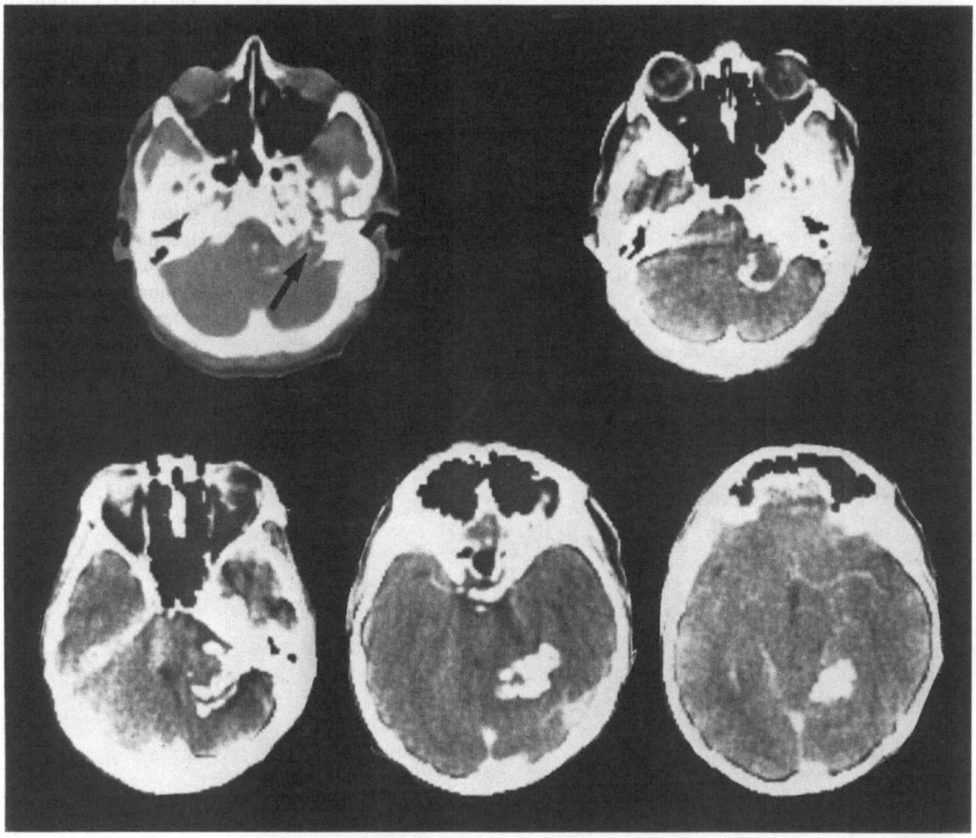

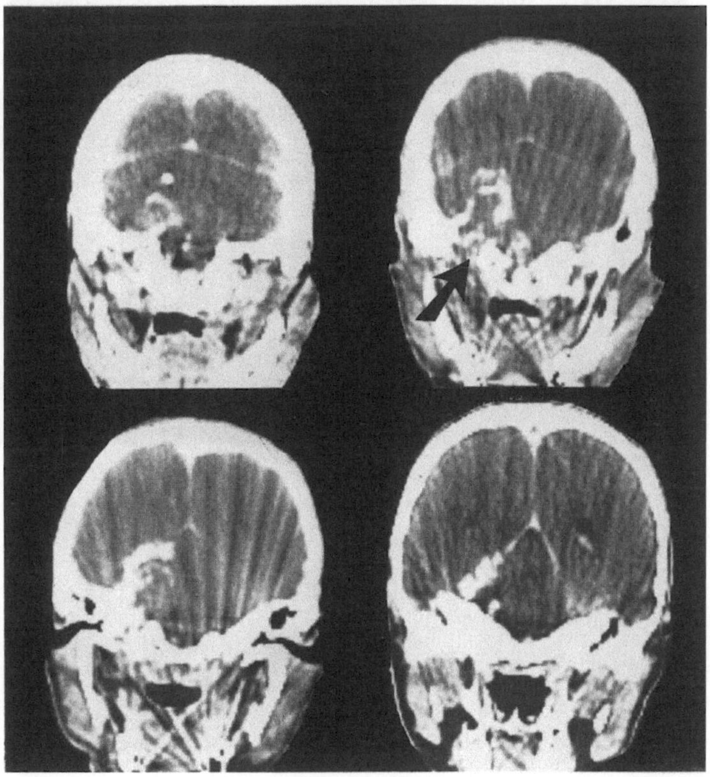

**Fig. D7.4.** Large chondroma in the region of the right cerebellopontine angle and the right cerebellar hemisphere with extension to the tentorium (coronary projections) in a 20-year-old man. Destruction of the petrous bone (arrows). Many irregularly shaped zones of calcification. Postcontrast study

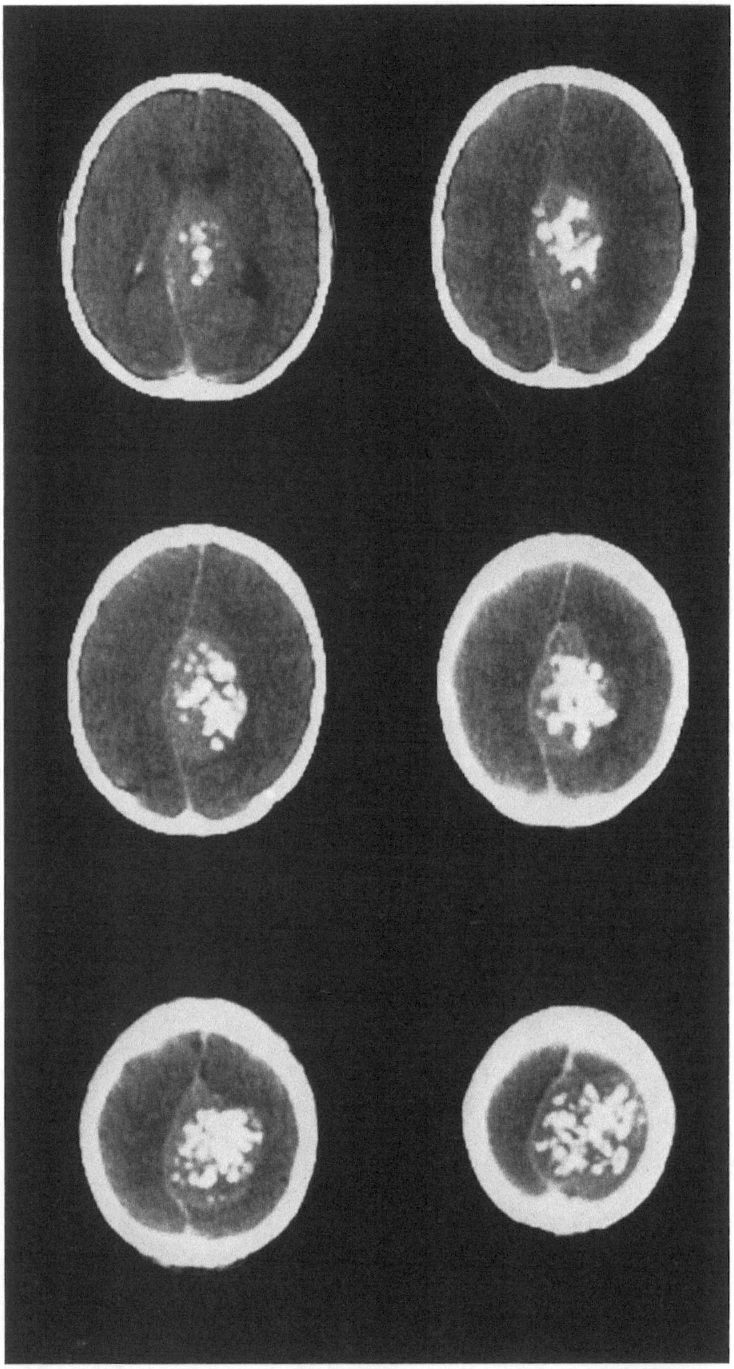

**Fig. D7.5.** Chondroma adjacent to the falx in the middle third of the superior sagittal sinus in a 49-year-old male with focal and generalized seizures. The tumor contains speckled calcifications resembling the trabeculation of enchondral ossification, which allows certain differentiation from meningioma at the same location (cf. Fig. D2.7). The solid noncalcified portions of the tumor demonstrate little increase in density after contrast enhancement. Considerable displacement of the falx. Postcontrast study. Window width 200 HU

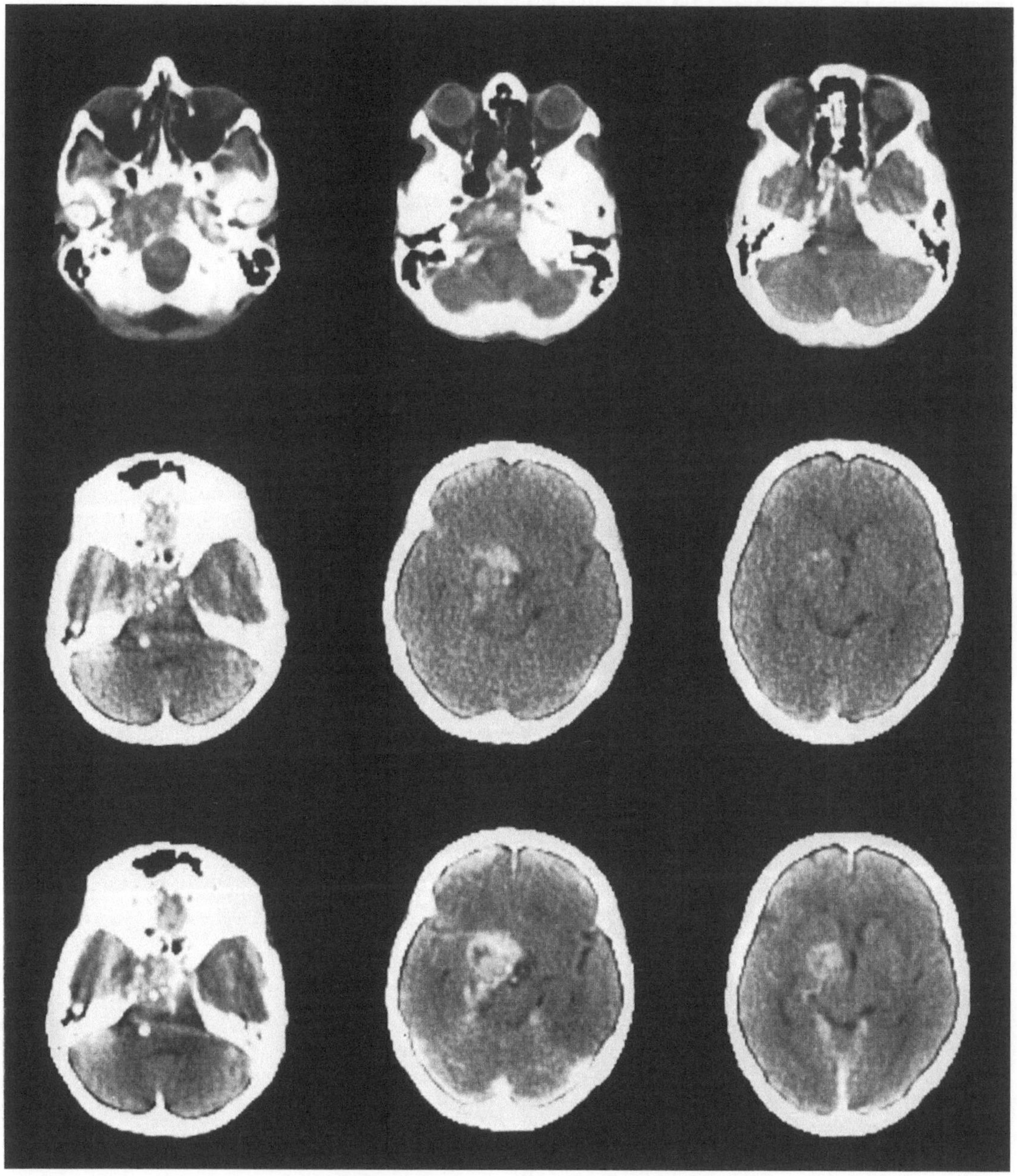

**Fig. D7.6.** Chordoma of the clivus with extensive destruction of the base of the skull (above) in 58-year-old female. Portions of the tumor within the cranial cavity appear hyperdense in the precontrast study (middle) and show an increase in density values after contrast enhancement (below). Fine specks of calcification within the tumor

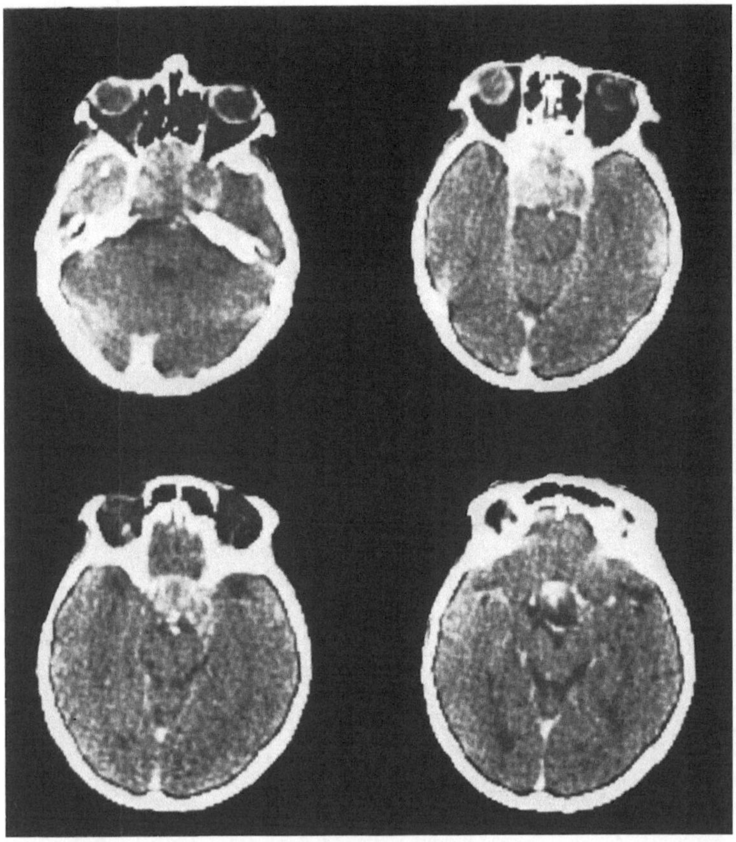

**Fig. D7.7.** Subsellar chordoma with extension to the sphenoid sinus and the skull cavity in a 65-year-old female. Inhomogeneous contrast uptake. Fine specks of calcification within the tumor. Postcontrast study

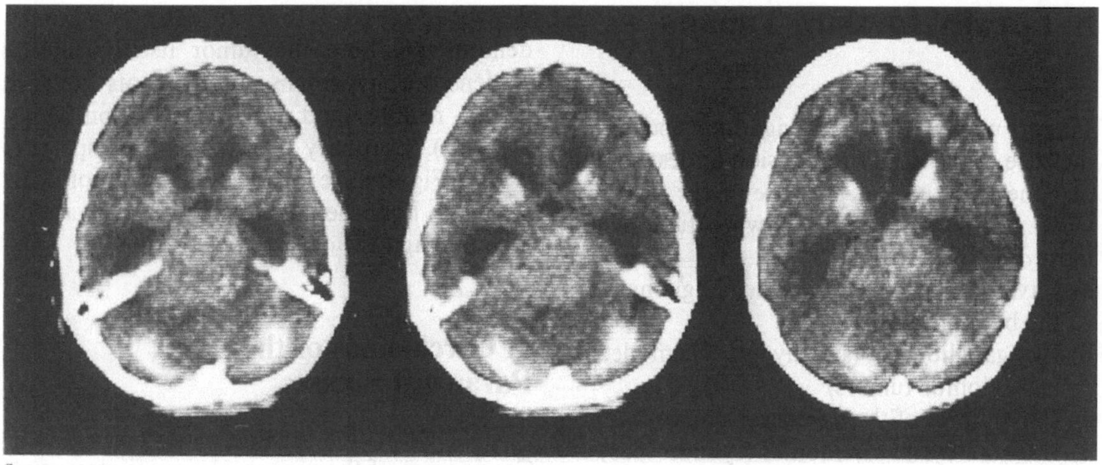

a

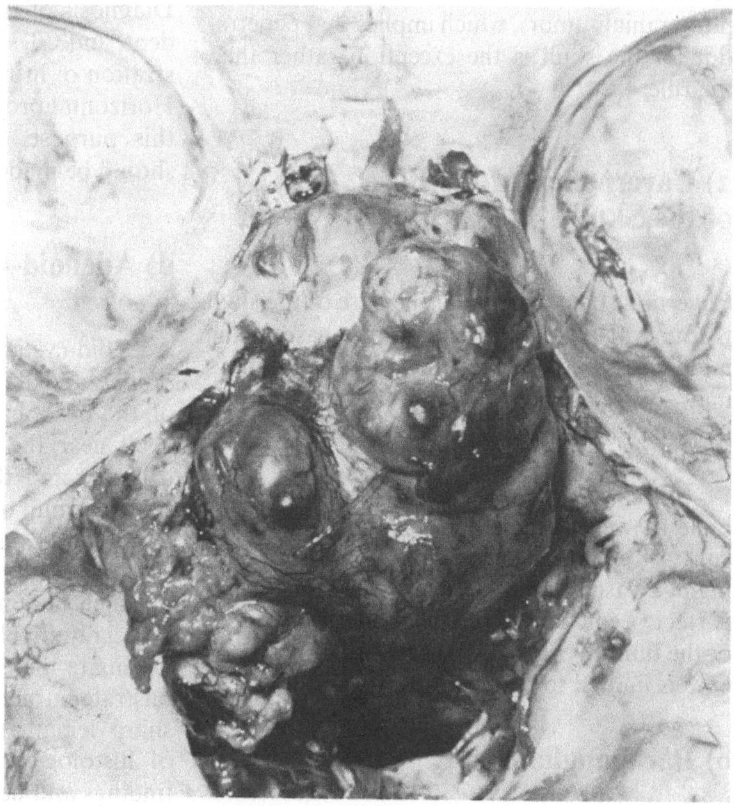

b

**Fig. D7.8** a, b. Clivus chordoma in a 66-year-old female. (**a**) The tumor appears as a hyperdense zone in the region of the caudal brain stem in precontrast studies. There are fine specks of calcification within the tumor. Initial diagnosis of brain stem tumor. Incidental finding of symmetrical paraventricular and cerebellar calcification due to a disorder of calcium metabolism. (Fahr's disease). (**b**) Autopsy specimen in the same patient. Nodular tumor originating in the clivus with significant narrowing of the foramen magnum. (Specimen courtesy of Priv.-Doz. Dr. B. Stampfl, Pathology Dept, Municipal Hospital, München-Harlaching)

# 8. Locally Invasive Tumors

Tumors with extracranial origins may penetrate the base of the skull with erosion or destruction of bone structures at the base of the skull (cf. Chap. E, p. 394). The following tumors are most often involved:

a) Cavernomas (cavernous hemangiomas) of the base of the skull
b) Paragangliomas (synonyms: chemodectomas, glomus tumors)
c) Carcinomas of the paranasal sinuses
d) Adenoid-cystic carcinomas (cylindromas)
e) Rhabdomyosarcomas
f) Aesthesioneuroblastomas

All of these tumors are much less common than intracranial tumors, which implies that penetration of the skull is the exception rather than the rule.

## a) Cavernomas of the Base of the Skull

Cavernous hemangioma of the base of the skull is found at the carotid siphon, the base of the middle fossa, and next to the sella. The tumors may cause hyperostosis, but the sclerotic margin of the tumor indicates its benign character.

In the *CT scan* one finds destruction of the bone as well as hyperdense zones with strong contrast enhancement (Fig. D8.1), a sign of a highly vascularized lesion. Nevertheless, a correct prediction of the histological character of the tumor is virtually impossible. Our experience is limited to two cases.

## b) Paragangliomas

*Tumors of the glomus tympanicum* and – more often – *glomus jugulare* – are called *paragangliomas* or *chemodectomas* (Helpap 1978). *The term glomus tumor is also used.* These tumors may grow along the jugular vein through the jugular foramen into the posterior fossa causing symptoms and signs of a cerebellopontine angle lesion, if the tumor is large enough. The diagnosis is usually made with plain skull films through demonstration of characteristic bone destruction (Figs. E16, 17, p. 390f.). *CT studies* demonstrate both the tumor itself, which is isodense or hyperdense and accepts contrast media readily, and bone destruction (Figs. D8.2, 3). Coronary projections are especially useful (Fig. D8.2 c–e). Demonstration of characteristic bone destruction permits an almost certain diagnosis of histological type.

## c) Carcinomas of the Paranasal Sinuses

Carcinomas of the paranasal sinuses may cause bone destruction at the base of the skull and penetrate into the orbits or the cranial cavity. Diagnosis of the primary tumor is usually evident, and CT studies are performed for demonstration of intracranial extension of the tumor. Horizontal projections are often insufficient for this purpose, and additional coronary slices should be made (Fig. D8.4).

## d) Adenoid-Cystic Carcinomas

Adenoid-cystic carcinomas are also called *cylindromas* and are found at two locations. Tumors of the nasopharynx penetrate the base of the skull near the midline, especially at the oval foramen and the Gasserian ganglion, while a second group of tumors invades the orbits. The first group causes circumscribed destruction at the base of the skull with widening of the oval foramen in some cases. Cranial nerve deficits, especially involving the third and fifth nerves, dominate the clinical picture. CT studies demonstrate intracranial portions of the tumor with sharp demarcation from brain tissue. Diagnosis of histological type is based on radiological findings and neurological deficits.

Cylindromas originating in the lacrimal gland penetrate from the orbit to the skull cavity (Fig. D8.5).

## e) Rhabdomyosarcomas

Rhabdomyosarcomas are malignant tumors of striated muscle which may penetrate the cranial cavity after destruction of the base of the skull in rare cases, where they may attain enormous proportions (Fig. D 8.6). These rare tumors are most often found in children (see also p. 395 and p. 485).

## f) Aesthesioneuroblastomas

Aesthesioneuroblastomas – neuroblastomas of the olfactory nerve – originate in the olfactory region and may penetrate from the upper part of the nasal cavity to the anterior fossa. The tumors are highly vascular and grow slowly, though they may infiltrate and destroy adjacent tissues or even produce metastases. Penetration of the orbit has been reported. CT findings in aesthesioneuroblastomas resemble those in other locally invasive tumors of the anterior fossa (s. Fig. D 8.7). Similar findings may be observed in subsellar chordomas (s. Fig. D 7.7).

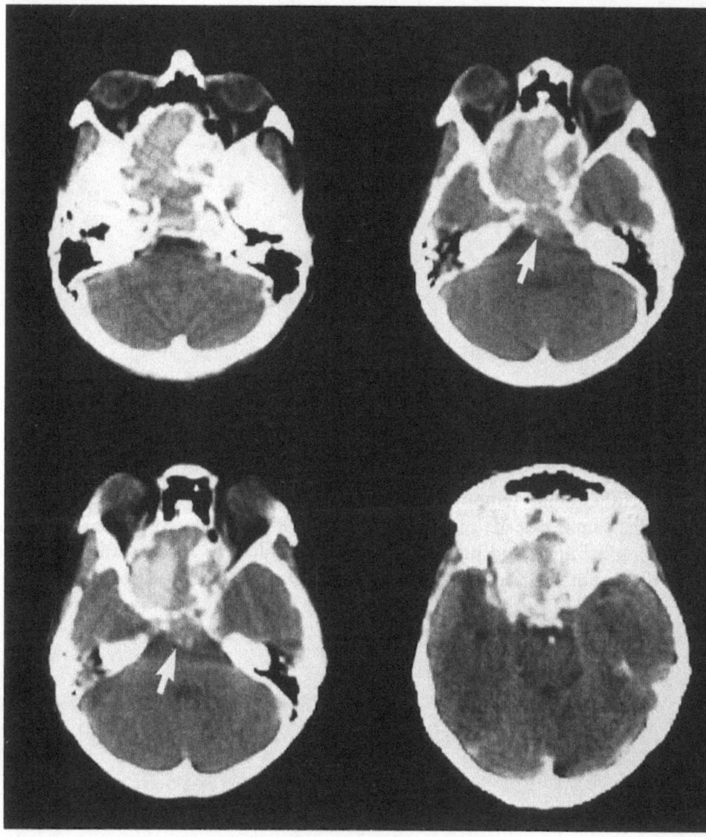

**Fig. D8.1.** Cavernous hemangioma originating in the sphenoid sinus in a 58-year-old patient. The tumor extends from the sphenoid sinus into the cranial cavity, where growth is most pronounced along the clivus (arrow). The tumor demonstrates strong contrast uptake (below). Sclerosis at the margins of the tumor suggests a histologically benign lesion

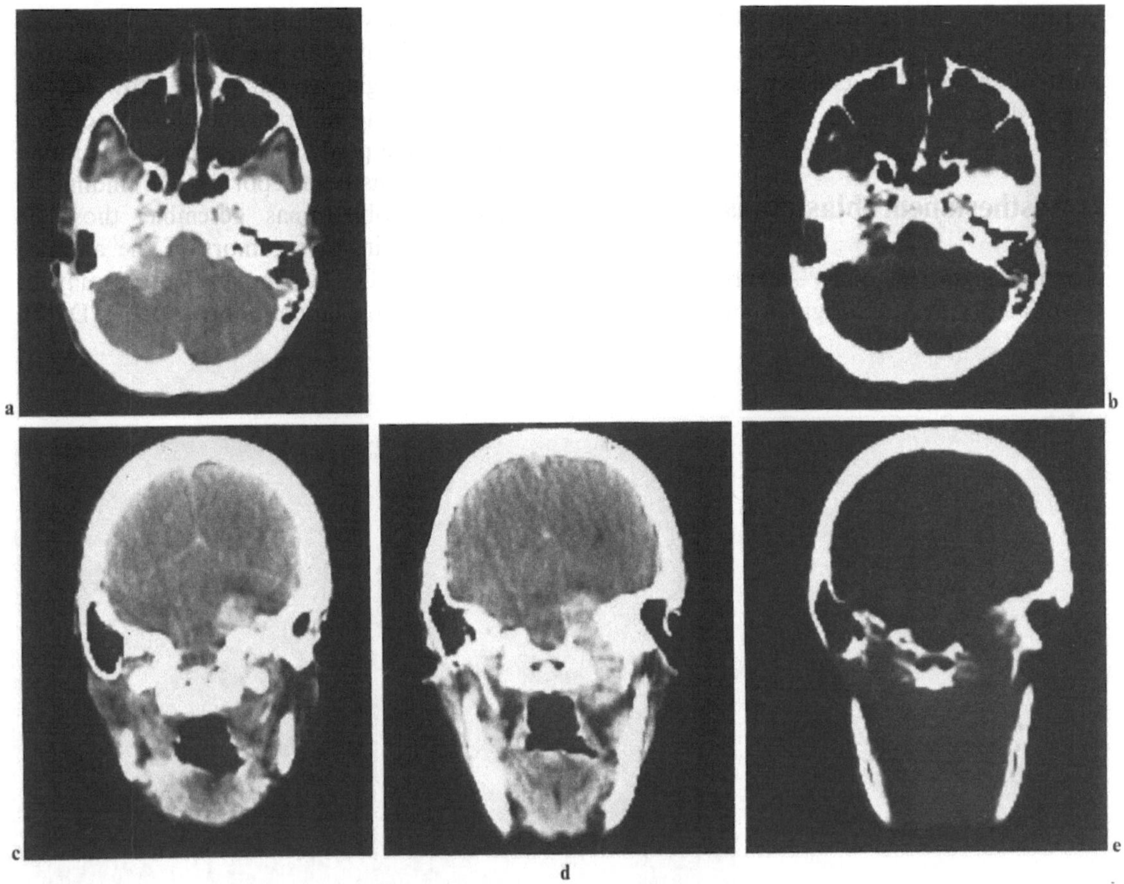

**Fig. D8.2.** (**a**) Glomus tumor on the left in a 50-year-old patient. The tumor extends into the skull cavity at the left cerebellopontine angle and jugular foramen. Clear delineation of the tumor after contrast enhancement. Destruction of the tip of the left petrous bone (**b**). Coronary projections (**c–e**) demonstrate the full extent of the tumor from below the base of the skull into the cranial cavity. Improved demonstration of characteristic bone destruction with this projection (**d, e**)

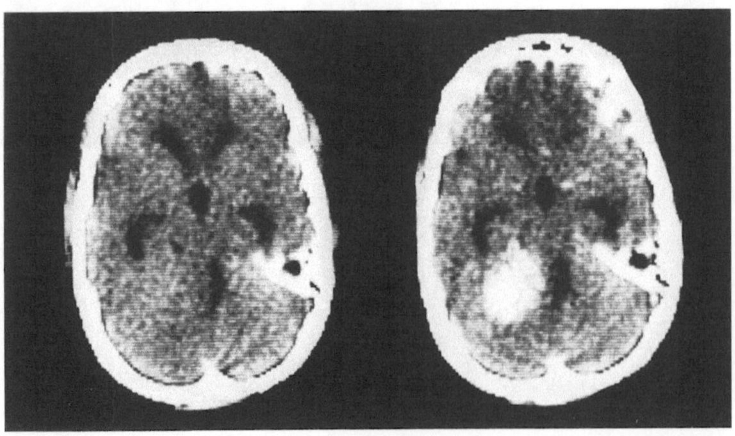

**Fig. D8.3.** Large glomus tumor at the left cerebellopontine angle with penetration of the base of the skull. Displacement and dilatation of the fourth ventricle in the precontrast study suggest the presence of a space-occupying lesion in the posterior fossa on the left. Very strong contrast uptake within the tumor indicating vascularity. Twenty-eight-year-old patient with signs of cerebellar dysfunction and a history of resection of a glomus tumor penetrating to the middle ear

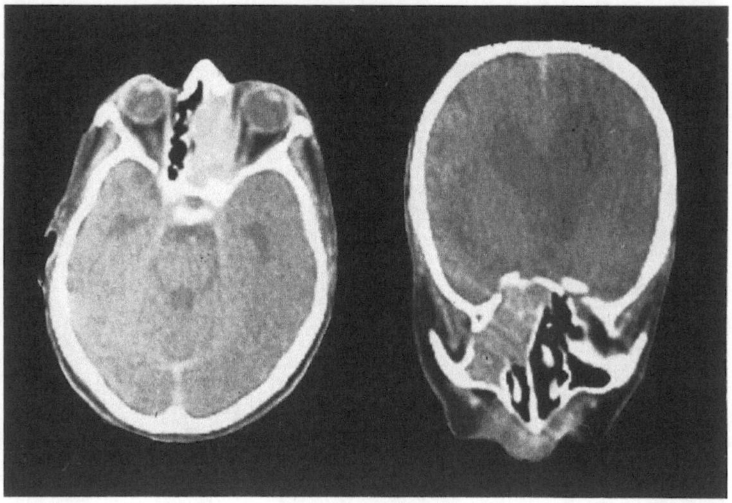

**Fig. D8.4.** Inverted papilloma with carcinomatous portions in the right maxillary sinus, the nasal cavity, and the ethmoid bone in a 71-year-old patient. The coronary projection shows that the tumor has caused thinning of the planum sphenoidale and rostral displacement of the right anterior clinoid process (arrow). Penetration of the skull cavity is imminent

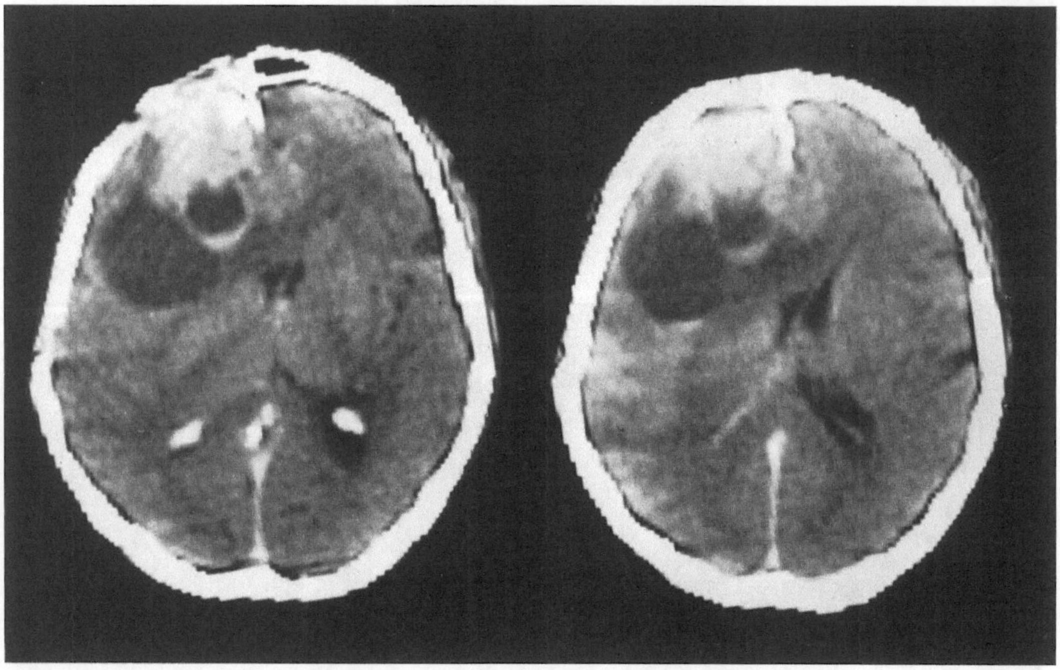

**Fig. D8.5.** Cylindroma originating in the nasal sinuses with extension into the skull cavity where solid and cystic tumor elements are found in the left frontal lobe with extension to the temporal region. Previous resection of a tumor penetrating the cranial cavity (missing bone flap in the left frontal region)

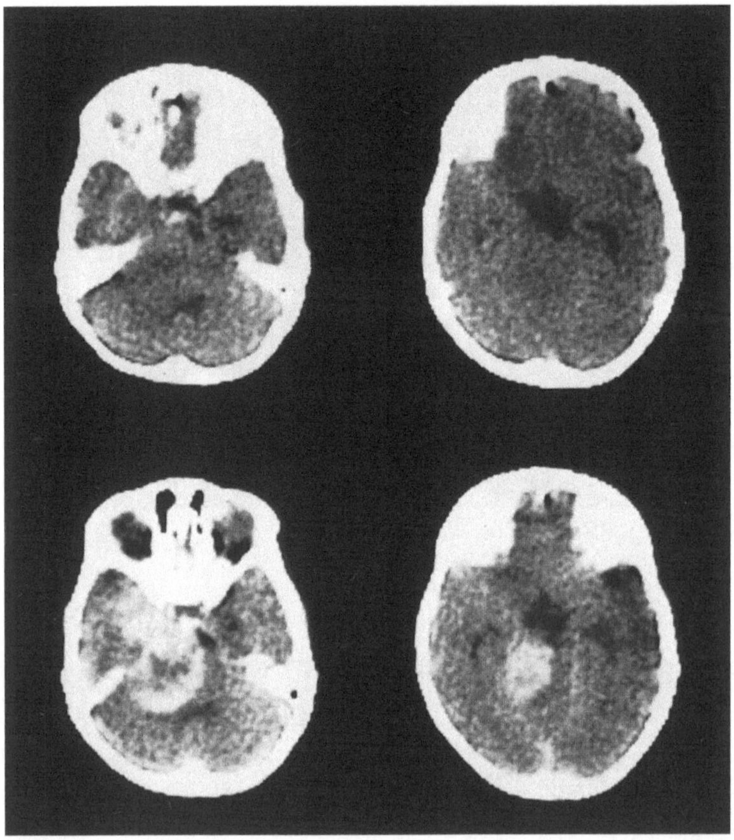

**Fig. D8.6.** Rhabdomyosarcoma with extension to the middle and posterior fossa in a $6^1/_2$-year-old boy. The tumor appears isodense in the precontrast study (above), but deformation of the pentagon and displacement of the fourth ventricle suggest the presence of a space-occupying lesion. Contrast enhancement reveals a very large inhomogeneous tumor extending from the base of the middle fossa through the tentorium to the right cerebellopontine angle, where the tumor crosses the midline (below)

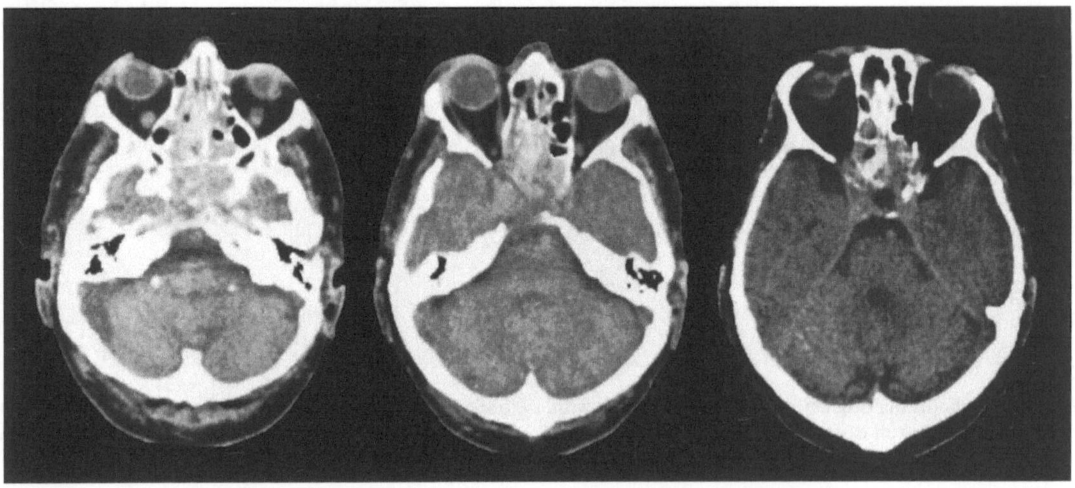

**Fig. D8.7** Aesthesioneuroblastoma with extension at the base of the anterior and middle fossae in a 59-year-old male with multiple cranial nerve lesions. The tumor has destroyed bone structures in the base of the skull. The normally air-filled paranasal sinus has the same density as soft tissue. (Courtesy of Prof. FELIX, Dept. of Radiology, Klinikum Charlottenburg, FU Berlin)

# 9. Intracranial Metastases

1. Very small tumors with extensive perifocal edema should raise suspicion of metastasis. Differentiation between a solitary intracranial metastasis and an autochthonous brain tumor is rarely possible, especially if there is no evidence of a primary tumor to suggest the diagnosis. CT may rarely provide information suggesting the histological type of the primary tumor (hemorrhage in metastases of melanoma or choriocarcinoma, for example).
2. When metastases are suspected, the posterior fossa should receive special attention, since metastases in the cerebellum are often isodense. The cortical regions of the parietal lobe deserve attention for the same reason
3. CT studies without contrast administration are inadequate when metastase are suspected
4. Demonstration of a solitary tumor in the CT scan does not exclude the possibility of multiple metastases (diameter of 5 mm is minimum for demonstration of metastatic tumor)
5. Multiple intracranial space-occupying lesions are not necessarily multiple metastases, since multifocal glioblastomas, brain abscesses, and primary cerebral malignant lymphomas may present with similar findings
6. An intracranial space-occupying lesion in a patient with a known malignant neoplasm does not necessarily represent a metastasis of this tumor in the brain

The literature contains widely varying reports on the incidence of intracranial metastases. ZÜLCH reported metastases in 7.1% of 9,000 brain tumors, CUSHING 3.2%, OLIVECRONA 3.8%, RUBINSTEIN (1972) 15%–25%, while PERCY et al. (1972) reported up to 41% in autopsy statistics from large general hospitals. Metastases accounted for 15.3% of all tumors in our series, a considerably higher proportion than that reported by the first three authors, who collected neurosurgical cases for the most part. This may be explained by the fact that the three participating CT laboratories in the present study work in close cooperation with a number of oncology departments.

*Bronchogenic carcinoma, carcinoma of the breast, melanoma, and hypernephroma* have a predilection for metastases to the brain and make up 62% of all intracranial metastases. Incidence is highest between the ages of 40 and 70 years, as is the case with the primary carcinoma.

### General Considerations in Computed Tomography of Intracranial Metastases

Computed tomography is the most important noninvasive method for demonstration of intracranial metastases, because it is more sensitive than all other diagnostic procedures including cerebral angiography and brain scintigraphy. *CT is capable of demonstrating brain metastases of 5 mm in diameter or larger in almost 100% of cases.* Studies in the posterior fossa demand special care in analysis, since bone structures at the base of the skull may produce artifacts which obscure portions of the cerebellum, with the result that tumors with approximately the same density as adjacent brain tissue may escape detection (Fig. D9.2 a, b). *Contrast enhancement is necessary in all cases.* Metastases smaller than 5 mm in diameter escape detection in computed tomograms with the present generation of CT scanners if perifocal edema is not present.

*Multiple metastases* are more often demonstrated in CT studies than with classic neuroradiological techniques. Visualization of a soli-

**Table 5.** CT findings in 338 patient with intracranial metastases

| Diagnosis | *n* | Appearance after contrast enhancement | | | | | |
|---|---|---|---|---|---|---|---|
| | | Ring | Nodule | Ring + nodule | Only hypodense zone | Solitary metastasis | Multiple metastases |
| Bronchogenic carcinoma | 113 | 48 | 31 | 30 | 4 | 60 | 53 |
| Breast cancer | 62 | 13 | 41 | 6 | 2 | 25 | 37 |
| Malignant melanoma | 34 | 3 | 21 | 8 | 2 | 21 | 13 |
| Hypernephroma | 22 | 8 | 10 | 4 | – | 16 | 6 |
| Carcinomas of the gastrointestinal tract | 16 | 7 | 7 | 2 | – | 9 | 7 |
| Other metastases of carcinoma (including 65 cases with unknown primary tumor) | 91 | 14 | 40 | 33 | 4 | 43 | 48 |
| Total | 338 | 93 | 150 | 83 | 12 | 174 | 164 |
| Percent | 100 | 27.5 | 44.4 | 24.6 | 3.5 | 51.5 | 48.5 |

tary tumor does not exclude multiple metastases (Fig. D9.4).

Table 5 illustrates frequency of solitary and multiple metastases in 338 patients with metastatic intracranial tumors. Multiple metastases were most often found in patients with carcinoma of the breast (59.7%), followed by bronchogenic carcinoma (46.9%). Multiple lesions were found in 38% of patients with malignant melanoma and in 27.3% of patients with hypernephroma.

Multiple metastases may be overlooked when only a single region of the intracranial cavity – the cerebellar or supratentorial region, for example – is studied on the basis of neurological signs which suggest tumor at this location. *Careful investigation of all intracranial structures, from the foramen magnum to the apex* – including contrast enhancement – *is required,* if the diagnostic potential of the CT technique is to be fully realized. Multiple metastases may appear in all conceivable combinations (Figs. D9.5–10).

*Very small metastases often escape direct detection in the CT scan.* Large metastases are sometimes demonstrated in CT studies, while additional smaller lesions are detected at autopsy (Fig. D11). Delayed contrast enhancement after rapid high-dose intravenous contrast infusion may show even very small metastatic lesions as Shalen et al. (1981) demonstrated. However, correlations between CT findings and postmortem examinations are not always accurate, since a long period of time may elapse between CT studies and death of the patient.

## Computed Tomography (Figs. D9.1–42)

### Precontrast Study

*Intracranial metastases do not demonstrate uniform absorption characteristics* (Figs. D9.1–42). High attenuation values were found in a large number of cases (33.8%). Metastases of melanomas are almost always hyperdense and the tumor is easily recognized in the precontrast CT scan.

Intracranial metastases are also visible in the plain CT scan when perifocal edema visualizes isodense lesions. Very high density values suggest hemorrhage within the tumor (Figs. D9.14, 15). Mixed absorption values are found in an additional third of all intracranial metastases; the inhomogeneous pattern is due to central necrosis. Approximately one-sixth of all intracranial metastases are isodense or hypodense in the precontrast study.

*Perifocal edema is very common in intracranial metastases.* Five hundred of our 575 patients (87%) demonstrated perifocal edema, surpassed only by glioblastoma, with edema in 91.7% of cases. Perifocal edema in brain metastases often covers a large portion of an entire hemisphere, and we found grade II or III edema

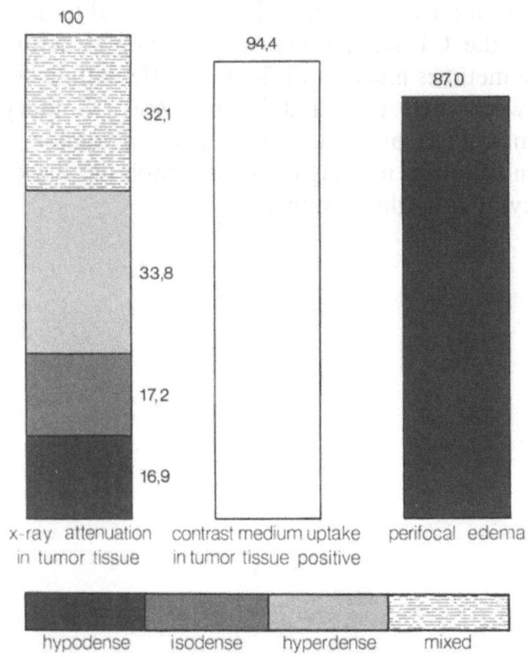


**Fig. D9.1.** X-ray attenuation, contrast medium uptake, and frequency of perifocal edema in intracranial metastases (percent)

in 57% of metastatic tumors with edema. It should be emphasized that small metastases measuring 15–20 mm in diameter may produce edema which encompasses the white matter of an entire cerebral hemisphere (Figs. D9.12, 13).

### Postcontrast Study

Contrast enhancement was positive in 94.4% of cases with intracranial metastases. The cases in which contrast enhancement was absent included metastases with hemorrhage, which had such high density values initially that no further increase in density was possible (Fig. D 9.14). In other cases, the metastases were so small that they were suspected on the basis of extensive perifocal edema even though they were not directly visualized (Fig. D9.16).

*Metastases vary considerably in appearance after contrast administration, and ring structures, nodular tumors, and combinations of the two* may be found (Figs. D 9.17–19, see Table 5). Rim enhancement usually represents spherical tumors with central necrosis. A single patient may have multiple metastases with various CT patterns. Appearance of the metastases after contrast enhancement is related to size, with small metastases generally appearing as solid tumors and large metastases demonstrating ring figures with central necrosis.

Ring enhancement predominates in *metastases of bronchogenic carcinoma* (42.5%) (Figs. D9.20, 21; Table 5). Ring structures were found in 69% of all patients with metastases of bronchogenic carcinoma, including cases with a combination of ring and solid tumor nodule.

*Metastases in carcinoma of the breast* (Figs. D9.22–26) are most often nodular tumors (66%). Solid tumors predominate in *metastases of malignant melanoma* as well (Figs. D9.27, 28), and *hemorrhage is a characteristic feature* (Figs. D9.14, 29, 30) found in one-third of our patients with metastases of melanoma. Ring structures are uncommon in melanoma (Fig. D9.31). Solid tumors and metastases with central necrosis are equally common in *hypernephroma* (Figs. D9.32–34); a spherical lesion with a small central necrosis is typical of this tumor (Fig. D9.33).

*Adenocarcinomas* also present with a variety of findings (Figs. D9.35–39; Table 5). In some cases we observed garland-like enhancement of the metastatic tumor otherwise found only in glioblastoma.

*Metastases of choriocarcinoma* usually present as intracerebral hemorrhage (Fig. D9.42). Differentiation between hemorrhage into a metastasis and spontaneous hemorrhage in an angioma or aneurysm is not possible if clinical findings and history do not suggest the presence of a metastatic tumor.

### Differential Diagnosis

Multiple intracranial metastases of known primary tumors usually do not present serious problems in differential diagnosis. However, the presence of a solitary intracranial mass lesion does not exclude the possibility of a second (autochthonous) brain tumor, especially when a long period has elapsed between the two illnesses.

*Multiple intracranial space-occupying lesions* in patients without a history of metastatic disease may represent intracranial metastases as well as *multiple brain abscesses* (Fig. F9, p. 410), *multiple meningiomas* (Fig. D2.26, p. 213), *multifocal lymphomas* (Fig. D1.216, p. 170) *or glioblastomas* (Figs. D1.94–97,

p. 85f.), *tuberculomas and parasitic disease* (Fig. F45, p. 431). The possibility of simultaneous occurrence of two different brain tumors must also be considered (Fig. D1.98, p. 88).

*A small solitary tumor with central necrosis or extensive brain edema should always raise suspicion of intracranial metastasis.* There are no other reliable criteria for differentiation between metastases and other intracranial tumors in the CT scan. Presence of a ring structure sometimes makes it difficult to differentiate between metastasis and brain abscess. Solitary metastasis of an unknown primary tumor is most often misdiagnosed as anaplastic astrocytoma or glioblastoma.

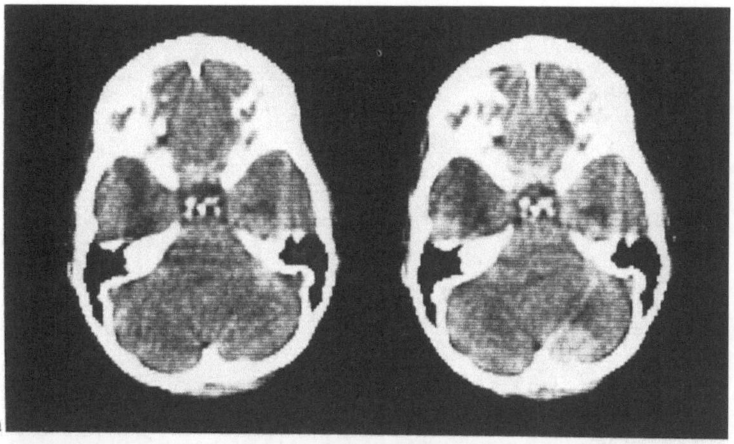
a

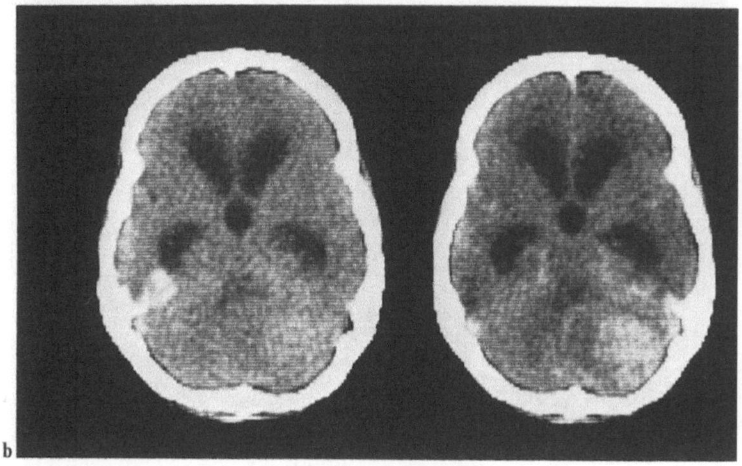
b

**Fig. D9.2** a, b. Isodense cerebellar metastases. (**a**) Metastasis of bronchogenic carcinoma near the cortex of the right cerebellar hemisphere in a 46-year-old female. The precontrast study (left) shows slight displacement of the fourth ventricle to the left. Density values in cerebellar tissue appear normal. Contrast enhancement (right) reveals the metastasis. (**b**) Metastasis of pancreatic carcinoma in the right cerebellar hemisphere of a 29-year-old female. The precontrast study shows deformation and narrowing of the fourth ventricle in its lateral recess on the right and significant hydrocephalus, suggesting the presence of a space-occupying lesion in the posterior fossa (left). Postcontrast studies demonstrate an inhomogeneous tumor in the right cerebellar hemisphere (right)

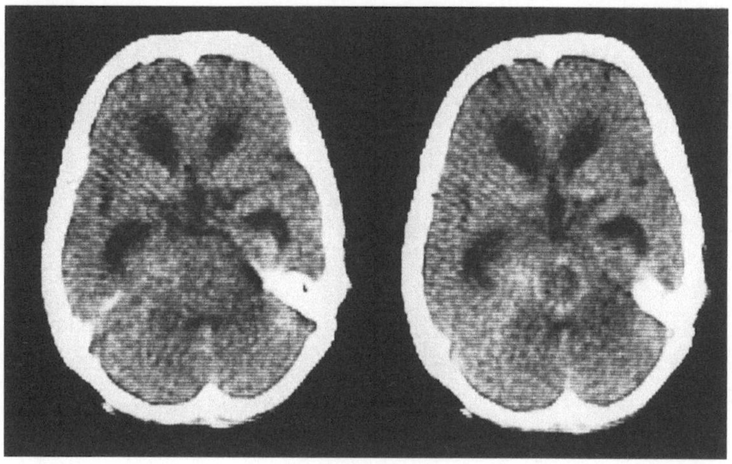

**Fig. D9.3.** Metastasis to the pons in a 75-year-old female. The precontrast study demonstrates distension of the pons with some dorsal displacement of the fourth ventricle. Slightly hypodense absorption values (left). Contrast enhancement demonstrates a ring figure in the metastasis (right), which has caused blockage of the aqueduct, resulting in hydrocephalus

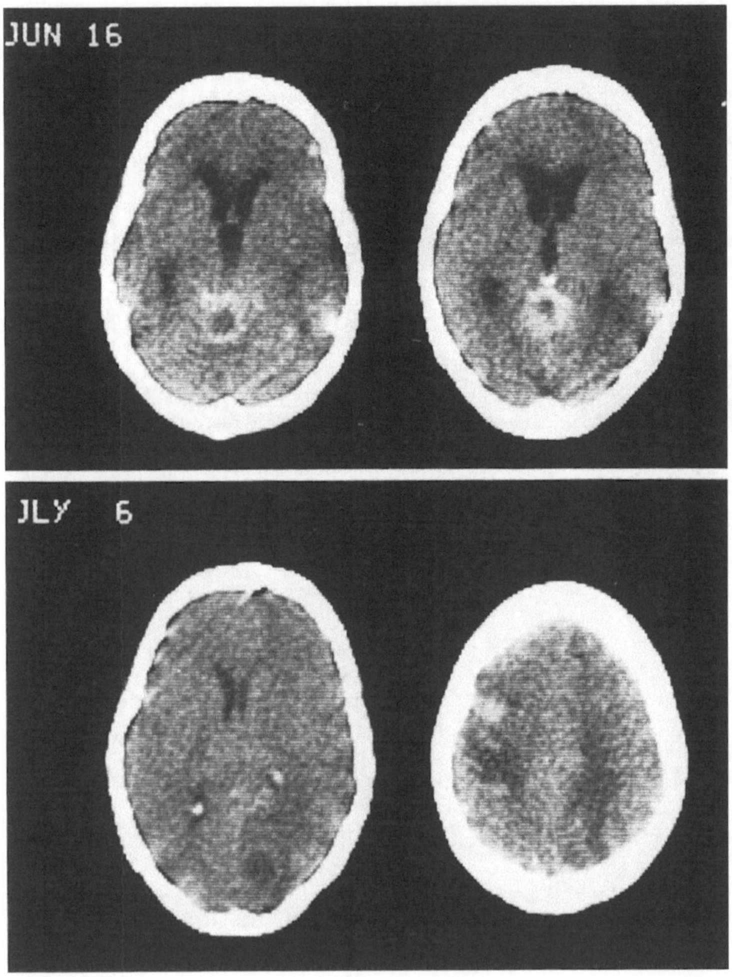


**Fig. D9.4.** Metastasis of malignant melanoma to the superior portion of the cerebellar vermis and the quadrigeminal cistern in a 33-year-old female. Initial CT studies (June 16) demonstrated a tumor, which proved to be a metastasis of melanoma at operation. The immediate postoperative course was uneventful until right hemiparesis and homonymous left hemianopsia developed 3 weeks later. Repetition of CT studies on July 6 demonstrated two additional metastases in the left precentral and right occipital regions which had not appeared, even after contrast enhancement, at the first examination. Postcontrast studies

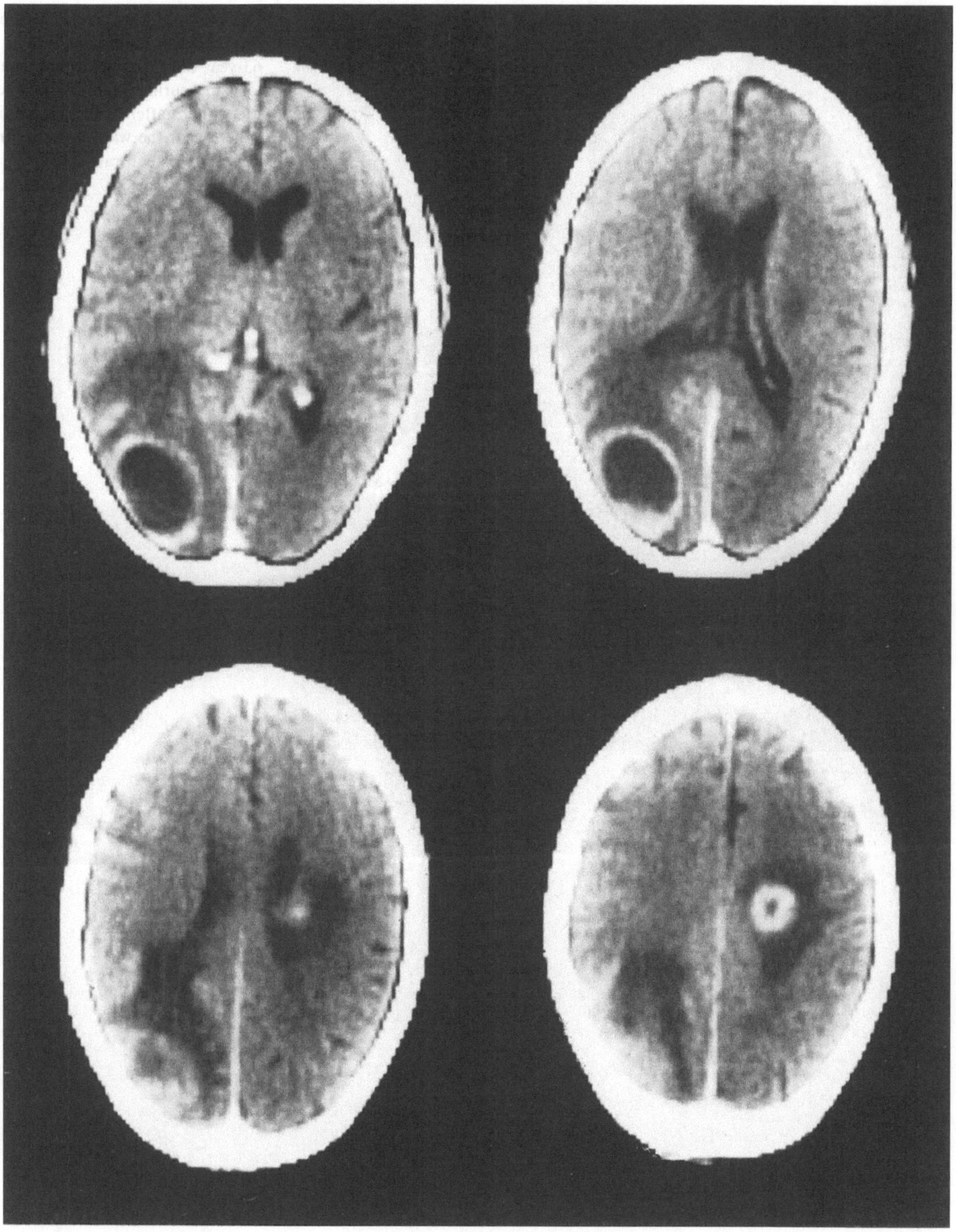

**Fig. D9.5.** Metastases of bronchogenic carcinoma in both cerebral hemispheres in a 60-year-old male. Both tumors – even the small one – have central zones of low density due to necrosis and appear as ring figures in the CT scan. This CT appearance is found only in intracranial metastases and abscesses. Postcontrast study

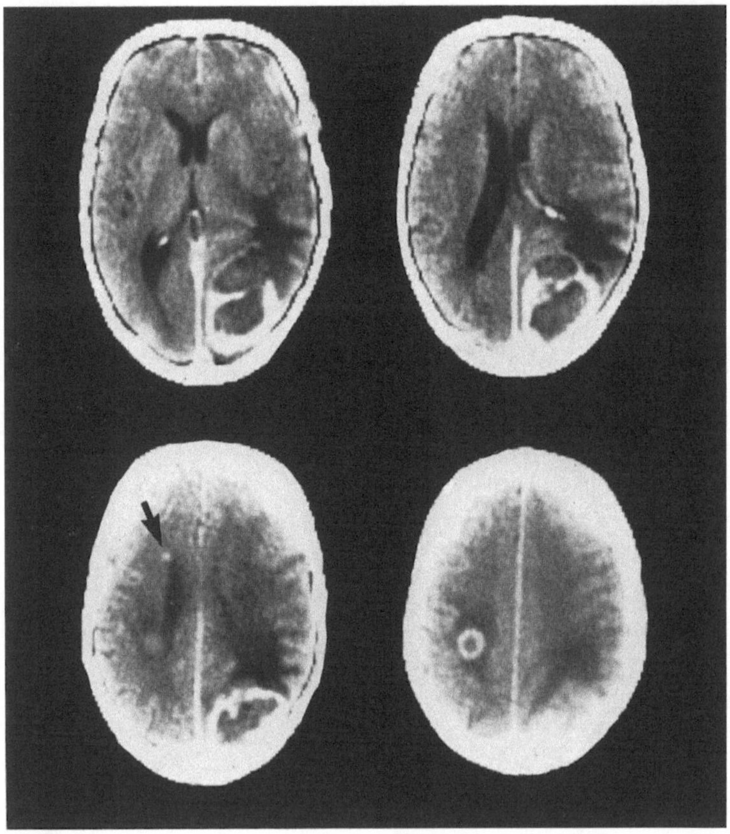

**Fig. D9.6.** Multiple metastases of bronchogenic carcinoma in a 63-year-old man. Below left: metastasis measuring 5 mm in diameter in the white matter of the left hemisphere near the wall of the ventricle (arrow). Postcontrast study

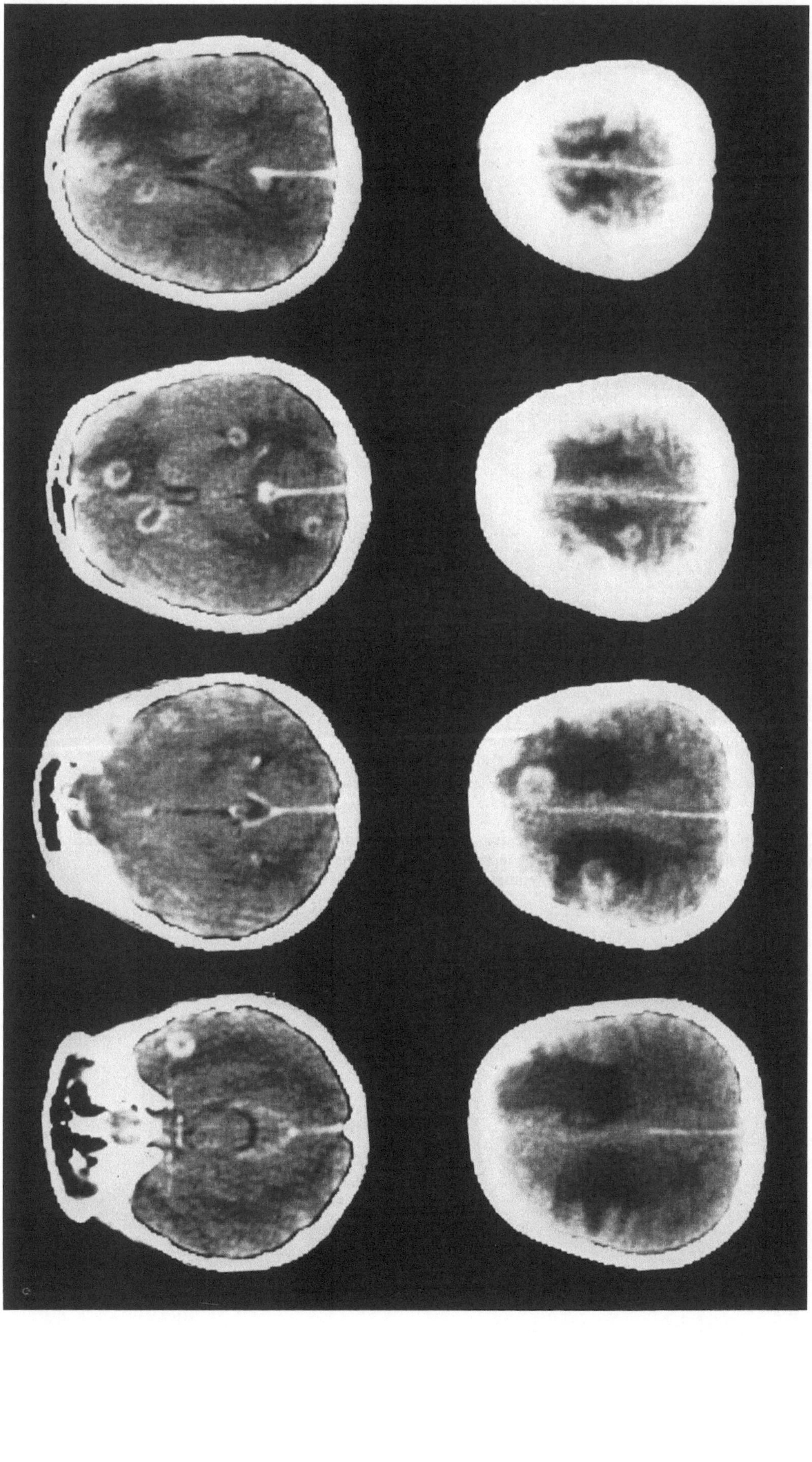

**Fig. D9.7.** Multiple metastases of adenocarcinoma of unknown origin in a 26-year-old female. All ten metastases visible in the CT scan demonstrate central hypodense zones representing necrosis. Pronounced edema in the white matter bilaterally. Postcontrast study

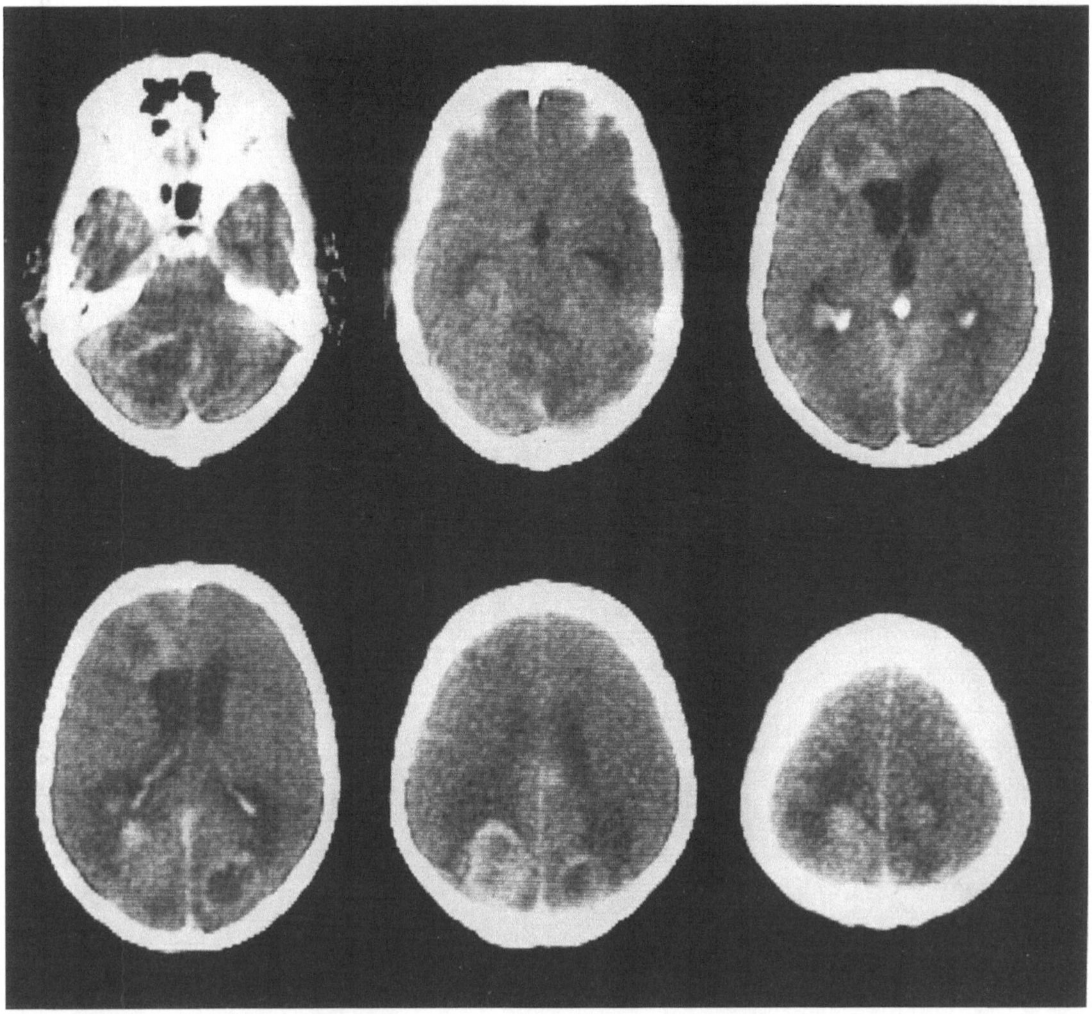

**Fig. D9.8.** Multiple metastases of bronchogenic carcinoma in a 60-year-old male. In addition to a number of supratentorial metastases a large tumor with marginal contrast uptake is demonstrated in the left cerebellar hemisphere. Postcontrast study

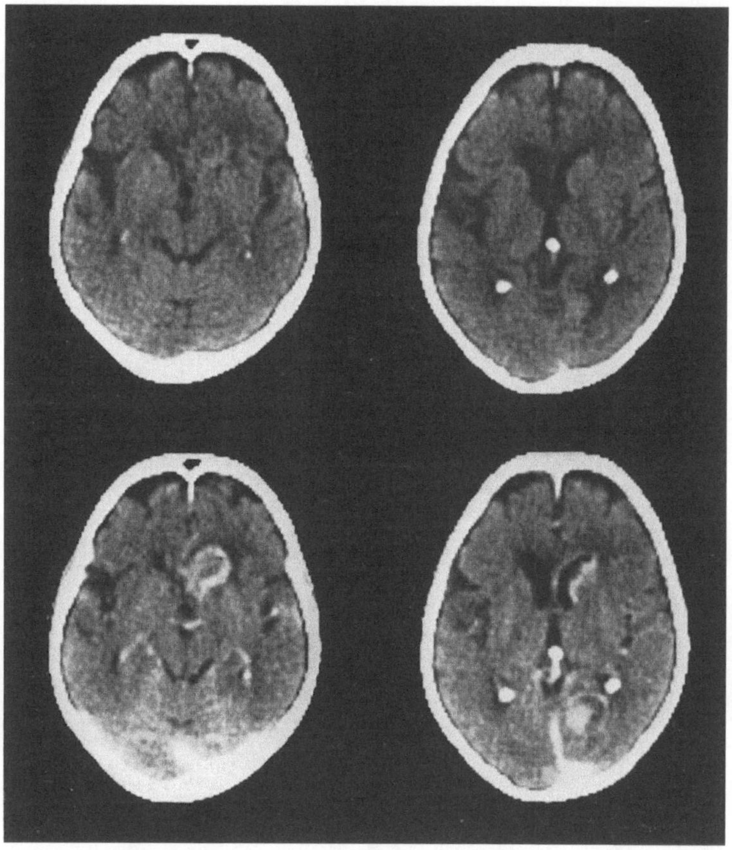

**Fig. D9.9.** Multiple metastases of bronchogenic carcinoma in a 68-year-old female. Above, precontrast studies; below, postcontrast studies. Demonstration of a metastasis in the right occipital region as well as an intraventricular metastatic tumor in the right anterior horn with growth along the ventricle wall (below right)

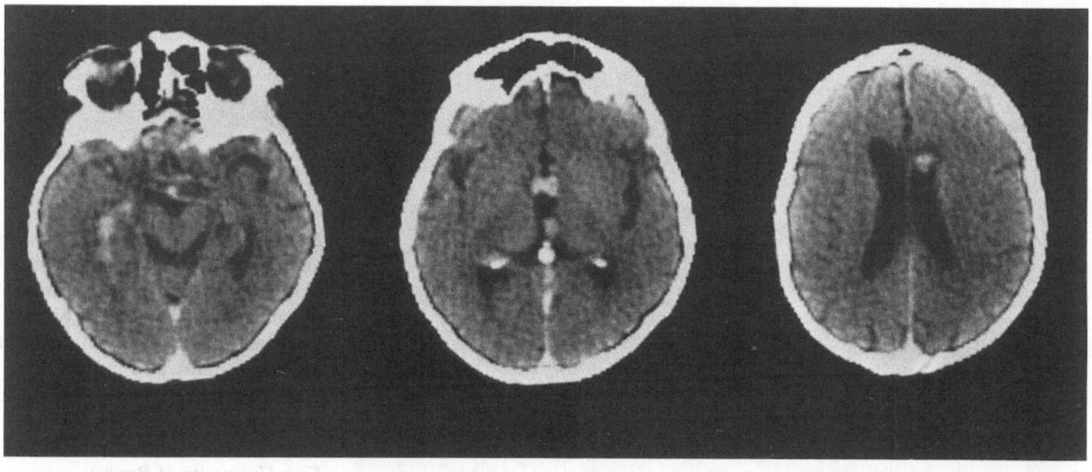

**Fig. D9.10.** Multiple intraventricular metastases of seminoma in the left inferior horn, the third ventricle (two), and the cella media region on the right. Postcontrast study

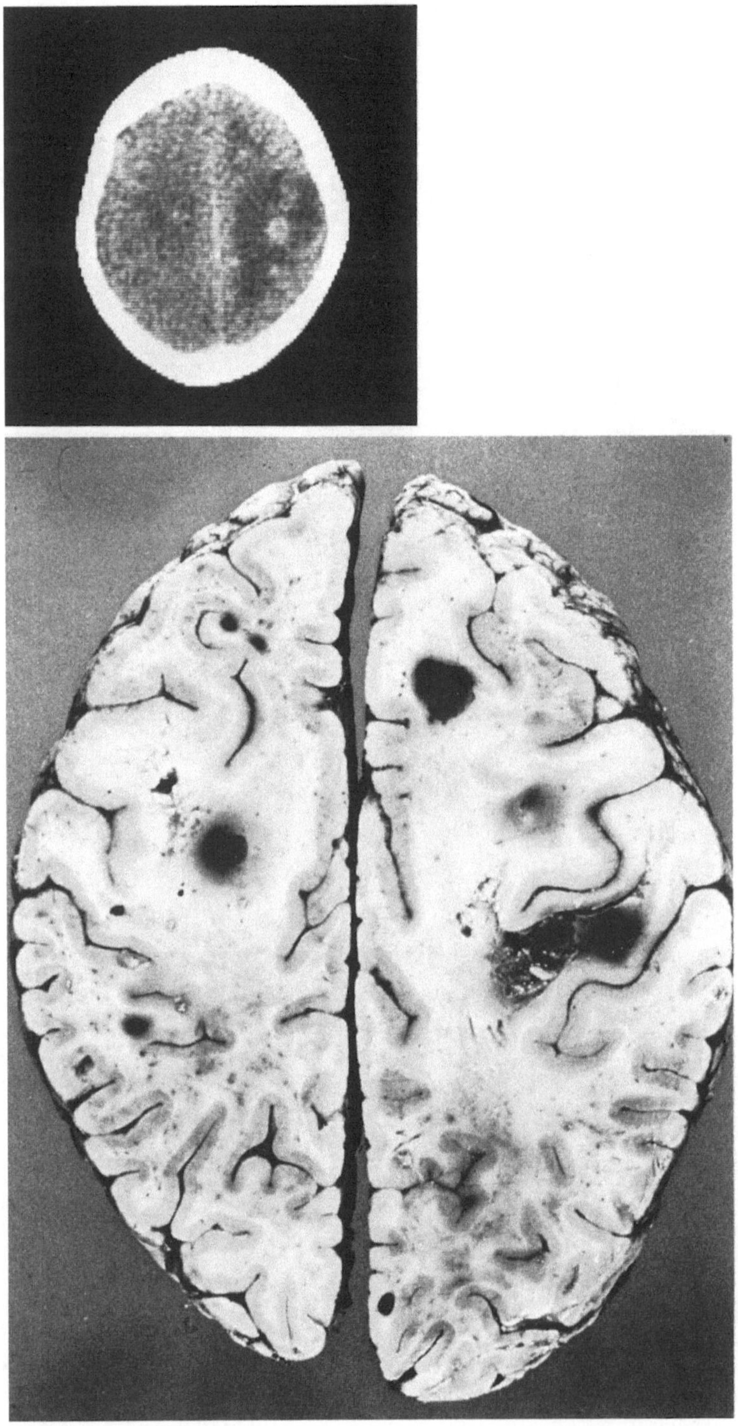

**Fig. D9.11.** Comparison of CT scan and autopsy specimen in a 57-year-old female with multiple metastases of carcinoma of the breast. Metastases smaller than 5 mm in diameter are not demonstrated in the CT scan. Postcontrast study. (Specimen courtesy of Priv.-Doz. Dr. G. EBHARDT, Neuropathological Institute, Free University of Berlin)

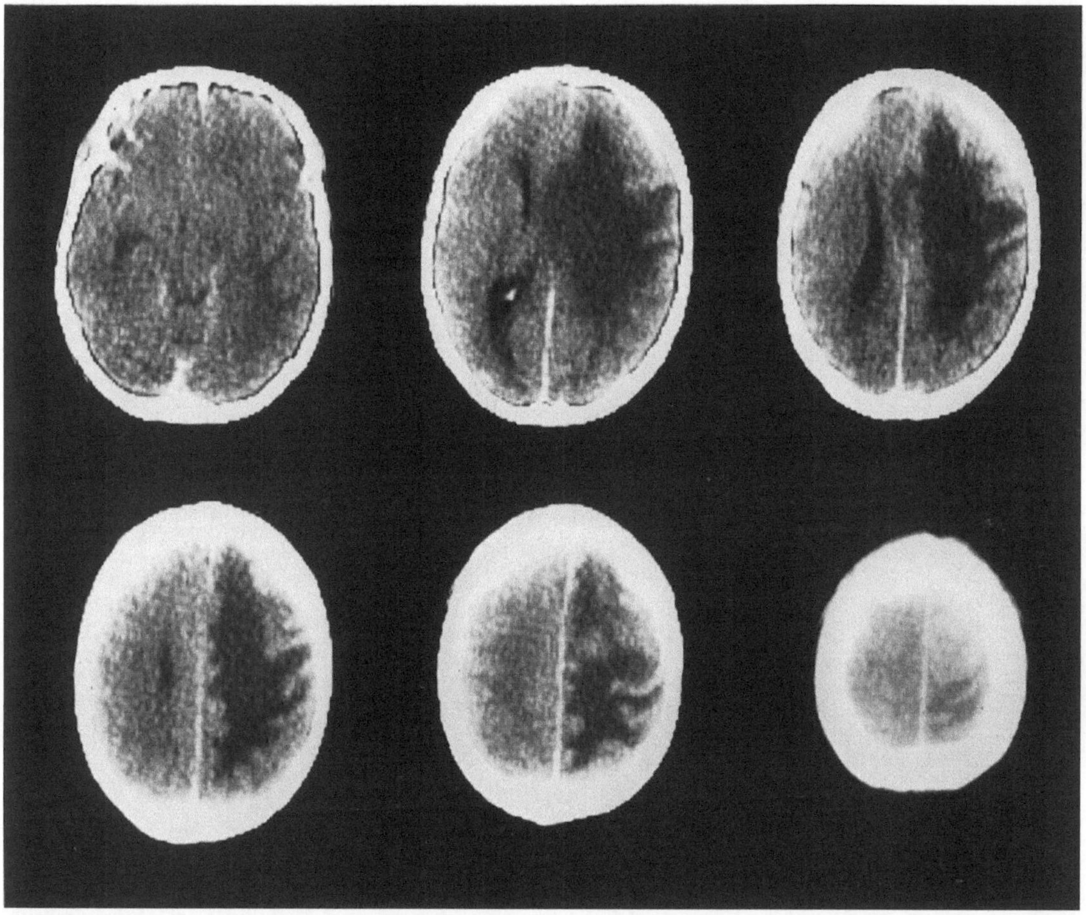

**Fig. D9.12.** Metastasis of carcinoma of the rectum in the right parasagittal region with grade III edema in a 39-year-old patient. Conspicuous discrepancy between the size of the lesion and extent of perifocal edema. This finding suggests metastasis. Postcontrast study

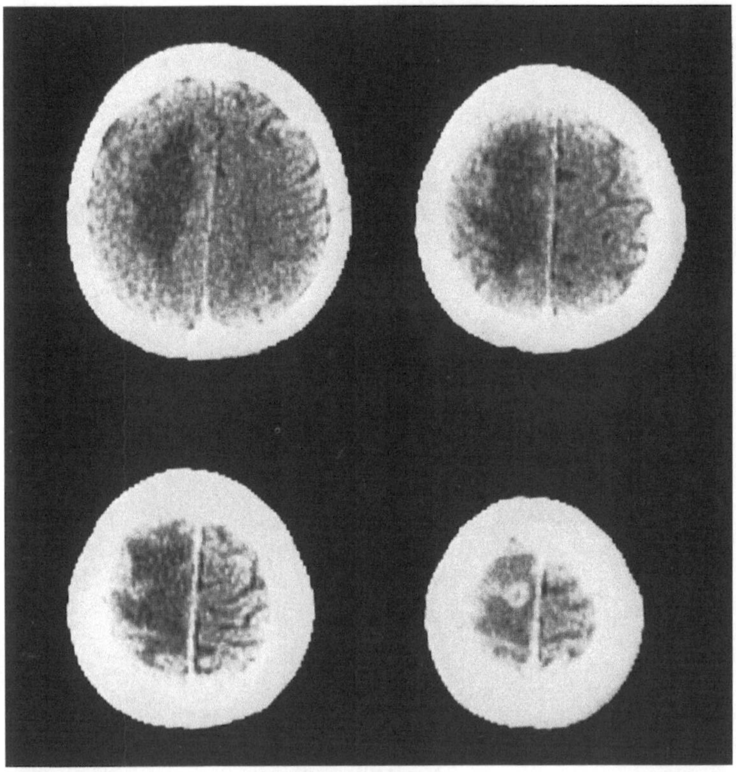

Fig. D9.13. Metastasis of renal carcinoma in the left parietal region in a 61-year-old female. Extensive (grade II) edema in the white matter, a characteristic finding in such a small intracranial metastasis (10 mm in diameter). Postcontrast study

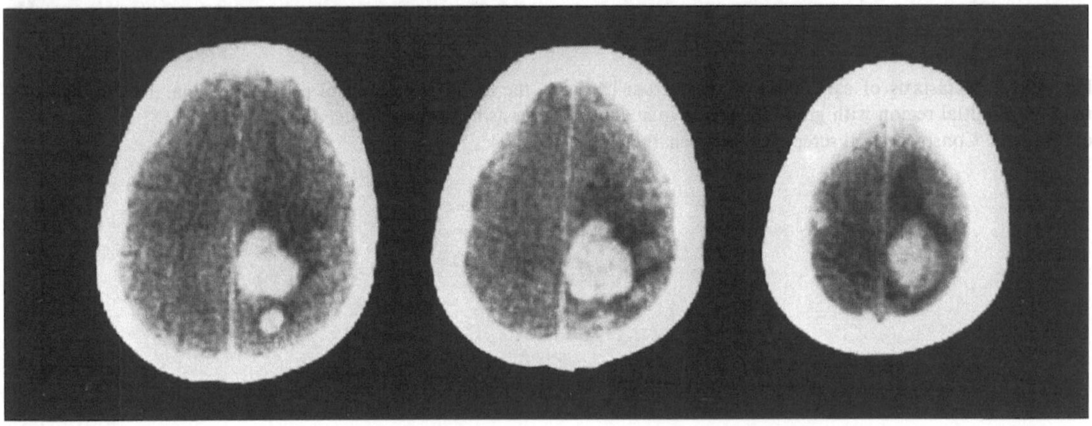

Fig. D9.14. Metastasis of malignant melanoma with recent hemorrhage in the right parietal region in a 57-year-old patient. No increase in absorption values after contrast enhancement because of very hyperdense values due to coagulated blood. Postcontrast study

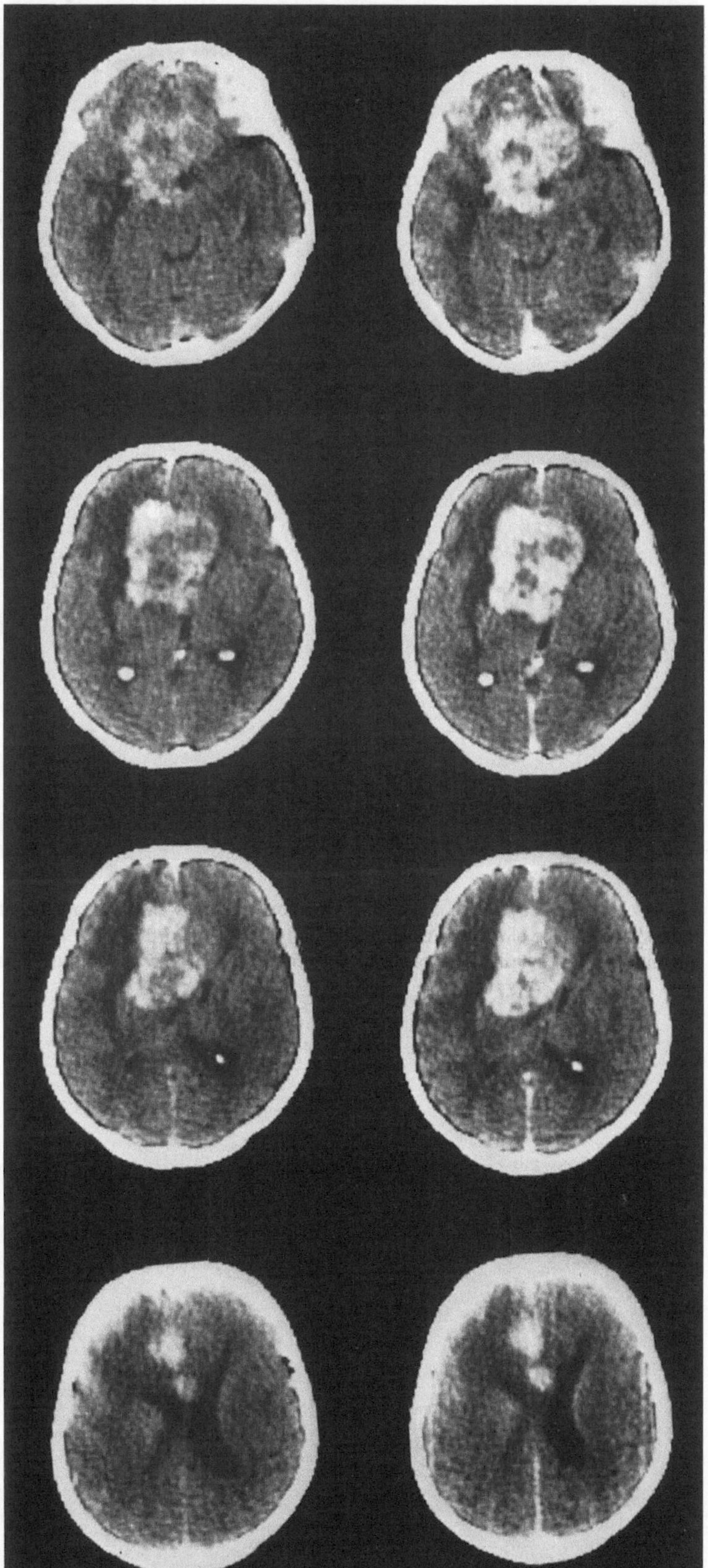

**Fig. D9.15.** Large metastasis of rectal carcinoma in the left frontal lobe with extension to the right in a 64-year-old female. Extensive hemorrhage in the tumor, which demonstrates a further increase in density values only in some portions after contrast enhancement. Typical funnel-shaped zone of edema in the left frontal lobe. Major displacement of the right anterior horn indicating the origin of the tumor in the left frontal lobe. Left, precontrast studies; right, postcontrast studies

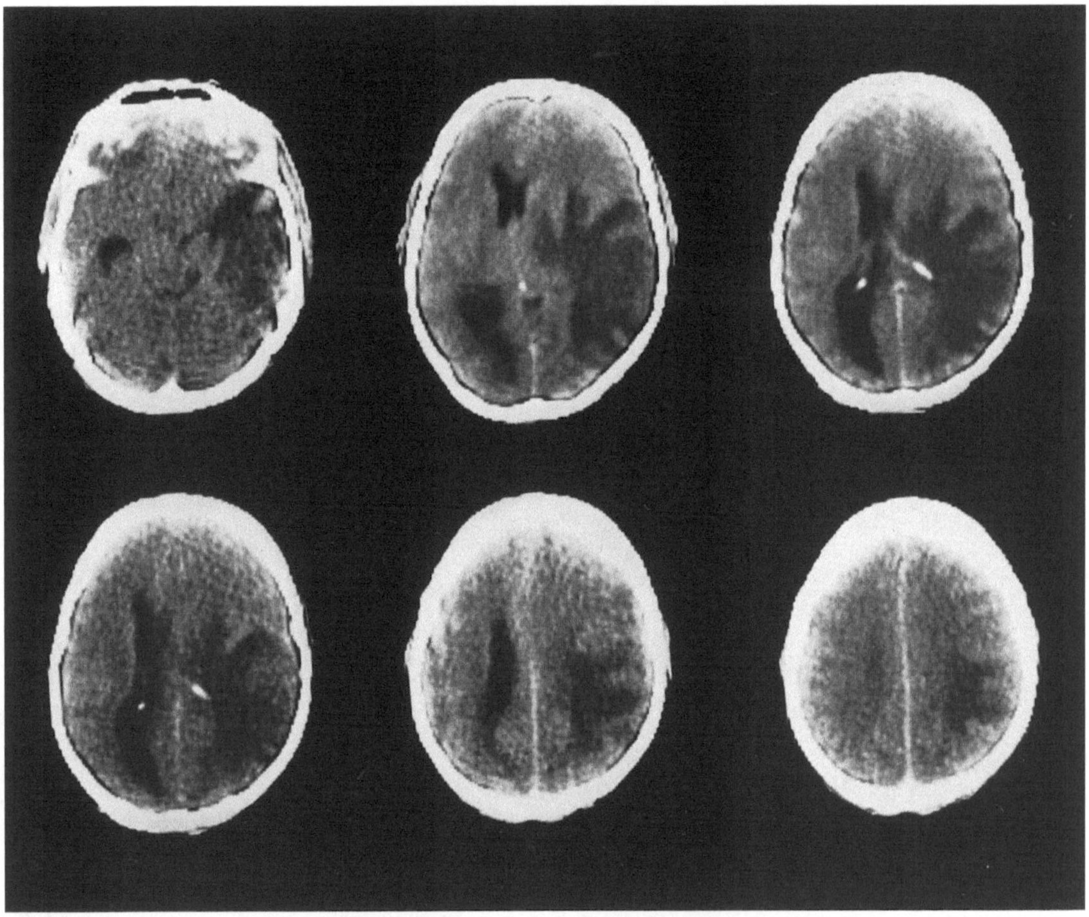

**Fig. D9.16.** Metastasis of squamous cell carcinoma in the right temporal lobe of a 40-year-old male. CT studies demonstrate only an extensive zone of edema with characteristic finger-shaped configuration, conforming to the structure of the white matter. The tumor itself is not visualized, even after contrast enhancement

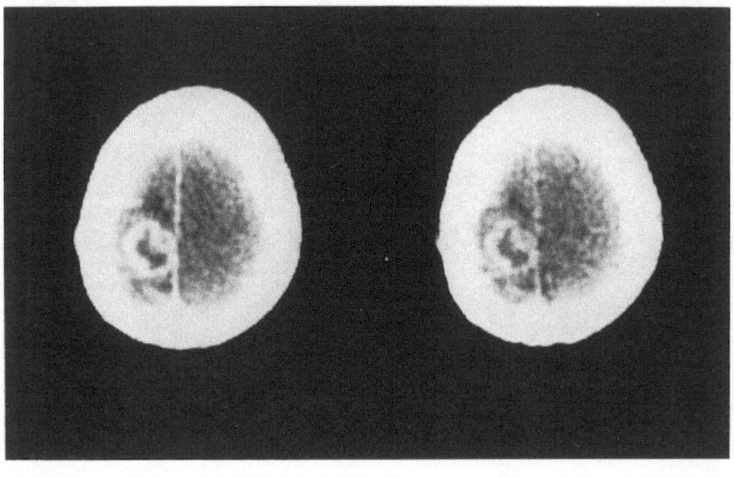

**Fig. D9.17.** Ring figure following contrast enhancement in metastasis of renal carcinoma in a 48-year-old male. Differentiation between this lesion and glioblastoma is not possible with the CT scan alone. Knowledge of the primary tumor suggested a diagnosis of metastasis

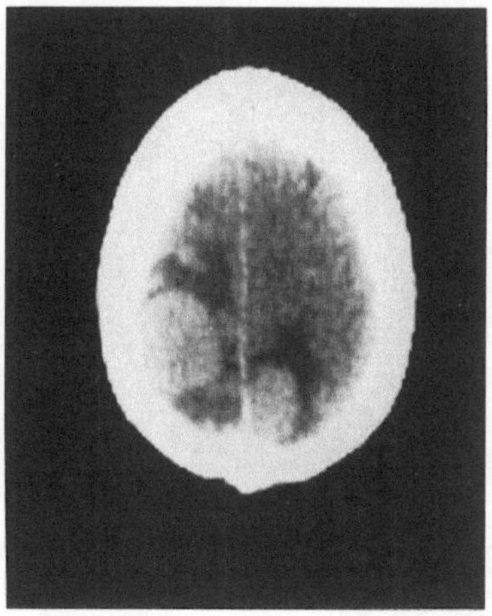

**Fig. D9.**18. Multiple metastases of testicular teratoma in a 41-year-old patient. The lesions appear as homogeneous knots of tumor. Postcontrast study

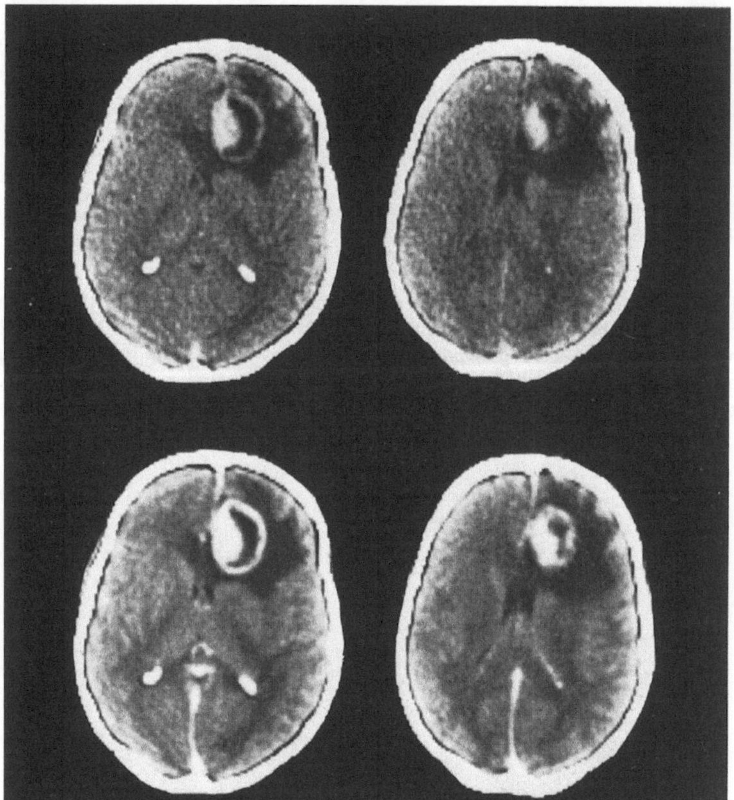

**Fig. D9.**19. Metastasis of malignant melanoma in the right frontal lobe with characteristic frontal edema which extends to the left frontal lobe as well. The precontrast study shows hyperdense values due to hemorrhage in the tumor and a ring figure (above). Strong contrast uptake within viable portions of the tumor (below)

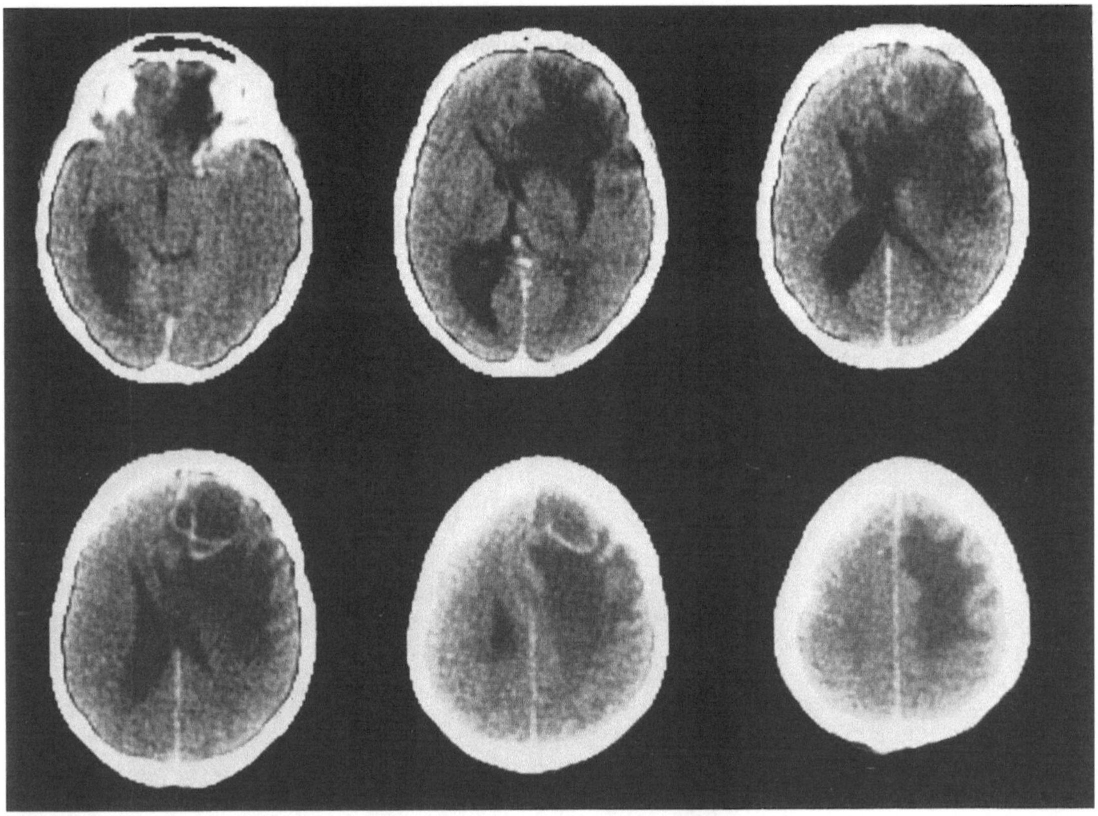

**Fig. D9.20.** Metastasis of bronchogenic carcinoma in the right frontal lobe in a 55-year-old female. Contrast enhancement produces rings and garland figures in viable portions of the tumor, with hypodense areas representing central zones of necrosis. Grade III perifocal edema extending through the white matter of almost the entire right hemisphere. Major displacement of midline structures with disruption of the CSF passage in the left lateral ventricle, which is extremely dilated in its posterior section. Postcontrast study

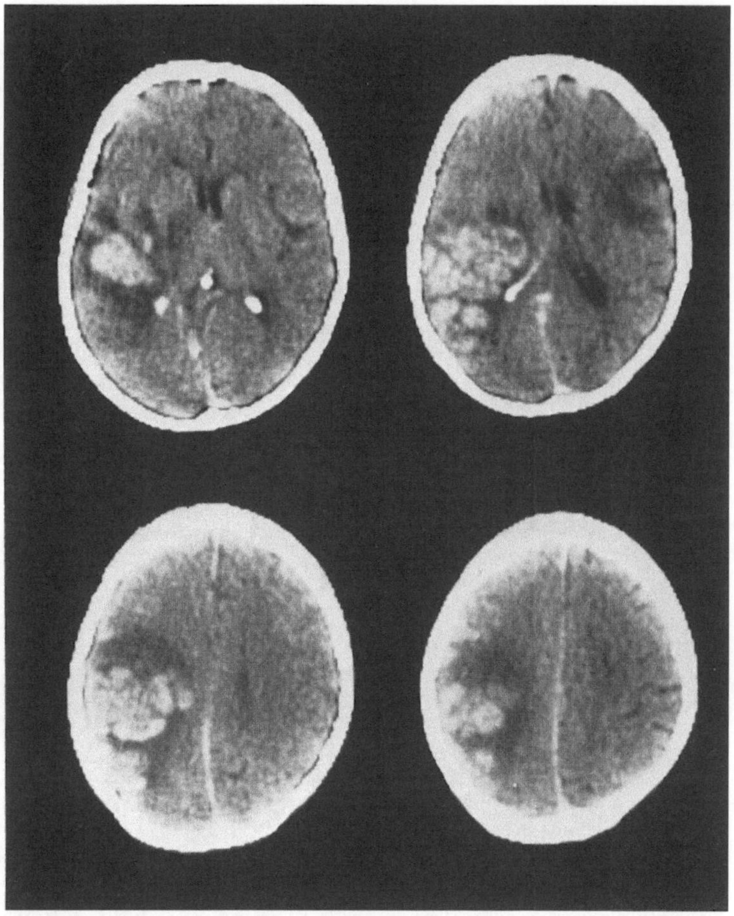

**Fig. D9.21.** Multiple metastases of bronchogenic carcinoma in a 68-year-old patient. The middle and posterior sections of the left cerebral hemisphere demonstrate a number of tumor nodules of various sizes. Additional frontotemporal metastasis on the right (edema). Postcontrast study

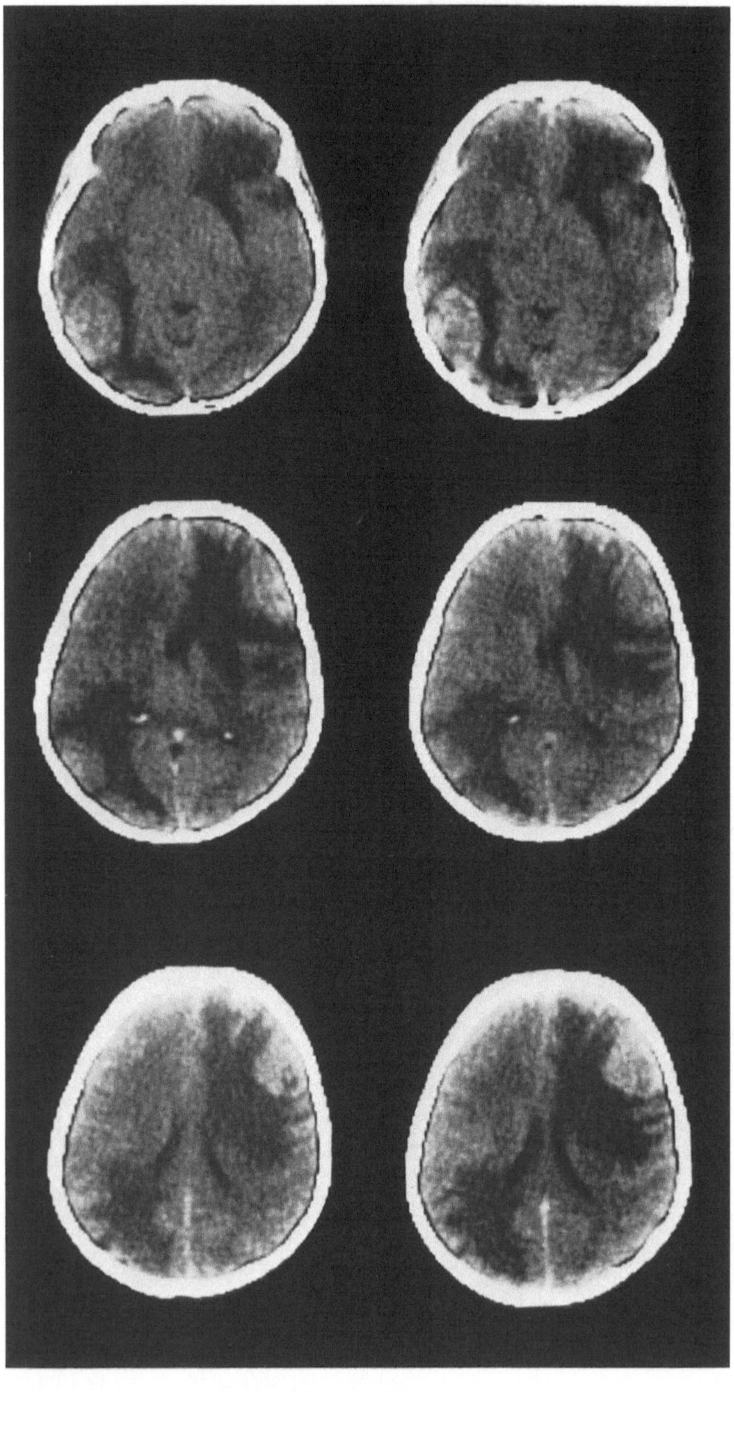

**Fig. D9.22.** Nodular metastases in both cerebral hemispheres in a 34-year-old patient with breast cancer. Grade II perifocal edema surrounding both tumor nodules. Left, precontrast study; right, postcontrast study

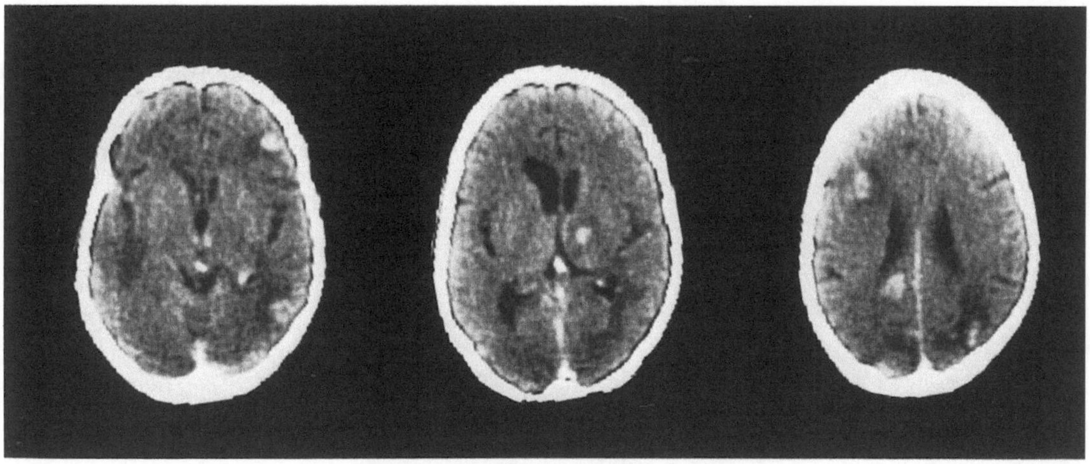

**Fig. D9.23.** Multiple metastases of breast cancer in a 67-year-old female. All tumor nodules demonstrate homogeneous contrast uptake, a finding characteristic of metastases of breast cancer. Postcontrast study

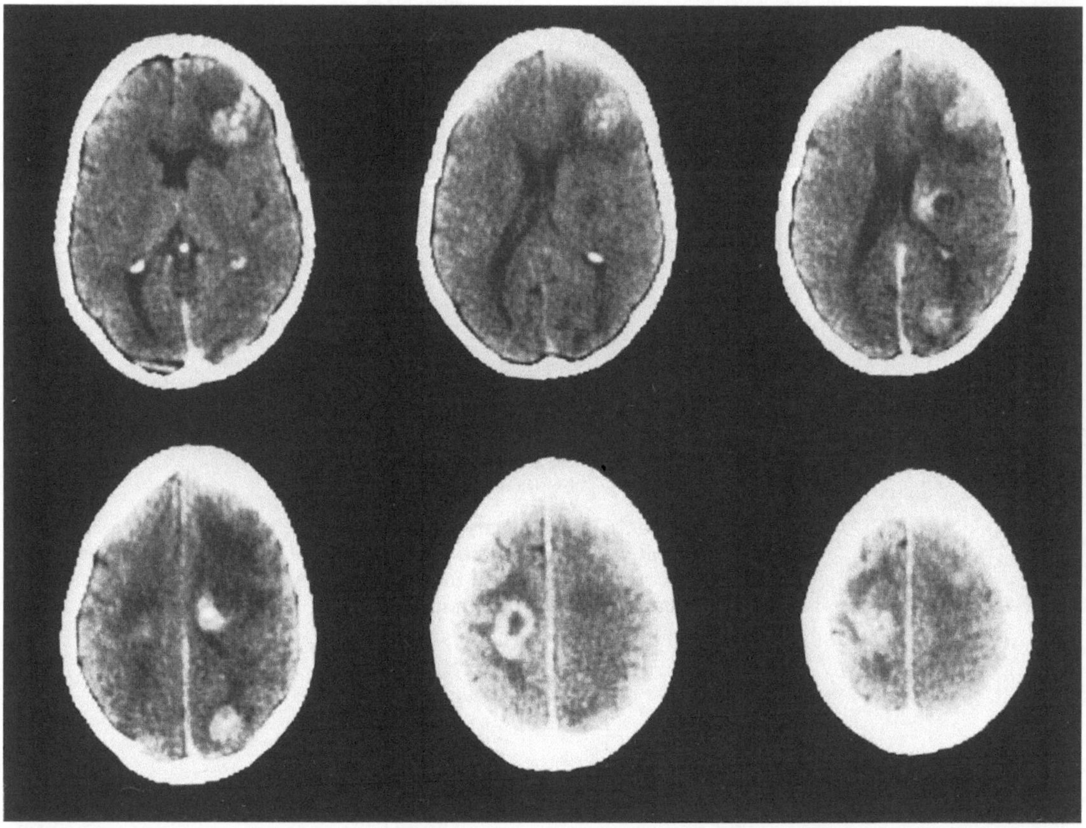

**Fig. D9.24.** Multiple metastases of breast cancer in a 53-year-old patient. Two of the four metastases demonstrate ring figures in at least one slice after contrast enhancement, while the remaining two metastases show homogeneous contrast uptake. Postcontrast study

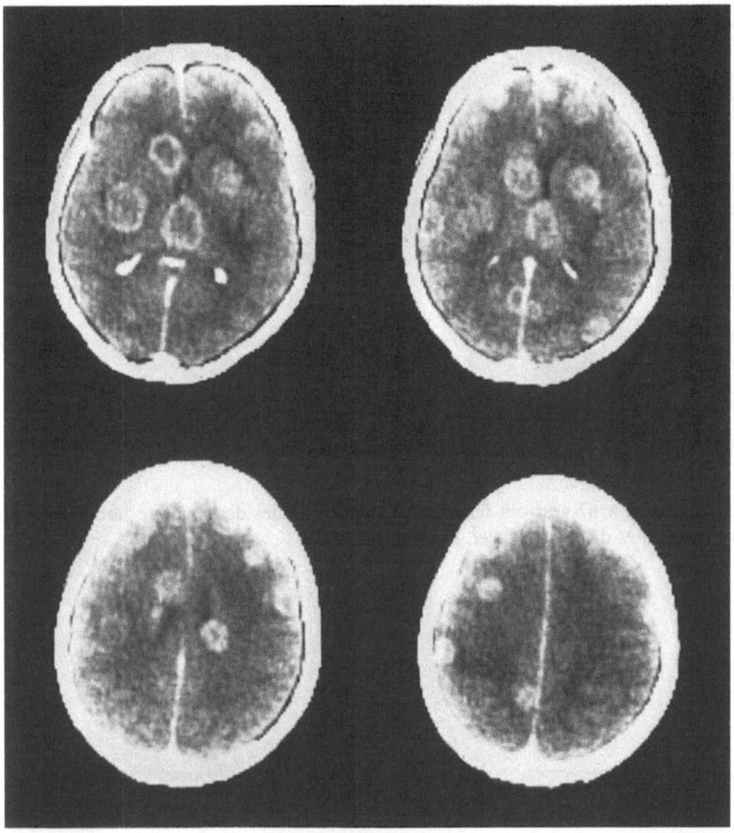

**Fig. D9.25.** Multiple metastases throughout both cerebral hemispheres in a 44-year-old patient with breast cancer. The larger metastases demonstrate ring figures, while the smaller lesions appear as solid tumor nodules after contrast enhancement. Postcontrast study

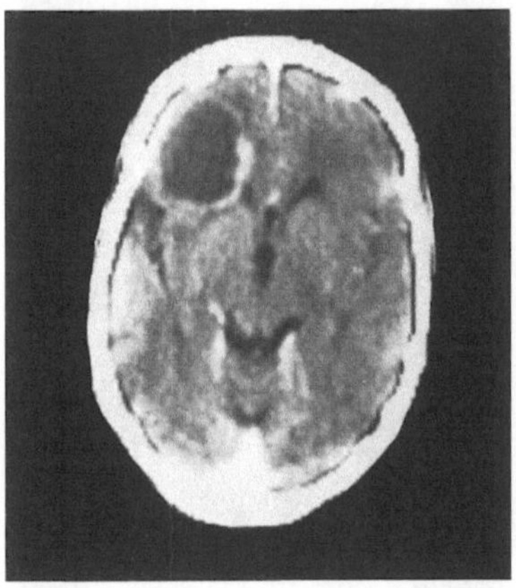

**Fig. D9.26.** Large solitary metastasis in the left frontal lobe of a 39-year-old patient with breast cancer. Demonstration of a ring figure after contrast enhancement. Large central zone of necrosis. Atypical appearance of metastasis of breast cancer. Postcontrast study

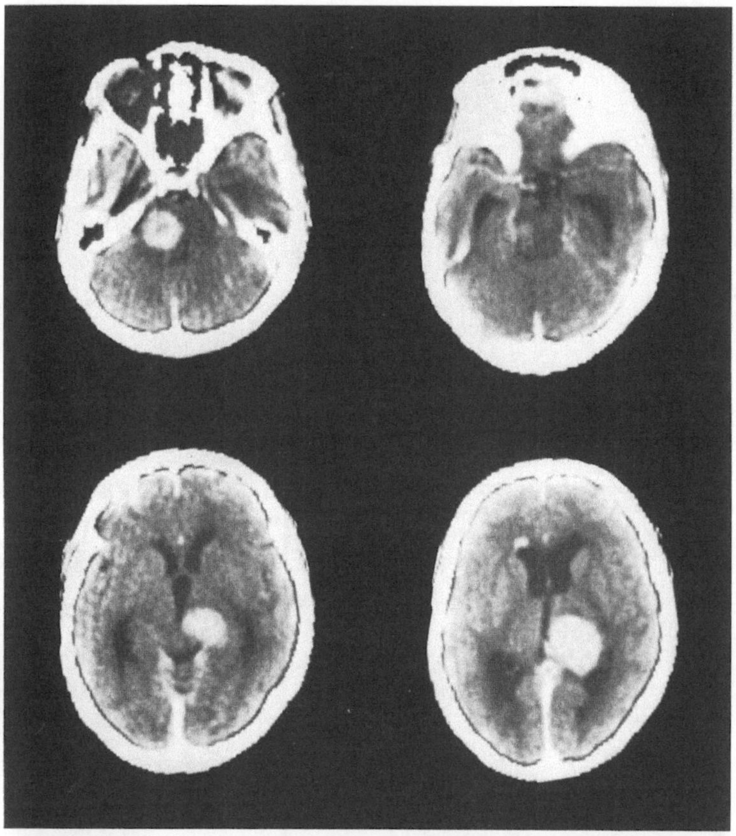

**Fig. D9.27.** Multiple metastases of malignant melanoma in 36-year-old patient. Tumor nodules with strong contrast uptake in the right thalamus, at the left cerebellopontine angle, and in the left anterior horn. Hyperdense values in the precontrast study

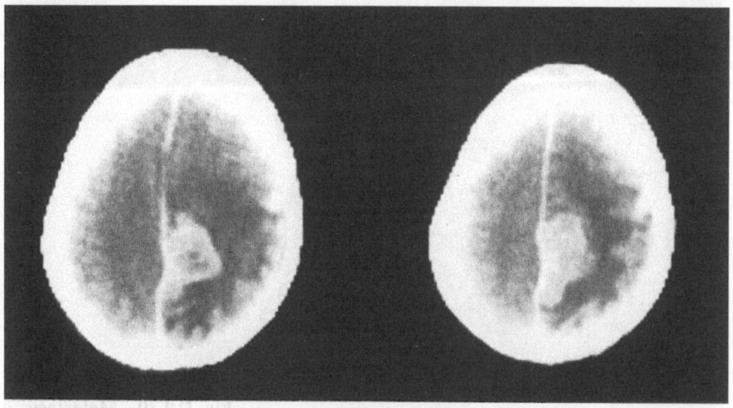

**Fig. D9.28.** Metastasis adjacent to the falx in a 52-year-old female with malignant melanoma. Location and homogeneous contrast uptake suggested a diagnosis of meningioma, but the history of a malignant melanoma favored a diagnosis of metastasis. Postcontrast study

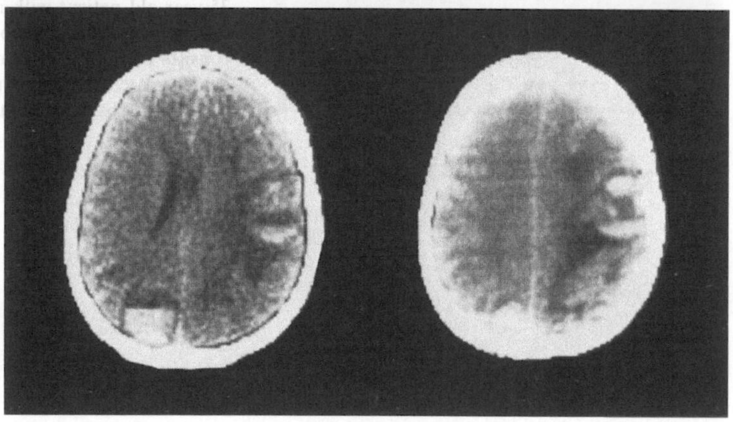

**Fig. D9.29.** Multiple metastases of melanoma in a 44-year-old patient. Recent hemorrhage in the tumor nodules with a horizontal fluid level due to sedimentation effect

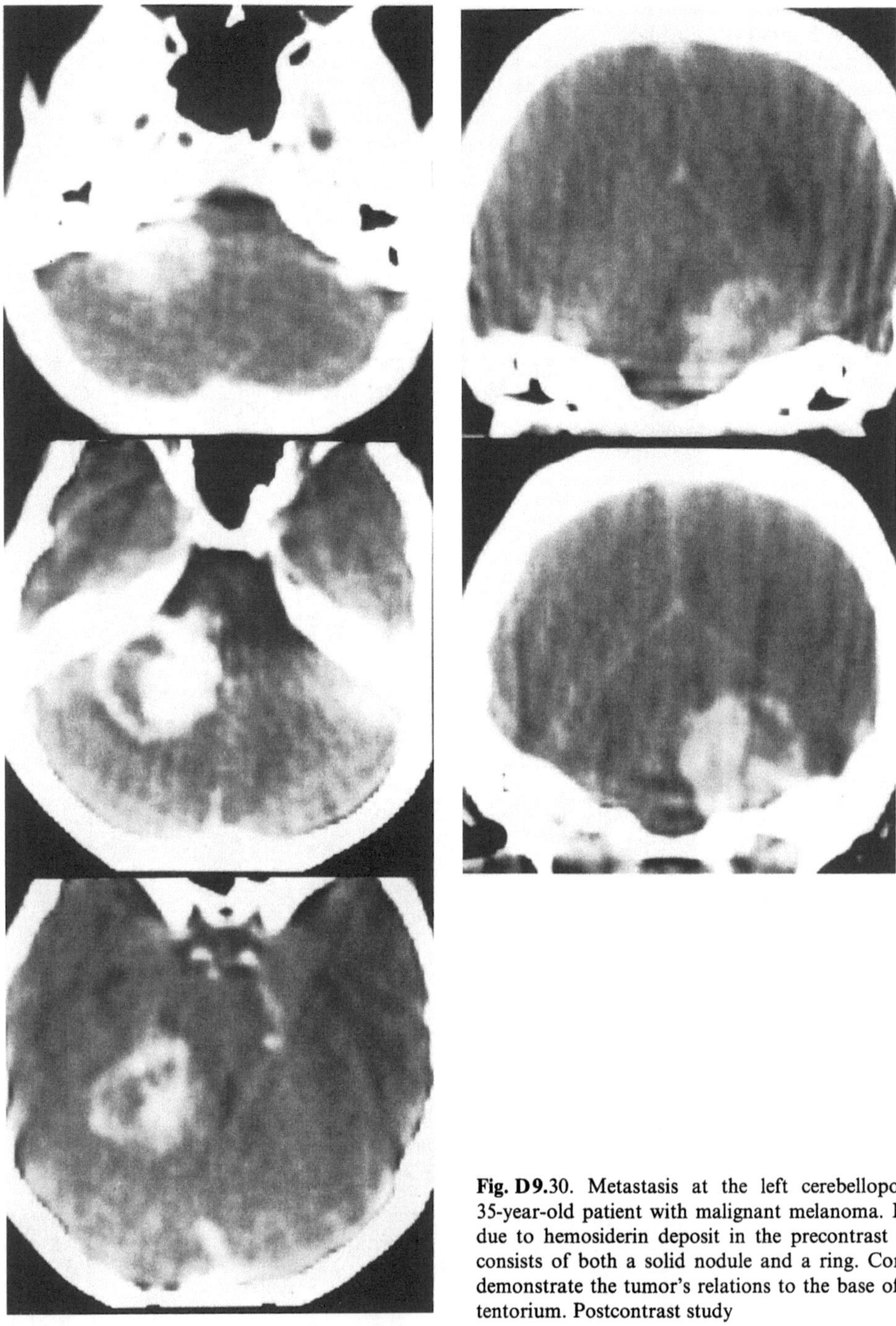

**Fig. D9.30.** Metastasis at the left cerebellopontine angle in a 35-year-old patient with malignant melanoma. Hyperdense values due to hemosiderin deposit in the precontrast study. The tumor consists of both a solid nodule and a ring. Coronary projections demonstrate the tumor's relations to the base of the skull and the tentorium. Postcontrast study

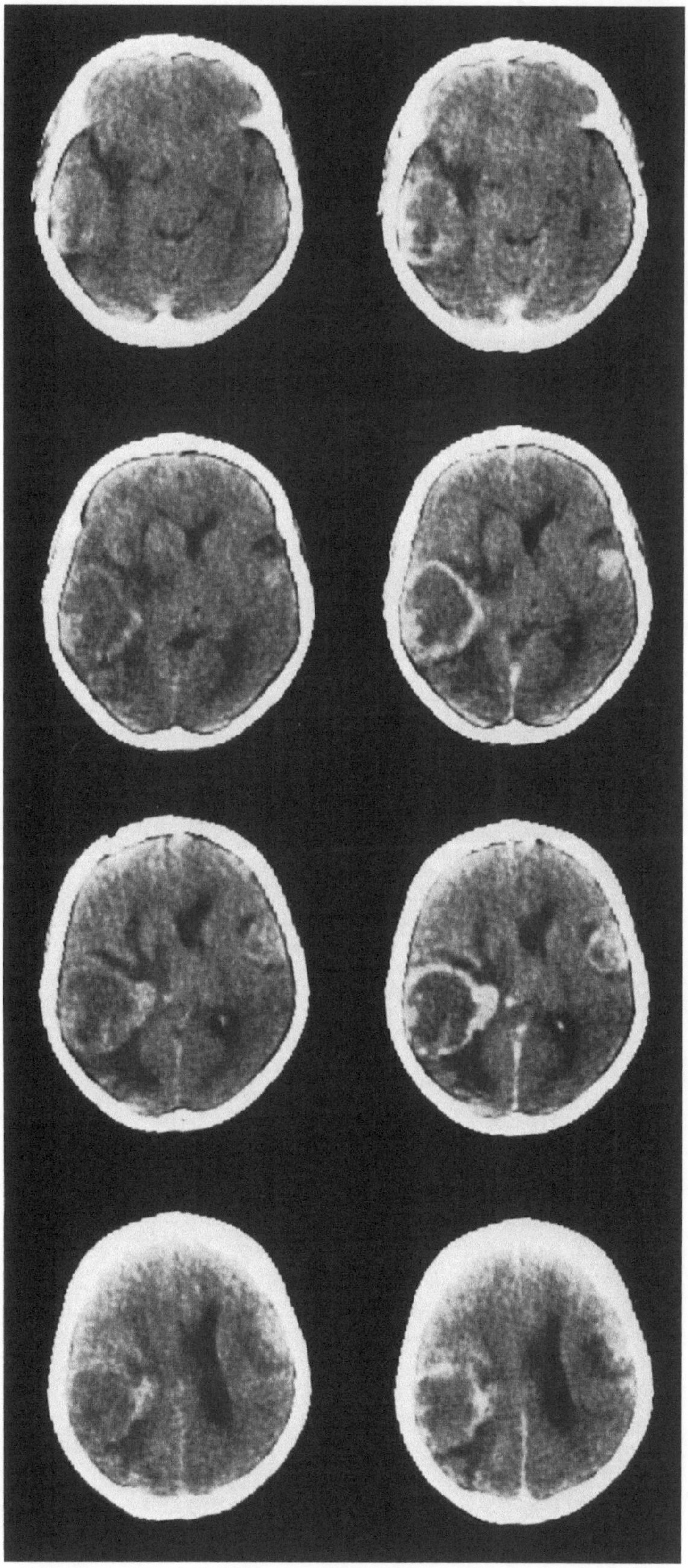

**Fig. D9.31.** Multiple metastases in a 56-year-old female with malignant melanoma. Left, precontrast studies; right, postcontrast studies. The tumor on the left shows extensive central necrosis, a rare finding in metastasis of melanoma

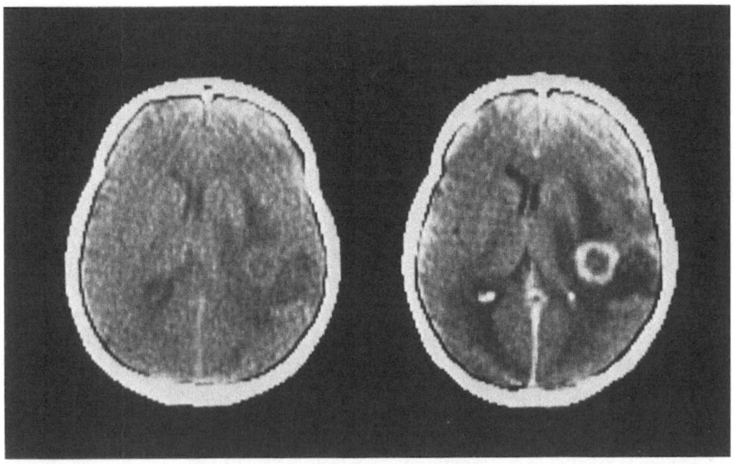

**Fig. D9.**32. Metastasis deep in the right temporale lobe of a 56-year-old female with renal carcinoma. Spherical tumor nodule with central zone of necrosis. Grade II perifocal edema. Approximately half of all metastases of renal carcinoma demonstrate identical or similar findings (cf. Fig. D9.33). Left, precontrast study; right, postcontrast study

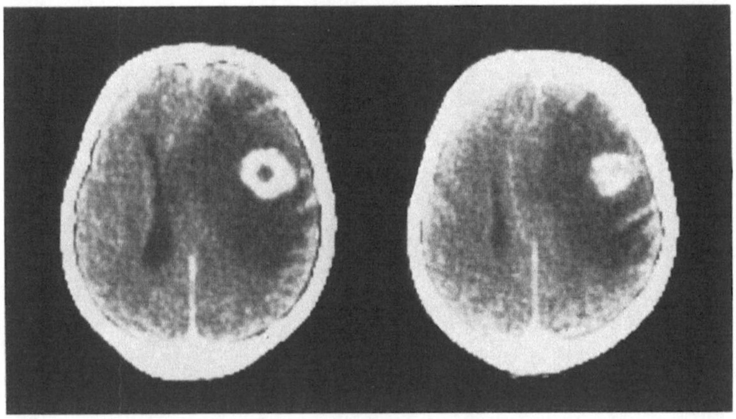

**Fig. D9.**33. Metastasis in the right precentral region of a 53-year-old patient with renal carcinoma. Spherical tumor nodule with small central zone of necrosis. Grade III perifocal edema, which has caused major midline displacement. Postcontrast study

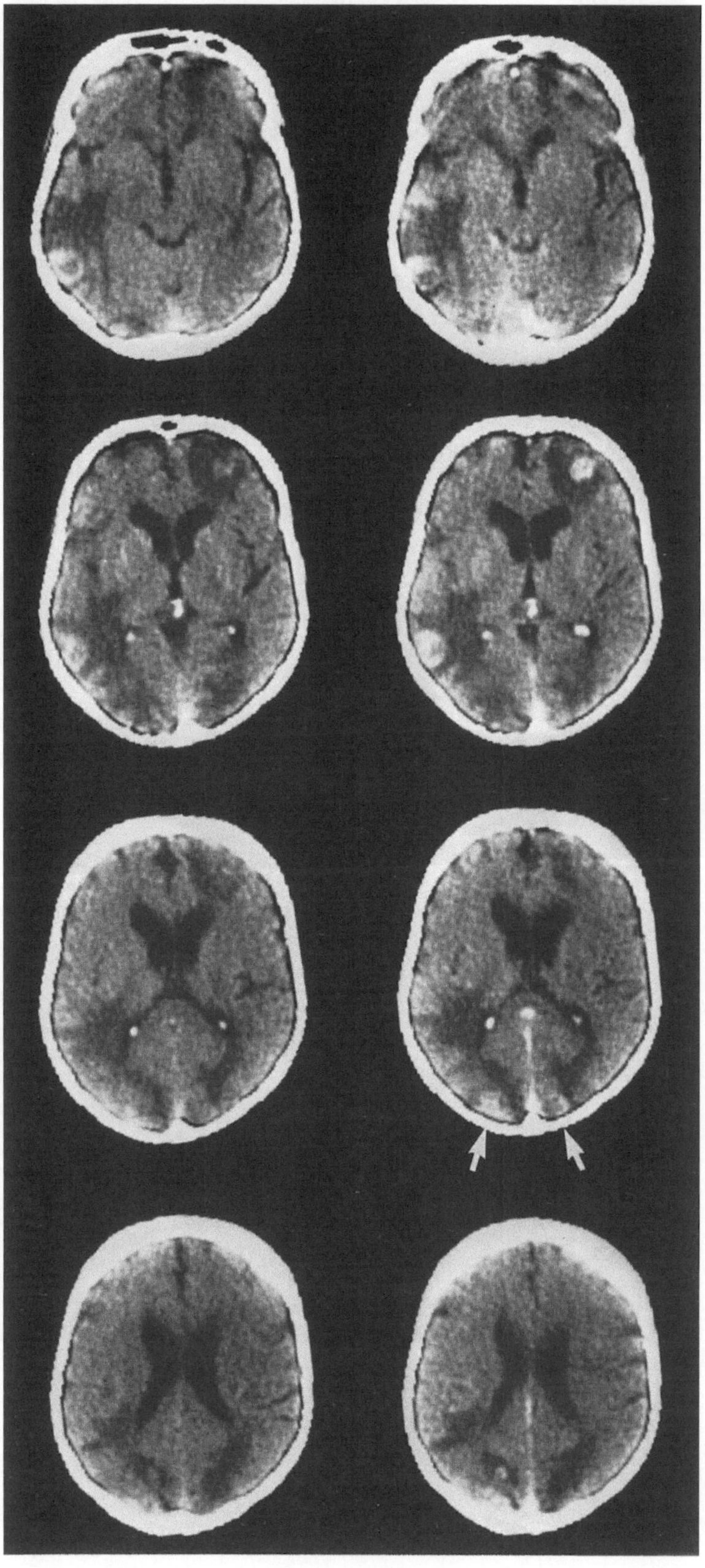

**Fig. D9.34.** Multiple metastases of renal carcinoma in a 59-year-old patient. Left, precontrast studies; right, postcontrast studies. Homogeneous contrast uptake in the small tumor in the right frontal lobe; demonstration of a central zone of necrosis in the larger lesion in the posterior portion of the left temporal region. Demonstration of additional metastases near the vault in both occipital lobes after contrast enhancement (arrows). Edema in the white matter of the occipital lobes in the precontrast studies suggests the presence of tumors at this location

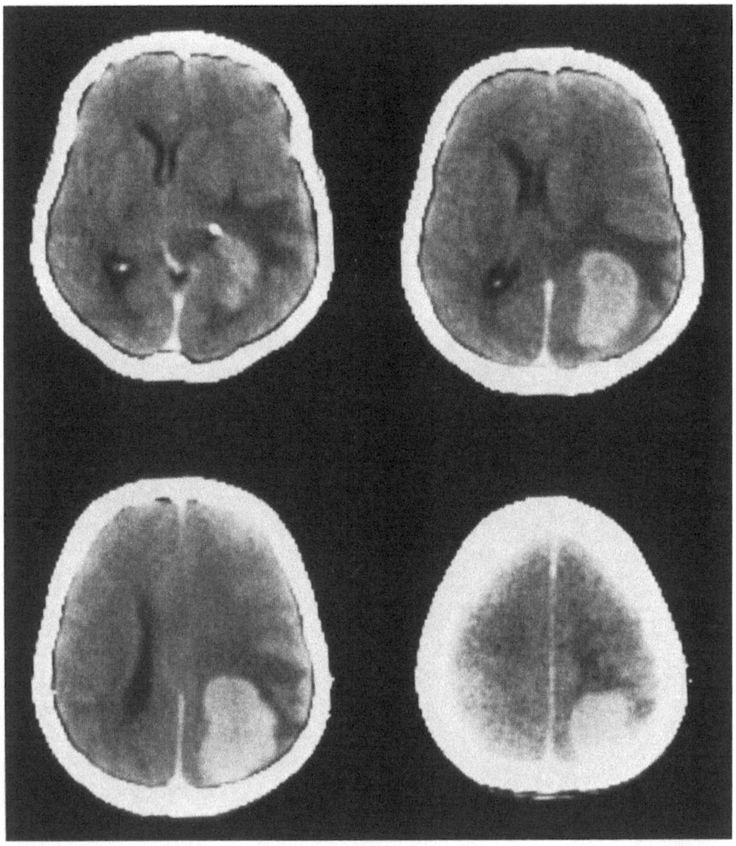

**Fig. D9.35.** Metastasis in the right parieto-occipital region in a 55-year-old female with bronchoalveolar adenocarcinoma. Homogeneous contrast uptake within the metastasis resembles that found in meningiomas and malignant lymphomas. Postcontrast study

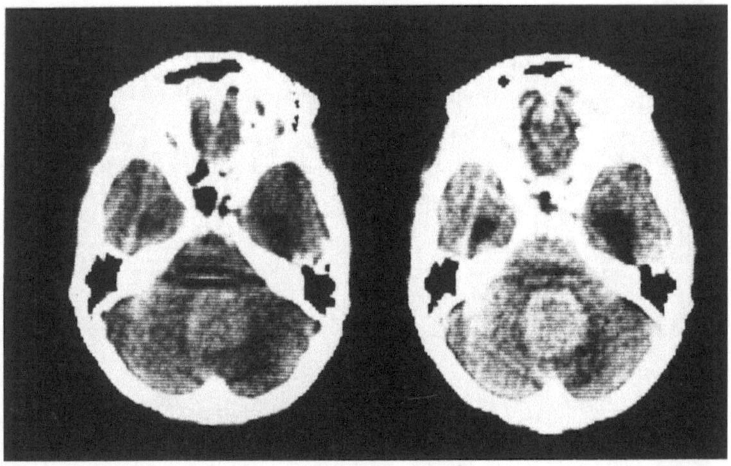

**Fig. D9.36.** Metastasis in the cerebellar vermis in a 64-year-old man with carcinoma of the rectum. Hyperdense values in the precontrast study (left) with slight increase in density values after contrast enhancement (right)

**Fig. D9.**37. Cerebellar metastasis in a 65-year-old patient with carcinoma of the cecum. Strong contrast uptake at the margins of the tumor with slight increase in density values at the center of the lesion. The history provided decisive evidence for a diagnosis of metastasis

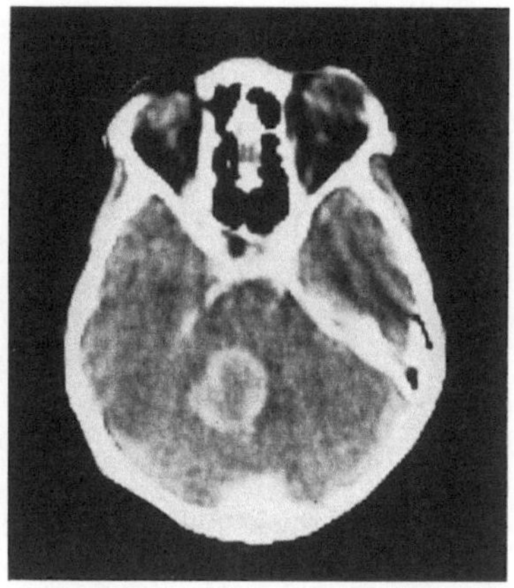

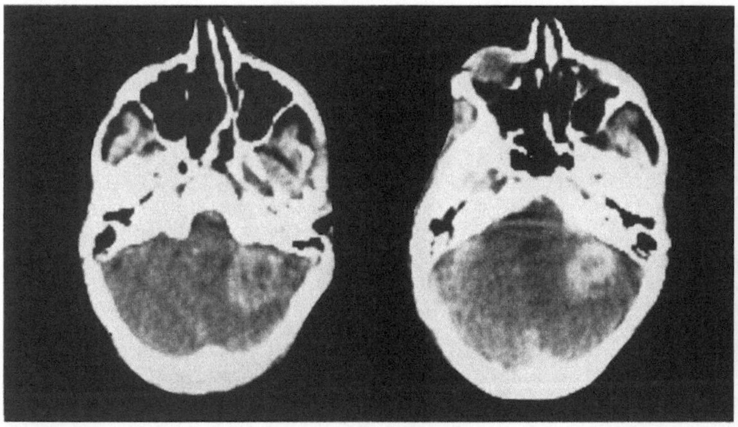

**Fig. D9.**38. Metastasis in the right cerebellopontine region with extension to the right cerebellar hemisphere in a 37-year-old patient with adenocarcinoma (location of primary tumor unknown). Inhomogeneous contrast uptake due to areàs of necrosis

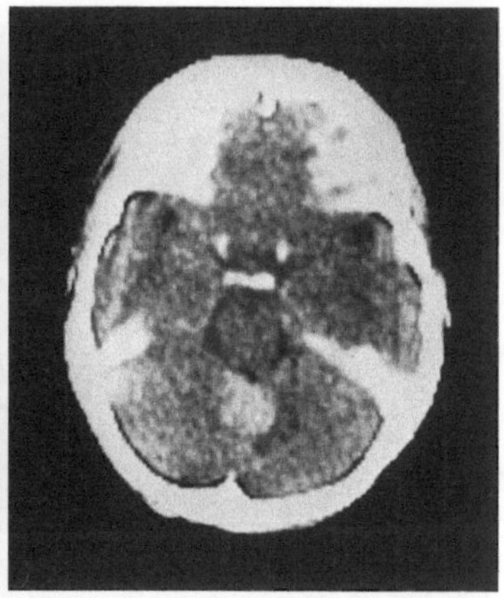

**Fig. D9.**39. Metastasis in the cerebellar vermis of a 28-year-old female with undifferentiated adenocarcinoma (location of primary tumor unknown). Postcontrast study

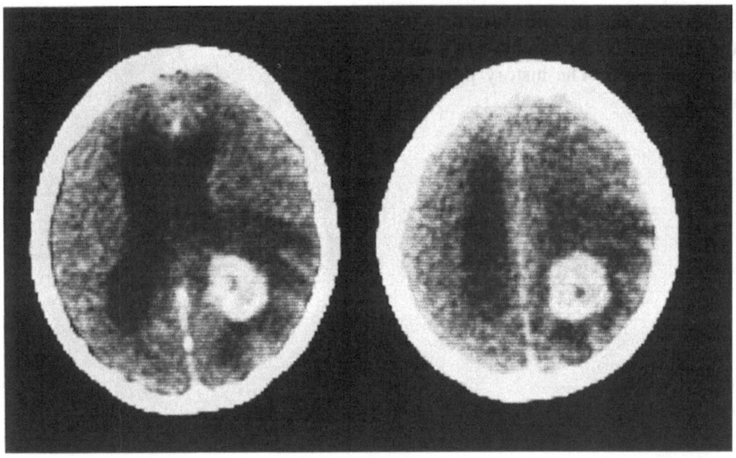

**Fig. D9.40.** Metastasis with strong contrast uptake in the right parietal region in a 55-year-old patient with uterine carcinoma. Central zone of necrosis. Pronounced hydrocephalus due to a second metastasis in the cerebellum

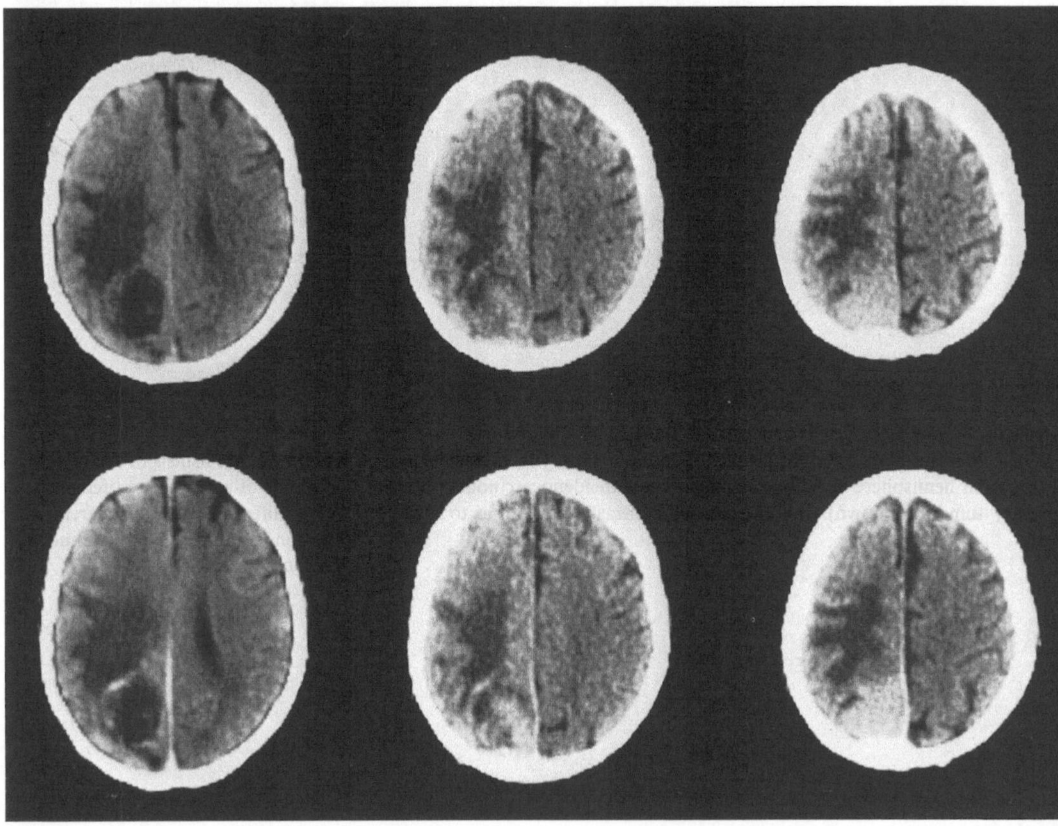

**Fig. D9.41.** Osteoplastic metastasis in a 68-year-old patient with prostatic carcinoma. The primary tumor had not been diagnosed at the time of the first CT study. Initial diagnosis of meningioma with marginal cyst (left) at the angle of the dura mater and the falx (cf. Figs. D2.17, D2.21). Hypodense values in the precontrast study (above) and significant thickening of the skull vault (right). Slight increase in density values after contrast enhancement (below)

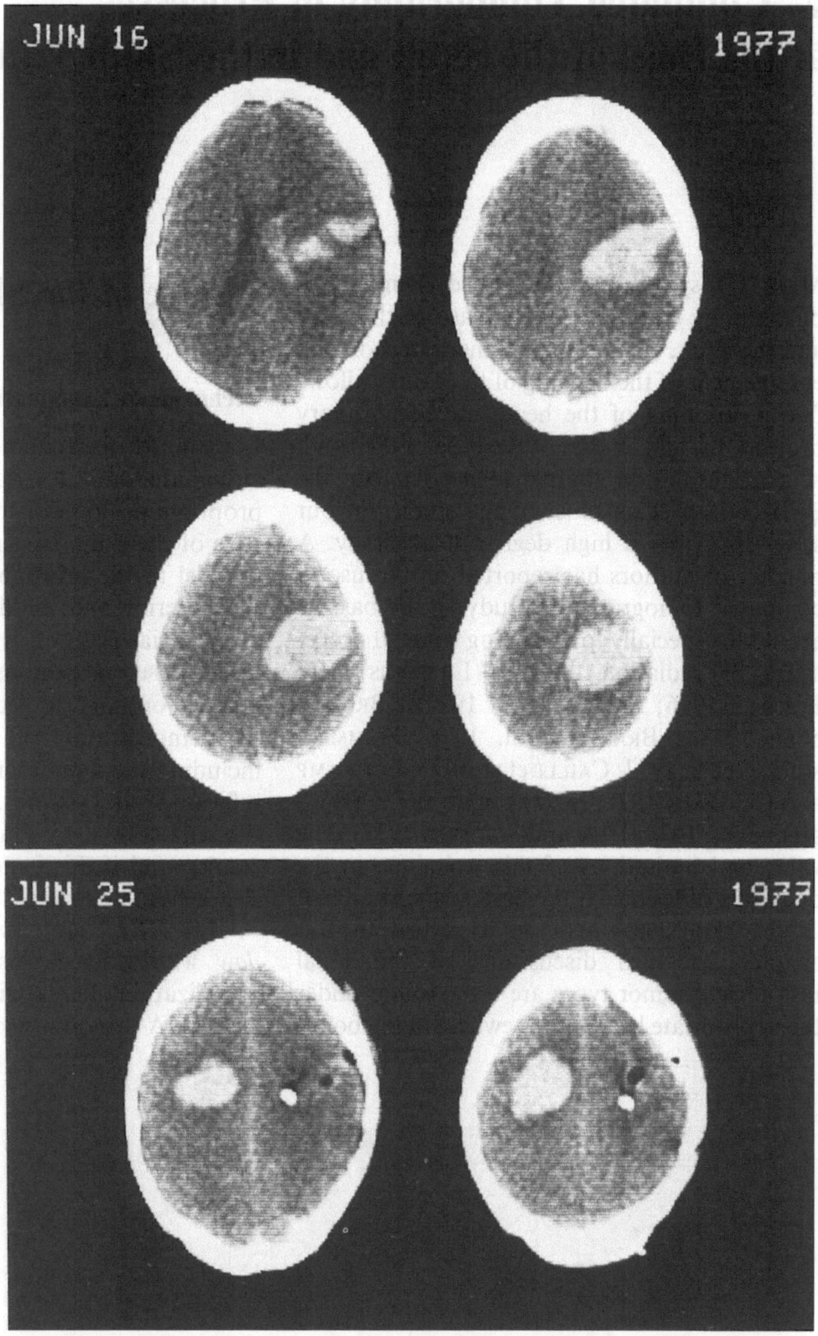


**Fig. D9.42.** Serial CT studies in a 37-year-old female with multiple intracranial metastases of choriocarcinoma. Admission to hospital on June 16 after acute onset of left hemiparesis and deterioration of the level of consciousness. Extensive hemorrhage in the white matter of the right hemisphere with penetration of the right lateral ventricle. Tissue removed from the margin of the hematoma at operation proved to be choriocarcinoma. Uneventful postoperative course until a sudden loss of consciousness accompanied by right hemiparesis supervened. CT study on June 25, 1977 with demonstration of a second metastasis, again with hemorrhage. The second lesion was not identifiable in the first CT examination, which did not include postcontrast studies. White speck in the region of initial tumor resection represents the tip of a silicon-rubber catheter implanted for external drainage of the lateral ventricle in order to prevent retention of CSF in the operative cavity

# E. Computed Tomography in Processes at the Base of the Skull and in the Skull Vault

Many CT systems allow detailed examination of the bony structures of the base of the skull and the vault. Elimination of the waterbox and enlargement of the opening of the gantry allows free positioning of the head, use of coronary projections, and studies of the base of the skull. A high-resolution matrix (320 × 320 for the EMI 5005 used in most of the studies in our series) provides a high degree of accuracy. A number of authors has reported on the use of computed tomography in studying the base of the skull, especially for planning surgical procedures or radiation therapy (LILIEQUIST and FORSELL 1976; BRADAC et al. 1977b; BRADAC et al. 1977c; BRADAC et al. 1978; HAMMERSCHLAG et al. 1977; CAILLÉ et al. 1977; LOHKAMP and CLAUSSEN 1977; BECKER et al. 1978; WEINSTEIN et al. 1978; HUK and SCHIEFER 1978). The value and limitations of this technique in the diagnosis of lesions at the base of the skull and in the skull vault will be described in this chapter. Detailed discussions of individual histological tumor types are to be found under the appropriate headings elsewhere in the book.

## 1. Base of the Skull

### Technique of Examination

Location of the pathological process and individual anatomical variations determine the appropriate position of the head in studies of the base of the skull. In general, slices are oriented parallel to the orbitomeatal line for studies of the anterior and middle cranial fossae, while a half-axial position with anteroflexion of the head is used in demonstration of the posterior fossa. Coronary projections are most suitable for demonstration of a number of structures including the lamina cribosa, the superior and inferior orbital fissures, the optic foramen, and the sella (Fig. E 1). Thin slices provide the best results, and if this is not possible, overlapping slices should be made.

*The CT picture is analyzed with a large window width,* since this permits simultaneous visualization of great differences in X-ray attenuation. A window width of at least 400 HU

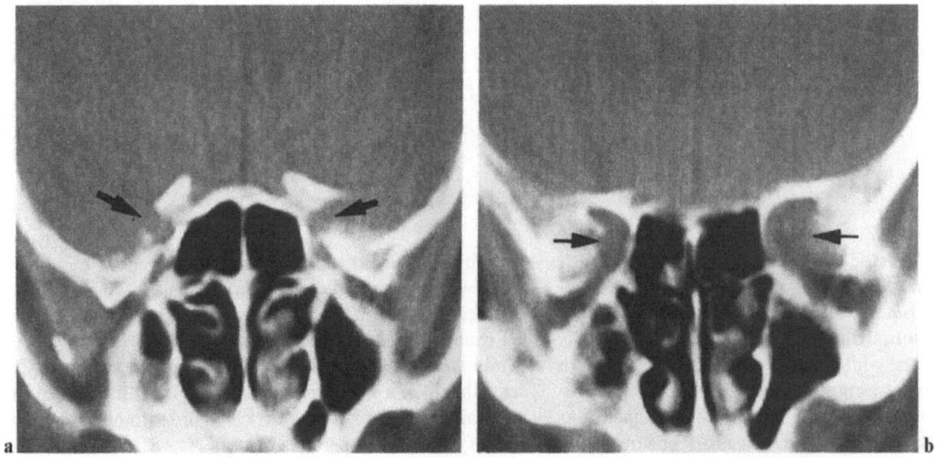

**Fig. E1** a, b. Normal findings in a coronary projection demonstrating the normal optic foramen (**a**, arrow) and the superior and inferior orbital fissures (**b**). The lateral border of the optic foramen is not visible since the foramen stands at a 45°-angle to the plane of the coronary projection

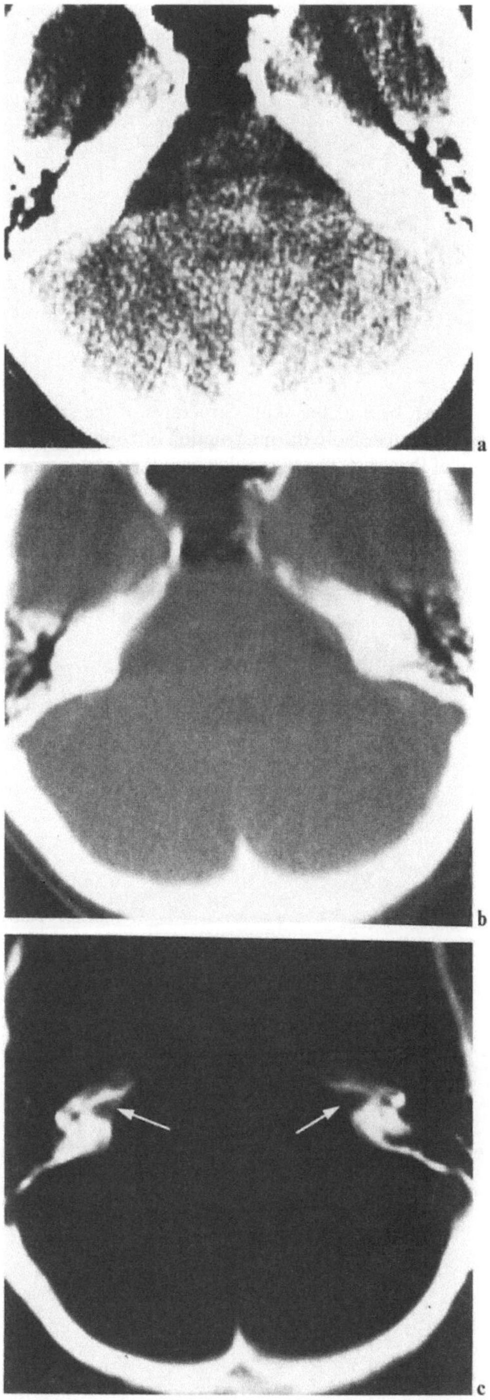

Fig. E2 a–c. Influence of window level on demonstration of various structures. (a) Demonstration of parenchyma with small window width. (b) Demonstration of bone structure with large window width (400 HU). (c) Demonstration of very dense bone without parenchyma with very high window level and the same window width as in b. Note the clear demonstration of the internal acoustic meatus, which is only visible with this setting (arrows)

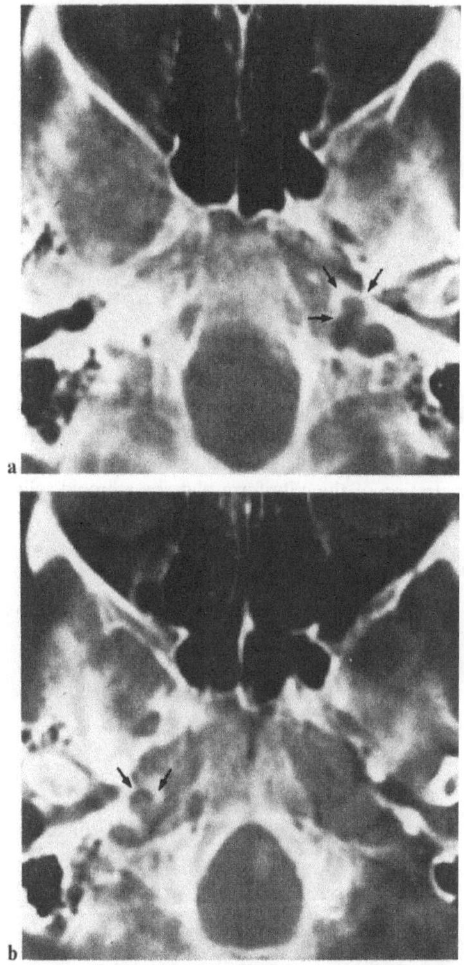

Fig. E3a, b. Example of asymmetrical demonstration of the jugular foramina related to head position: (a) Demonstration of the foramen on the right: the medial portion (arrows) appears distended. These findings are not pathological, since a lower slice (b) demonstrates that the foramen on the left is similar in appearance. Note that the crista is not as clearly demonstrated as on the right side. This is not necessarily pathological, as findings in another patient demonstrate (Fig. E6a)

has proven most suitable for this purpose. Window level is variable and a function of the density of the structures in question. Compact bone structures are demonstrated at very high window levels (Fig. E 2).

## Normal Structures of the Base of the Skull

The normal structures of the base of the skull are usually well visualized. Several slices with different head positions are necessary for com-

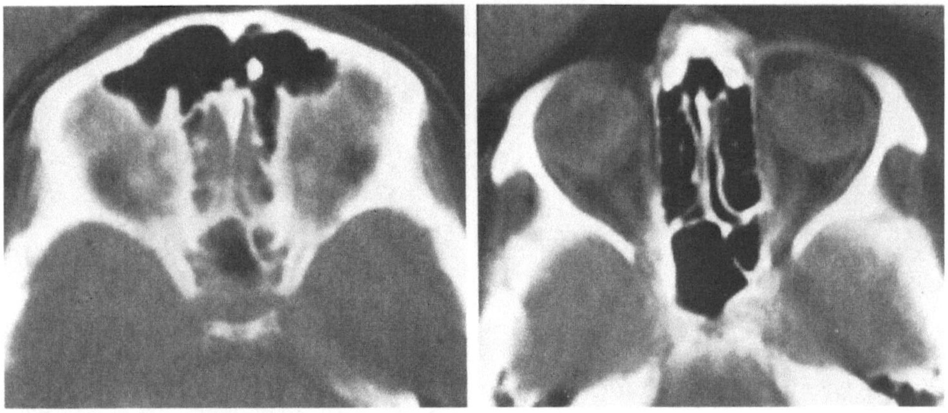

**Fig. E4.** Normal structures in the anterior cranial fossa. Clear demonstration of the roof of the orbit; the crista galli and the cribriform plate are visible in the midline; apparent penetration of the cribriform plate by ethmoid cells is due to the uneven base of the skull. Structures of the sella are well demonstrated. Note the interruption of bone structures at the tip of the orbit. The border between the optic foramen and the superior orbital fissure is not clearly visible

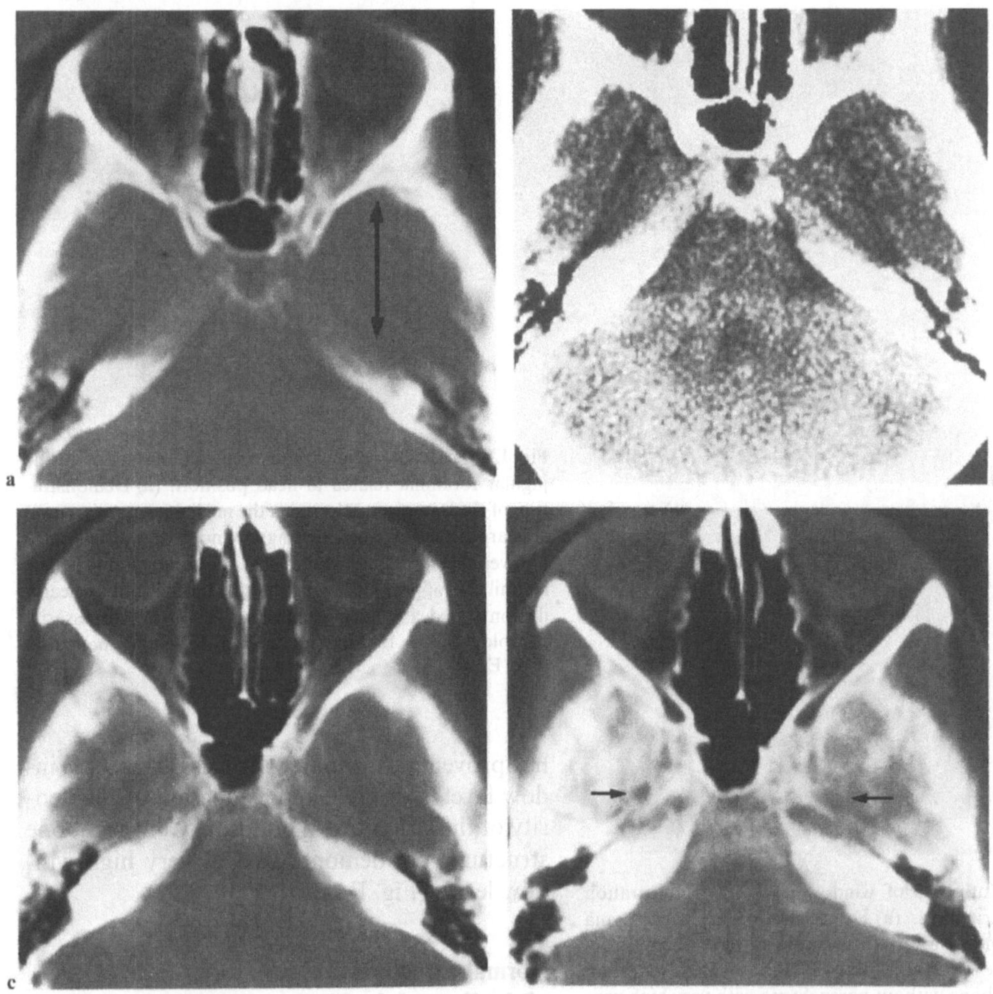

**Fig. E5a–d.** Demonstration of bone structures in the middle cranial fossa: **(a)** The sphenoid bone constitutes the rostral border, the pyramid (double arrow) the dorsal borders of the middle fossa. **(b)** The same slice is used for demonstration of soft tissue structures. **(c, d)** Lower slices demonstrate the bone structures of the middle fossa. Demonstration of the oval foramen bilaterally (arrows)

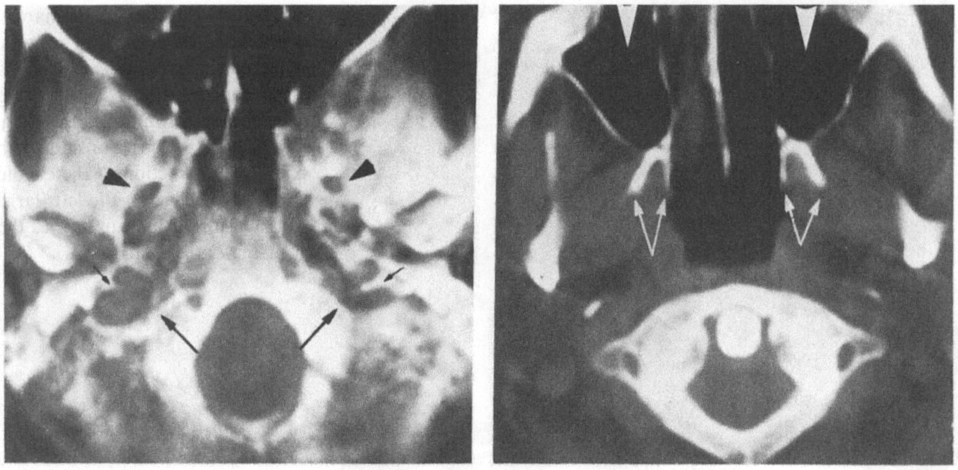

Fig. E6a, b. Structures of the base of the skull. (**a**) Base of the skull at the level of the middle and posterior fossae. Clear demonstration of the oval foramen (black arrow tips) and the jugular foramen with anatomical asymmetry (large arrows). Note the asymmetry of the crista separating the medial and lateral parts of the jugular foramen (small arrows). Foramen magnum in the middle. (**b**) Lower slice. The maxillary sinus (white arrow tips) is visible in the anterior portion. Pterygopalatine fossa between the lateral wall of the maxillary sinus and the lateral wall of the maxillary sinus and the lateral pterygoid process. Typical demonstration of the medial and lateral pterygoid processes (double arrows). Atlas and odontoid process visible in the posterior section

plete demonstration of all the structures at the base of the skull. This entails increased radiation exposure, which is a disadvantage of the method.

CT studies of the base of the skull often reveal a *certain degree of asymmetry in the structures at the base, though this is not necessarily a pathological finding,* since individual variation and as well as position of the patient's head produce such results (Fig. E 3). One must guard against misinterpretation of a normal anatomical variant as a pathological finding in analysis of such CT pictures. This is especially true when the structure in question is located in the area of the presumed lesion – for instance in evaluation of the internal auditory canal in cases of suspected acoustic neurinoma. Variation in appearance of bone structures at different settings of window width and level is caused by the fact that the auditory canal is incompletely or irregularly surrounded by bone structures in certain slices. This is due to the partial volume effect in most cases and may lead to misinterpretation (BROOKS and DICHIRO 1976).

Figures E 4–6 are additional examples of normal findings of the structures at the base of the skull.

# Pathological Findings

Pathological alterations in structures of the base of the skull are found in a number of different processes. Practical considerations suggest the following classification.

## a) Intracranial Space-Occupying Lesions Involving the Base of the Skull

Pituitary adenomas, perisellar meningiomas, trigeminal neurinomas, acoustic neurinomas, cerebellopontine angle meningiomas, glomus tumors, chondromas, chordomas, infraclinoidal giant aneurysms, gliomas, and craniopharyngiomas.

These lesions resulted in one or more of the following pathological findings in the CT scan in almost all of our patients:

**Bone destruction;**

**Deformation of structures of the skull base** – enlargement of the sella or of foramina;

**Extension to neighboring cavities** – to the sphenoid sinus in sellar tumors, for example;

**Hyperostosis or sclerosis** (only found in meningioma).

These four types of pathological findings may be observed singly or in various combinations. Figures E 7–13 provide typical examples.

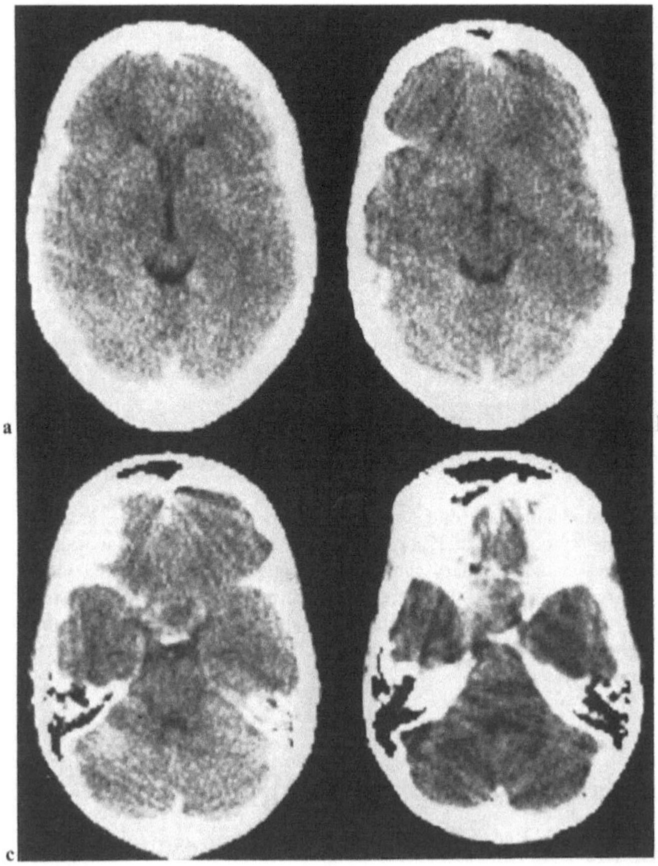

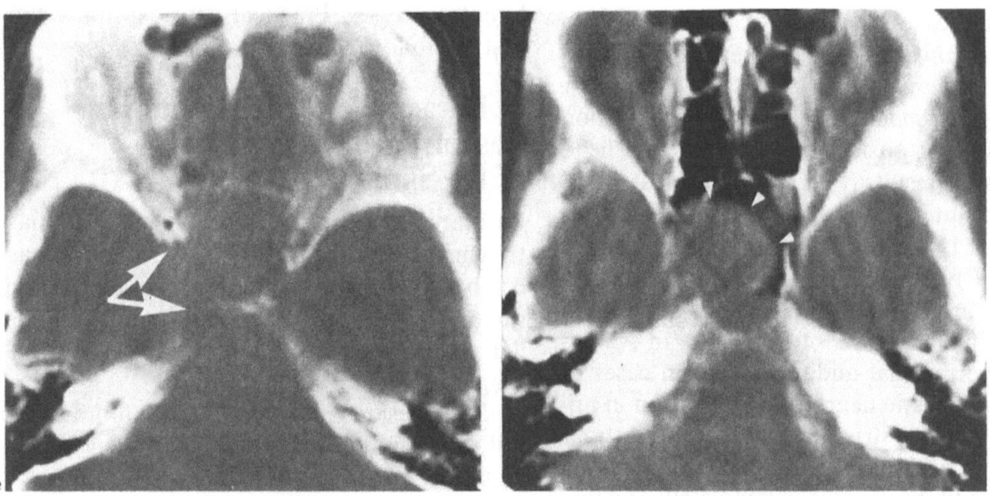

**Fig. E7** a–f. Pituitary adenoma with some suprasellar extension and major penetration of the sphenoid sinus. (**a–d**) Ventricular system normal. Slight contrast uptake in a suprasellar and intrasellar tumor, more pronounced on the left. (**e, f**) CT study of the structures at the base of the skull. (**e**) Destruction of the clinoid process and the dorsum sellae on the left (large arrows). (**f**) Extension of the tumor into the sphenoid sinus (small arrow tips)

A few observations of *bone destruction* are noteworthy. In some cases, bone destruction was more extensive than the tumor itself appeared to be; the destruction demonstrated the true size of the lesion (Fig. E 14).

Evidence of bone destruction was absent in the CT scan in one case in which such changes would have been expected. Conventional tomographic studies demonstrated destruction at the apex of the petrous bone, although CT findings were normal. The tumor was a small meningioma at the apex with limited extension to the cerebellopontine angle. Angiographic studies also revealed pathological findings in this case (Fig. E 15).

Bone destruction constituted the only

pathological CT finding in a few cases of glomus tumor. (Figs. E 16, 17).

Problems in diagnosis of *small tumors at the cerebellopontine angle* are discussed in Chap. D 3, but a few additional remarks are in order. It is usually not possible to demonstrate small neurinomas directly (DAVID et al. 1976; KAZNER et al. 1976; BRADAC et al. 1977a), though widening of the internal meatus often provides indirect evidence of the tumor (HATAM et al. 1979; Fig. E18). This finding should be confirmed by conventional tomographic studies. *Questionable CT findings of a widened internal auditory canal have no diagnostic value if they are not confirmed by conventional radiological studies* (see also the section on normal structures of the skull base).

It should be emphasized that other small tumors were demonstrated only by means of conventional neuroradiological techniques such as angiography and pneumoencephalography (BRADAC et al. 1977a; Fig. E17). In fact, direct demonstration of such tumors in the CT scan was not possible until very recently. SORTLAND made a major contribution to the solution of this diagnostic problem when he introduced combined air cisternography and computed tomography in 1978. A detailed description of the procedure is to be found in Chap. D3 on p. 258 and 265ff.

*Diagnosis of purely intrasellar pituitary adenomas* is discussed in detail in another section of the book (see Chap. D4, p. 272). It is sometimes possible to demonstrate intrasellar adenomas directly in the CT scan if the tumors are large enough (Fig. E19). However, diagnosis is also possible on the basis of alterations in bone structures, although it must be borne in mind that not every enlargement of the sella implies the presence of an intrasellar tumor (cf. empty sella p. 272 and 283).

Bone destruction caused by large infraclinoidal aneurysms is virtually identical to that caused by neoplasms (Fig. E20).

## b) Metastases in the Base of the Skull

CT findings in patients with metastases at the base of the skull were unequivocal in our cases. *Bone destruction* was easily recognized in the CT scan, and *sclerosis of adjacent bone* was observed in some cases. Unexpected bone metas-

(Continuation see p. 394)

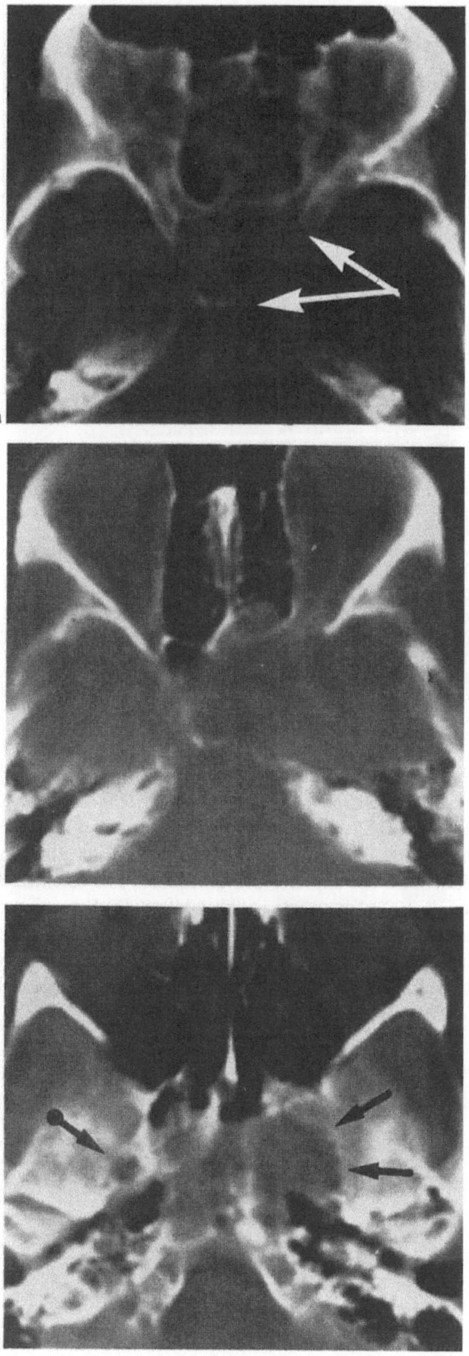

a b c

**Fig. E8a–c.** Intrasellar and parasellar pituitary adenoma. (**a**) Destruction of the right sphenoid process and the dorsum sellae (double arrow). (**b**) Extension of the tumor to the sphenoid sinus. (**c**) Destruction of parasellar bone structures on the right (black arrows). The oval foramen is not demonstrated on the right but is clearly visible on the left (black arrow with dot)

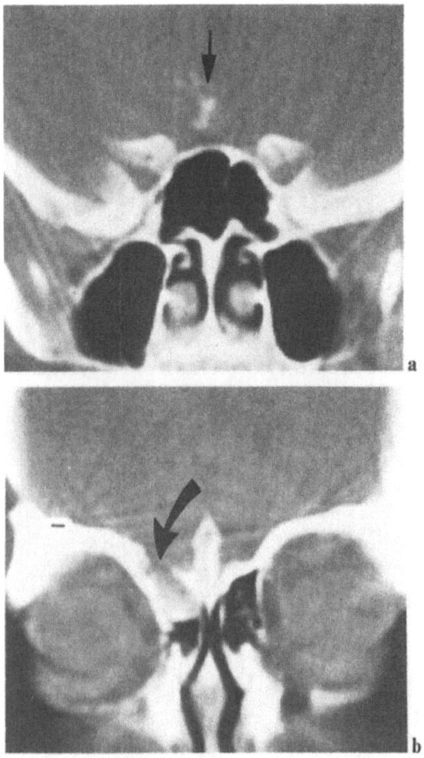

Fig. E9a, b. Destruction of the skull base in the anterior fossa by recurrence of craniopharyngioma. Coronary projection. (a) Slice at the level of the sphenoid plane; note the normal appearance of the clinoid processes, the sphenoid plane, and the superior orbital fissure. The calcified tumor (small arrow) is visible in the midline. (b) Extension of the tumor in the rostral direction with destruction of the cribriform plate and penetration of the ethmoid cells (large arrow). Partial destruction of the medial wall of the orbit

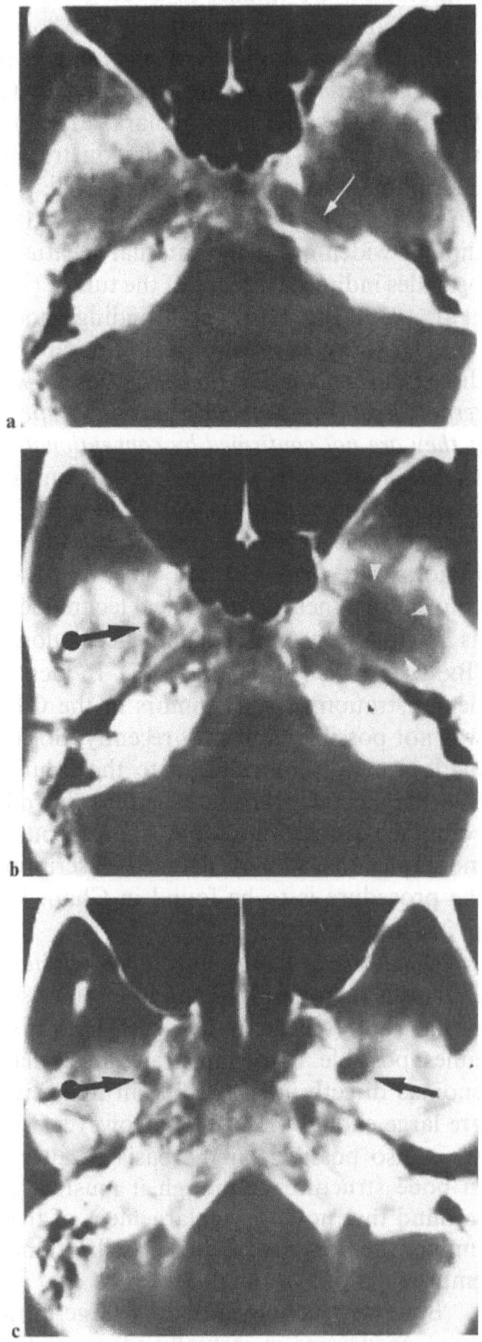

Fig. E10a–c. Trigeminal neurinoma on the right. (a) Destruction of the anterior edge of the pyramid. (b) Major widening of the right oval foramen (small arrow tips). Note the normal oval foramen on the left (black arrow with dot). (c) A slice 6 mm lower than (b) shows that the oval foramen is not as wide as in (b) since the tumor ends with a conic portion at the level of the foramen

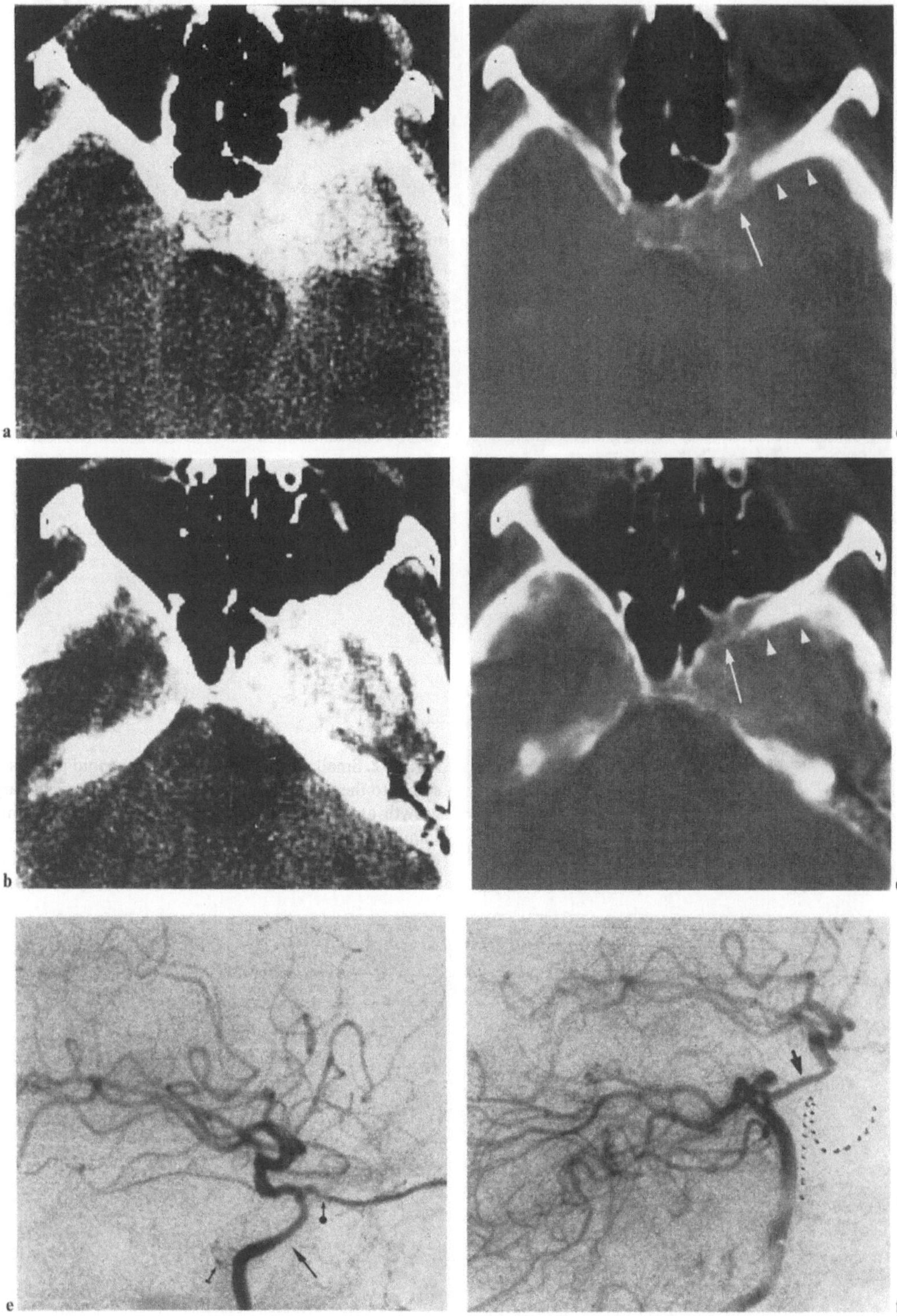

**Fig. E11** a–f. Large parasellar meningioma on the right. (**a**, **b**) Demonstration of the tumor after contrast enhancement. (**c**, **d**) Demonstration of bone structures with destruction of the clinoid process and the tip of the right orbit (arrow). Hyperostosis of the sphenoid wing (arrow tips). (**e**) The carotid angiogram demonstrates narrowing of the internal carotid artery (large arrow) as well as of the ophthalmic artery (arrow with dot). Note the pathological vessels (small arrow with bar) (**f**) Vertebral angiogram with demonstration of the internal carotid circulation fed by the posterior communicating artery (large arrow). The collateral circulation between the vertebral and carotid arteries is the result of stenosis in the internal carotid artery caused by the tumor

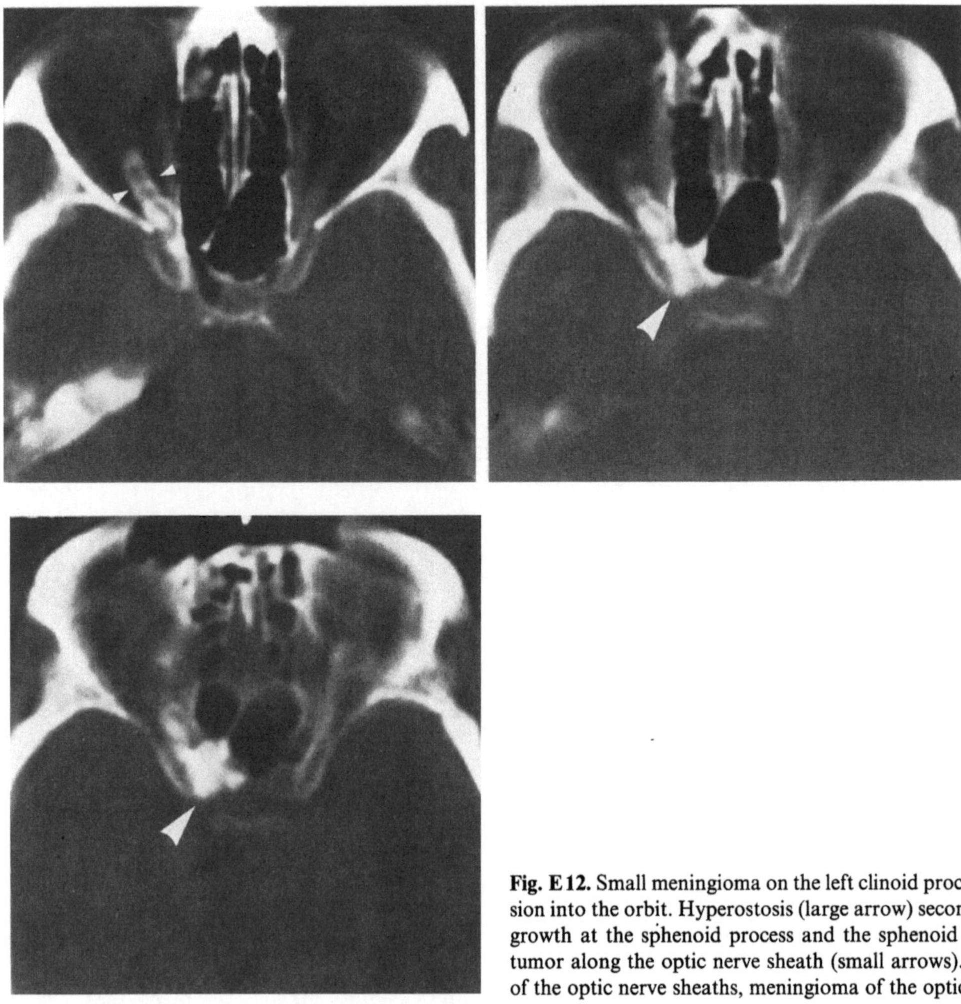

**Fig. E 12.** Small meningioma on the left clinoid process with extension into the orbit. Hyperostosis (large arrow) secondary to tumor growth at the sphenoid process and the sphenoid sinus. Cuff of tumor along the optic nerve sheath (small arrows). (Meningioma of the optic nerve sheaths, meningioma of the optic foramen)

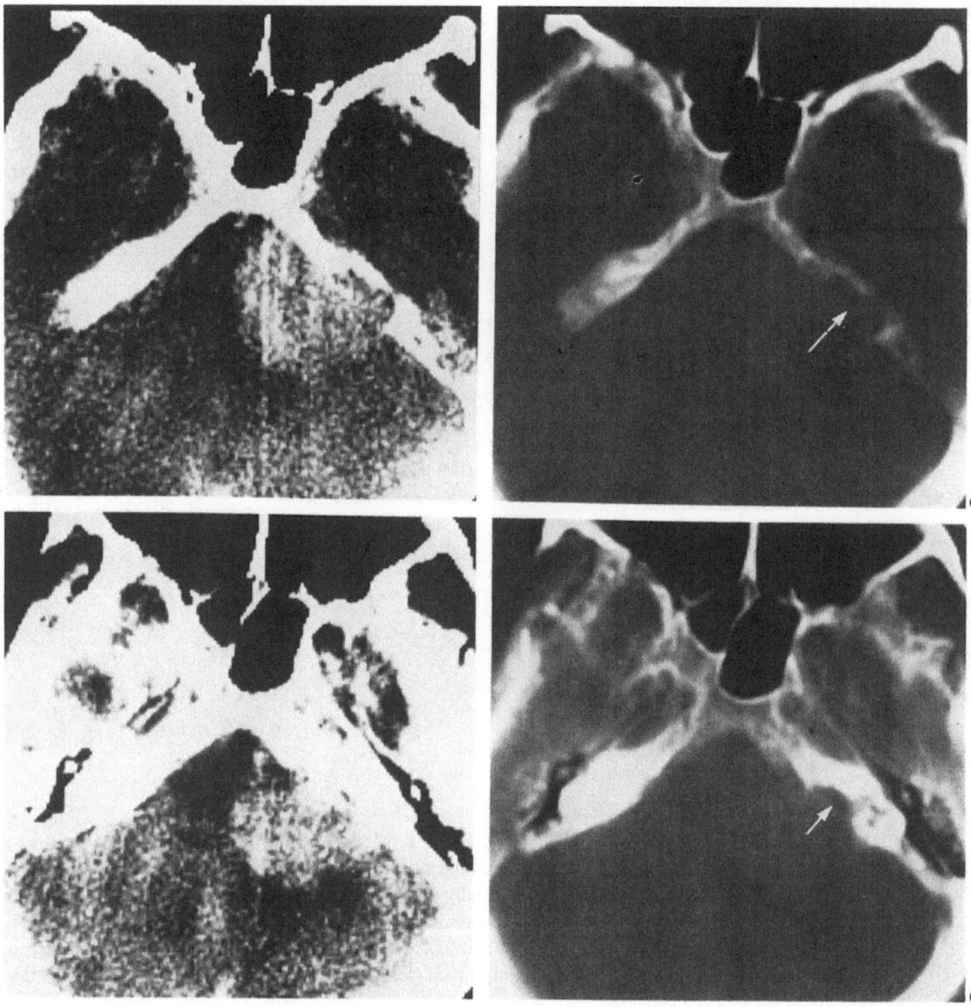

**Fig. E13**a–d. Acoustic neurinoma on the right. (**a, b**) Direct demonstration of the tumor after contrast enhancement. (**c, d**) The same slices at different window settings with demonstration of the pyramids. Destruction of the right pyramid is evident

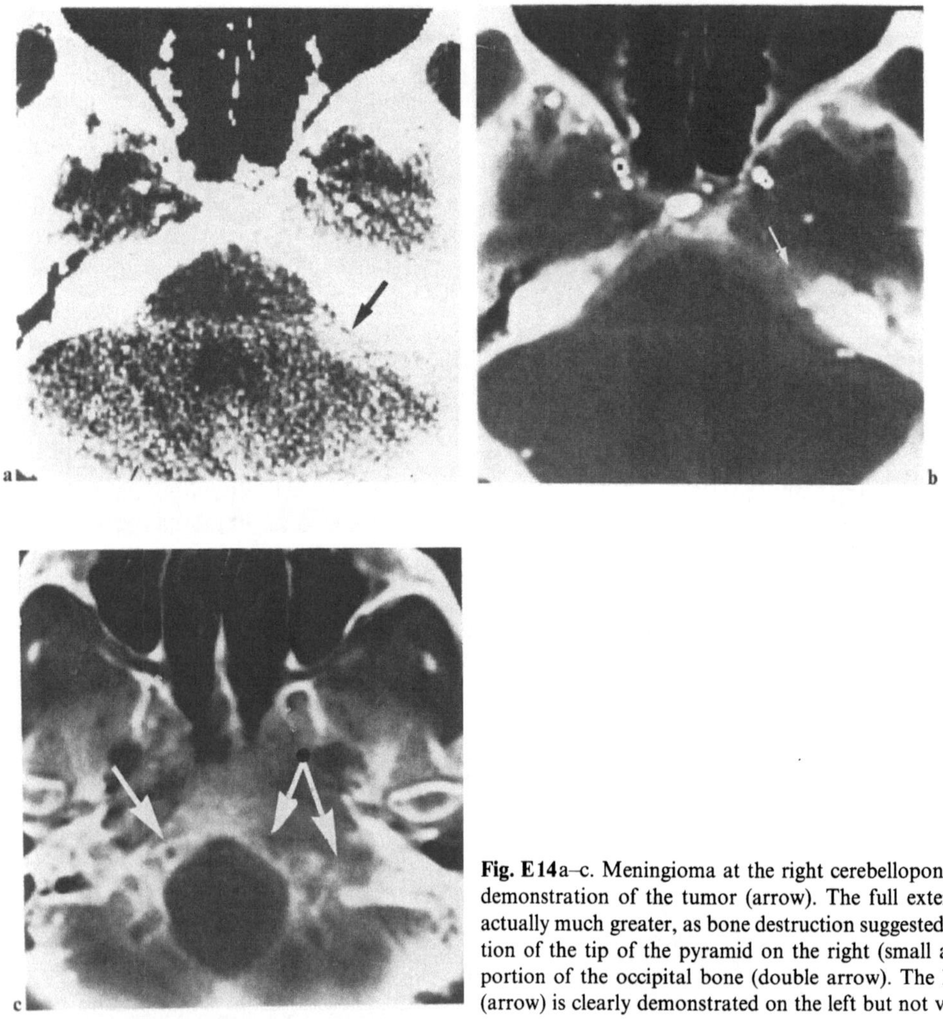

**Fig. E14a–c.** Meningioma at the right cerebellopontine angle. (**a**) Direct demonstration of the tumor (arrow). The full extent of the tumor was actually much greater, as bone destruction suggested. (**b, c**) Total destruction of the tip of the pyramid on the right (small arrow) and the basal portion of the occipital bone (double arrow). The hypoglossal foramen (arrow) is clearly demonstrated on the left but not visible on the right

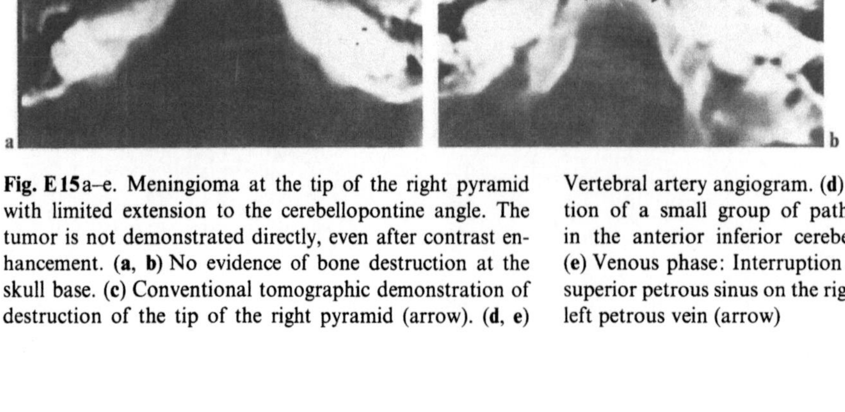

**Fig. E15a–e.** Meningioma at the tip of the right pyramid with limited extension to the cerebellopontine angle. The tumor is not demonstrated directly, even after contrast enhancement. (**a, b**) No evidence of bone destruction at the skull base. (**c**) Conventional tomographic demonstration of destruction of the tip of the right pyramid (arrow). (**d, e**) Vertebral artery angiogram. (**d**) Arterial phase: Demonstration of a small group of pathological vessels originating in the anterior inferior cerebellar artery (small arrows). (**e**) Venous phase: Interruption of the petrous vein and the superior petrous sinus on the right (arrow with bar). Normal left petrous vein (arrow)

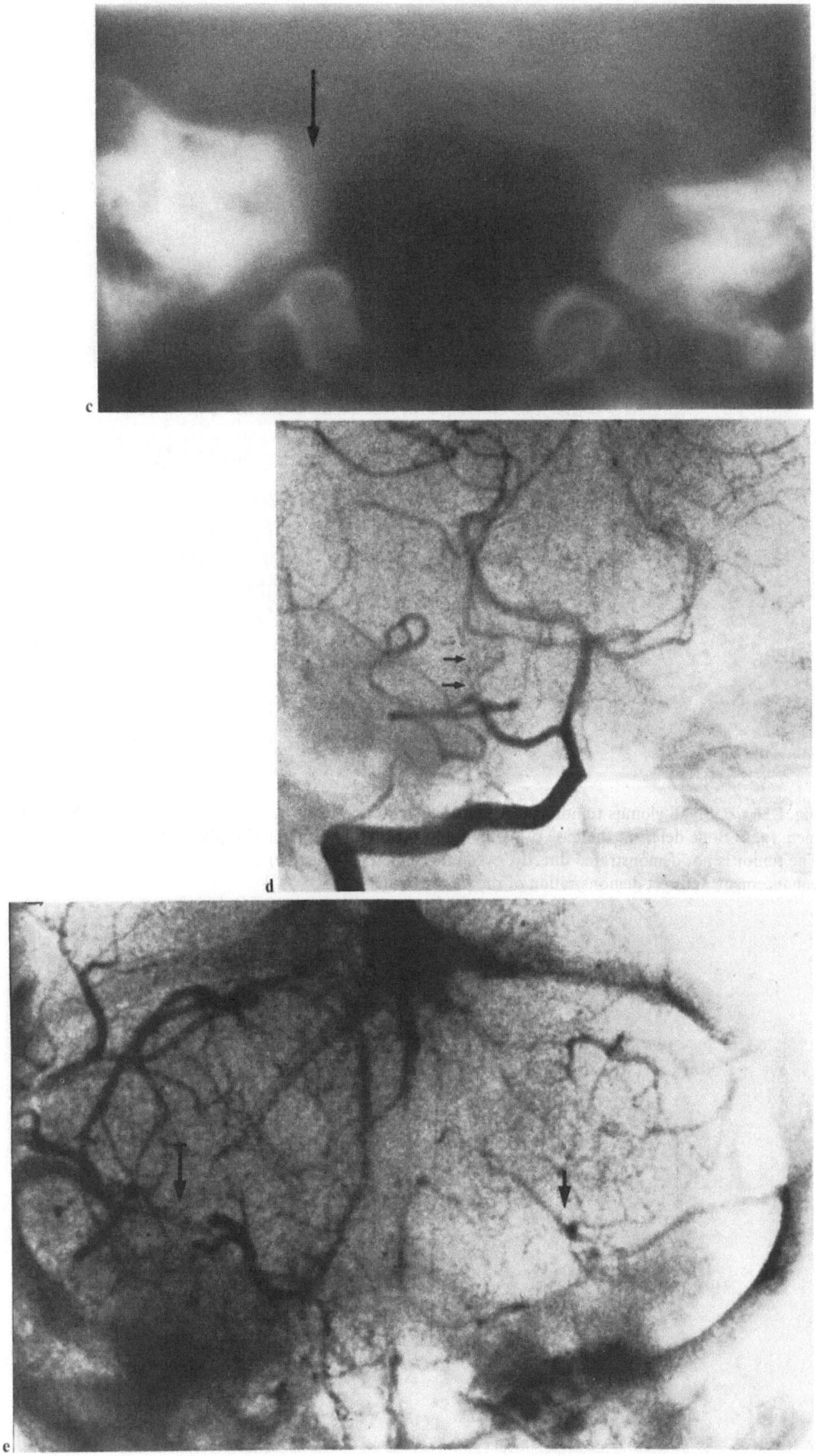
c
d
e

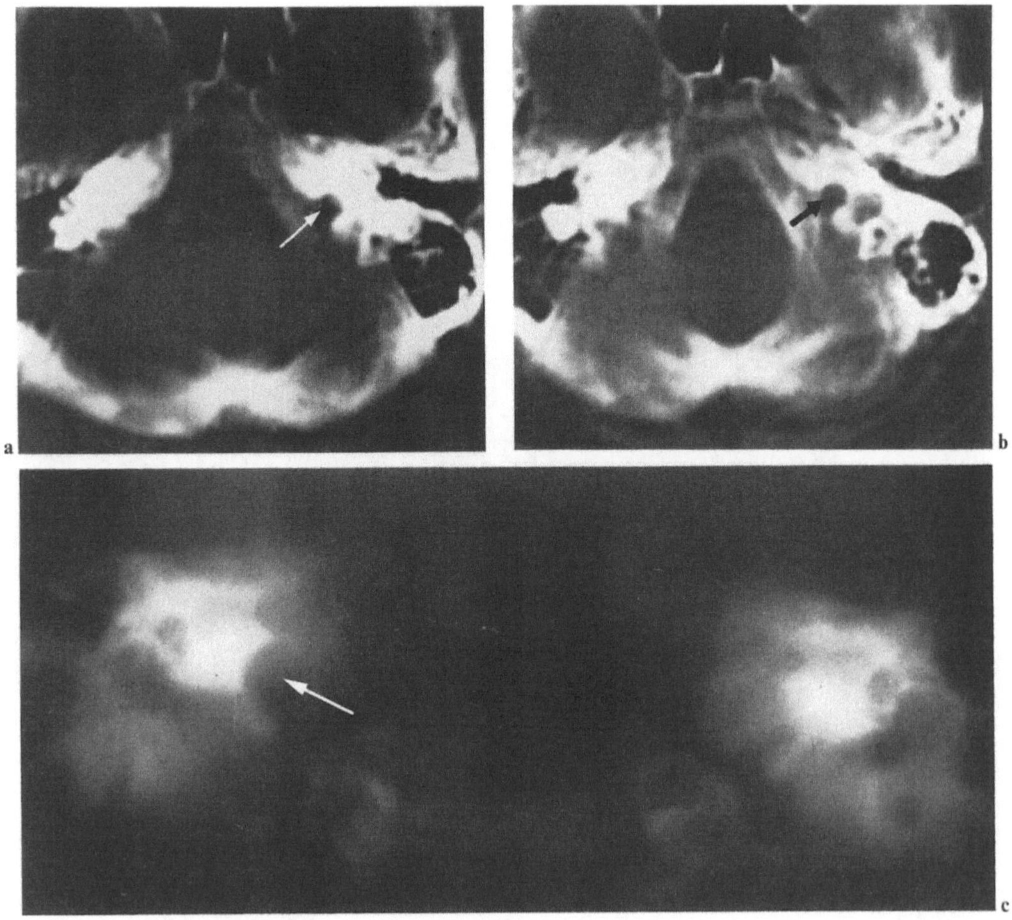


**Fig. E16** a–c. Small glomus tumor at the right jugular foramen. (**a**, **b**) Bone defect at the base of the pyramid (arrow). The tumor is not demonstrated directly, even after contrast enhancement. Indirect demonstration of the tumor by bone destruction. (**c**) Conventional X-ray tomography demonstrates a sharply delineated defect at the base of the pyramid (arrow)

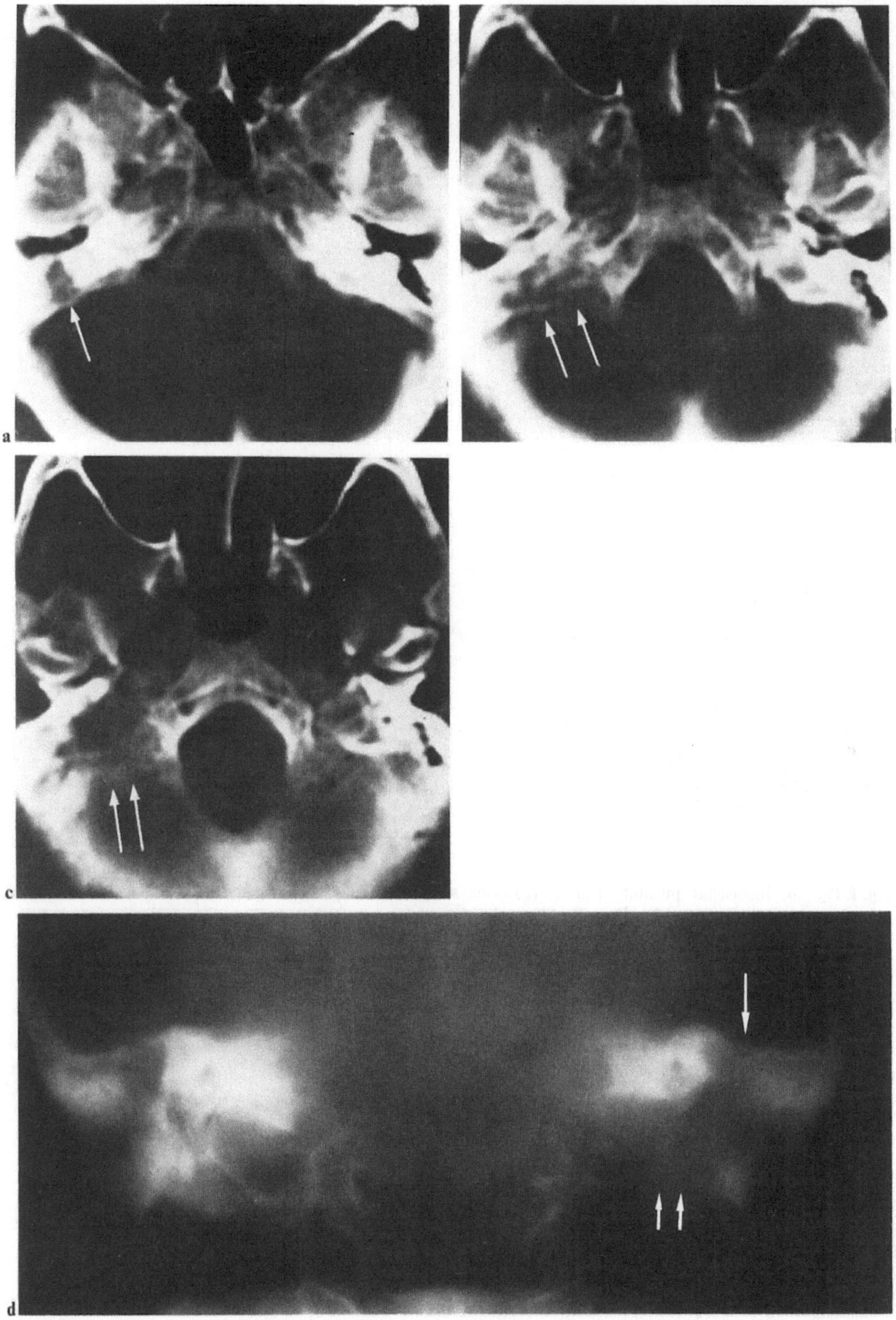

**Fig. E17**a–d. Glomus tumor at the left jugular foramen. The tumor demonstrates rostral extension into the pyramid (**a**) as well as lateral and dorsal extension with destruction of the pyramid and the occipital bone (**b**, **c**). The tumor is not demonstrated directly, even after contrast enhancement. (**d**) Conventional tomographic demonstration of bone destruction at the jugular foramen (two arrows) with extension of the tumor into the pyramid (arrow)

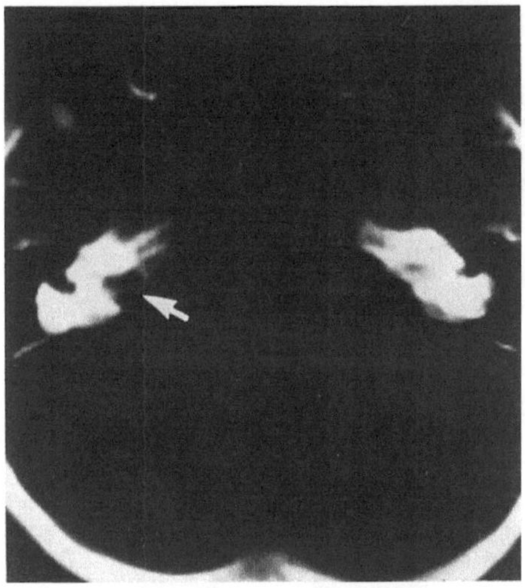

**Fig. E18.** Small intracanalicular acoustic neurinoma. The tumor itself is not demonstrated in CT studies. Asymmetry of the internal acoustic meatus, with dilatation on the left (arrow). Demonstration of a widened pore in conventional tomographic studies

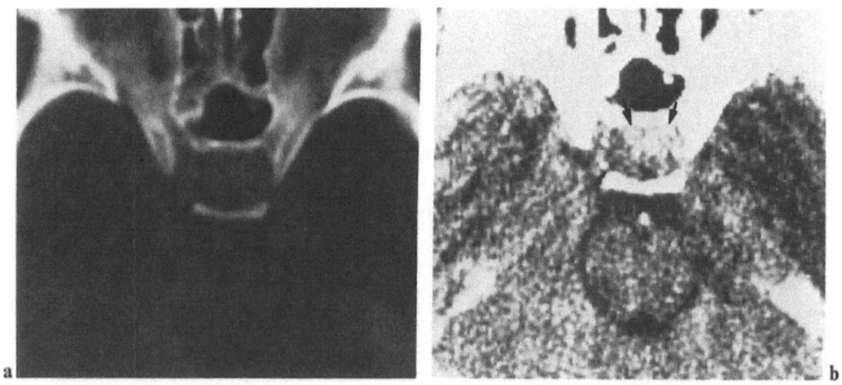

**Fig. E19a, b.** Intrasellar pituitary tumor. (**a**) Bone structures: Slight enlargement of the sella. (**b**) The tumor appears as a hyperdense structure within the sella after contrast enhancement (arrows)

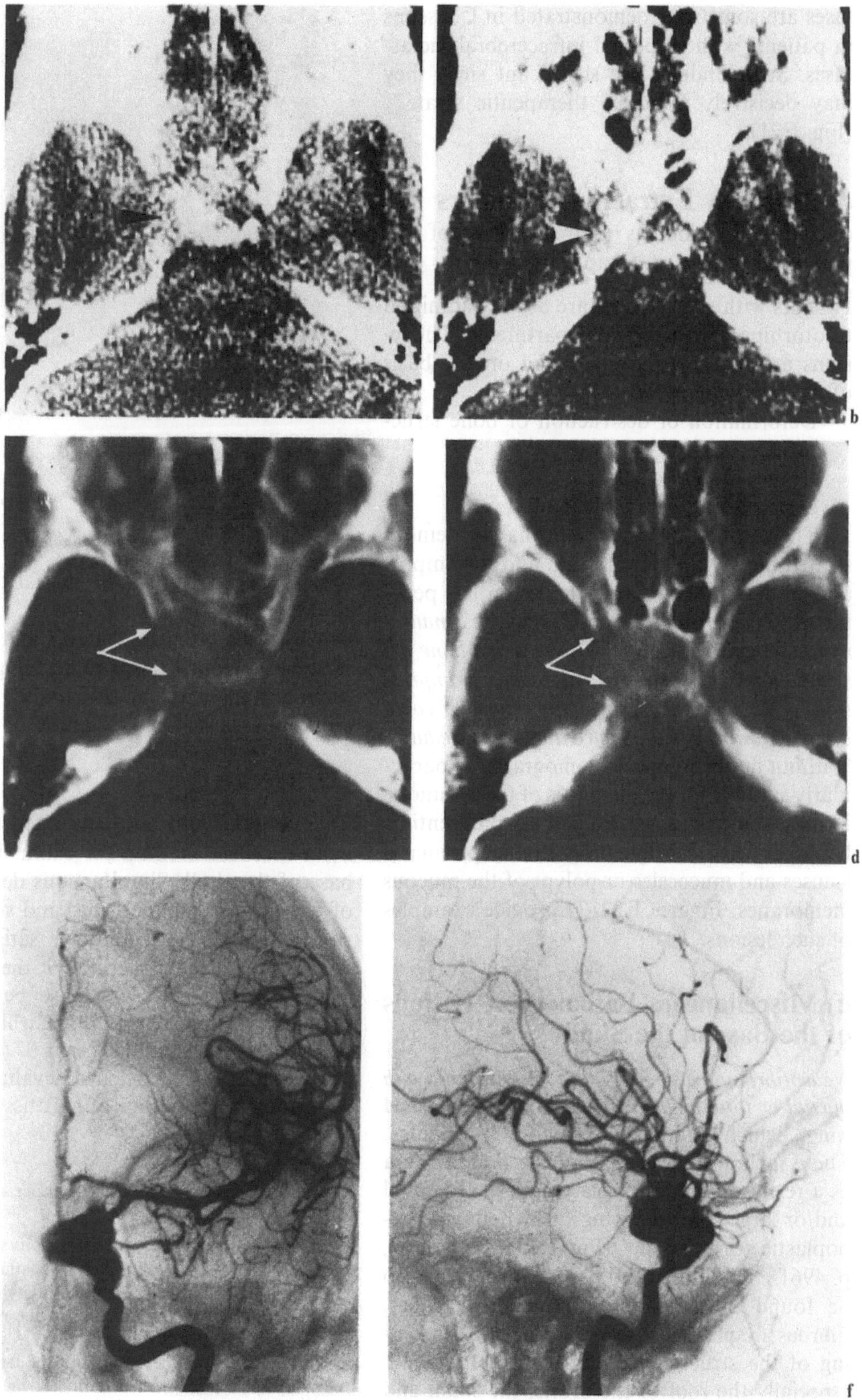

**Fig. E20** a–f. Large aneurysm of the infraclinoidal segment of the left carotid artery. (**a**, **b**) Hyperdense zone within the sella and in the parasellar region (arrow). (**c**, **d**) Partial destruction of the clinoid process and the dorsum sellae on the left (arrows). (**e**, **f**) Carotid angiogram

tases are sometimes demonstrated in CT scans in patients with suspected intracerebral metastases. Such findings are significant since they may decisively influence therapeutic strategy (Fig. E21).

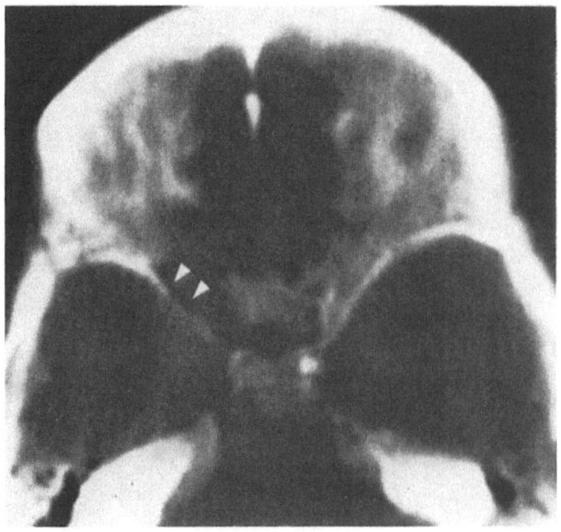

**Fig. E21.** Destruction of the left sphenoid wing by metastasis of breast cancer (arrow tips)

## c) Primarily Extracranial Tumors

(including carcinomas and sarcomas of the paranasal sinuses, cf. Chap. D8, p. 342)

Patients with such tumors are usually admitted to otorhinolaryngological departments. The lesions are most easily recognized on the basis of the following indirect signs:

Deformation or destruction of bone structures;

Obliteration of cavities;

Sclerosis of adjacent structures.

The soft tissue of the tumor may be demonstrated directly in the CT scan, and it is important to determine whether the lesion has penetrated to the orbit or the cranial cavity. *Simultaneous demonstration of soft tissues and bone destruction provides a more comprehensive impression of the extent of the tumor than one could otherwise attain with conventional procedures.* Without doubt computed tomography is particularly suitable for the diagnosis of these tumors. It may sometimes be difficult to differentiate between tumors originating in the paranasal sinuses and mucoceles or polyps of the mucous membranes. Figures E22–24 provide examples of such lesions.

## d) Miscellaneous Pathological Lesions of the Base of the Skull

*Neurofibromatosis may be associated with partial or total unilateral* **aplasia of the sphenoid wing,** which produces typical CT findings. These include enlargement of the middle fossa as a result of ventral displacement of the small and/or large sphenoid wings, which may be hypoplastic or aplastic (Fig. E25, Fig. G44, p. 496f.). Additional soft tissue lesions may also be found in the face and the facial bones. **Fibrous dysplasia** causes considerable thickening of the structures at the base of the skull, especially the roof of the orbits, the small and large sphenoid wings, and base of the middle cranial fossa. This may result in compression and displacement of orbital structures as well as narrowing of the foramina at the base of the skull (Fig. E26). Differential diagnosis includes other extracranial tumors, though these usually cause bone destruction, and osteoplastic meningiomas of the sphenoid wing, which are often accompanied by soft tissue tumor in the adjacent areas (Figs. E27 and G4, p. 468).

*Conclusions*

There is no doubt that computed tomography is an excellent method for examination of the base of the skull. Simultaneous demonstration of bone, brain parenchyma, and soft tissue lesions is possible. Technically satisfactory CT studies depict the structures of the base of the skull. Some of the latter are better demonstrated in coronary projections, while others appear best in horizontal slices.

CT studies are particularly valuable in demonstrating the presence of soft tissue lesions in

---

▶

**Fig. E22a–c.** Carcinoma of the nasal cavity with penetration of the maxillary sinus and the pterygopalatine fossa. (**a**) Penetration of the tumor from the nasal cavity to the maxillary sinus on the left with destruction of the medial wall and partial destruction of the lateral wall (arrow). (**b**) One slice (5 mm) higher: Total destruction of the lateral wall of the maxillary sinus (arrow). Penetration of the tumor into the sphenoid sinus. (**c**) Increased density values in the ethmoid cells on the left (arrow with dot) and in the wall of the upper part of the sphenoid sinus (small arrow). These findings are probably not directly related to the tumor but result from swelling of the mucous membranes

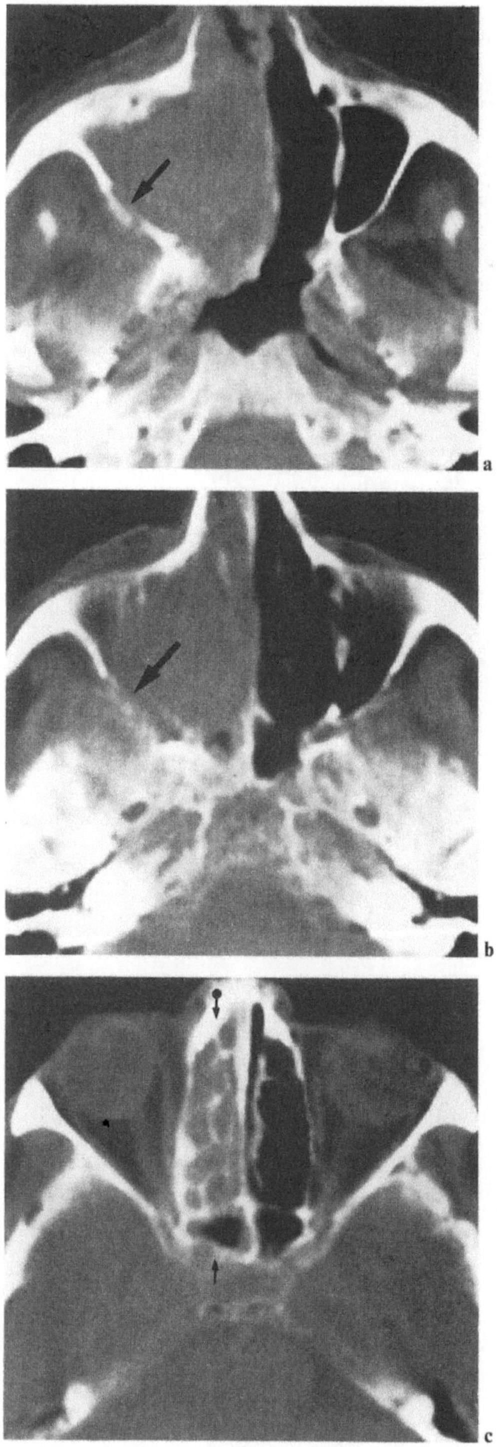

Fig. E 22

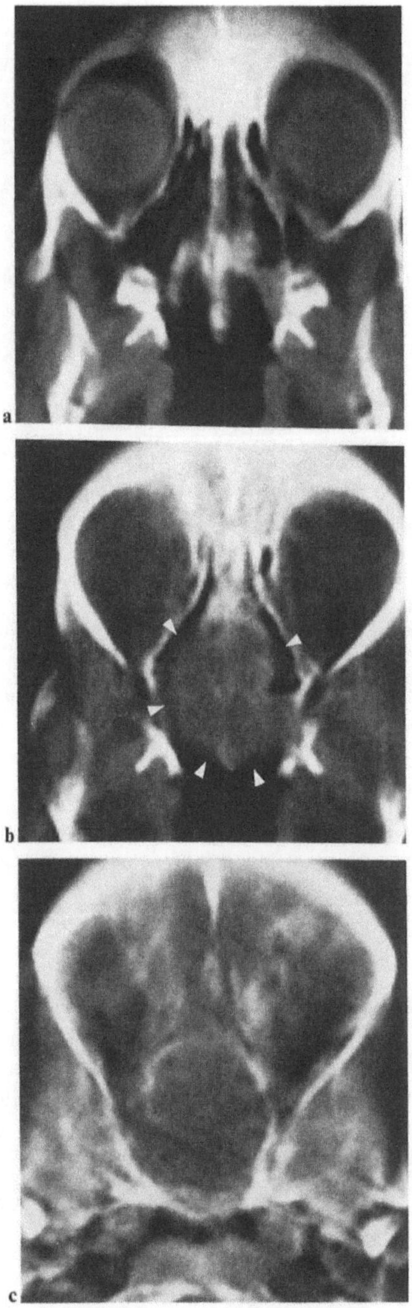

**Fig. E23** a–c. Rhabdomyosarcoma of the nasopharynx. **(a)** CT scan at the level of the caudal nasopharynx with normal findings. (Anteflexion of the head) **(b)** The nasopharynx is completely filled with tumor (arrow tips). Destruction of the vomer. **(c)** Extension of the tumor to the anterior fossa

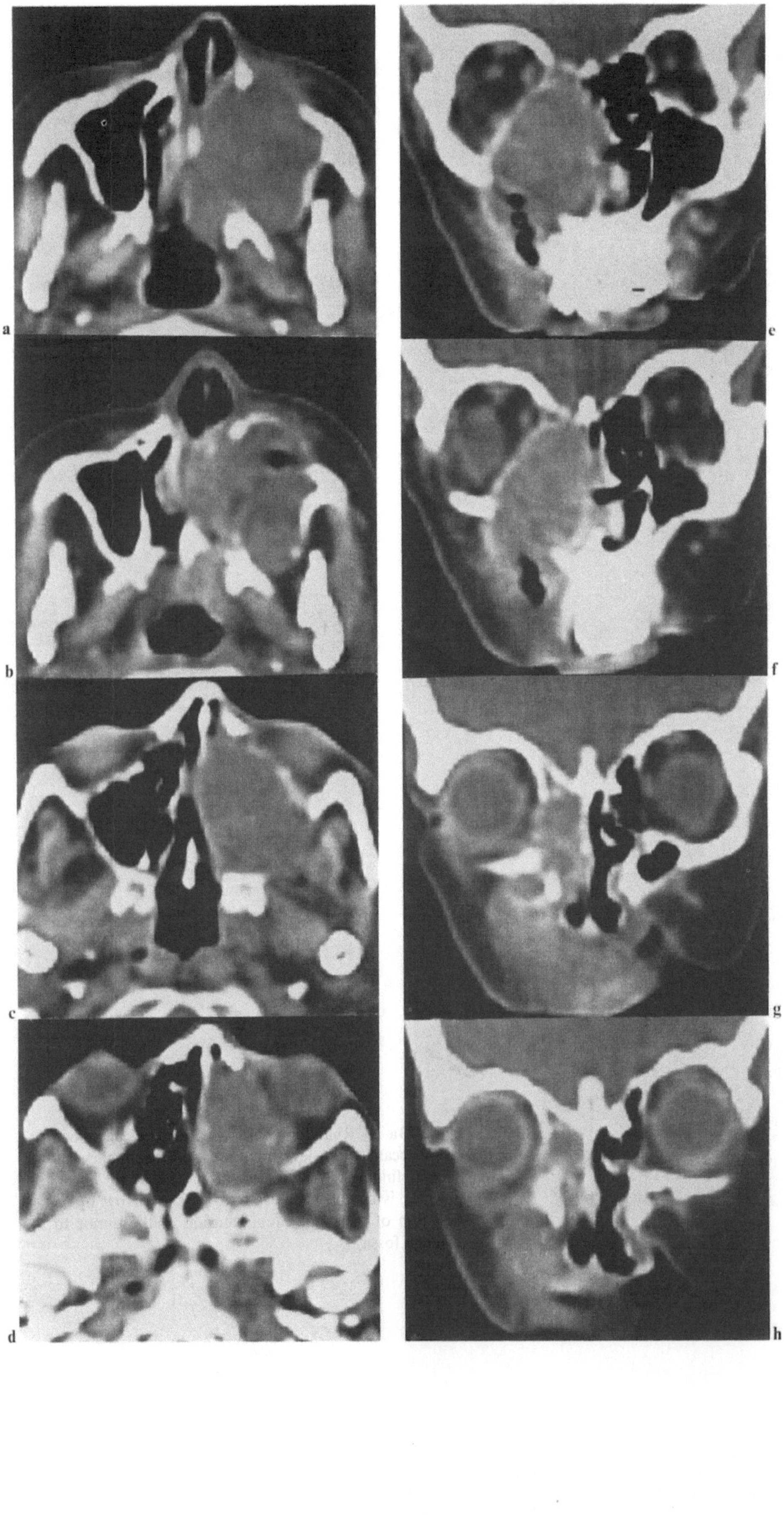
a
b
c
d
e
f
g
h

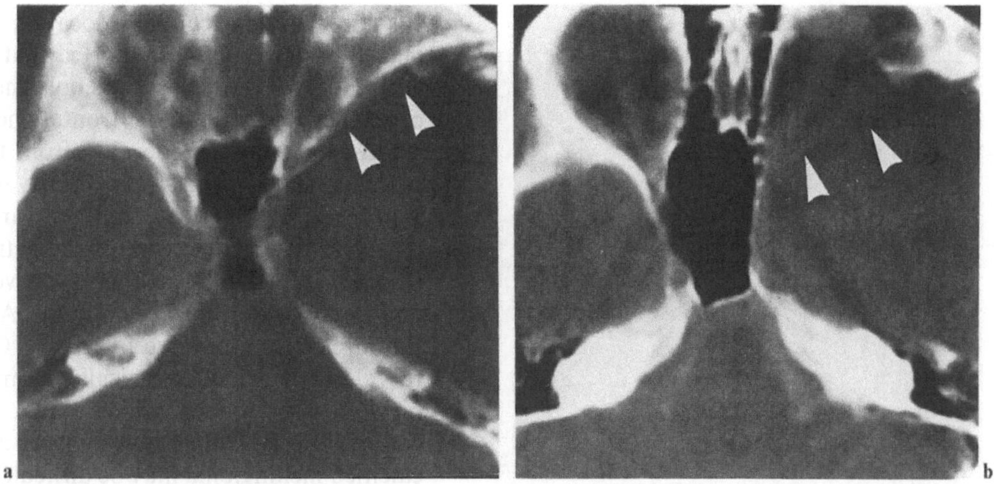

Fig. E25a, b. Neurofibromatosis. (a) Enlargement of the middle fossa on the right resulting from anterior displacement of the lesser sphenoid wing (arrows). (b) Aplasia of the greater sphenoid wing on the right (arrows)

association with changes of bone structures. In addition, computed tomography shows the structures at the base of the skull and their pathology in a completely new dimension.

Small tumors in or near the base of the skull may escape detection in the CT scan. Demonstration of bone destruction is therefore extremely important for diagnosis in these cases. Bone destruction may be the only pathological CT finding in some larger tumors not directly visible in the CT scan. Special techniques are necessary in these cases.

*Computed tomography and conventional tomographic studies are complementary.* The advantages of computed tomography are evident; however, at present fine detail in bone structures is best revealed with conventional tomography, especially since small defects may escape detection in the CT scan. However, new CT systems with even better resolution will probably allow demonstration and analysis of very small bone defects. CT studies will then attain or surpass the accuracy of conventional X-ray tomography.

◄ Fig. E24a–h. Cylindroma in the right maxillary sinus of a 58-year-old female. Horizontal projections show that the right maxillary sinus is entirely filled with tumor. Destruction of the walls of the maxillary sinus. Penetration of the tumor into the right nasal cavity, the epipharynx, and the right orbit (a–d). Coronary projections demonstrate the tumor in its craniocaudal extension. The soft tissue mass is clearly visible together with the bone destruction caused by the tumor (e–h)

There are some questionable findings which require confirmation in conventional tomographic studies. There is no doubt that computed tomography is not an adequate substitute for invasive neuroradiological techniques, especially cerebral angiography. This procedure often provides important additional, even decisive findings which may save the neurosurgeon from unpleasant surprises. A balanced combination of the different diagnostic techniques provides the most accurate preoperative diagnosis.

## 2. Skull Vault

*Diagnosis of neoplastic changes in the skull vault is still the domain of the plain skull film and of conventional tomographic studies. CT studies may provide supplementary evidence,* especially by demonstrating soft tissue associated with the bone lesions in question.

The following tumors may cause alterations in bone structures visible in the CT scan:

- Osteomas;
- Hemangiomas of the vault;
- Epidermoid and dermoid cysts;
- Meningiomas and malignant meningiomas;
- Malignant lymphomas;
- Plasmocytomas;
- Metastases of carcinoma and other malignant neoplasms (including neuroblastoma, for example).

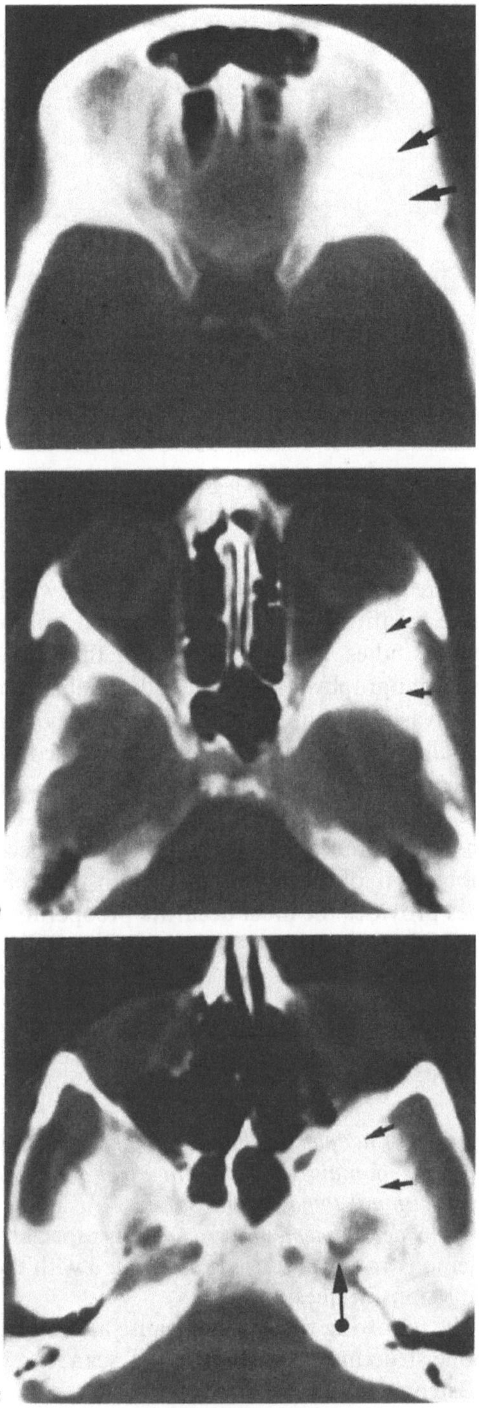

a b c

**Fig. E26**a–c. Fibrous dysplasia involving the bone structures of the anterior and middle cranial fossae. (**a**) Thickening of the roof of the orbit (arrows). (**b**) Thickening of the greater and lesser sphenoid wings. In (**b**) displacement of orbital structures (proptosis). (**c**) Narrowing of the oval foramen (arrow with dot)

The skull is a common location for **osteomas.** SCHWARTZ (1940) reported that the latter account for 1% of all skull neoplasms. In most cases they originate in the frontal and ethmoid sinuses but may also develop from the diploe of the skull vault (cf. Chap. osteomas, Fig. D7.1, p. 336). Osteomas of various sizes may originate at the apex of the petrous bone (Fig. D7.2, p. 336). Osteomas grow very slowly and rarely cause clinical symptoms. As a result, they are often discovered by chance. CT studies reveal their characteristically homogeneous high density values which equal those of compact bone. Differentiation from an entirely calcified meningioma may be difficult or impossible.

**Capillary and cavernous hemangiomas of the skull vault** produce characteristic radiological findings. CT studies reveal distension of the skull bone as well as a trabecular structure within the vascular tumor (Fig. E28).

**Epidermoid and dermoid cysts** may produce such characteristic changes in bone structures that the diagnosis is made with the plain skull film alone. The actual tumor appears as a hypodense zone in the CT scan (Figs. D6.41–43). Epidermoids originating in the diploe deserve special mention here. Dermoid cysts in the fronto-orbital or temporal regions are associated with typical bone changes. These tumors develop from ectopic embryonic ectodermal material and are most often found in the cleft lines of the skull (Figs. D6.45–47, p. 330f.).

**Meningiomas** are often associated with bone changes such as extensive thickening of the vault above the tumor (Fig. D2.22) or so-called enostosis (Figs. D2.20, 21, p. 210f.). Some meningiomas spread within the skull vault and may cause considerable distension of the bone (Fig. D2.47). CT studies usually demonstrate the soft tissue tumor quite clearly. Small meningiomas of the vault cause circumscribed swelling (Fig. E29). An intracranial soft tissue lesion is usually present in these cases as well.

**Malignant meningiomas and meningeal sarcomas** are also often associated with changes in bone structures, which may range from disruption of the bone texture to massive distension which always demonstrates lower attenuation values than normal bone.

**Malignant lymphomas** may originate in the skull vault. This usually causes destruction of normal bone structures in the presence of a soft

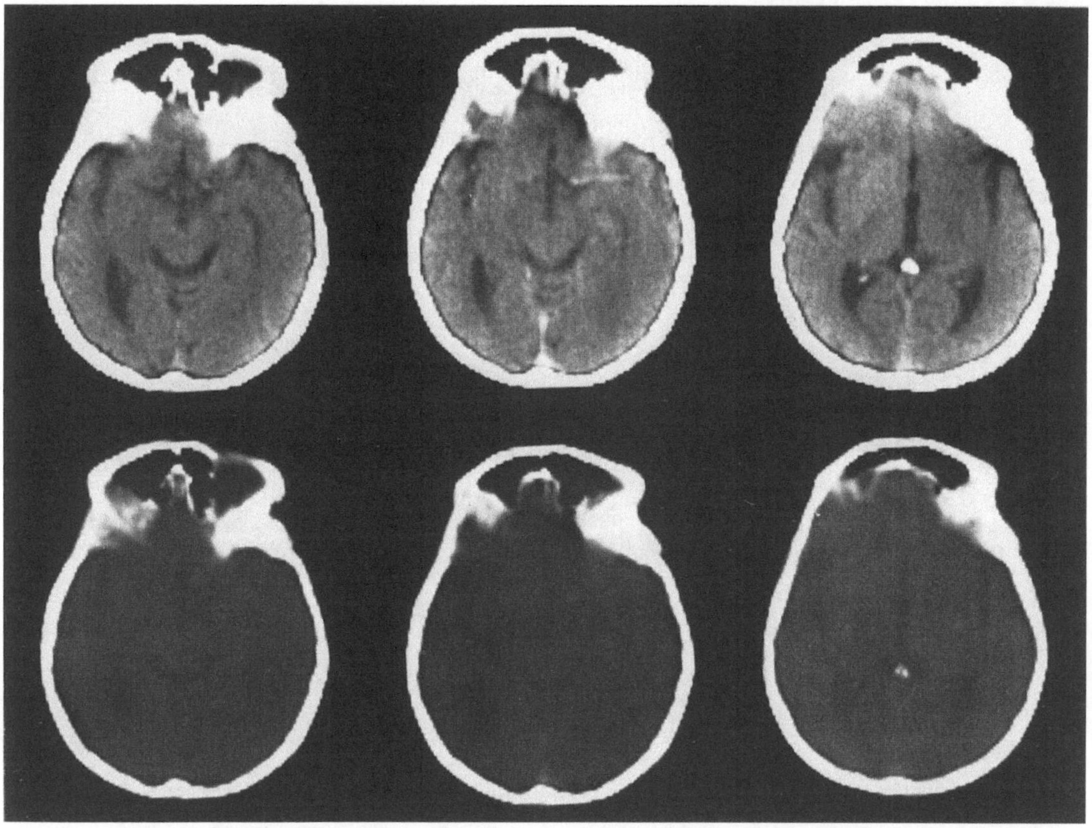

**Fig. E27.** Recurrence of osteoplastic meningioma on the sphenoid wing in a 27-year-old female. Distension of the right sphenoid wing by the tumor. Studies with normal window level do not demonstrate significant differences between the right and the left sides (above left). Greater window width allows clear demonstration of the osteoplastic tumor. The structure with bone density in the greater sphenoid wing on the left proves to be the normal sphenoid wing and the roof of the orbit

tissue lesion which may extend to both the scalp and the intracranial cavity, where the tumor is usually delineated by the meninges (Fig. E30). **Plasmocytoma** results in a similar picture, with destruction of normal bone texture and a lens-shaped soft tissue lesion located between the rather well-demarcated extremes of the bone defect (Fig. E31). **Metastases of carcinoma** destroy normal bone tissue and replace it with neoplastic tissue. Osteolytic lesions usually demonstrate blurred borders in plain skull films with similar findings in CT scans, which also demonstrate the metastasis itself (Figs. E32–35). Metastases in the skull vault may be solitary, but multiple metastases are more common and may result in extensive bone destruction (Fig. E34). Osteolytic metastases in the skull vault are especially characteristic of bronchogenic carcinoma, hypernephroma, carcinoma of the breast and the thyroid. Conventional radiography is clearly superior to computed tomography in demonstration of small multiple metastases in the skull. Plain skull films in two projections usually provide the diagnosis with less effort than that required for CT studies.

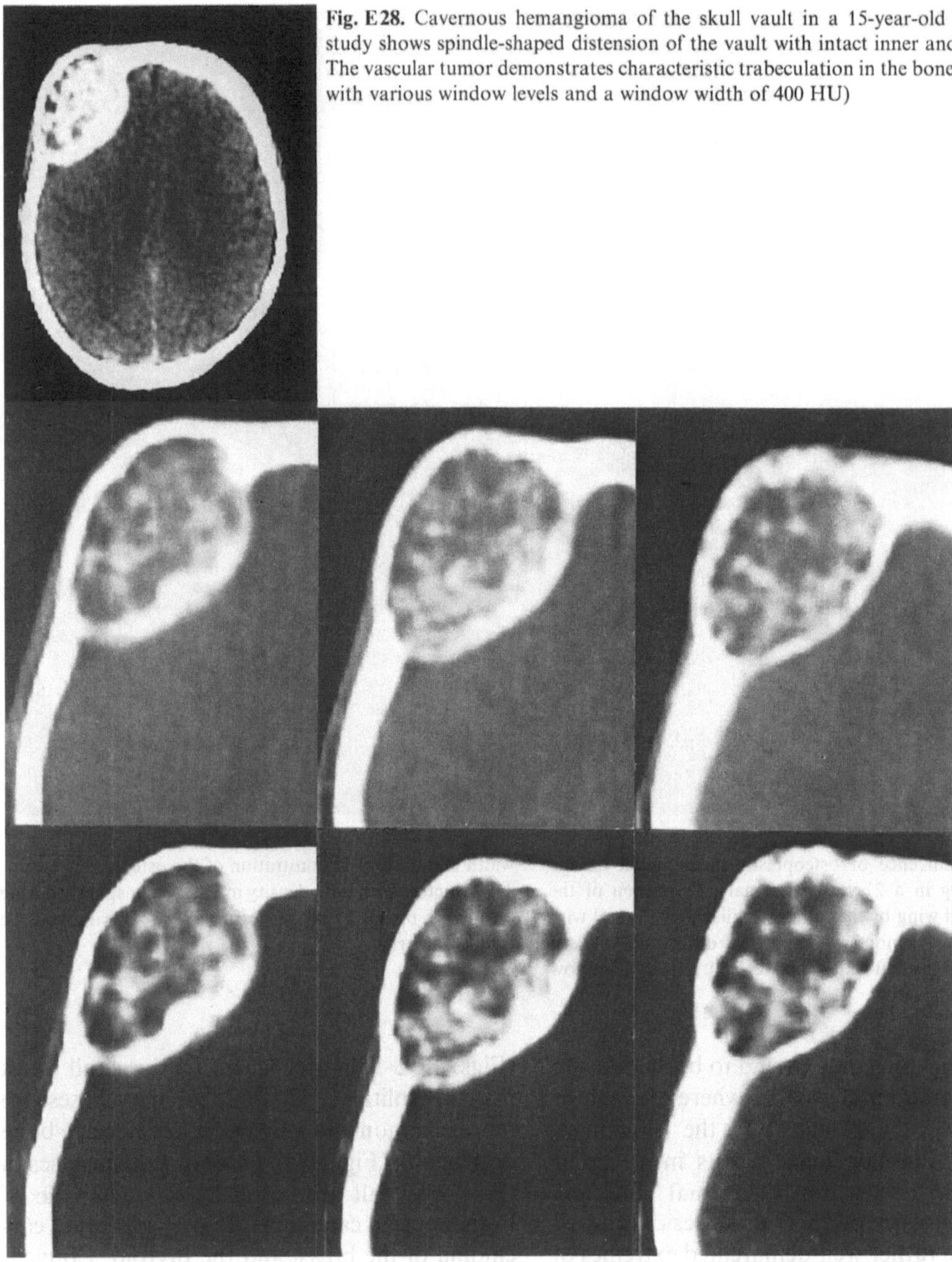

**Fig. E28.** Cavernous hemangioma of the skull vault in a 15-year-old boy. The CT study shows spindle-shaped distension of the vault with intact inner and outer tables. The vascular tumor demonstrates characteristic trabeculation in the bone (enlargement with various window levels and a window width of 400 HU)

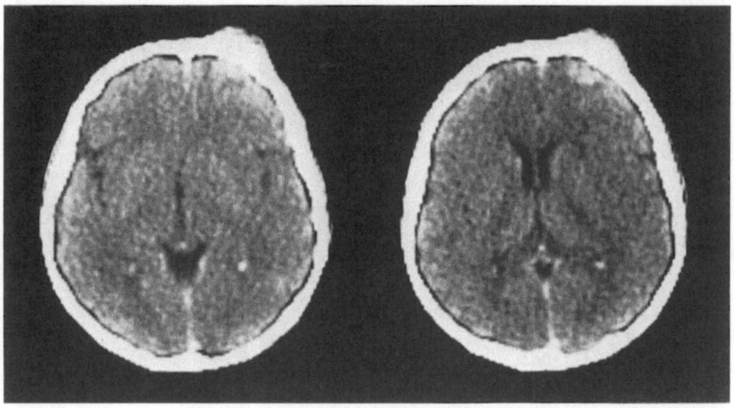

**Fig. E29.** Small meningioma with some osteoplastic growth in the right frontal bone. Distension of the vault with protrusion of the right forehead. Contrast enhancement shows a small soft tissue tumor with intracranial extension. 52 year-old male with swelling of the forehead on the right side

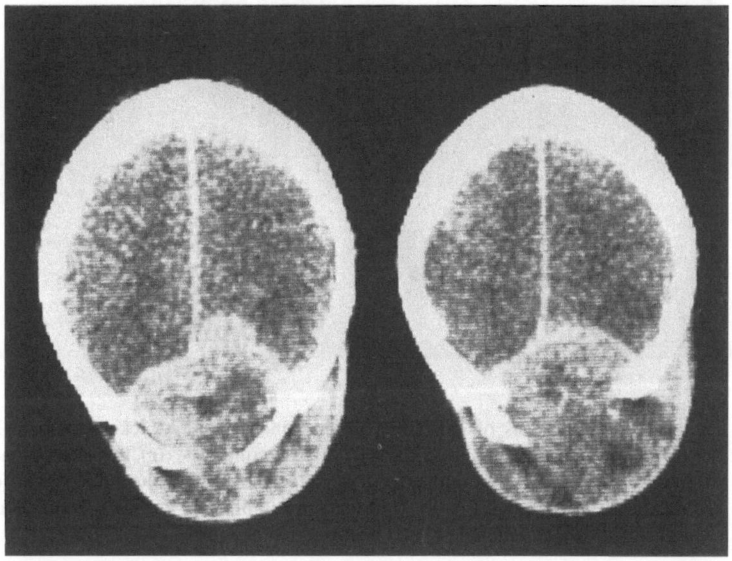

**Fig. E30.** Centroblastic lymphoma in a 56-year-old patient with extreme protrusion of the occipital bone. CT studies demonstrate extensive destruction of the vault and an inhomogeneous soft tissue lesion in the skull and the cranial cavity. The intracranial portion of the tumor is separated from brain tissue by dura mater. The lymphoma has penetrated the dura mater at one point next to the falx

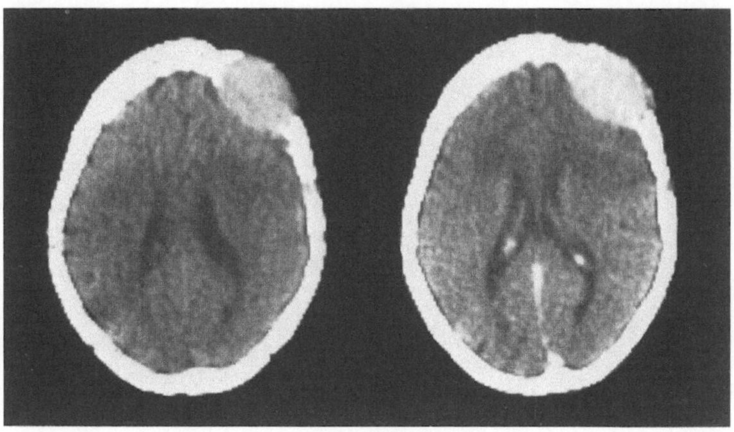

**Fig. E31.** Plasmocytoma in the vault of a 64-year-old female. Sharply demarcated destruction of the frontal bone on the right. A spindle-shaped soft tissue lesion with strong contrast uptake is visible in the bone defect. Left, precontrast study; right, postcontrast study

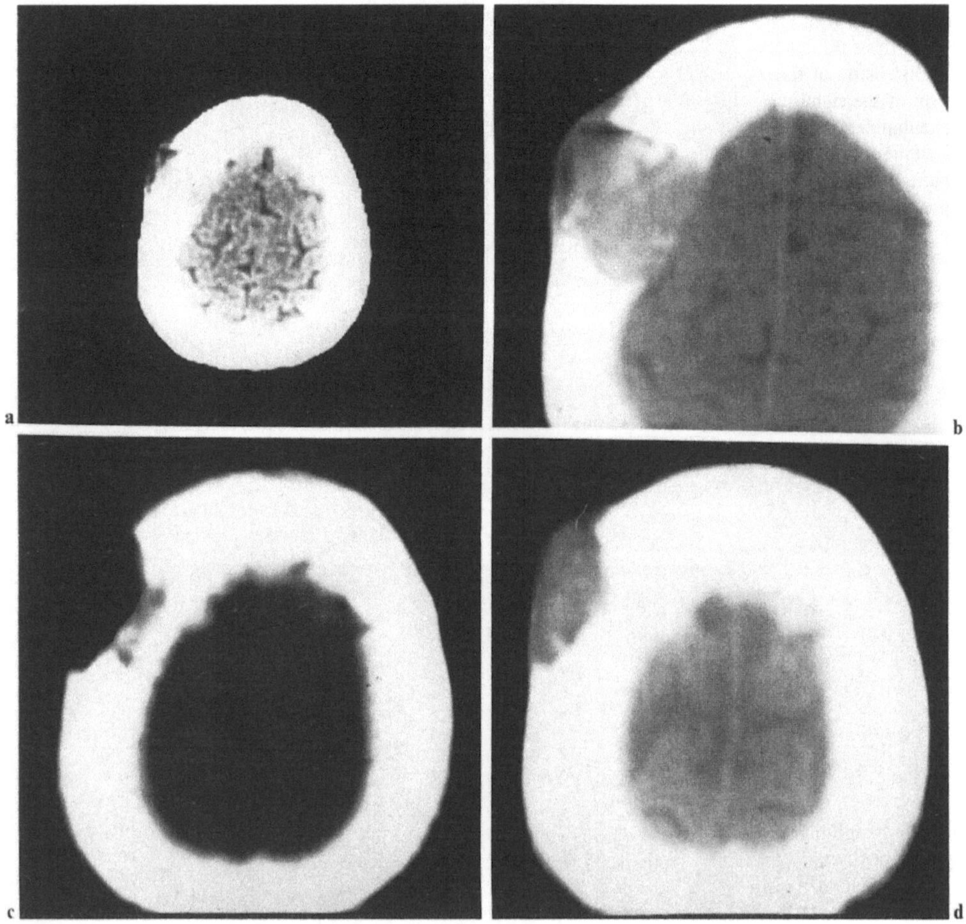

**Fig. E32** a–d. Metastasis of carcinoma at the junction of the frontal and parietal bones on the left. (**a**) The contour of the vault in the left frontoparietal region is slightly blurred in the standard CT scan. (**b**) Enlargement of the same slice with wider window (400 HU) shows that the full thickness of bone has been widely replaced by tumor tissue. (**c**) The next higher slice shows the bone defect with its blurred margins. (**d**) Demonstration of the soft tissue lesion in the subcutaneous layer with a lower window level

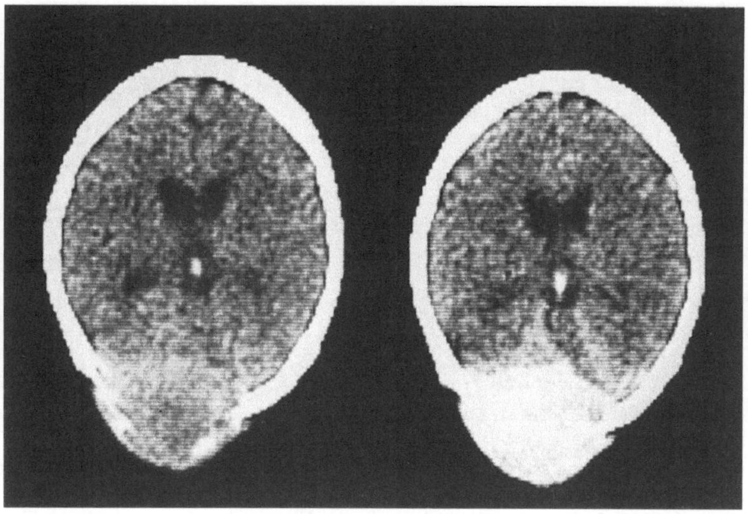

**Fig. E33.** Very large metastasis to the vault in a 71-year-old patient with thyroid carcinoma. Extensive bilateral destruction of the occipital bone. The soft tissue lesion has penetrated the skull cavity, and there is no sharp line of demarcation against normal brain structures (left, precontrast study). Contrast enhancement (right) produces a strong increase in density values and delineates the tumor against normal brain tissue

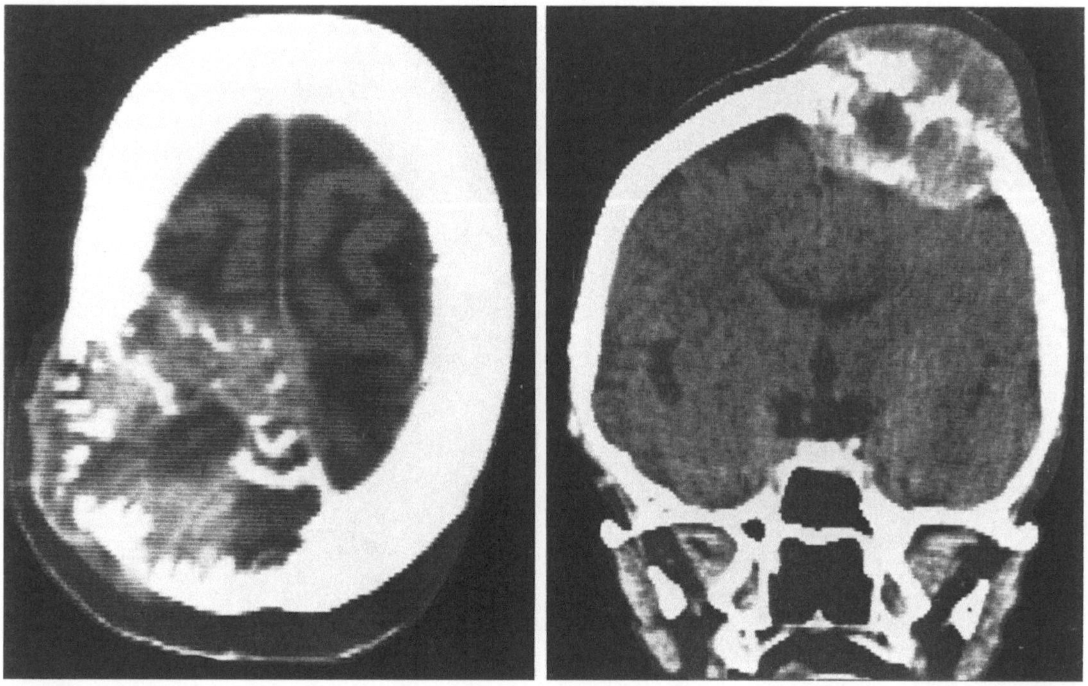

**Fig. E34.** Metastasis in the skull vault of 62-year-old patient with thyroid carcinoma. Extensive bone destruction in the left parietal region with expansive tumor growth. The coronary projection demonstrates the full extent of intracranial spread of the tumor, which is sharply delineated against normal brain tissue. The dura mater was intact at operation

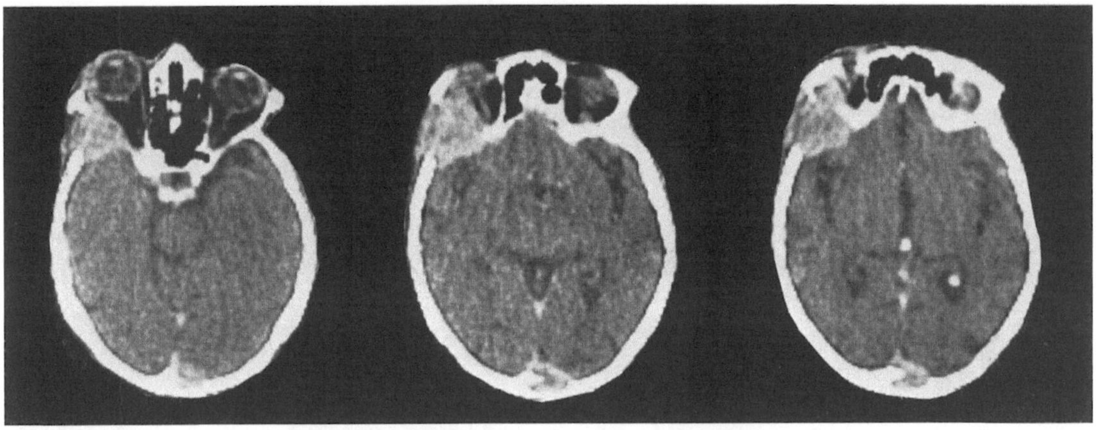

**Fig. E35.** Multiple metastases in the skull of a 71-year-old patient. Extensive destruction in the greater sphenoid wing with a visible soft tissue lesion which is clearly delineated against normal brain structures after contrast enhancement. Demonstration of an additional metastasis in the occipital bone near the midline. The outer table is intact

# F. Computed Tomography in Nonneoplastic Space-Occupying Intracranial Lesions

A number of nonneoplastic intracranial space-occupying lesions may resemble neoplasms in the CT scan, and definitive diagnosis is not possible with CT studies alone in many cases. Misinterpretations are possible, even when all clinical data are considered in the interpretation of the CT scan. However, the most accurate possible preoperative diagnosis is a prerequisite for decisions on therapeutic strategy and surgical approach. Therefore some cases may require the full range of conventional neuroradiological techniques and careful consideration of clinical findings for correct interpretation of the CT scan with its consequences for therapy. Table 6 summarizes the most common alternatives in differential diagnosis of brain tumors. *Inflammatory disease and granulomatous lesions* constitute the critical group of diseases which may simulate neoplastic lesions. *Cystic malformations* are also important alternatives in differential diagnosis. *Parasites* associated with intracranial lesions are rare in Europe and North America, but they must be considered as possibilities in the differential diagnosis of intracranial space-occupying lesions, especially in Central and South America.

*Acute intracranial hemorrhage of any etiology* does not usually cause problems in diagnosis with CT since attenuation values within the hemorrhage and the history almost always suggest the correct diagnosis. So-called *chocolate cysts* – older, encapsulated intracerebral hematomas – may present problems, especially if there is no history suggestive of acute hemorrhage.

Type III *chronic subdural hematomas* (GRUMME et al. 1976) with isodense contents may appear as space-occupying lesions which do not allow precise diagnosis in the precontrast CT scan.

*Giant arteriovenous malformations and aneurysms* may also simulate tumors.

*Brain infarction with disruption of the blood-brain barrier* and contrast uptake is a special

**Table 6.** Nonneoplastic intracranial space-occupying lesions in the differential diagnosis of brain tumors

1. **Inflammatory lesions**
   Brain abscess
   Subdural empyema
   Meningoencephalitis
   Radiation necrosis
   Primary stenosis of the aqueduct and occlusion of the foramina of Luschkae and Magendie
2. **Acute demyelinating diseases**
   Disseminating encephalomyelitis
   Diffuse sclerosis
3. **Granulomas**
   Gummas
   Tuberculomas
   Granulomas in sarcoidosis
   Other granulomas
4. **Cysts**
   Arachnoid cysts
   Dandy-Walker syndrome
   Other cysts
5. **Parasites**
   Cysticercosis
   Echinococcosis
6. **Intracranial hematomas**
   Spontaneous intracerebral hematomas
   Old liquefied hematomas ("chocolate cysts")
   Chronic subdural hematoma (isodense)
7. **Vascular malformations**
   Arteriovenous malformations
   Sturge-Weber syndrome (encephalotrigeminal syndrome)
   Giant aneurysms
   Basilar artery ectasia
8. **Brain infarction (arterial and venous)**
   Space-occupying edema of infarction
   Brain infarction with disruption of the blood-brain barrier
   Space-occupying hemorrhage secondary to infarction
   Thrombosis of cerebral veins or sinuses with edema and/or hemorrhage

diagnostic problem. Misinterpretation as tumor is not rare in such cases. *Thrombosis of venous sinuses* may also simulate a space-occupying lesion in the CT scan.

These problems in differential diagnosis occurred in 108 patients observed in a series of 7,543 consecutive CT studies (KAZNER et al. 1978). This constitutes an incidence of 10.6% of a total of 1,017 histologically verified brain tumors in this series, illustrating the frequency of such problems in the differentiation of brain tumors and nontumorous space-occupying intracranial lesions. Intracerebral hemorrhage was not included in these statistics since clotted blood can easily be recognized. Hemorrhage within a tumor is an uncommon event which may pose diagnostic difficulties.

# 1. Inflammatory Processes

## a) Brain Abscesses

Brain abscesses can be demonstrated in the CT scan with high accuracy (AULICH et al. 1976; CLAVERIA et al. 1976; KAZNER 1976; SCHIEFER and HUCK 1976; MOSLEY et al. 1977). Single or multiple rings appear in most cases (Figs. F 1–11). *Differentiation between brain abscess and glioblastoma with central necrosis – which also demonstrates rim enhancement – may be difficult or impossible, especially in adults without a history and signs of previous inflammatory disease* (Figs. D 1.60, F 5). Experience shows that presence of a narrow ring, spherical shape, and multiplicity are unreliable criteria of brain abscess. Demonstration of gas within a ring structure is the only pathognomonic indicator of abscess (Fig. F 10). Differentiation between glioblastoma and brain abscess by means of attenuation measurements in the abscess contents and intensity of contrast uptake in the ring (MAUERSBERGER 1981) is not sufficiently reliable for certain diagnosis. Our studies show that the contents of an abscess do not necessarily have lower absorption values than the central necrosis in glioblastoma; we found attenuation values between 19 and 23 HU in both lesions. However, this is not true in all cases (cf. Chap. glioblastoma, p. 60ff.). Attenuation in the contents of an abscess is a function of time. A newly developed abscess has approximately the same density as brain edema or tumor necrosis, while older abscesses may demonstrate lower density values which may attain 16 HU.

*Biopsy must be performed to exclude brain abscess* in an unclassifiable space-occupying lesion which demonstrates a ring structure after contrast enhancement and which is located in a region of the brain where surgical therapy of a tumor would be contraindicated (Fig. F 3).

Carotid angiography may provide decisive evidence for diagnosis through demonstration of the abscess capsule or pathological vessels typical of glioblastoma. Kinetics of contrast enhancement and serial brain scintigraphy do not provide specific evidence for differentiation between abscess and brain tumor.

Anaplastic astrocytomas and brain metastases in the cerebral hemispheres may also show ring enhancement while pilocytic astrocytoma must be considered in the differential diagnosis of an abscess in the posterior fossa.

A *chambered brain abscess* may also demonstrate findings similar to those in glioblastoma (Figs. F 7, 8). *Multifocal brain abscesses* must be differentiated from multiple metastases, though multiple glioblastomas are sometimes found (Fig. D 1.94–97, p. 85f.). Multiple brain lesions are also found in *cysticercosis* (Fig. F 45).

*Perifocal edema in brain abscess* may vary considerably in extent, depending on the stage of the abscess. Lesions in the early phase are almost always accompanied by extensive perifocal edema.

### Additional Possibilities in Differential Diagnosis

*Ring enhancement may be observed in the early postoperative phase following resection of a brain tumor.* This is usually due to a temporary disorder of the blood-brain barrier and to development of granulation tissue at the margin of the operative site (Fig. F 12). CT studies do not always allow certain differentiation between postoperative abscess and normal postoperative healing after resection of a brain tumor if ring enhancement is present. Clinical deterioration due to retention of secretions in the surgical cavity may present with CT findings suggestive of brain abscess (Figs. F 13, 14). Blood or xanthochromic fluid is usually found at a second operation in such cases. Perifocal edema is often observed in these lesions and leads one to suspect brain abscess. However, edema is not helpful in evaluation of such findings.

**Radiation necrosis** may present with CT findings similar to those found in abscess and glioblastoma (Fig. F15). One usually encounters a hypodense zone of necrosis surrounded by a dense ring after contrast enhancement. We have also observed **radiation fibrosis** with homogeneous contrast uptake resembling that found in a solid brain tumor.

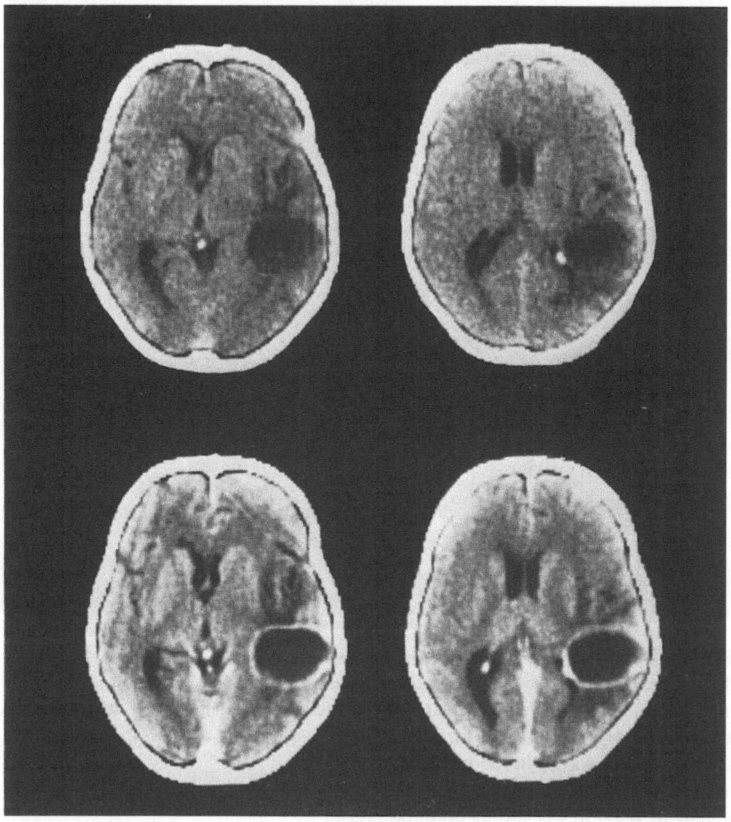

**Fig. F1.** Brain abscess in the posterior portion of the right temporal region in a 65-year-old female. Circumscribed hypodense zone with a finger-shaped area of edema in the white matter (above, precontrast study). Contrast enhancement produces a narrow hyperdense ring figure representing the capsule of the abscess (below). Differential diagnosis: glioblastoma, metastasis

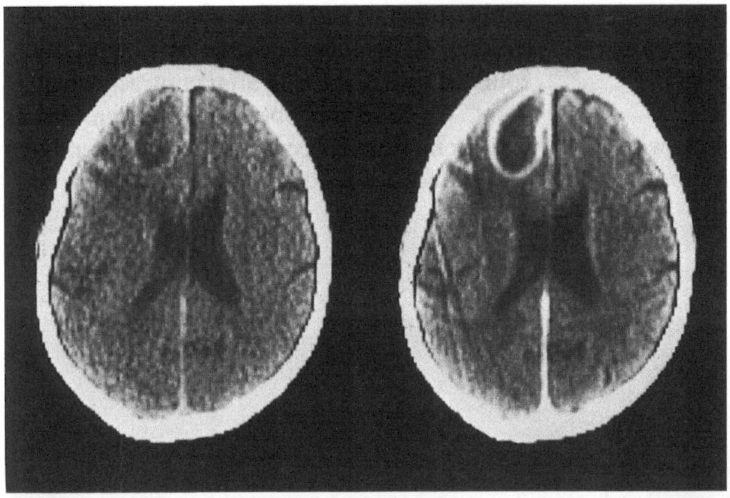

**Fig. F2.** Brain abscess in the left frontal region in a 64-year-old patient. Origin of the lesion is the frontal sinus. Strong contrast uptake in the abscess capsule. Perifocal edema. Left, precontrast study, right, postcontrast study. Differential diagnosis: glioblastoma

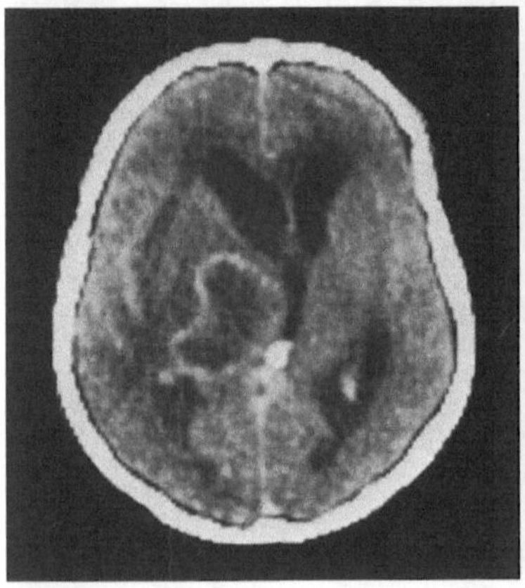

**Fig. F3.** Kidney-shaped brain abscess in the left thalamus with contrast uptake in the capsule in a 46-year-old man with a history of sepsis. Extensive finger-shaped zone of edema in the white matter. Density values in the abscess are similar to those in edematous brain tissue (22–24 HU). Differentiation between abscess and glioblastoma is not possible on the basis of CT findings alone

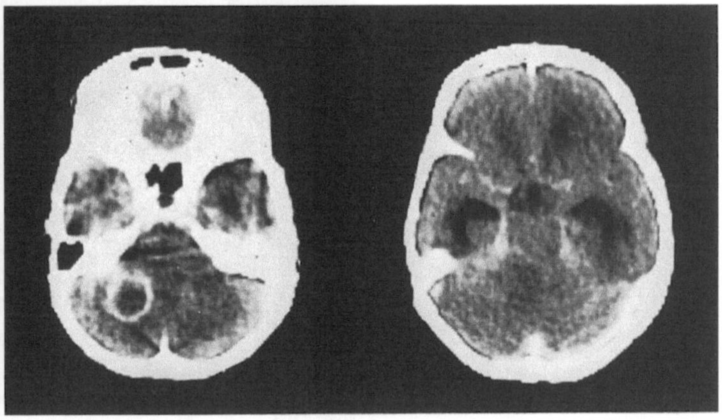

**Fig. F4.** Abscess in the left cerebellar hemisphere in a 53-year-old female without a history of infection. Strong contrast uptake in the abscess capsule, perifocal edema, and extensive hydrocephalus with periventricular lucency. Initial CT diagnosis of cerebellar tumor

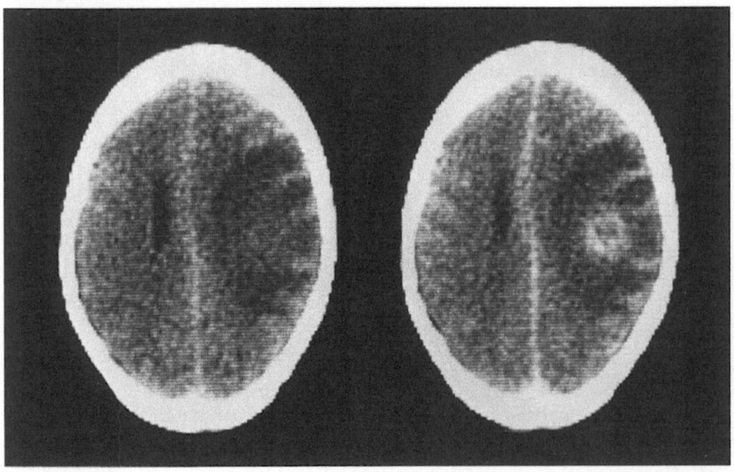

**Fig. F5.** Small brain abscess in the parietal region with extensive perifocal edema in a 51-year-old man without a history of infection. Initial CT diagnosis of glioblastoma or metastasis. Left, precontrast study; right, postcontrast study

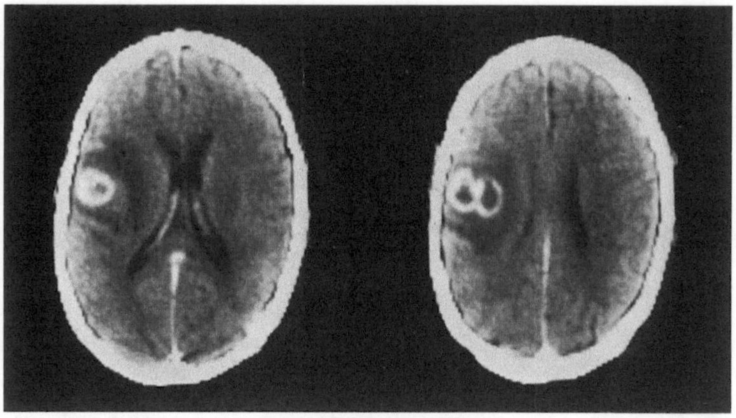

**Fig. F6.** Chambered brain abscess in the left temporoparietal region of a 62-year-old female. The individual capsules blend into one another. Perifocal edema. Strong contrast uptake in the choroid plexus in both lateral ventricles is a normal finding

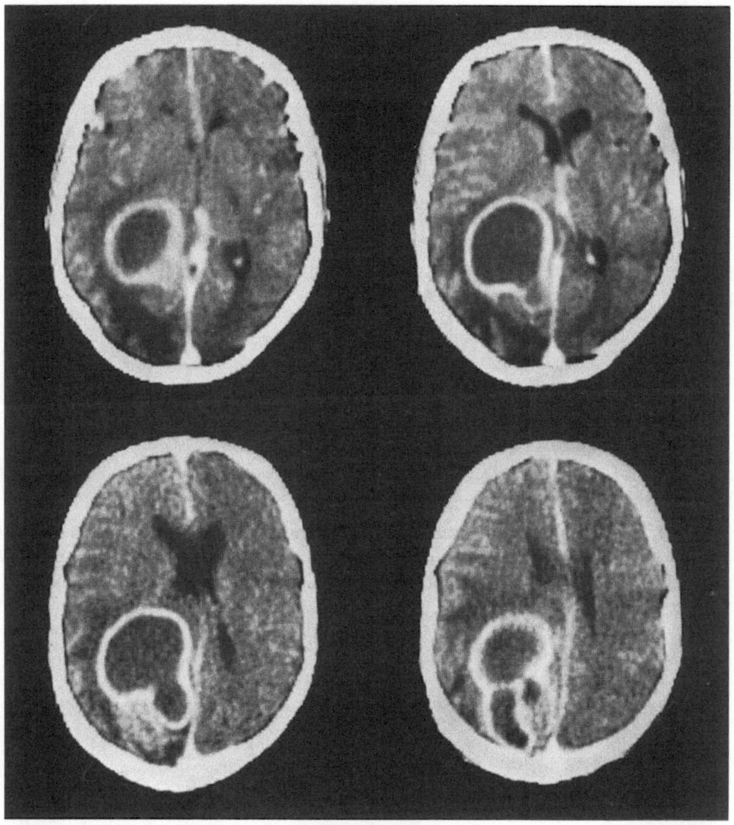

**Fig. F7.** Multichambered abscess in the left parieto-occipital region of a 14-year-old boy. Postcontrast study

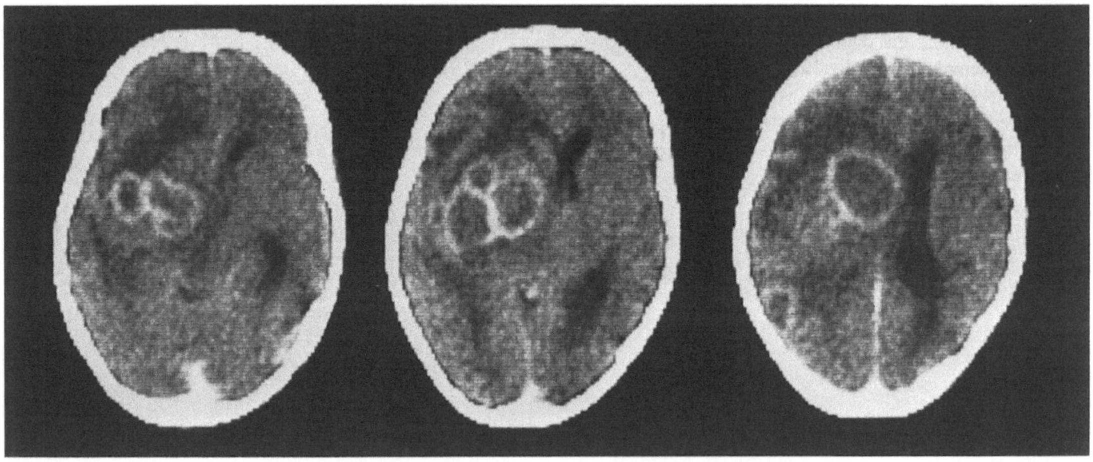

**Fig. F8.** Multichambered abscess deep in the left cerebral hemisphere as far as the basal ganglia, combined with a subcortical abscess extending to the left parieto-occipital region (right) in a 12-year-old boy. Postcontrast study

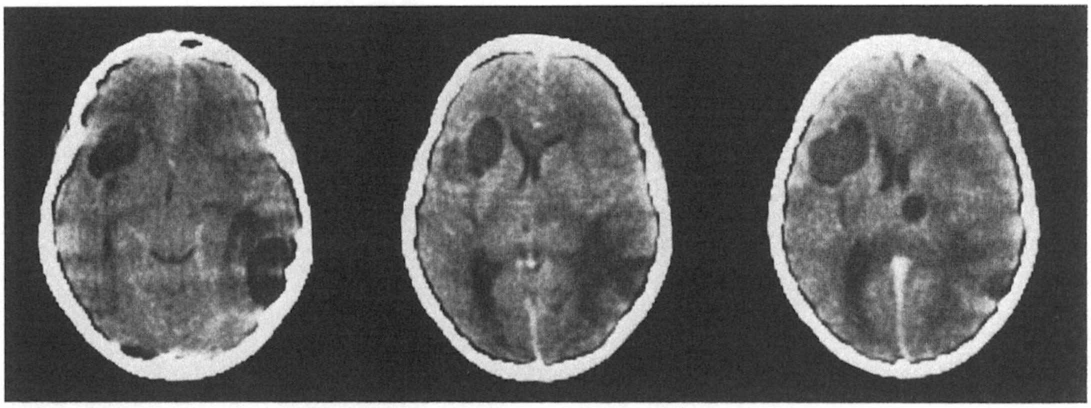

**Fig. F9.** Multilocular brain abscesses and a subdural abscess in the posterior portion of the right temporal region in a 12-year-old boy. Contrast enhancement of the abscess capsules is no longer demonstrable after several weeks of therapy with steroids and antibiotics. Postcontrast study

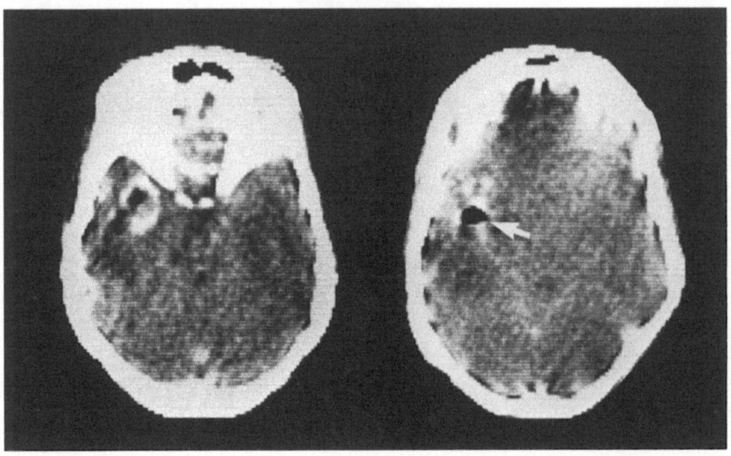

**Fig. F10.** Brain abscess containing gas at the tip of the left temporal lobe in a 40-year-old female with sinusitis. Artifacts result from the great difference in density values between gas and the abscess capsule (computer overswing, arrow). Postcontrast study

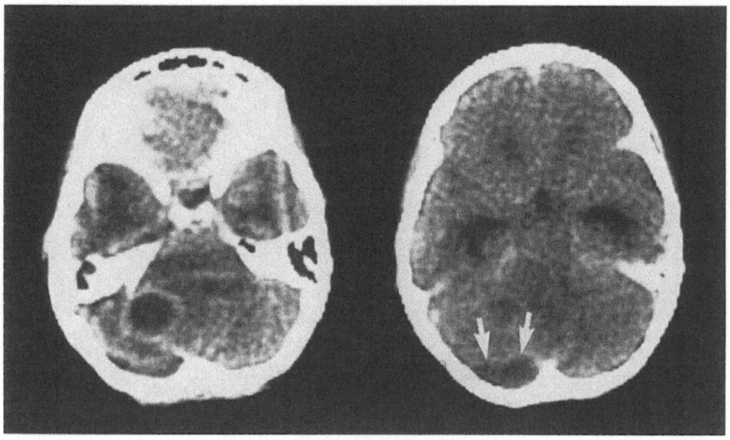

**Fig. F 11.** Cerebellar abscess on the left with a ring structure after contrast enhancement in 25-year-old male. Subdural empyema over the left cerebellar hemisphere with contrast uptake in the visceral membrane of the inflammatory lesion (arrows). Extensive edema in the cerebellar white matter

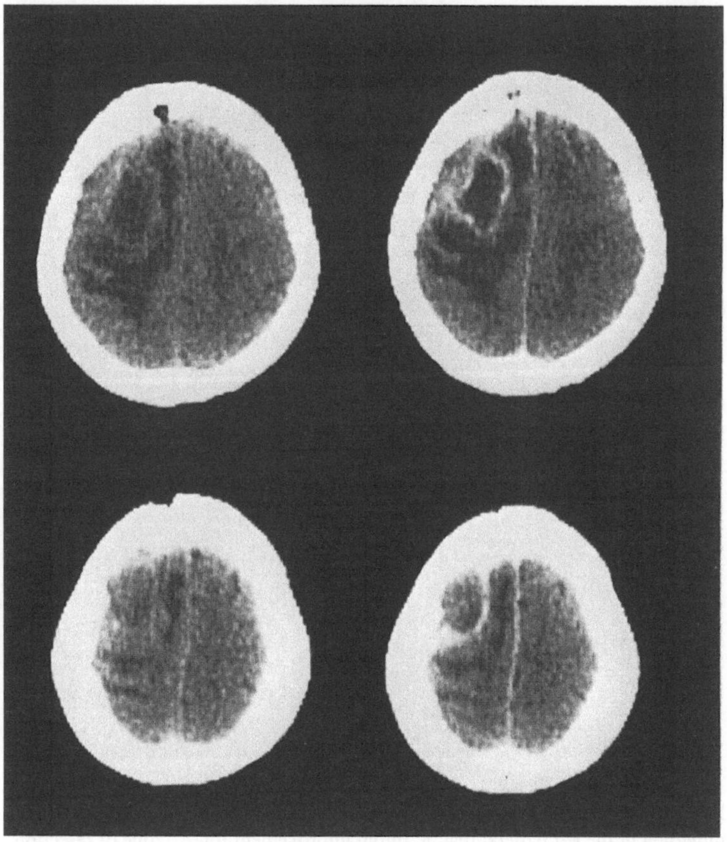

**Fig. F 12.** Temporary disorder of the blood-brain barrier $4^1/_2$ weeks after resection of meningioma in the left precentral region of a 68-year-old female. Garland figure at the margin of the zone of resection following contrast enhancement suggesting brain abscess

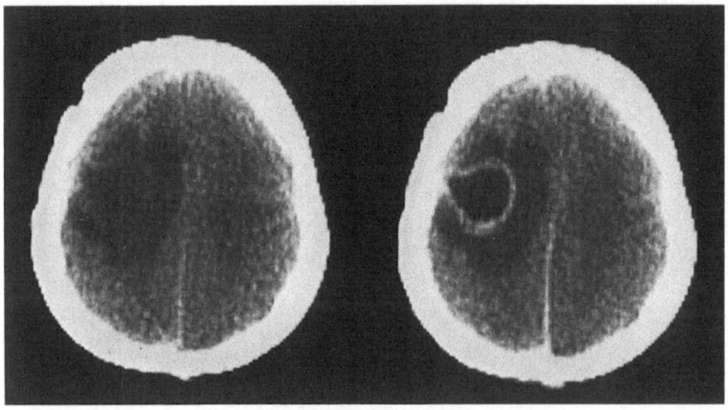

**Fig. F 13.** CT findings $3^1/_2$ weeks after total resection of a circumscribed astrocytoma (grade II) in the left precentral region of a 37-year-old female with a progredient speech disorder and epileptic seizures (cf. Fig. D 1.5). Demonstration of a space-occupying lesion with a ring figure following contrast enhancement and perifocal edema in the zone of resection. Postoperative abscess suspected. At operation a collection of secretions was found, but there was no evidence of inflammation

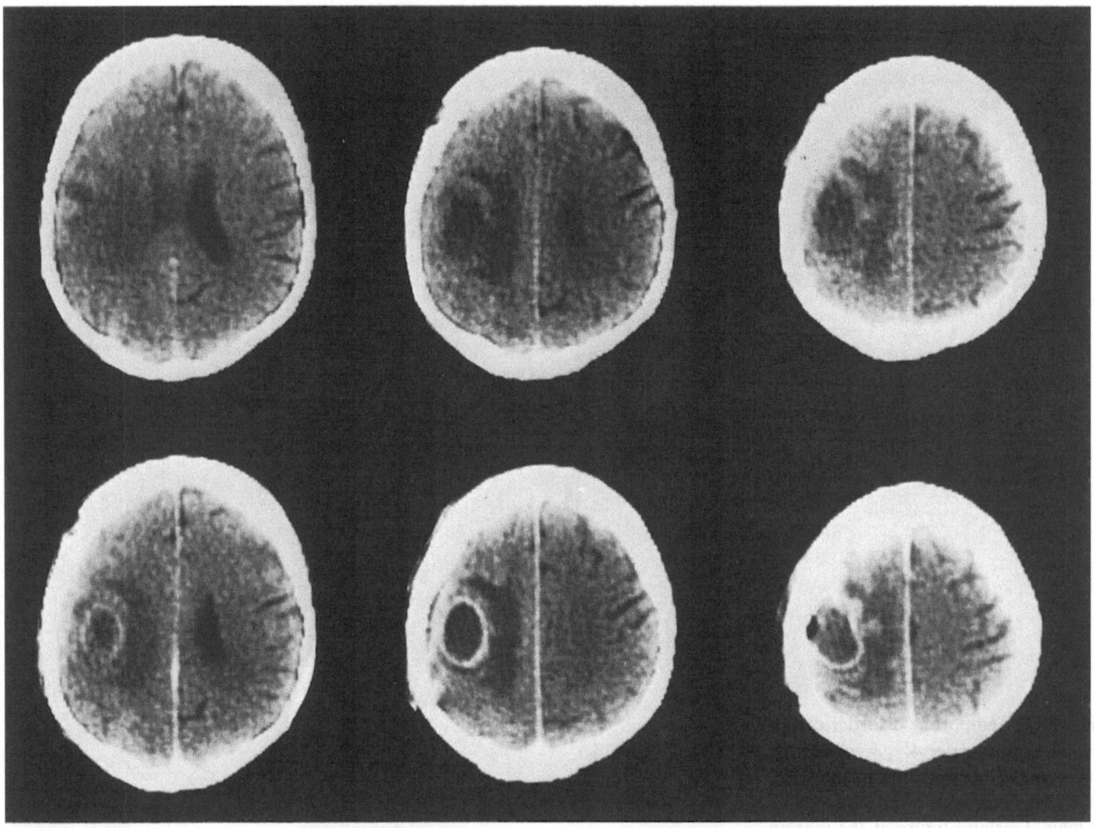

**Fig. F 14.** CT findings 1 month after resection of meningioma in the left parietal region. Initial improvement followed by progredient paresis of the right arm. Demonstration of a ring figure and perifocal edema in the zone of resection, raising suspicion of abscess. Residual air in the zone of resection. A second operation revealed a cavity containing brownish-green secretions without evidence of bacterial infection. Granulation tissue in the wall of the lesion

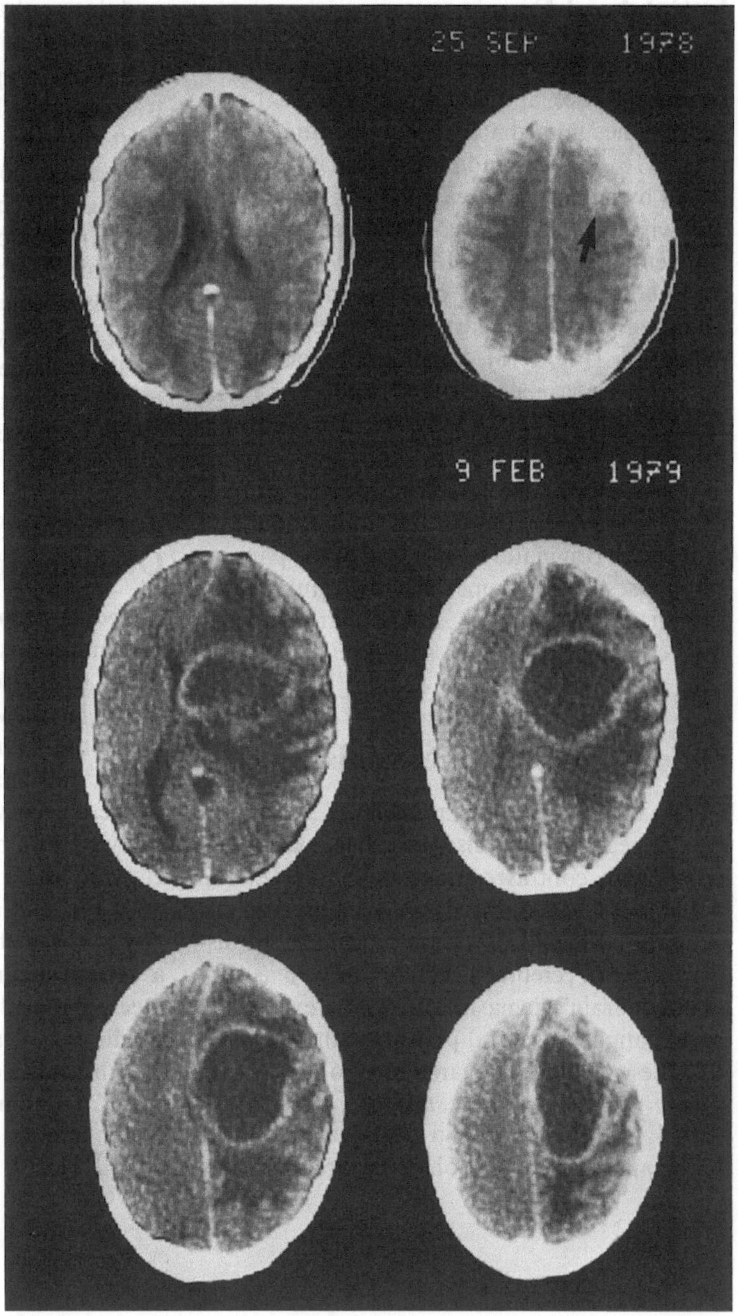


**Fig. F15.** Radiation necrosis in a 15-year-old boy. Preoperative CT findings (September 15, 1978): slightly hyperdense tumor in the white matter of the right precentral region (arrow). An anaplastic oligodendroglioma was resected at operation; subsequent irradiation with 5,000 rad. Two months after completion of radiation therapy a severe organic brain syndrome and left hemiparesis developed. Follow-up CT study (February 9, 1979): large hypodense zone in the white matter in the right hemisphere with marginal contrast uptake and extensive perifocal edema. Significant displacement of midline structures. Acute radiation necrosis was found at operation

## b) Subdural Empyemas

Subdural empyemas are in fact abscesses in the subdural space and usually appear as hypodense zones immediately below the dura mater (Fig. F16). Contrast administration is often followed by a density increase in both the parietal and visceral membranes of the encapsulated empyema (Figs. F11, 16, 17).

Subdural empyemas on the convexity may attain enormous proportions and demonstrate loculation (Fig. F16). Small empyemas in the posterior fossa may be overlooked (Fig. F11). Abscess and empyema may occur in combination (Figs. F9, 11).

**Empyema of the interhemispheric fissure** is characteristic of children and adolescents and most often originates in infection of the paranasal sinuses or the upper eyelid. A tubular or lens-shaped lesion with strong marginal contrast enhancement is typical (Fig. F17).

## c) Focal Meningoencephalitis

Cerebral involvement in *bacterial meningitis* may appear as a circumscribed space-occupying lesion with contrast uptake in the cortex (cf. Aulich et al. 1976, Fig. F18). We observed circumscribed hypodense areas causing slight displacement of cerebral structures, as well as generalized brain edema in all regions except the basal ganglia in several patients with *encephalitis*. These findings appeared most often in children with *herpes simplex encephalitis* (Fig. F19). The lesions did not take up contrast material. Probst (1980) observed circumscribed nodular contrast enhancement in the CT scan of a patient with presumed viral focal encephalitis. Follow-up studies did not show any contrast uptake. The author assumes that a transient disorder of the blood-brain barrier was the cause of contrast enhancement. *Tuberculous meningitis* is characterized by ventricular dilatation. In one case we found diffuse edema of the white matter as well as a circumscribed hypodense zone in the right parietal region (Fig. F20). Severe encephalitis in children often results in large tissue defects with extensive hypodense areas resembling the distribution of major brain vessels (Kazner et al. 1976).

## d) Chronic Stenosis and Occlusion in the CSF Pathways

**Aqueduct stenosis** following meningeal infection or ventriculitis causes partial or total blockage of the CSF circulation. This leads to dilatation of the lateral ventricles and the third ventricle, while the fourth ventricle is normal in size, shape, and position. Contrast enhancement of the cerebellar vermis, which consists almost entirely of gray matter, may simulate a space-occupying lesion in this region (pseudotumor vermis, Fig. F22a; Fig. D1.187). Ventriculography is the method of choice in order to make a certain diagnosis in such cases (Fig. F22b). **Occlusion of the foramina of Luschka and Magendie** may lead to extreme dilatation of the fourth ventricle ("entrapped fourth ventricle") with CT findings similar to those in cystic cerebellar tumors or other forms of cystic disease (Fig. F21).

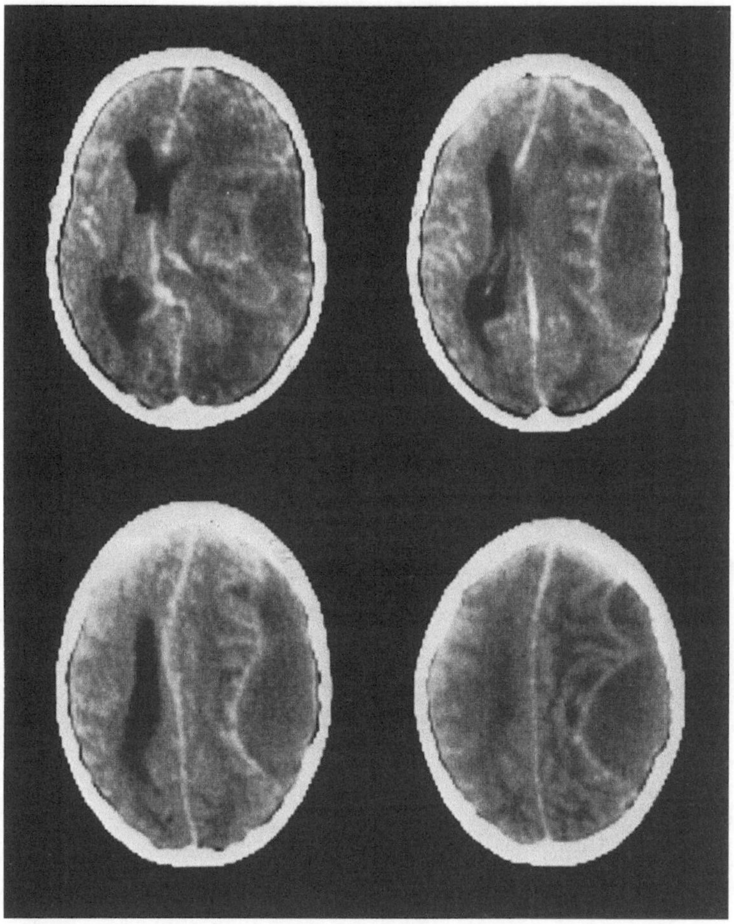

**Fig. F 16.** Extensive chambered subdural empyema above the right cerebral hemisphere in a 12-year-old boy. Edema in the white matter of the entire right hemisphere. Extreme displacement of midline structures. Contrast uptake in the visceral membrane of the capsule of the empyema. Postcontrast study

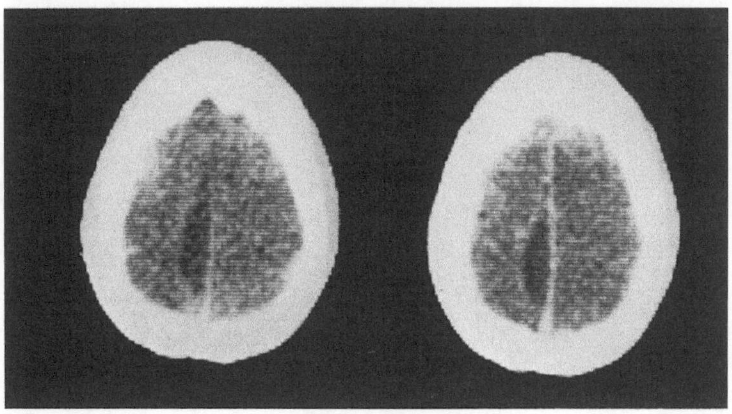

**Fig. F 17.** Subdural empyema in the interhemispheric fissure in a 14-year-old girl. Left, precontrast study. Right, postcontrast study

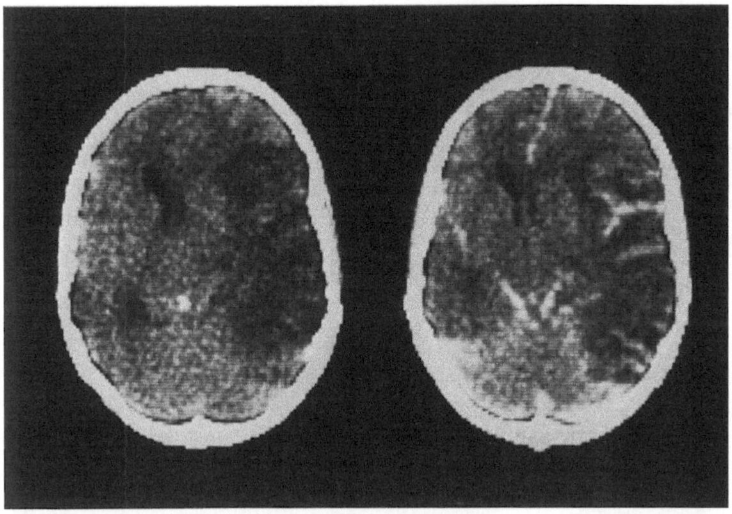

**Fig. F18.** Pyogenic meningoencephalitis in the right frontal and temporal lobes with space-occupying effect and contrast uptake in the sulci in an 18-year-old male. The pathogen was not identified. Left, precontrast study. Right, postcontrast study

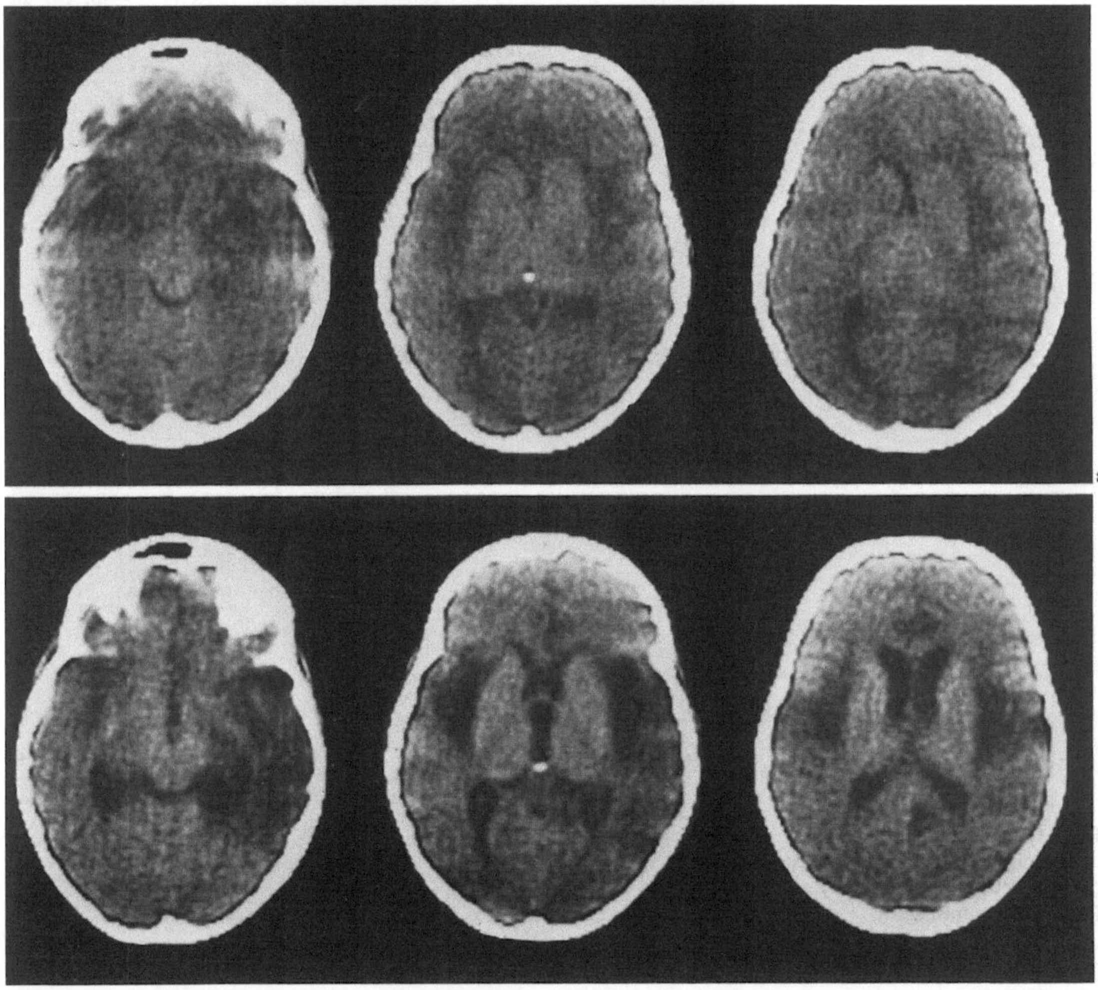

a

b

**Fig. F19a, b.** Herpes simplex encephalitis in a 15-year-old girl. (**a**) April 16, 1978: Diffuse edema in both cerebral hemispheres with exception of the basal ganglia and the midbrain. Compression of the lateral ventricles and the third ventricle. (**b**) Follow-up study on May 19, 1978: large hypodense zones in the insular region and the temporal lobes, more pronounced on the right, with dilatation of the ventricles. The findings were interpreted as tissue defects secondary to encephalitis

**Fig. F20.** Diffuse bilateral edema and a circumscribed hypodense zone in the right parietal region of a 19-year-old female with tuberculous meningitis

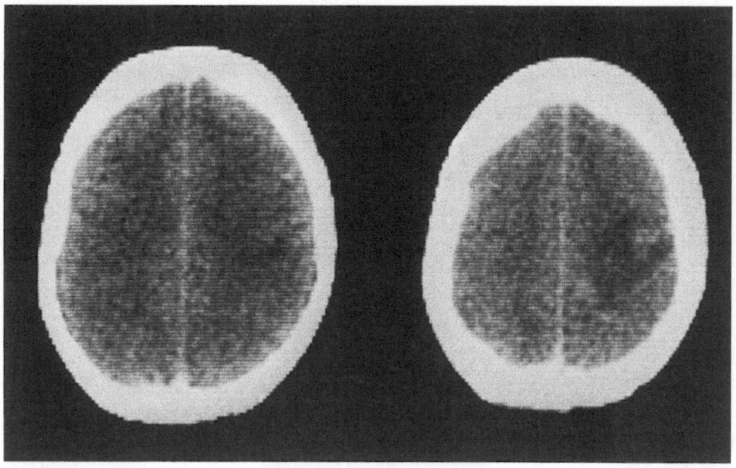

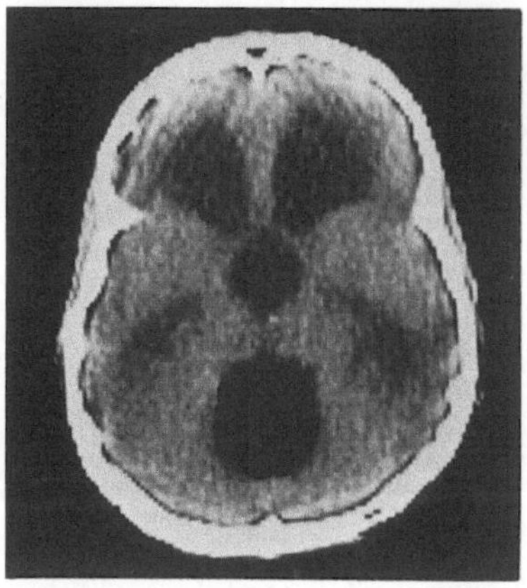

**Fig. F21.** Extreme dilatation of the fourth ventricle secondary to occlusion of the foramina of Luschka and Magendie following meningeal infection ("entrapped fourth ventricle"). Massive dilatation of the rest of the ventricular system. Thirty-four-year-old female with severe ataxia

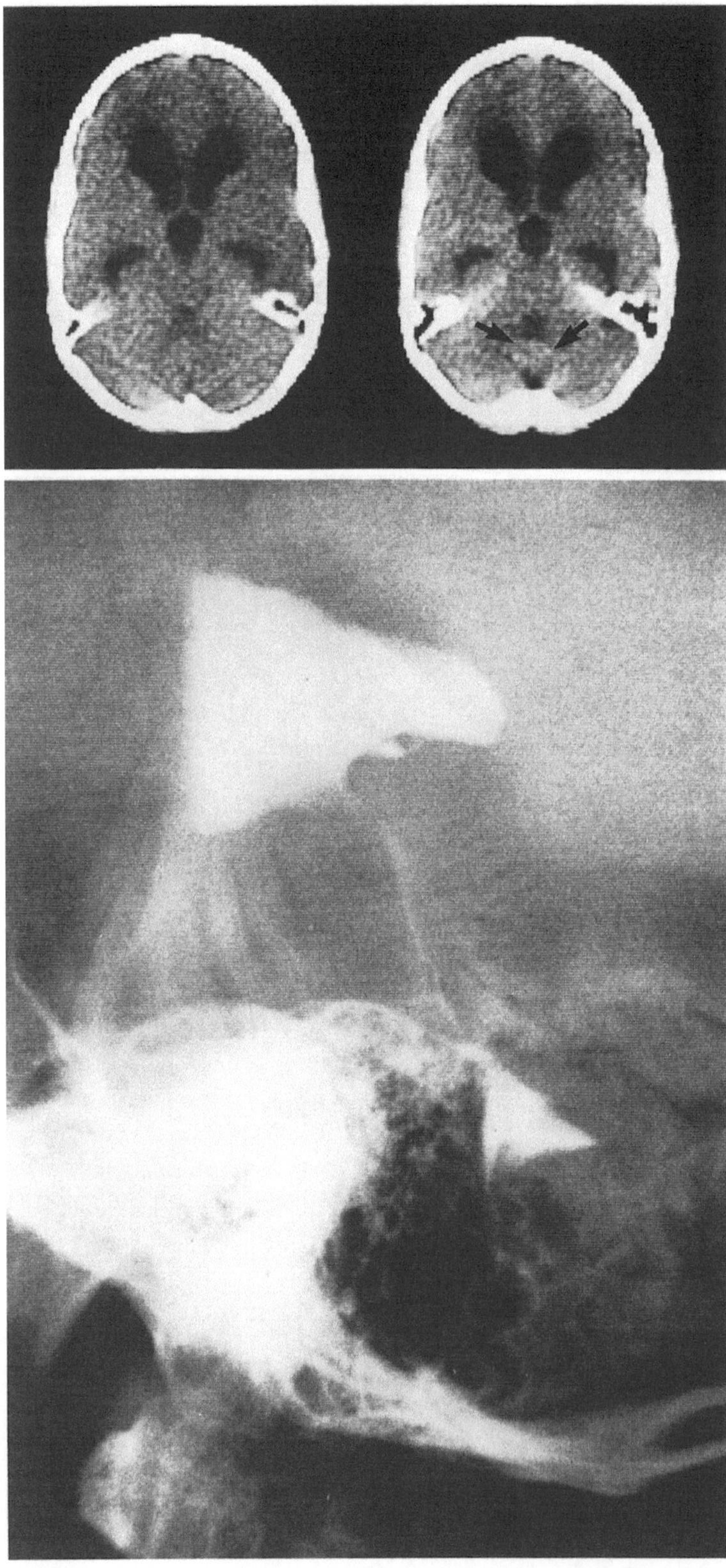

**Fig. F22** a, b. Aqueduct stenosis in a 13-year-old boy with signs of cerebellar dysfunction. (**a**) Massive hydrocephalus with periventricular lucency. Right: delicate contrast uptake in the cerebellar vermis suggesting a tumor (pseudotumor vermis, arrows). Definitive diagnosis established with positive ventriculography (**b**). Extreme narrowing of the aqueduct

## 2. Acute Demyelinating Diseases

WÜTHRICH et al. (1976) were the first to report contrast uptake in **multiple sclerosis** plaques. CT findings resembling tumor may develop during the acute phase of this disease. However, follow-up CT studies vary considerably with changing clinical symptoms in the course of the disease, as Fig. F23 demonstrates. A recent multiple sclerosis plaque does not always take up contrast media, and multiple low density lesions have also been observed (Fig. F24).

A disorder of the blood-brain barrier may occur in acute cases of **diffuse sclerosis,** which results in contrast enhancement in the involved cerebral region. Figure F25 demonstrates such a case showing a large irregular hypodense zone with marginal contrast uptake.

## 3. Granulomas

**Gummas and tuberculomas** are now so rare that diagnosis is usually made only at histological examination. There are no pathognomonic criteria in the CT scan. The few cases of gumma in our series demonstrated large hypodense zones with multiple small calcifications, a picture resembling that in epidermoid (Fig. F26). Tuberculomas are similar to brain abscesses in the CT scan (Fig. F27). Solid nodes of granulomatous tissue with homogeneous contrast enhancement, similar to that in brain tumors, may also be found.

Circumscribed granulomatous meningitis may occur in **sarcoidosis** with the development of large irregular granulomas which take up contrast material (Fig. F28). There seems to be a predilection for the Sylvian fissure, where we observed two such cases.

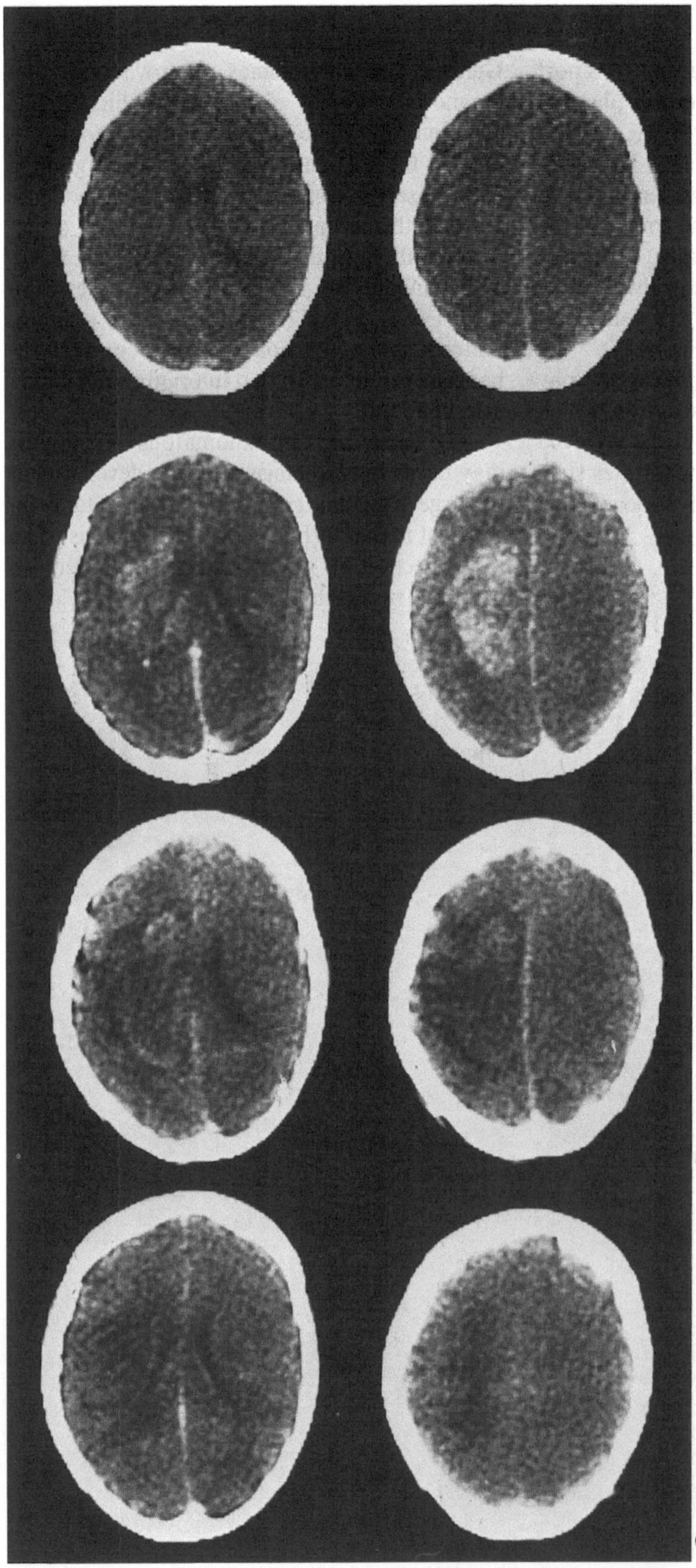

a

b

c

d

**Fig. F23**a–d. Follow-up studies in a 27-year-old female with a diagnosis of multiple sclerosis. Development of right hemiparesis over a period of several days accompanied by speech disorder. Normal findings in the first CT scan (**a**). A circumscribed lesion with strong contrast uptake was demonstrated in the white matter of the left hemisphere adjacent to the lateral ventricle 1 week later (**b**). The lesion does not correspond to the distribution area of a single vessel. Additional CT studies 2 weeks later show less pronounced contrast uptake (**c**), while a follow-up study after 4 more weeks (**d**) demonstrates a hypodense zone in the white matter of the left hemisphere. Postcontrast study

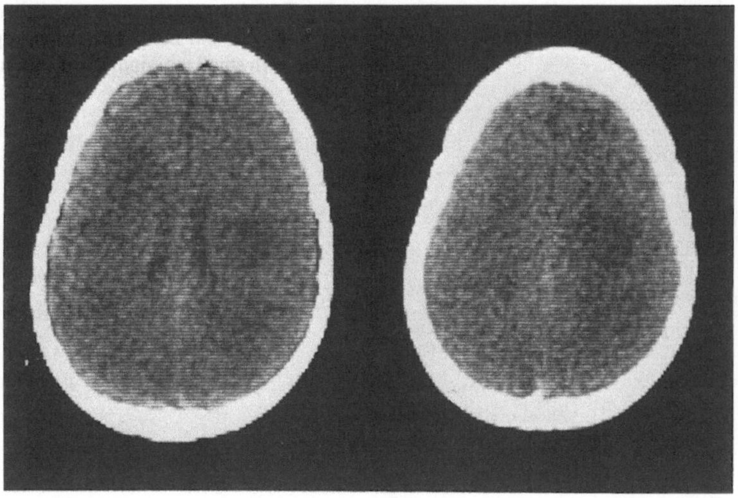

**Fig. F24.** Fresh plaques of multiple sclerosis in the white matter of both cerebral hemispheres in a 21-year-old patient. No contrast uptake in the lesions. Histological confirmation of the diagnosis at autopsy

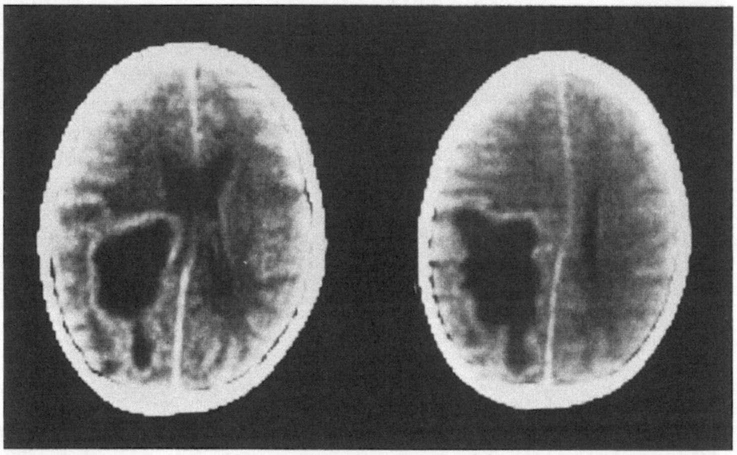

**Fig. F25.** Irregular low density zone in the middle and posterior sections of the left cerebral hemisphere in a 12-year-old boy. Marginal contrast uptake. Initial diagnosis of tumor. Histological diagnosis of acute diffuse sclerosis. (CT studies courtesy of Dr. BACKMUND, Neurology Department of the Max-Planck Institute of Psychiatry, Munich)

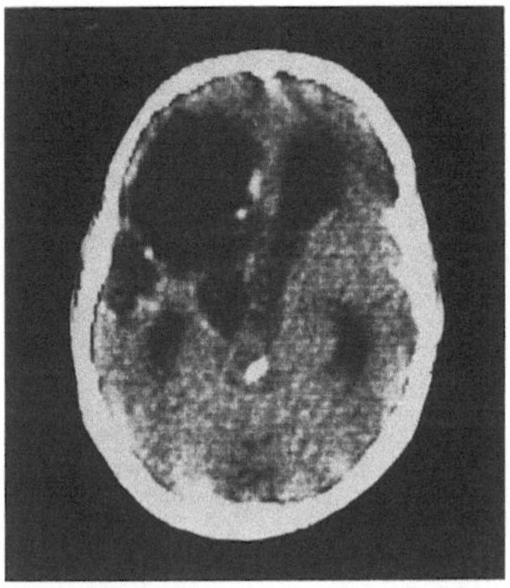

**Fig. F26.** Large gumma in the anterior section of the left cerebral hemisphere in a 48-year-old man. The lesion appears as a sharply delineated hypodense zone with small marginal calcifications. It could be mistaken for an epidermoid cyst

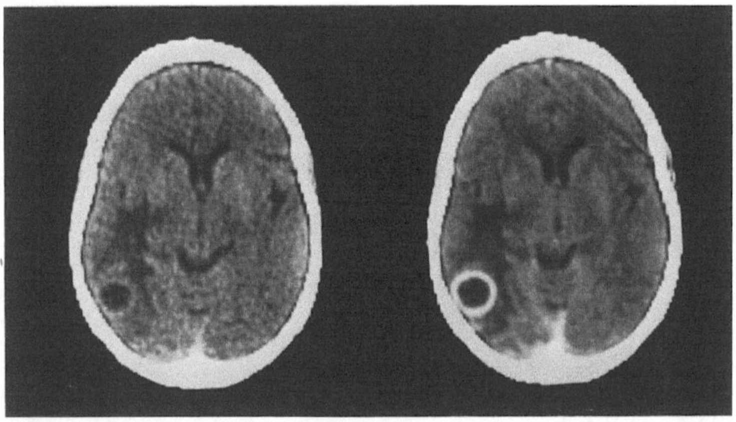

**Fig. F27.** Tuberculoma at the junction of the temporal and occipital lobes on the left in a 66-year-old patient. Grade II perifocal edema and appearance of a ring-like lesion after contrast enhancement. Differentiation from brain abscess is not possible with CT findings alone. No history of tuberculosis. Left, precontrast study; right, postcontrast study

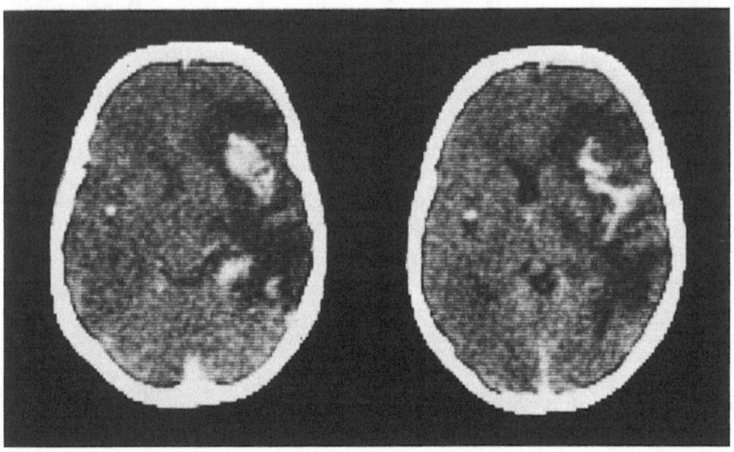

**Fig. F28.** Conglomerate granuloma in the right frontotemporal region in an 8-year-old boy with sarcoidosis. The lesion originates in the meninges of the Sylvian fissure and demonstrates extensive perifocal edema and strong contrast uptake

# 4. Cysts

## a) Arachnoid Cysts

So-called arachnoid cysts are the most common cystic lesions, often found in the temporal region (Figs. F29, 30). They are sometimes discovered when slight head injury forces the cyst fluid into the subdural space (Fig. F31). This occurs most often in children.

CT diagnosis of an arachnoid cyst is made on the basis of absorption values, which equal those of CSF, and of typical location and characteristic changes such as thinning and bulging of the vault above the cyst. The changes in the vault are also visible on plain skull films.

*Arachnoid cysts* are sometimes found in the *chiasmatic cistern,* where very large cysts may develop, especially in children (Fig. F32). These lesions may cause massive hydrocephalus and may be incorrectly diagnosed as an extremely dilated third ventricle.

The *quadrigeminal region* is another rare but typical location of *arachnoid cyst,* which may attain large size, especially in children (so-called supracollicular cysts, Fig. F34).

*Arachnoid cysts* are occasionally found *in the posterior fossa* (Fig. F35), though a large cisterna magna may also simulate an arachnoid cyst of the posterior fossa (Figs. F36, 37). They may also occur in the cerebellopontine angle (Fig. F38), and differentiation from cystic tumors such as angioblastoma may be difficult, if not impossible. Attenuation values are generally higher in the cyst contents of an angioblastoma than in the arachnoid cyst, which has the same density as CSF. These lesions may also be misinterpreted as epidermoid cysts if marginal calcification is not present. Arachnoid cyst in the posterior fossa in an infant may present special problems in diagnosis, since adjacent compressed cerebellar tissue may take up contrast media to a certain extent and simulate a tumor (Fig. F39).

Diagnosis of a *Dandy-Walker cyst* is usually not difficult, since this malformation demonstrates rather characteristic changes. The entire cerebellar vermis is usually missing, and one finds CSF over the entire length of the caudal brain stem from the floor of the fourth ventricle to the vault. The malformation appears rectangular in the middle cross-sections of the cerebellum and circular in the higher sections.

## b) Other Cysts

*So-called simple cysts* (Silverberg, 1971) are found in the posterior fossa, and their density values are not always identical to those of CSF. As a result, confusion with angioblastoma is possible (Figs. F40, 41).

Nonneoplastic cysts are sometimes found in the cerebral hemispheres; their etiology may vary considerably and sometimes remains unclear (Fig. F42). Calcification may occur so that the cyst simulates a tumor (Fig. F43).

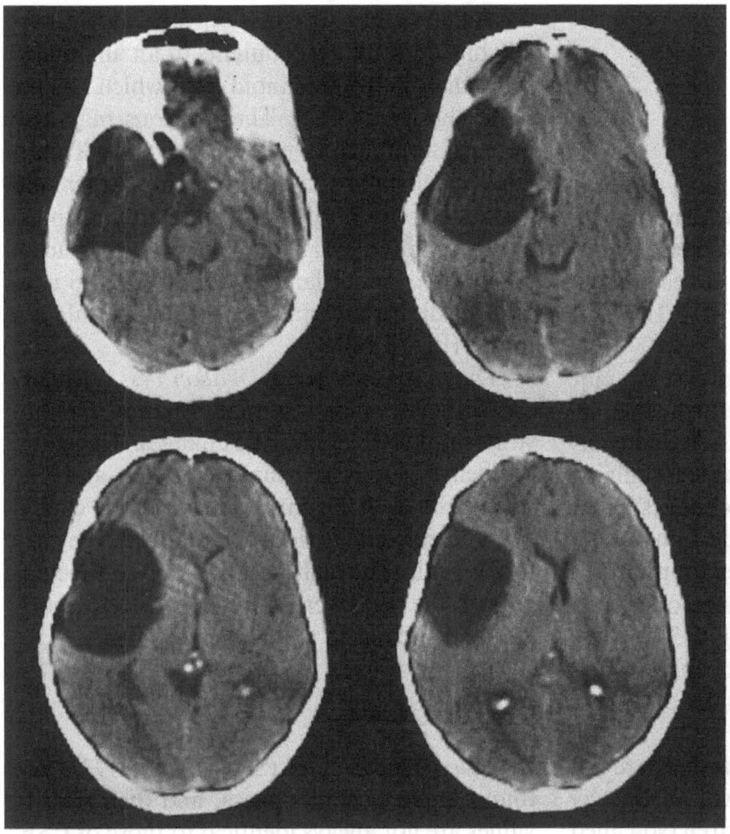

**Fig. F29.** Large arachnoid cyst in the left temporal region with bulging and thinning of the vault above the hypodense lesion (9–11 HU) visible in higher slices. Significant mass effect

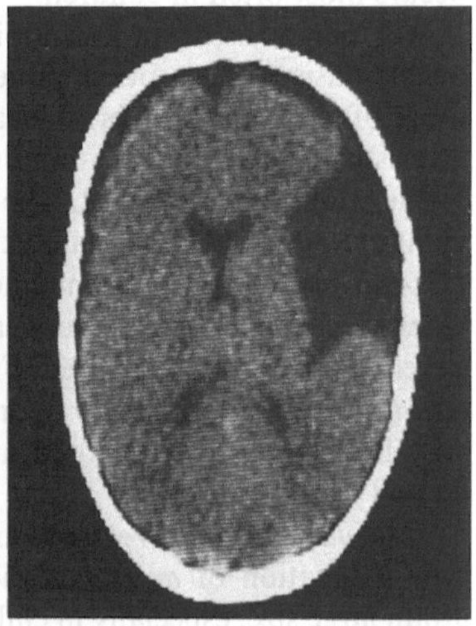

**Fig. F31.** Arachnoid cyst in the right temporal region of a 6-year-old child. Development of bilateral subdural effusions after slight trauma causing a tear in the membrane of the cyst. Precontrast study

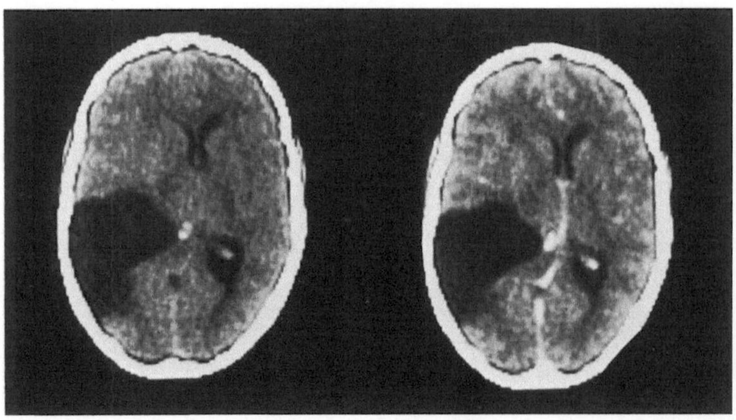

**Fig. F30.** Large arachnoid cyst at the junction of the temporal and occipital lobes on the left with significant mass effect in a 58-year-old female. Density values similar to those of CSF. No change following contrast enhancement. Left, precontrast study; right, postcontrast study

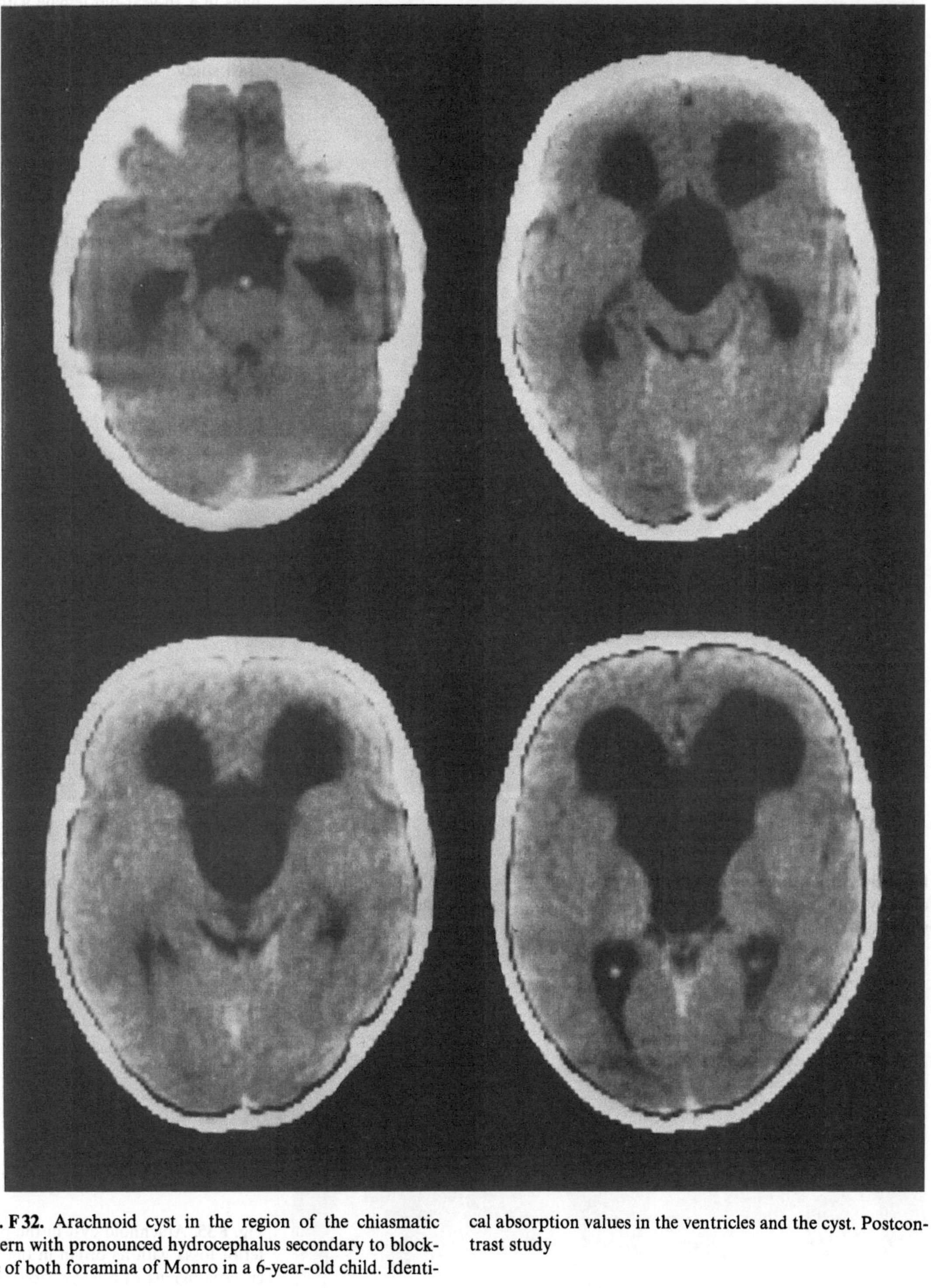

**Fig. F32.** Arachnoid cyst in the region of the chiasmatic cistern with pronounced hydrocephalus secondary to blockage of both foramina of Monro in a 6-year-old child. Identical absorption values in the ventricles and the cyst. Postcontrast study

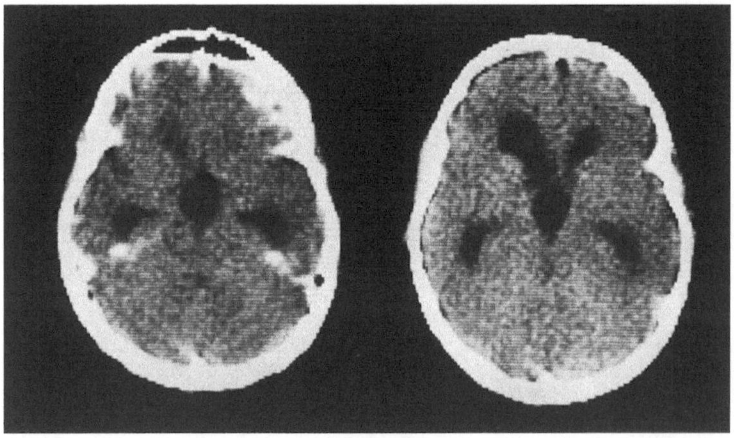

**Fig. F33.** Cyst of the lamina terminalis in a 16-year-old female with hyperprolactinemia and amenorrhea. Confirmation at operation. Precontrast study

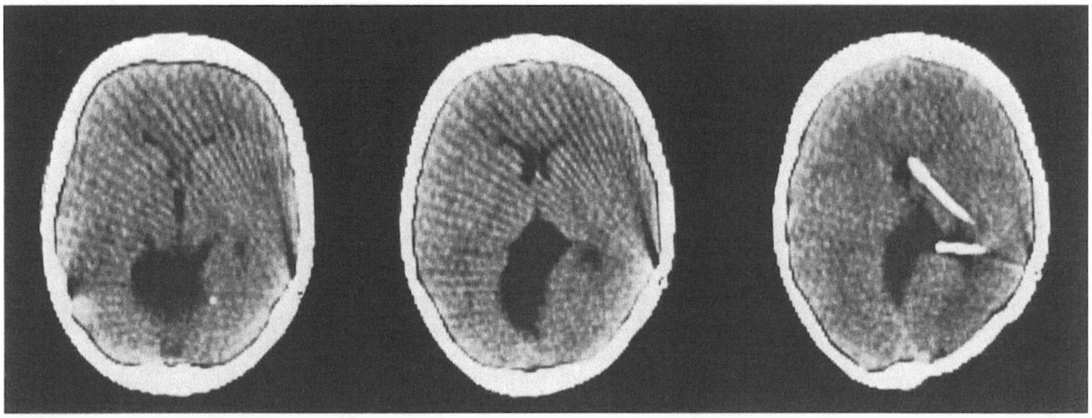

**Fig. F34.** Large supracollicular arachnoid cyst in a 3-year-old boy with hydrocephalus. Large space-occupying lesion with CSF density at the tentorial hiatus on the dorsal side of the midbrain. A CSF drainage system with the ends of the catheter in the cyst and the right anterior horn had been implanted previously

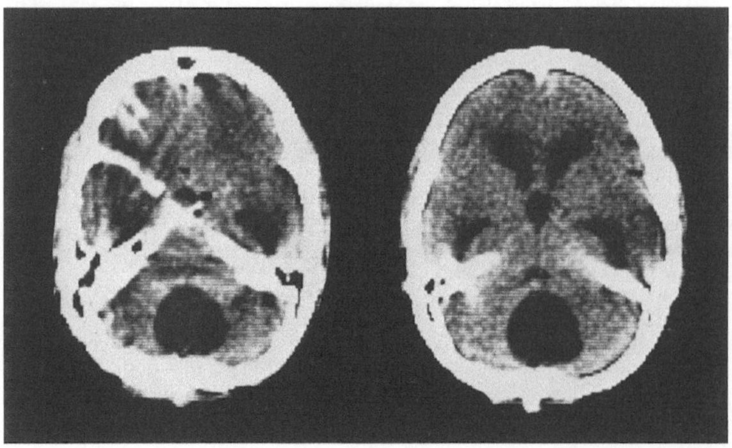

**Fig. F35.** Arachnoid cyst in the posterior fossa with its origin in the cisterna magna of a 50-year-old patient. Compression of the cerebellar vermis and the fourth ventricle with resultant hydrocephalus. Epidermoid cyst is an alternative in differential diagnosis; a hemangioblastoma can be excluded because of CSF density of the cystic lesion

**Fig. F36.** Arachnoid cyst in contact with skull bone in the posterior fossa of a 51-year-old patient. Characteristic changes in bone suggest the diagnosis

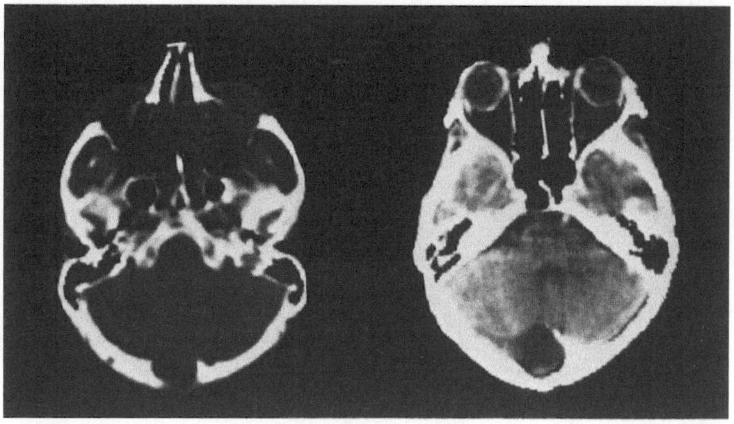

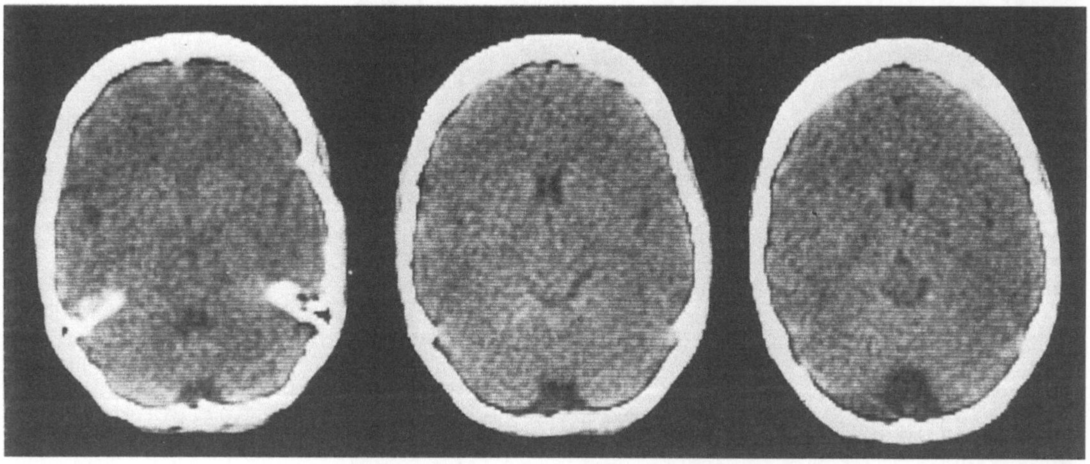

**Fig. F37.** Large cisterna magna which might be mistaken for a cystic lesion in the posterior fossa. 32-year-old female. Absence of space-occupying effect argues against a diagnosis of cystic malformation or tumor

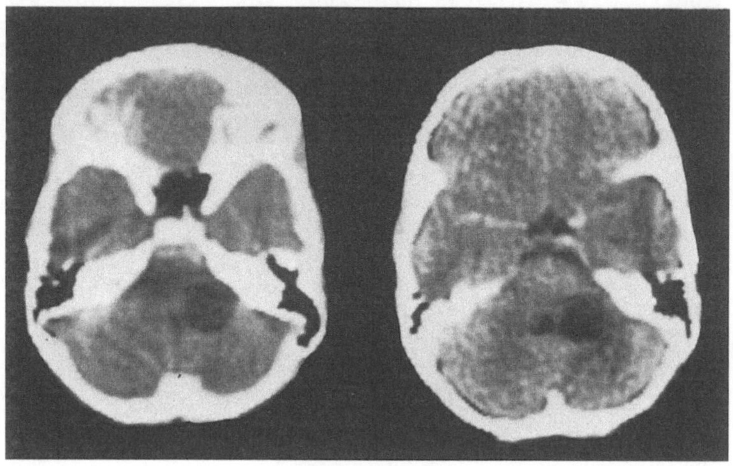

**Fig. F38.** Arachnoid cyst at the right cerebellopontine angle in an 8-year-old girl with signs of a lesion at the cerebellopontine angle. Postcontrast study

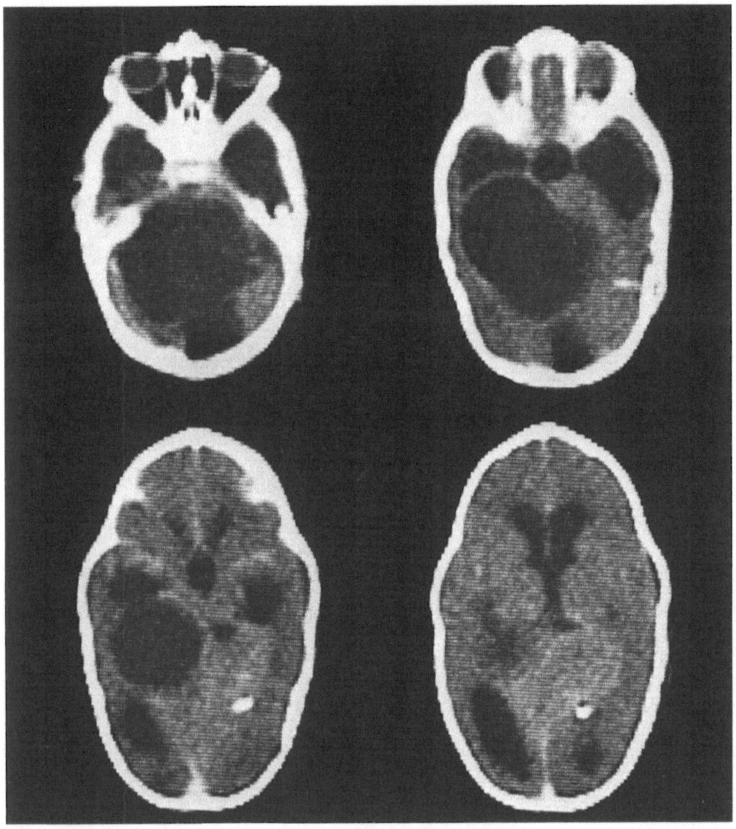

**Fig. F39.** Large arachnoid cyst in the posterior fossa of an 8-month-old child. The cyst extends through the tentorial hiatus to a position under the left temporal lobe and has caused torsion and rostral displacement of the cerebellum which appears as a slightly hyperdense zone next to the cyst on the right (lower pair of CT slices). Orthogradely cut tentorium simulates contrast uptake in the wall of the cyst (upper pair of CT slices, interpretation of the CT scan after operation). Postcontrast study

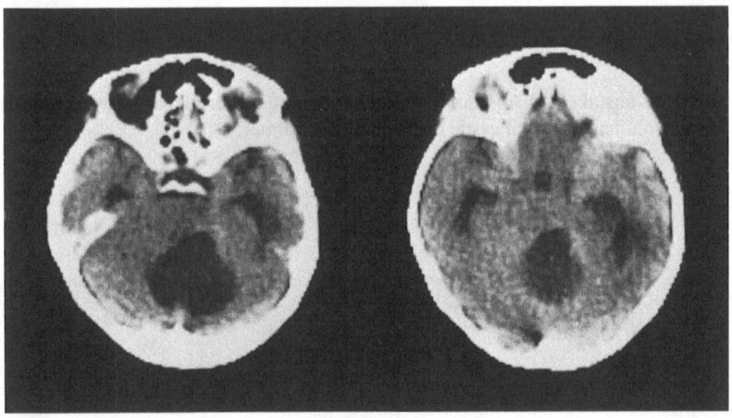

**Fig. F40.** So-called simple cerebellar cyst in the cerebellar vermis of a 69-year-old female with signs of cerebellar dysfunction. Density values in the cyst (18 HU) are significantly higher than those of CSF. Differentiation from cyst in hemangioblastoma is not possible with CT findings alone

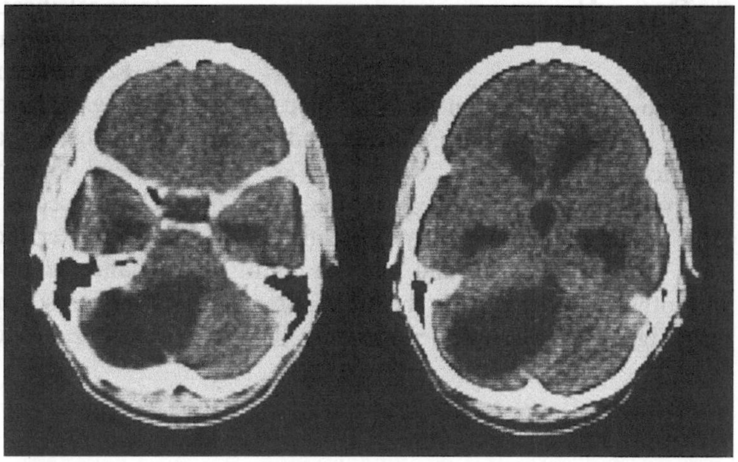

**Fig. F41.** Large so-called simple cyst in the left cerebellar hemisphere accompanied by occlusive hydrocephalus in a 26-year-old patient. Density values in the xanthochromic contents of the cyst only slightly higher than those of CSF, allowing differentiation from hemangioblastoma in this case

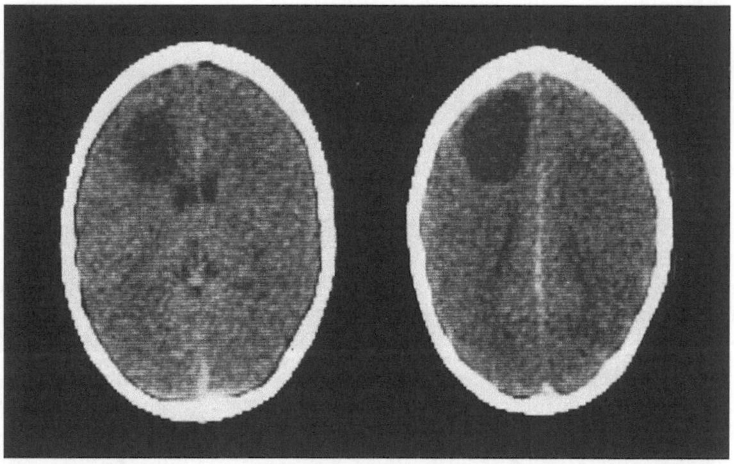

**Fig. F42.** Posttraumatic cyst in the left frontal lobe with compression of the left anterior horn in a 12-year-old boy with a history of craniocerebral injury (old liquefied intracerebral hematoma?)

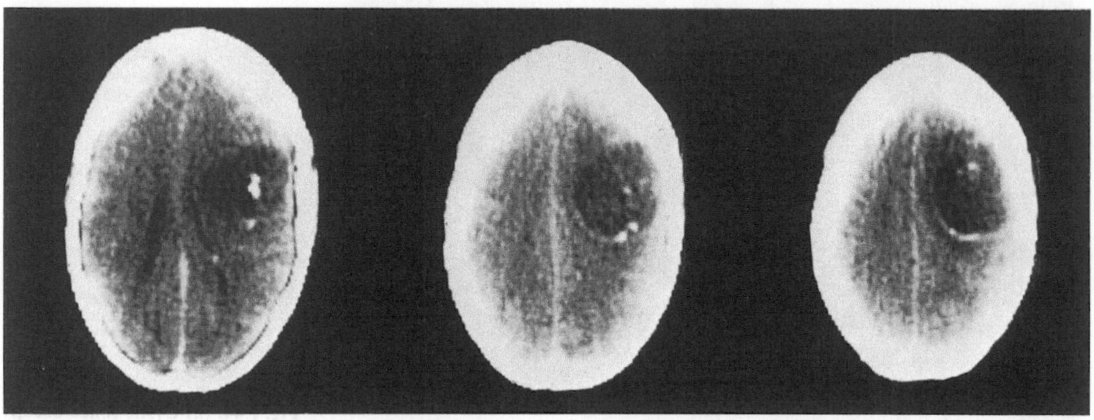

**Fig. F43.** Large cyst with fine specks of calcification in the right frontoprecentral region in a 36-year-old female. Initial misinterpretation of CT findings as oligodendroglioma. A smooth-walled cyst with intramural calcification was found at operation. Partially calcified fibers of fibrin were found in the cyst contents. Possibility of past hemorrhage. Postcontrast study

## 5. Parasites

Parasites are rare nonneoplastic space-occupying lesions in Western Europe and North America.

**Cysticercosis** may appear in the form of large single or multiple sharply delineated lesions with low density and may be confused with other types of cysts in the brain parenchyma (Fig. F44). Multiple lesions may demonstrate calcification, contrast enhancement, and/or cystic structures (Fig. F45).

**Echinococcosis** demonstrates similar CT findings. The correct diagnosis was suspected in one case of alveolar echinococcus in the left parietal lobe of a patient with a history of echinococcosis of the liver. CT findings were uncharacteristic (Fig. F46), and slight contrast enhancement was observed. This contrasts with other cases, where the lesions appeared as low density zones (cysts) without contrast uptake.

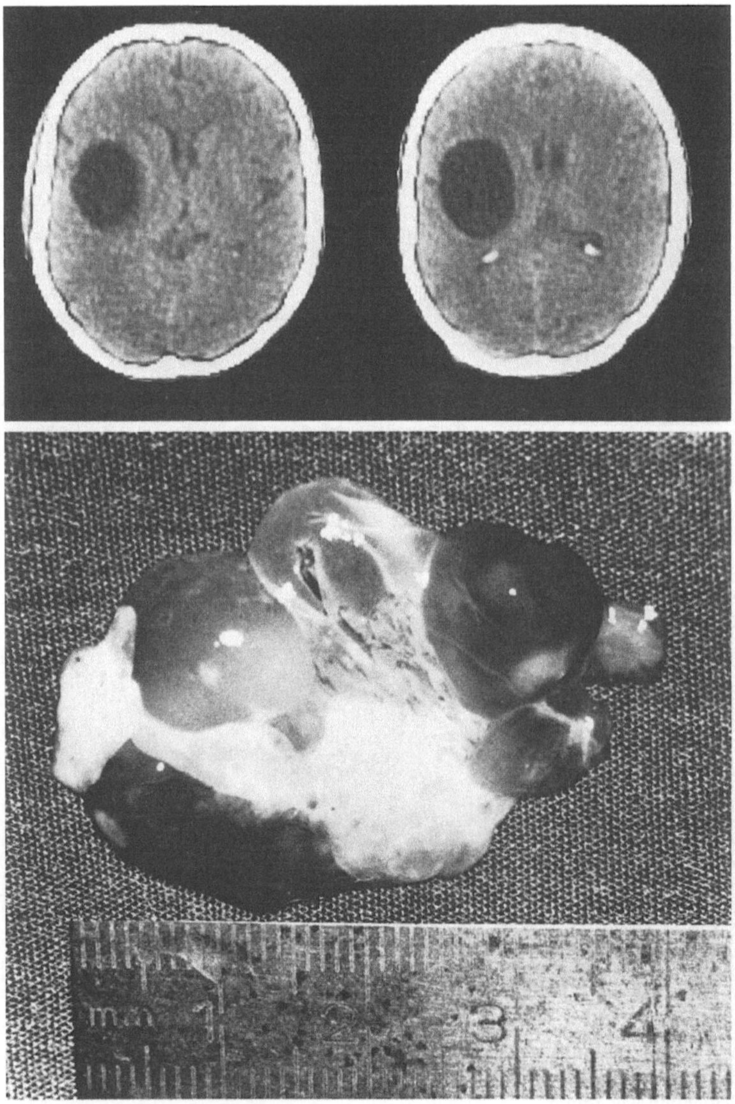

a b

**Fig. F44.** (**a**) Cystic space-occupying lesion deep in the left cerebral hemisphere. (**b**) At operation the lesion was found to contain cysticerci

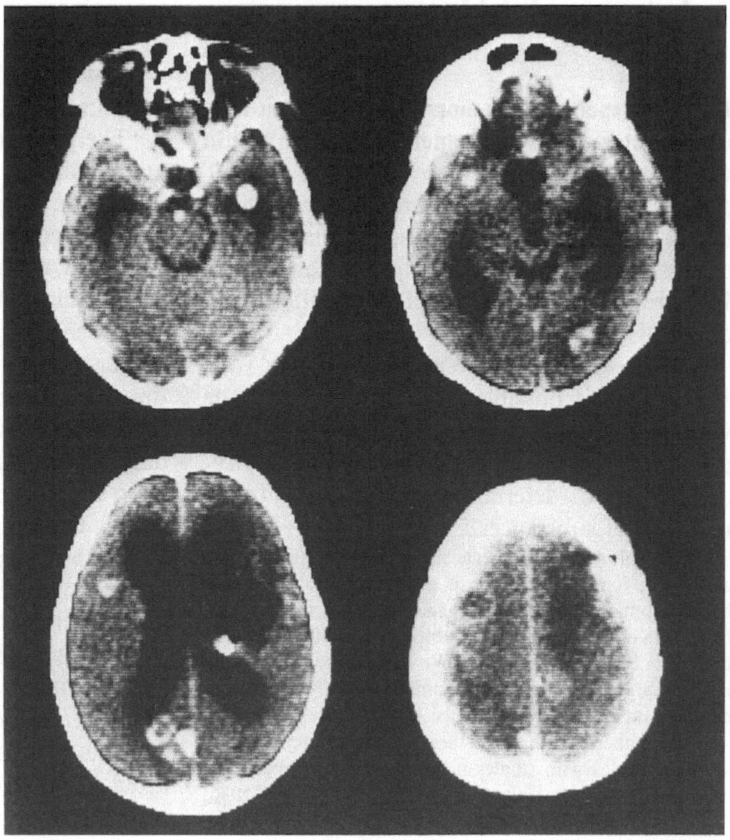

**Fig. F45.** Multiple mixed cystic and solid lesions with calcification and/or contrast uptake in a 54-year-old man with cysticercosis. Burr hole in the right temporal region for biopsy. Postcontrast study

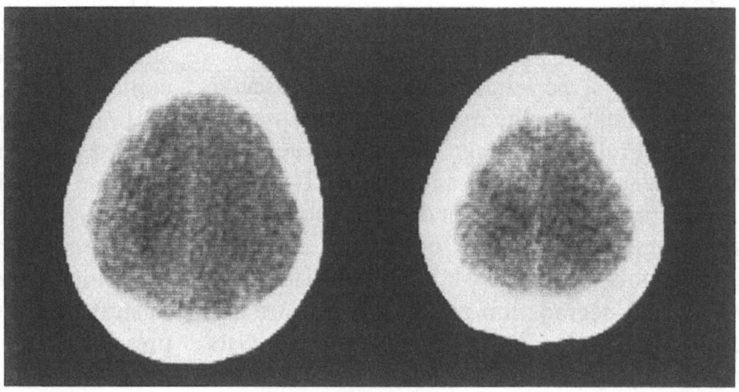

**Fig. F46.** Echinococcosis alveolaris in the left precentral region in a 43-year-old patient. Slightly hyperdense and isodense regions in the precontrast study (left); little contrast uptake (right). The diagnosis was suspected on the basis of known liver echinococcosis

# 6. Intracranial Hematomas

**Recent intracerebral hemorrhage** of any etiology is characterized by extremely high attenuation values ranging from 70 to 90 HU in the CT scan. CT diagnosis of intracranial hemorrhage is not difficult in most cases, especially when the history and clinical findings are considered. Intracranial calcification is the only alternative diagnosis.

*Differentiation between calcification and hemorrhage* is possible when studies are made with two different voltages. HOUNSFIELD proposed this technique, using 100 kV and 140 kV, as a means of determining the relative atomic numbers of substances.

Since photoelectric effects are greater at 100 kV than at 140 kV, X-ray attenuation is greater in substances with higher atomic numbers such as calcium. Therefore, a calcified lesion demonstrates higher absorption values in CT studies with 100 kV than at 140 kV. X-ray absorption in an intracerebral hematoma is determined primarily by electron density and not by the presence of substances with high atomic numbers. As a result, there is little difference in absorption values with studies made at different voltages in case of hemorrhage (PHELBS and COOL 1976; ZATZ 1976; GADO et al. 1977; MARSHALL et al. 1977; MCDAVID et al. 1977; NORMAN 1977; WENDE et al. 1980).

In *rare cases spontaneous intracranial hemorrhage may result from brain tumor* which is not apparent in initial CT studies. This is especially true in hemorrhage at atypical locations (Figs. D1.65, 68, 194).

Arterial *hypertension* and **cerebrovascular malformations** are the most common causes of intracerebral hemorrhage. So-called **chocolate cysts** are a special entity and develop from microangiomas which are not demonstrable in angiographic studies. The "cysts" are encapsulated pools of brownish fluid consisting of blood and degradation products which are not easily absorbed. CT studies of chocolate cysts reveal sharply delineated hyperdense zones (Figs. F47, 48) which do not take up contrast media. Chocolate cysts may persist for long periods of time and maintain high density values for years.

**Hematoma in the lateral pontine region** is another rare finding which simulates a "cerebellopontine angle tumor" in the CT scan. High density values, absence of contrast enhancement and sudden appearance of neurological deficits, usually of the fifth and eighth cranial nerves, allow the correct diagnosis. Microangiomas are usually the source of hemorrhage.

**Older liquified hematomas** may demonstrate hypodense values in rare cases (Fig. 49).

The presence of a sedimentation effect with high absorption values in the posterior part of the lesion suggests the diagnosis (Fig. F50). Perifocal edema may accompany older hematomas, and this may lead to a false diagnosis of tumor (Fig. F49).

At a certain stage of resorption the liquid contents of *a hematoma may demonstrate isodense absorption values,* with the result that the lesion is not demonstrable in the CT scan unless perifocal edema is present (Fig. F51). Ring enhancement may be observed in many cases. The ring structure represents the zone in which resorption takes place. As in all cases of rim enhancement tumor must be considered in the differential diagnosis (cf. Figs. F12–14). WEISBERG (1980) demonstrated that *ring enhancement is a common finding in patients with intracerebral hematomas* if one examines these patients systematically. A ring is visible 7 days after the acute event at the earliest and vanishes after a maximum of 2 months.

## Isodense Chronic Subdural Hematoma

Approximately one-third of chronic subdural hematomas are not directly demonstrable in CT studies because the X-ray absorption of the contents of the hematoma is the same as that of brain tissue. In a previous article we described indirect signs which allow diagnosis of isodense chronic subdural hematoma (GRUMME et al. 1976). These include compression of the ipsilateral ventricle, midline displacement, obliteration of the Sylvian fissure, failure to demonstrate the cortical gyri, and ipsilateral compression of the white matter. Studies with high density resolution usually demonstrate the space-occupying effect of an isodense chronic subdural hematoma, evident in narrowing of the white matter in the supraventricular CT slice (LANKSCH et al. 1978). We consider these findings definitive and no longer perform angiography to confirm the diagnosis.

Three of the 3,750 patients with brain tumors in our series showed *diffuse growth of a glioma extending throughout an entire cerebral hemisphere* which resulted in a great increase in brain volume without a change in tissue density (Figs. D 1.53, 54, p. 57f.). *A type III chronic subdural hematoma* was considered in the differential diagnosis of these cases. *Rapid infusion of a large dose of contrast medium* allows certain differentiation between the two lesions, since increase of density in the cerebral cortex and enhancement of the hematoma capsule are demonstrated in some cases of chronic subdural hematoma (Fig. F 52).

*Bilateral isodense chronic subdural hematomas* are characterized by a reduction in the distance between the tips of the anterior horns with an abnormally acute angle between these structures ("rabbit-ear phenomenon", MARCU and BECKER, 1977). The lateral ventricles are conspicuously narrow even in the cella media region in such cases (Fig. F 53).

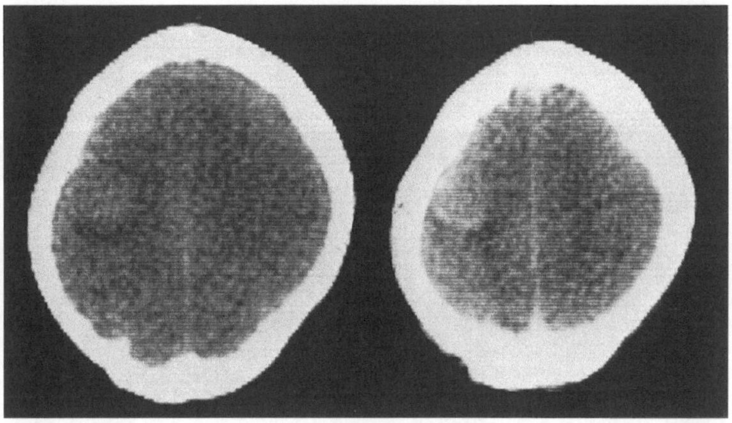

**Fig. F 47.** So-called chocolate cyst in the left parietal region, initially interpreted as tumor, in a 30-year-old patient. Histological diagnosis of microangioma with past hemorrhage. History of paresthesia in the right hand and focal seizures. Post-contrast study, no contrast medium uptake

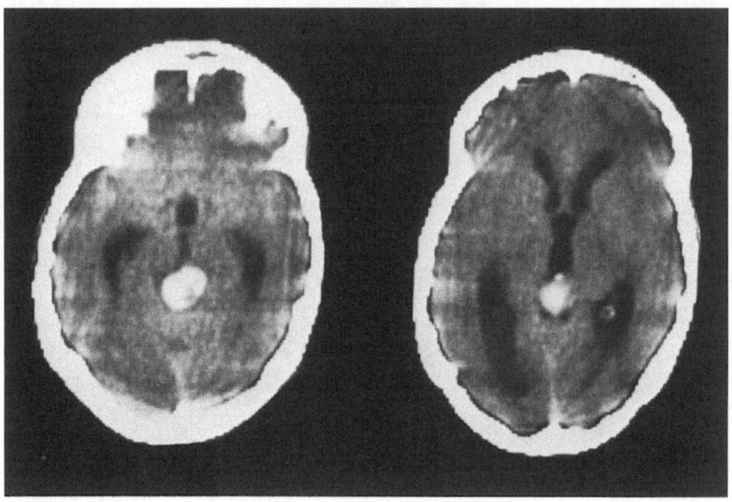

**Fig. F 48.** So-called chocolate cyst with microangioma in the midbrain of a 23-year-old patient with subarachnoid hemorrhage. CT findings do not allow differentiation from calcified pinealoma. (CT studies courtesy of Dr. BACKMUND, Max-Planck Institute of Psychiatry, Munich)

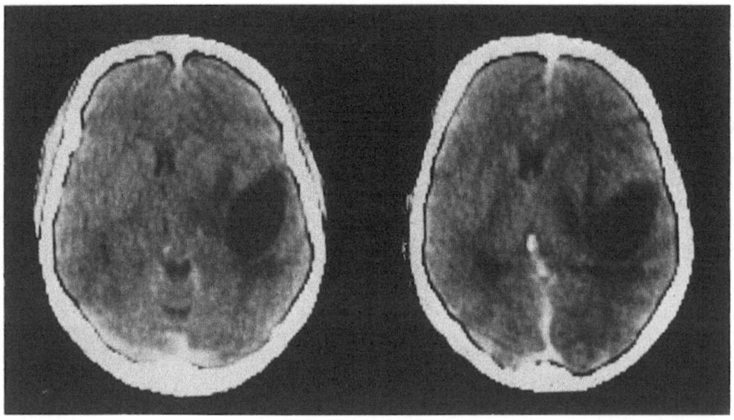

**Fig. F49.** Old liquefied hematoma in the right temporal lobe with space-occupying effect and finger-shaped perifocal edema in a 37-year-old patient. No contrast uptake in the lesion. CT findings similar to those in cystic astrocytoma. Postcontrast study

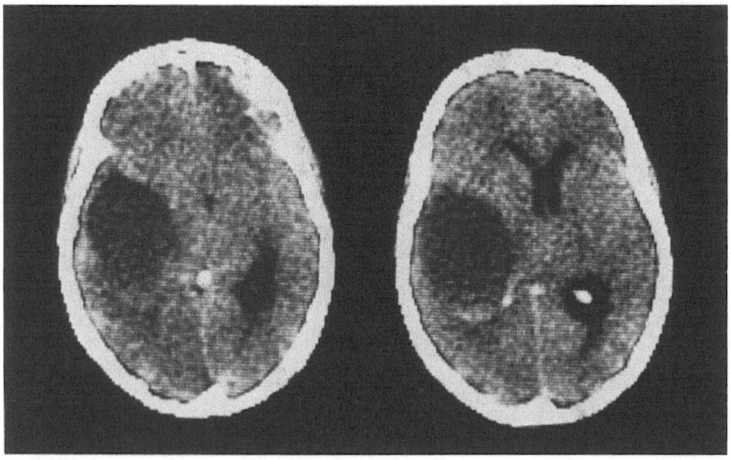

**Fig. F50.** Old liquefied intracerebral hematoma in the left temporal lobe of a 29-year-old patient with no history of an acute neurological disorder. Sedimentation effect in the lesion suggests the correct diagnosis (slightly hyperdense zone in the posterior segment of the hematoma cavity in the CT scan on the right). Appearance of the lesion unchanged after contrast enhancement. Initial diagnosis of astrocytoma with low-grade malignancy

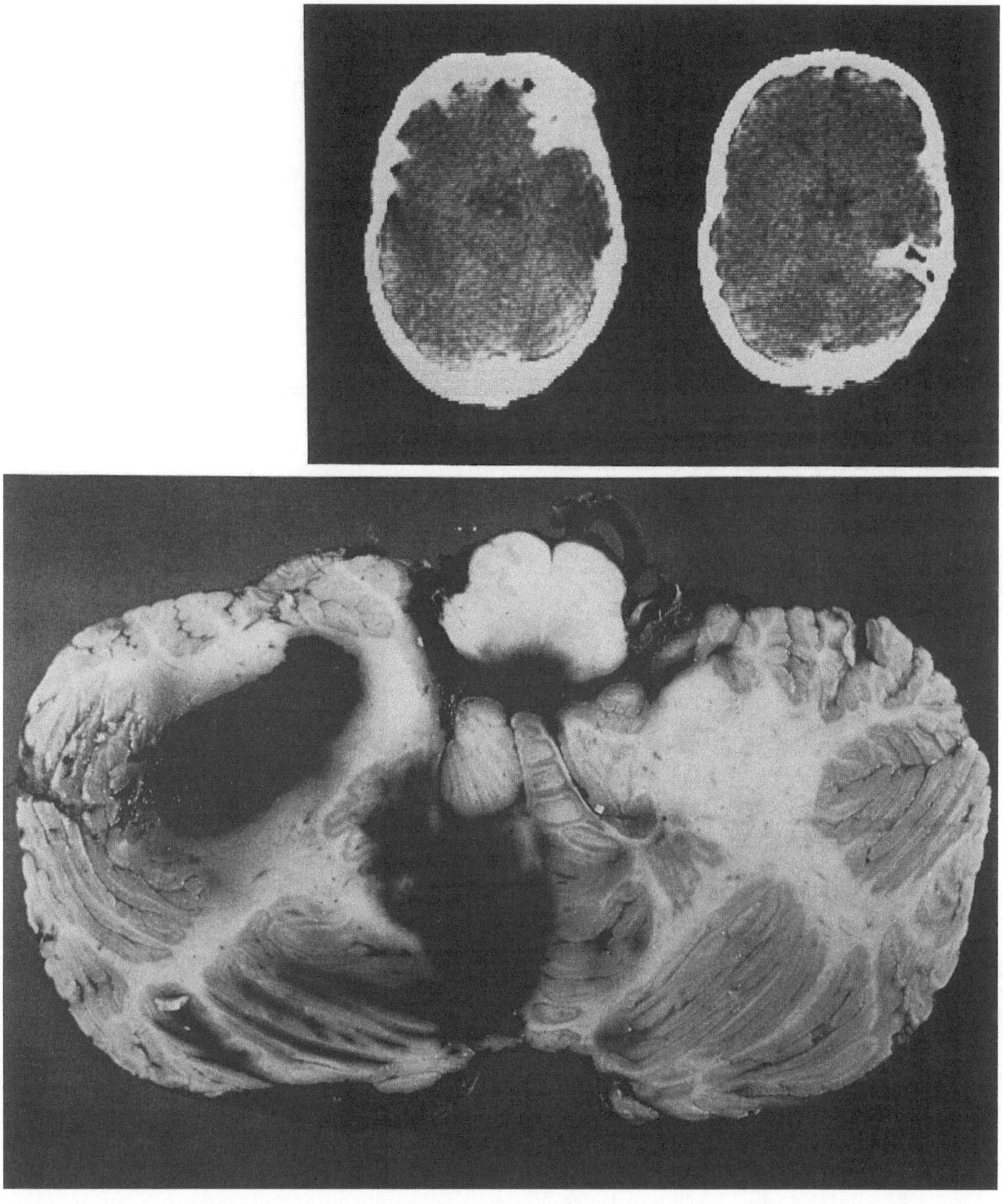

**Fig. F51.** Isodense hematoma in the left cerebellar hemisphere in a 59-year-old patient. Comparison with the autopsy specimen. Recent fatal hemorrhage in the dentate nucleus a short time after the CT study. (Specimen courtesy of Priv.-Doz. Dr. G. EBHARDT, Neuropathological Institute, Free University of Berlin)

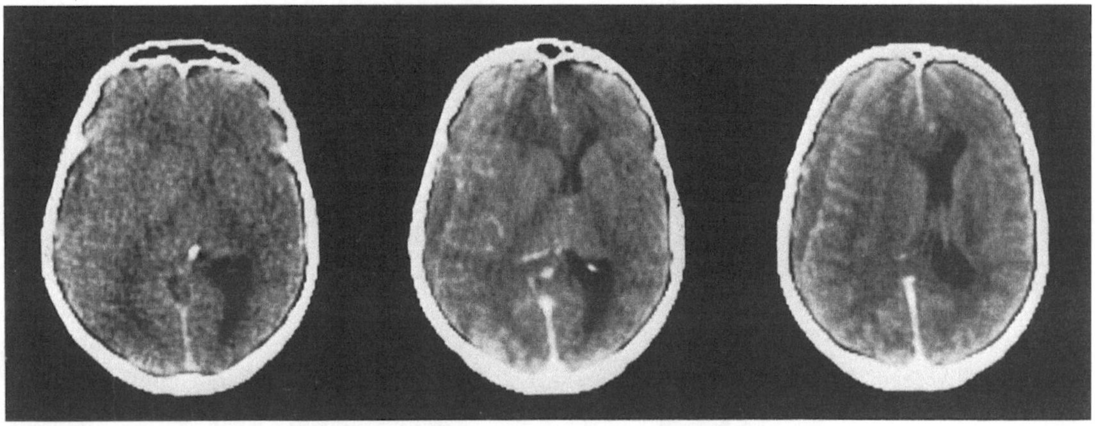

**Fig. F52.** Isodense chronic subdural hematoma above the left cerebral hemisphere in a 45-year-old female. Left, precontrast study; middle and right, postcontrast studies. Clear demarcation of the hematoma by contrast uptake in the cortex

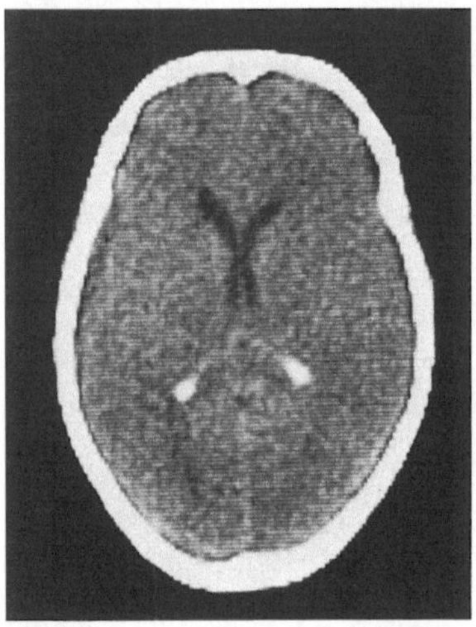

**Fig. F53.** Bilateral isodense chronic subdural hematoma in a 67-year-old male. Acute angle between the anterior horns resulting from bilateral compression ("rabbit ear phenomenon")

# 7. Vascular Malformations

**Large arteriovenous malformations** may have a space-occupying effect even in the absence of hemorrhage (Figs. F 54–56). These lesions are often characterized by homogeneous slightly hyperdense irregularly shaped zones in plain scans with great increases in density following contrast enhancement.

*Extensive calcification is often found in and around angiomas,* a phenomenon which facilitates diagnosis (Fig. F 57). The afferent and efferent vessels are often demonstrated as serpentine figures after contrast enhancement in large arteriovenous malformations. Angiomas in the midbrain or the caudal brain stem may simulate pontine tumors after contrast enhancement (Fig. F 58). As in all other cases of a-v malformation, definitive diagnosis is the preserve of cerebral angiography (cf. Fig. F 54).

**Sturge-Weber disease** (encephalotrigeminal syndrome) is characterized by garland-like calcification in the cerebral cortex, especially in the temporo-parieto-occipital region, though involvement of the frontal lobes may be observed in exceptional cases. These findings may be confused with tumor only if the typical port-wine naevus in the face is absent. Circumscribed brain atrophy with dilatation of the external CSF space and thickening of the skull vault above the involved brain region also suggest the diagnosis (Fig. F 59).

**Large suprasellar and parasellar aneurysms** may simulate pituitary adenomas or meningiomas (Fig. E 20, p. 393, F 60). Intense contrast uptake is always suggestive of a vascular lesion, especially when calcification is also present (Figs. F 61, 63). Differentiation between a large aneurysm and a tumor may also be difficult in lesions at other locations (Figs. F 64, 65, 67–71).

*A false diagnosis of tumor in a case of giant aneurysm* is especially likely when thrombosis involves a large portion of the aneurysm (Fig. F 67). Giant aneurysm should be suspected when density increases at the periphery and when a ring structure appears. Circumscribed calcification may be found in the capsule, and contrast uptake is present only in the portions of the vascular lesion containing circulating blood (Fig. F 67).

*Aneurysm of the vein of Galen* is a rare cause of hydrocephalus in children. The lesion may simulate a tumor in the pineal region in the precontrast CT study, but strong contrast enhancement usually permits the diagnosis (Fig. F 72). CT diagnosis of this type of vascular lesion does not pose problems even in cases with asymmetrical development (MARTELLI et al. 1980).

**Basilar artery ectasia** appears as a wide hyperdense band with a tortuous course which may reach as far as the cerebellopontine angle. The lesion may resemble a tumor in some CT projections (Figs. F 73–76). Ectasia of both internal carotid arteries may also occur (Fig. F 77).

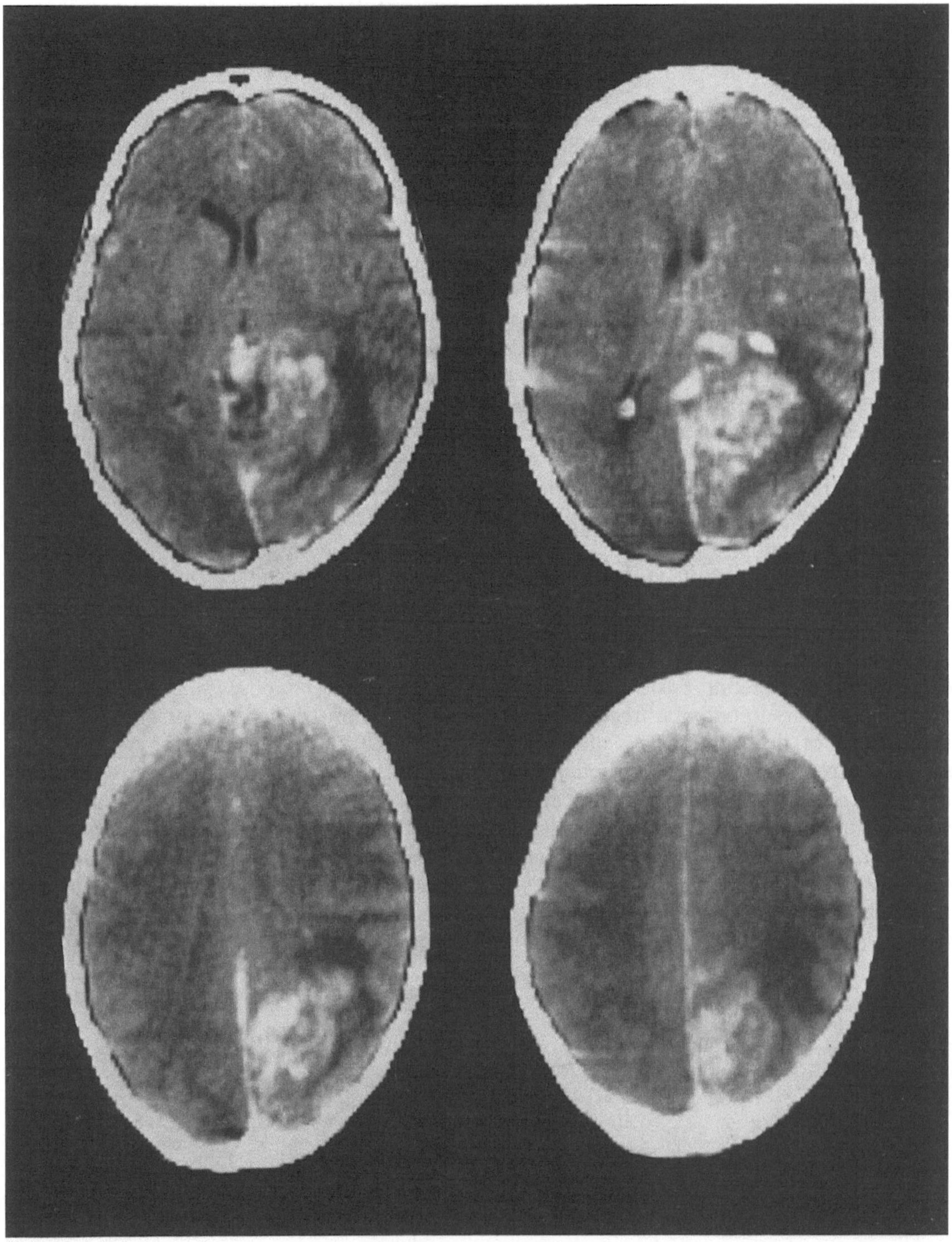

a

**Fig. F54**a–c. Large arteriovenous malformation in the right occipital lobe in a 48-year-old female. The vascular lesion is served primarily by the right posterior cerebral artery (**b**, **c**). Note the pronounced space-occupying effect (**a**). Anterior displacement of the choroid plexus, compression of the right posterior horn and perifocal edema. Misinterpretation as brain tumor is possible. Postcontrast study

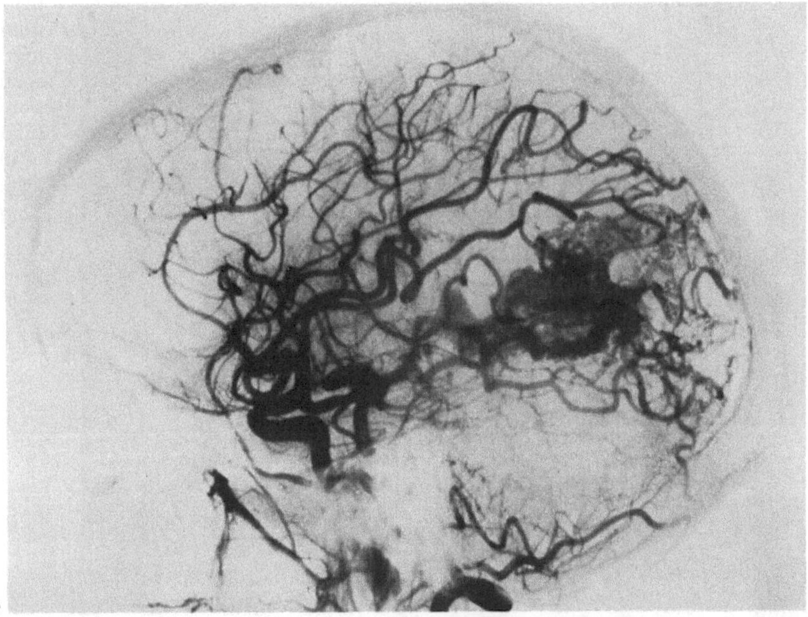

Fig. F 54 b

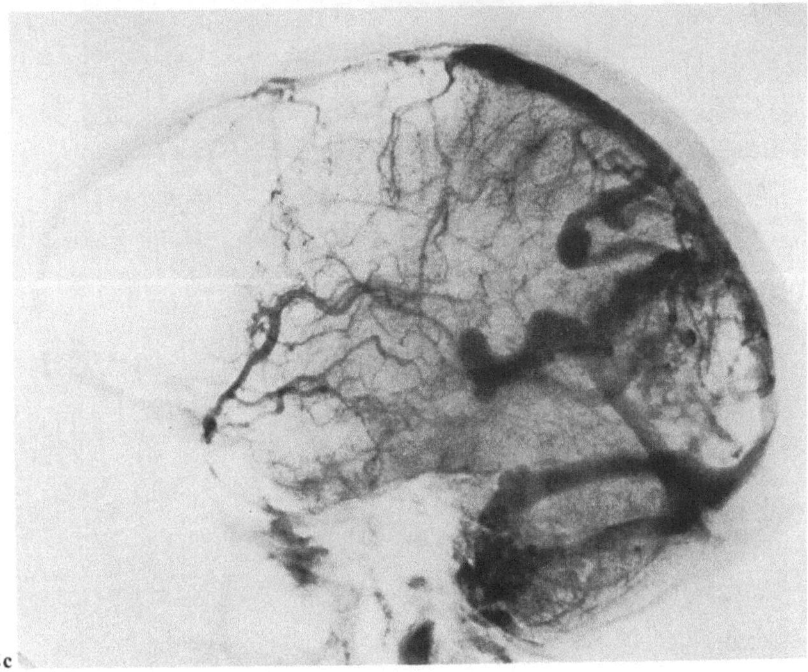

Fig. F 54 c

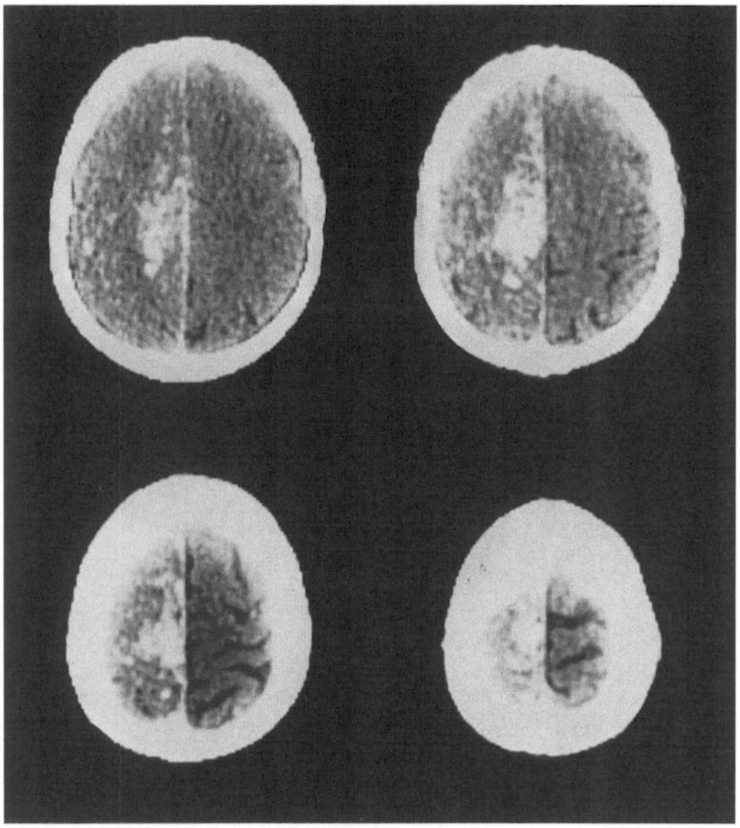

**Fig. F55.** Arteriovenous malformation in the left central region (postcontrast study). The irregular contour and speckled inhomogeneous contrast uptake in the vascular lesion are characteristic. The cortex is not demonstrated on the left due to the space-occupying effect of the angioma. Postcontrast study. 57-year-old female

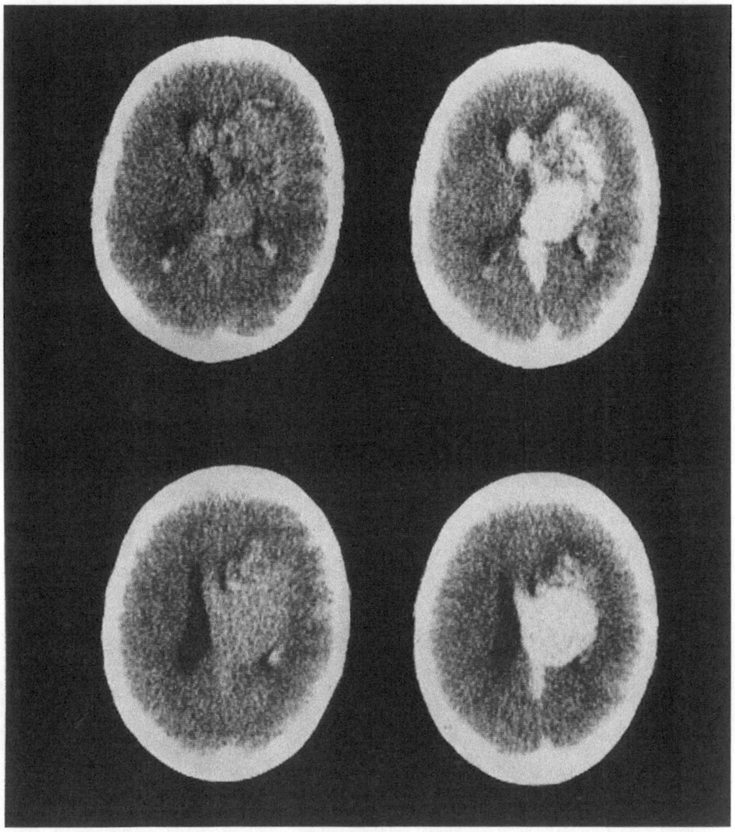

**Fig. F56.** Very large arteriovenous malformation in the right cerebral hemisphere with strong contrast uptake. Left, precontrast study; right, postcontrast study. (CT studies courtesy of Prof. Dr. J. LISSNER, Radiology Department, Klinikum Großhadern, Ludwig-Maximilian University, Munich)

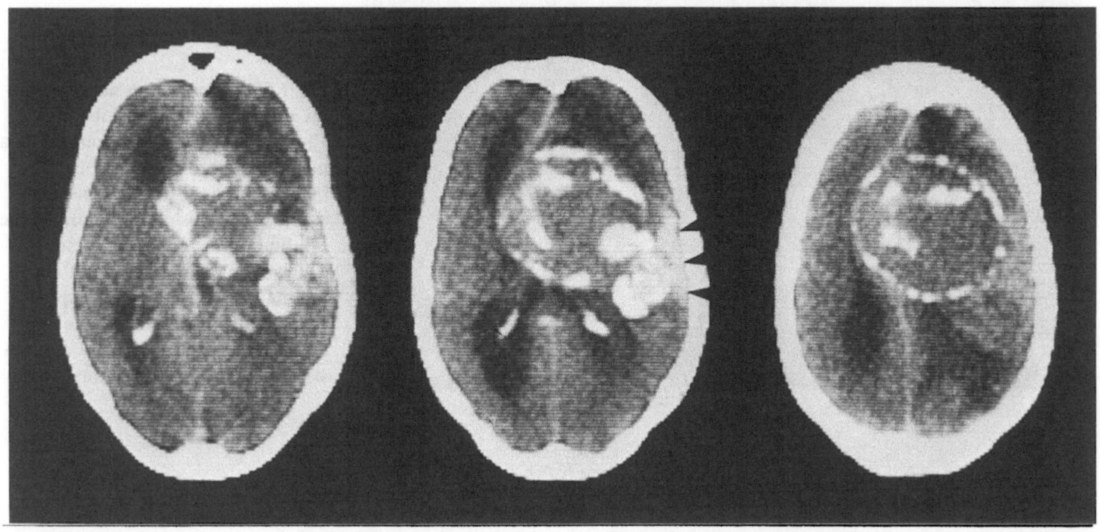

**Fig. F57.** Partially calcified arteriovenous malformation with past intracerebral hemorrhage (ring of marginal calcification) in a 55-year-old female. A meningioma with superficial growth pattern in the right temporal region was found unexpectedly at operation (black arrow tips). The lesion was not identified preoperatively in the CT scans. Postcontrast study

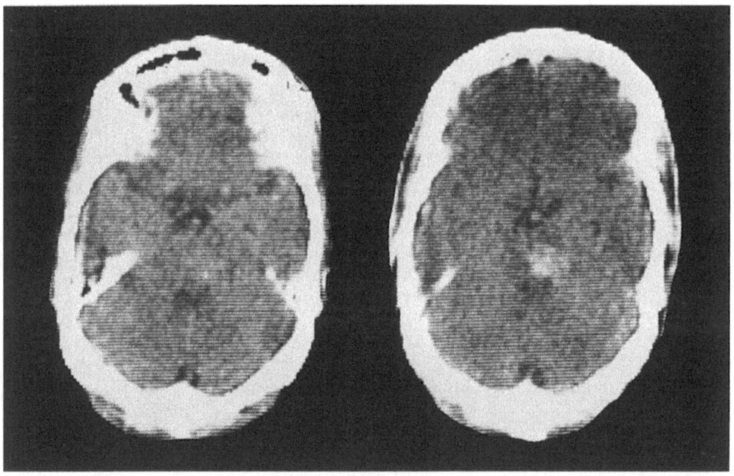

**Fig. F58.** Arteriovenous malformation in the right pontine region of a 43-year-old patient. The precontrast study shows a small calcification (left). Contrast enhancement reveals an irregular hyperdense zone, representing the vascular lesion (right)

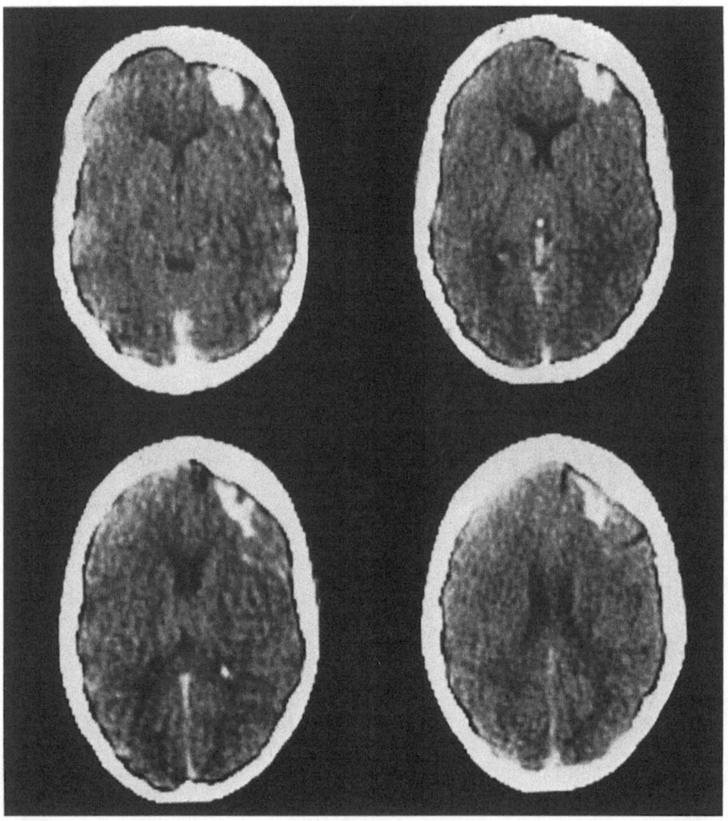

**Fig. F59.** Calcification near the cortex of the right frontal lobe in a 17-year-old female with seizures as a manifestation of encephalotrigeminal syndrome (Sturge-Weber disease). Initial misinterpretation of the CT findings as oligodendroglioma. Thickening of the skull vault above the malformation, circumscribed cortical atrophy, and absence of mass effects argue against a diagnosis of neoplasm. Postcontrast study

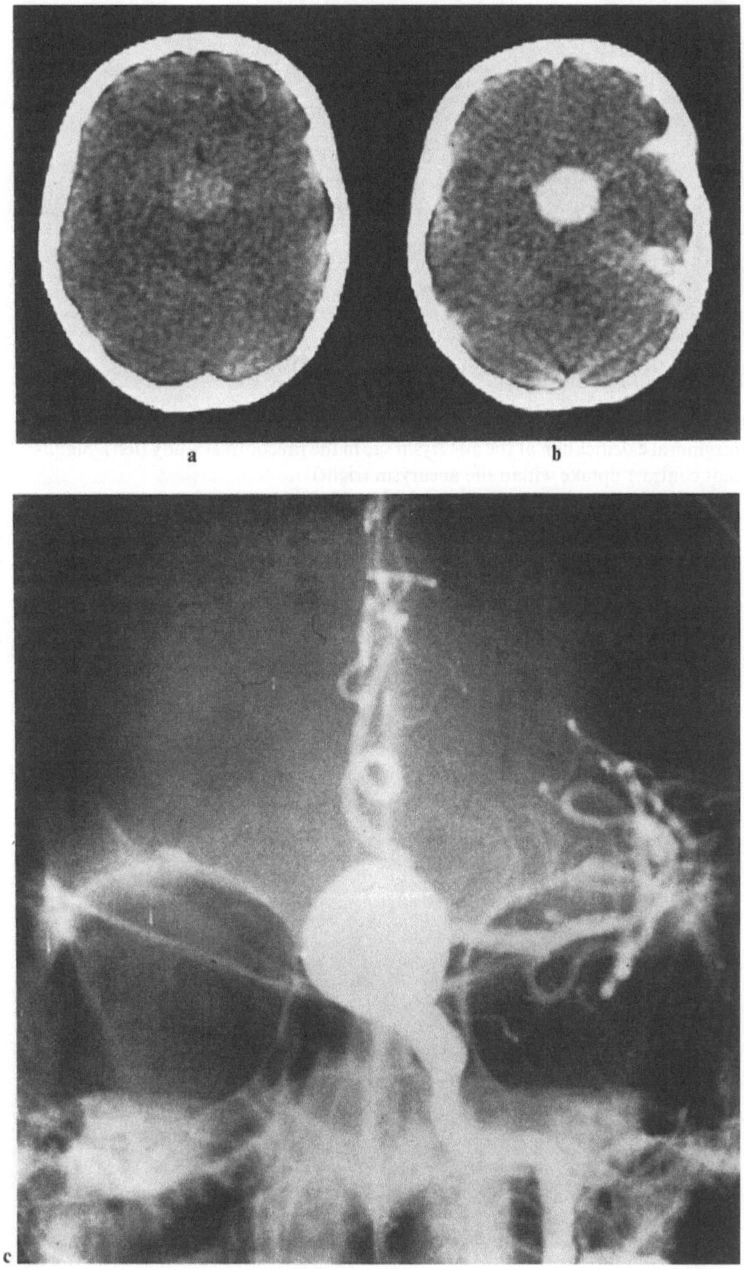

**Fig. F60** a–c. Very large so-called ophthalmic aneurysm of the left carotid artery in precontrast (**a**) and postcontrast studies (**b**) in a 58-year-old female. CT findings resemble those in suprasellar pituitary adenoma or meningioma of the tuberculum sellae. A major increase in density values after contrast enhancement suggests the presence of a vascular lesion (**b**). Angiography provides the definitive diagnosis (**c**)

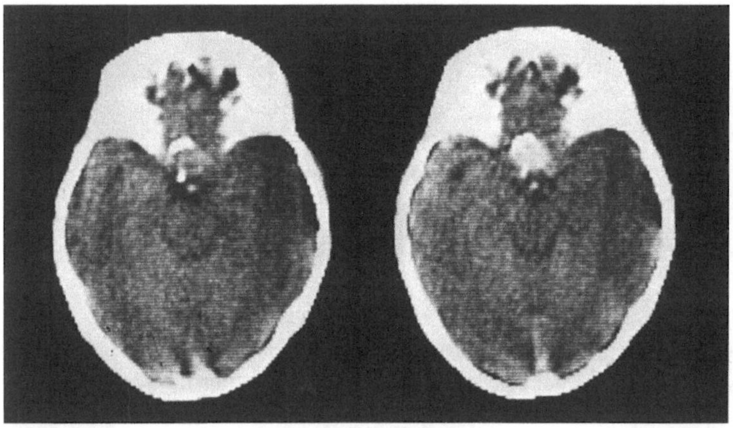

**Fig. F61.** Ophthalmic aneurysm of the left carotid artery in a 65-year-old female. Intramural calcification of the aneurysm sac in the precontrast study (left). Significant contrast uptake within the aneurysm (right)

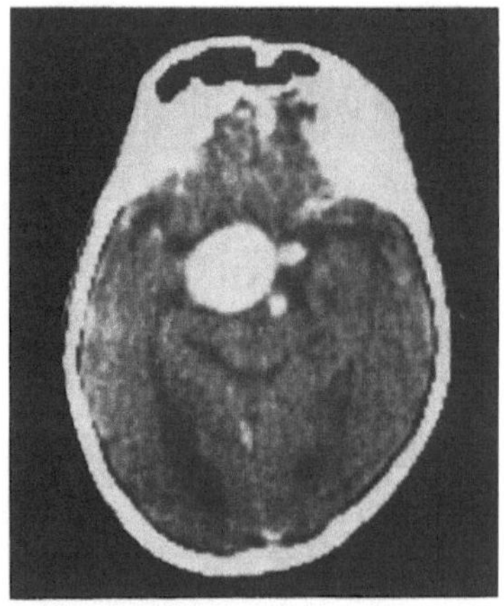

▲ a

**Fig. F62** a, b. Giant carotid aneurysm on the left in a 64-year-old patient. (**a**) Strong homogeneous uptake of contrast medium in the aneurysm as well as in the right internal carotid artery and the basilar artery, which are demonstrated on the right adjacent to the aneurysm. (**b**) Angiogram in the same patient

▼

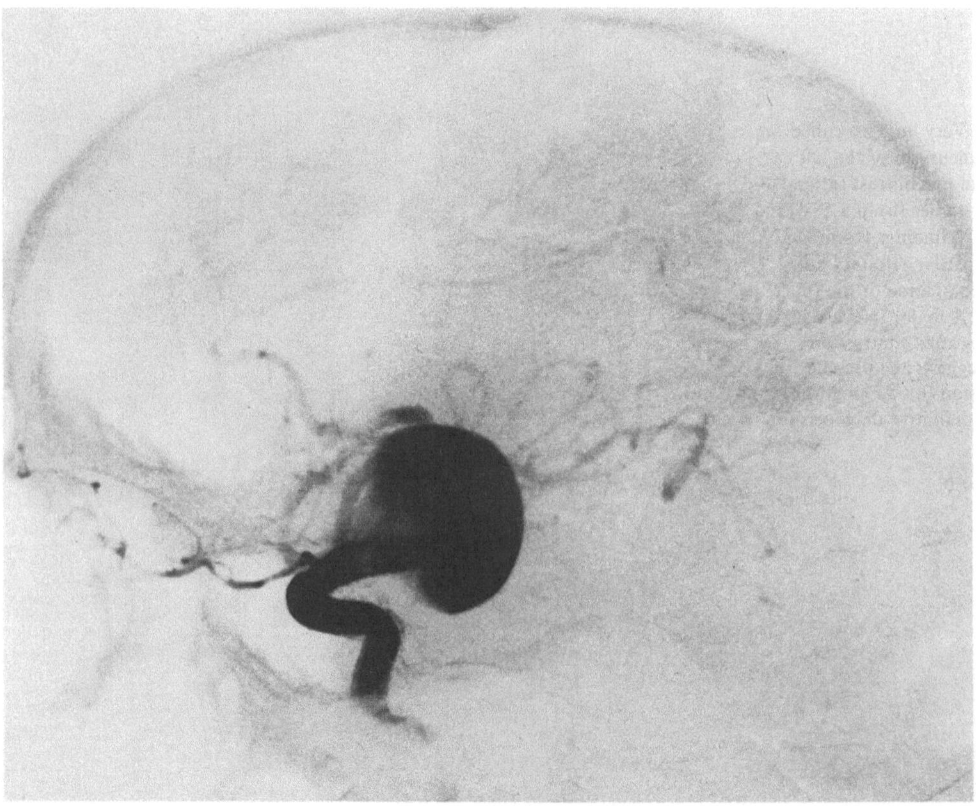

b

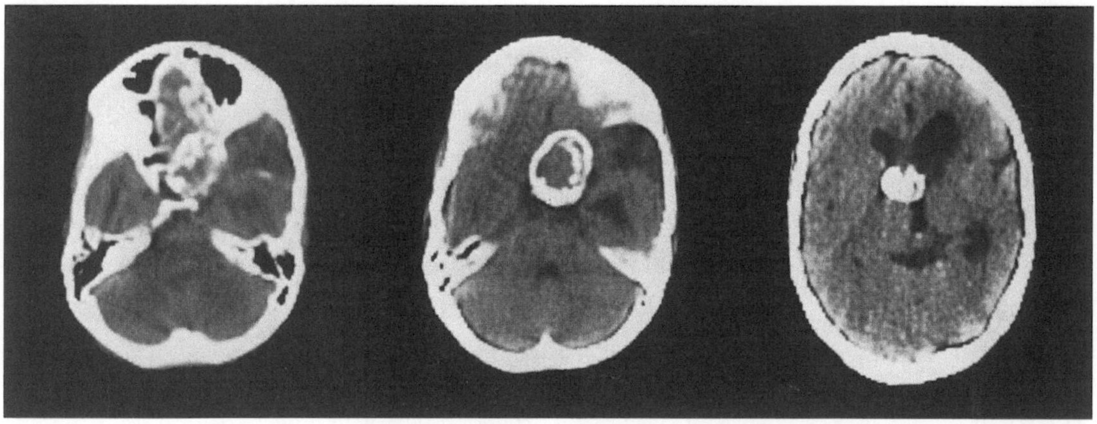

**Fig. F 63.** Large aneurysm of the right internal carotid artery in a 29-year-old patient. Demonstration of extensive calcification, primarily in the wall of the aneurysm, in several horizontal slices. This type of capsular calcification is characteristic of aneurysm

**Fig. F 64.** Aneurysm in the infraclinoidal segment of the left carotid artery in a 10-year-old boy. Strong contrast uptake in the aneurysm. Bone destruction in the left sphenoid wing and the tip of the left petrous bone. These findings argue against a diagnosis of meningioma. Postcontrast study

►

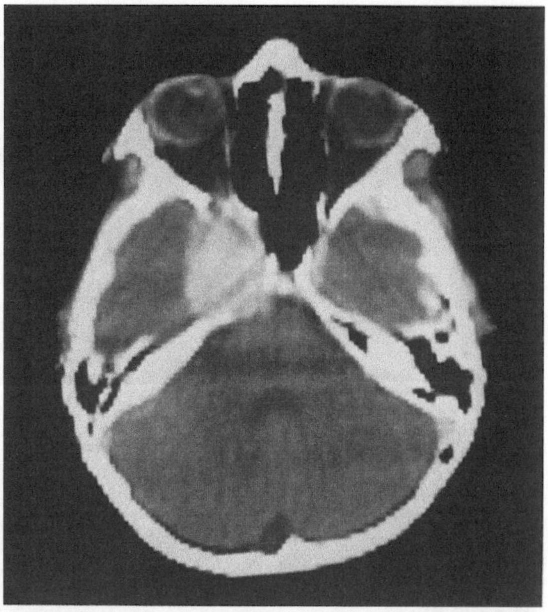

**Fig. F 65.** Saccular aneurysm at the carotid bifurcation on the right. Rostral extension with compression of the right anterior horn. Cone of edema from the tip of the right anterior horn to the external capsule. Bilateral calcification of the basal ganglia as an incidental finding. 52-year-old patient. Postcontrast study

▼

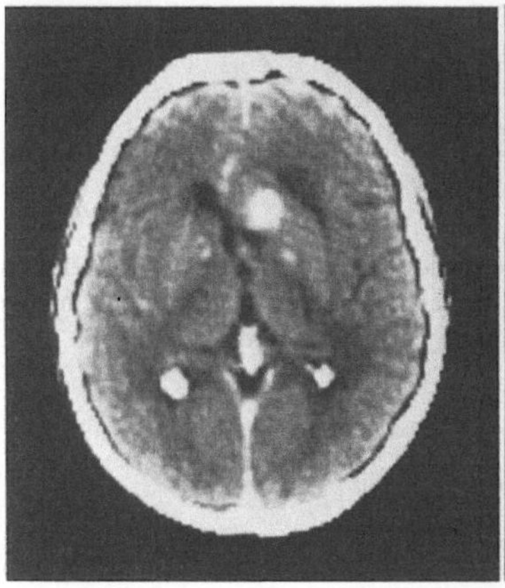

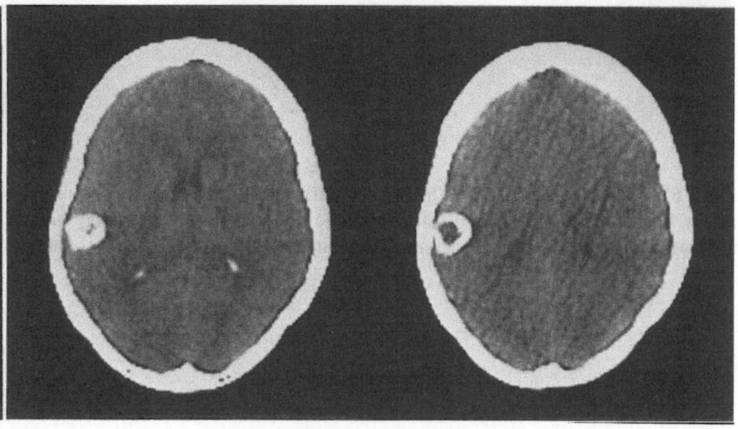

**Fig. F 66.** Aneurysm of a peripheral branch of the left middle cerebral artery with a ring of calcification in a 28-year-old female

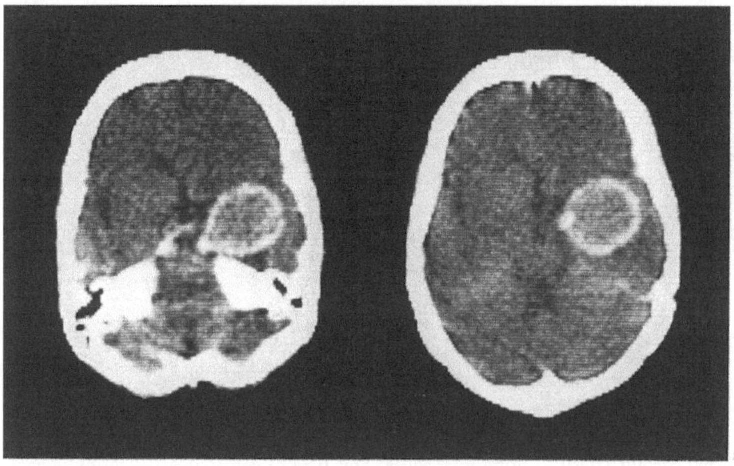

a

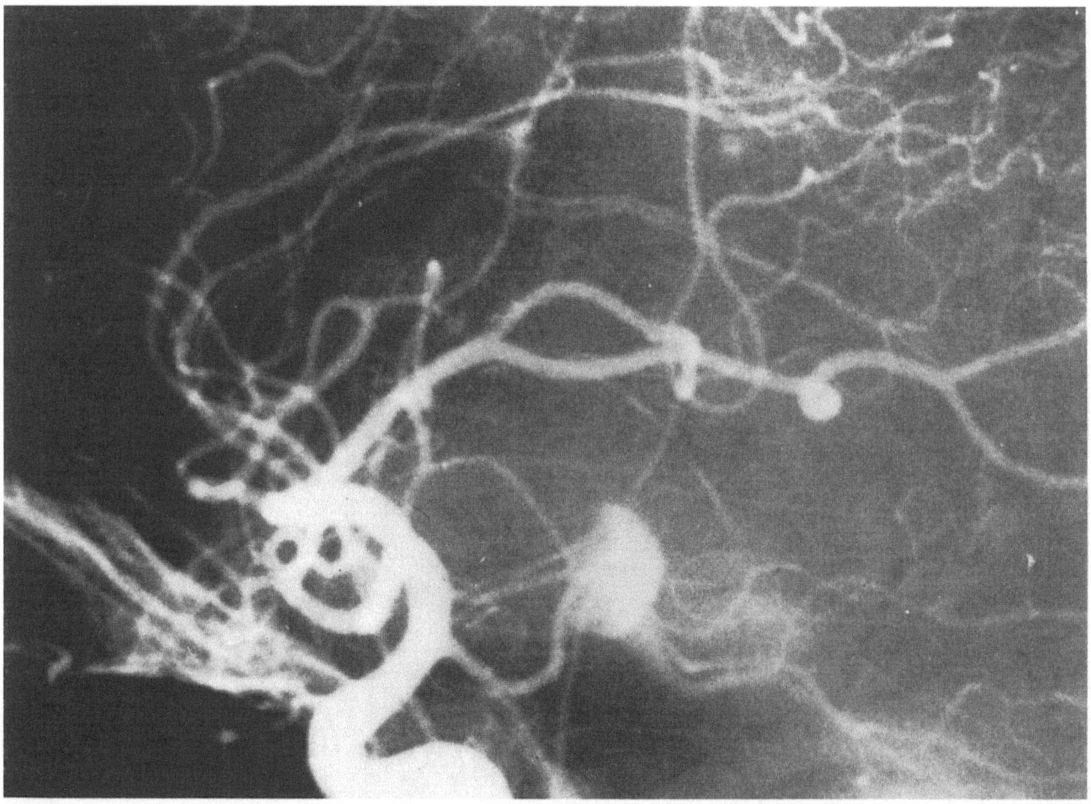

b

**Fig. F67** a, b. Giant aneurysm of the right posterior cerebral artery filled for the most part with thrombotic material in a 59-year-old female. The aneurysm is demonstrated as a rosette figure in the precontrast study. Contrast uptake on the medial wall of the aneurysm (**a**). Confirmation of the diagnosis by angiography (**b**) and at operation

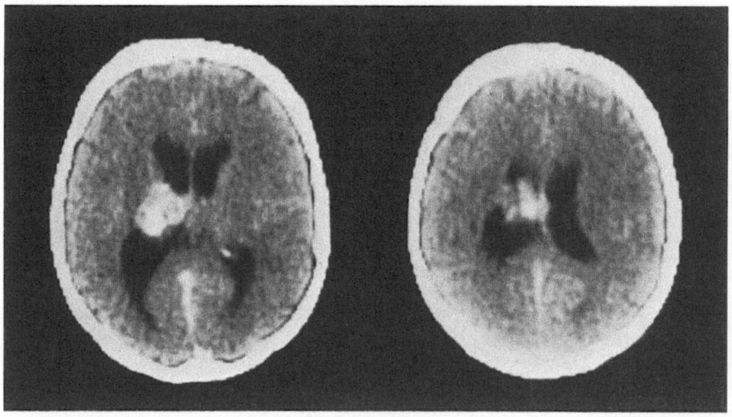

**Fig. F68.** Partially calcified aneurysm of the left posterior choroidal artery at an intraventricular location. These findings could be interpreted as a ventricular tumor such as plexus papilloma or meningioma. 47-year-old patient. Postcontrast study

a b c d
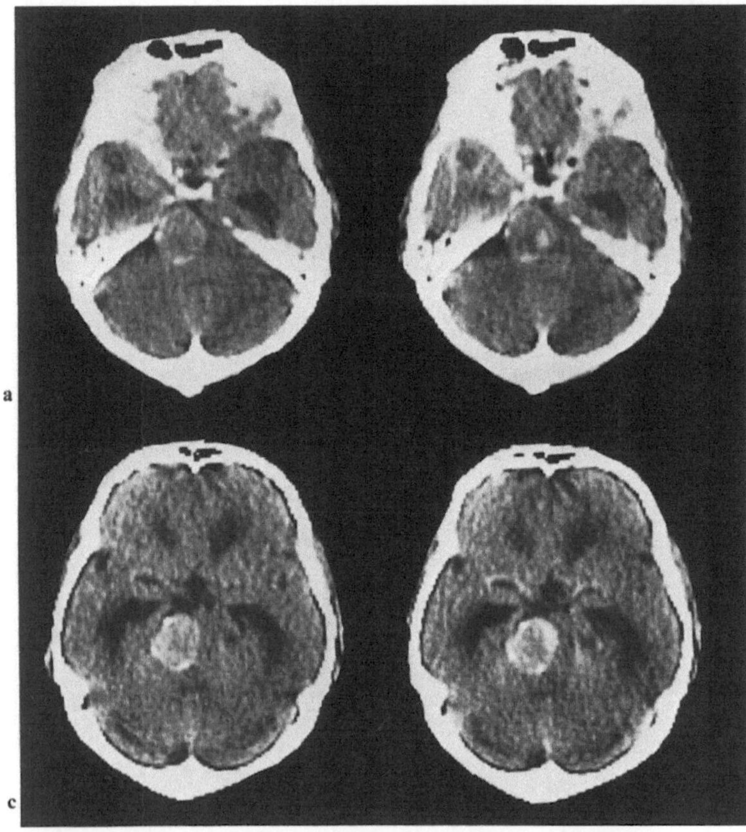

e
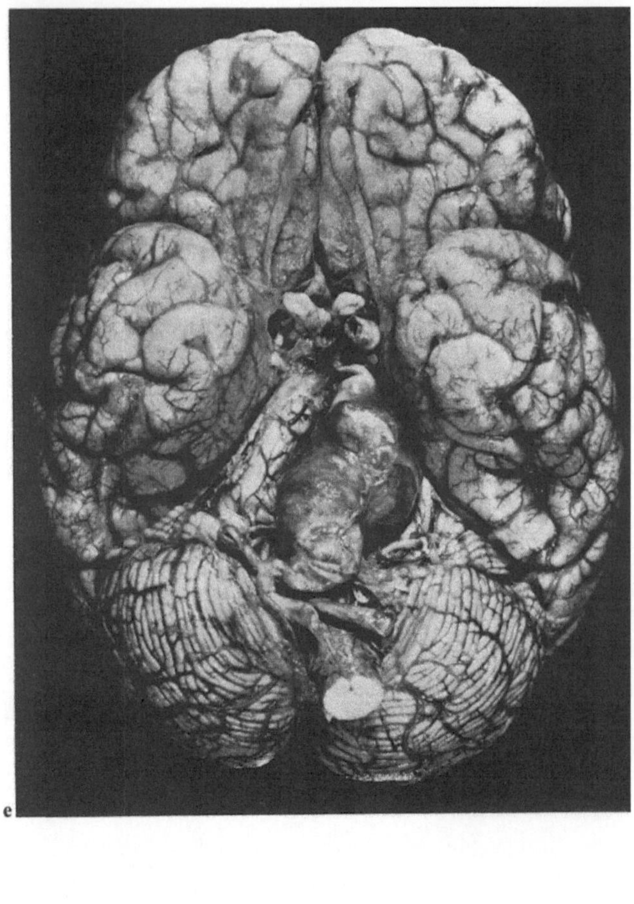

**Fig. F69** a–e. Very large arteriosclerotic aneurysm of the basilar artery in a 68-year-old patient with signs of increased intracranial pressure. (**a–d**) CT studies demonstrate a large space-occupying lesion at the tip of the left pyramid with marginal calcification and inhomogeneous contrast uptake. The suspected diagnosis of partially thrombosed aneurysm of the basilar artery was confirmed at autopsy 2 years after implantation of a CSF drain (**e**). Cause of death was total occlusion of the carotid artery

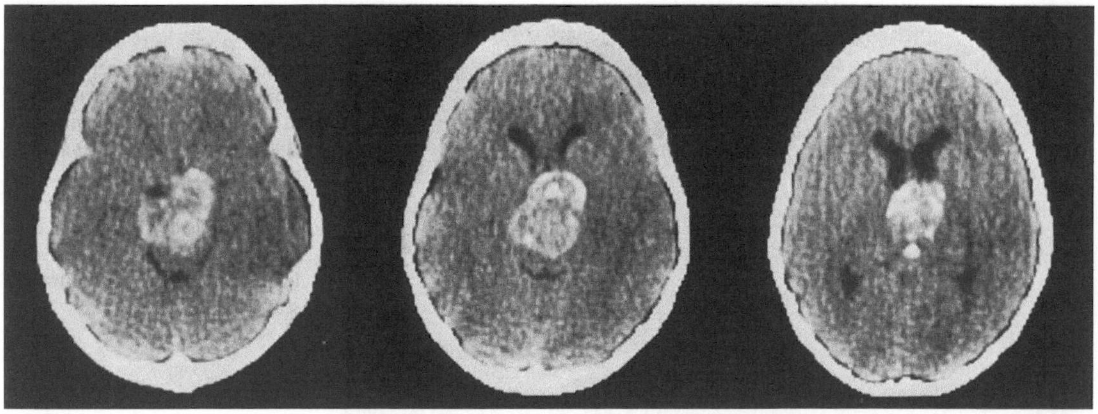

**Fig. F70.** Giant aneurysm of the basilar artery with projection to the midbrain in a 23-year-old patient. Intramural calcification typical of aneurysm. Definitive diagnosis only possible by angiography

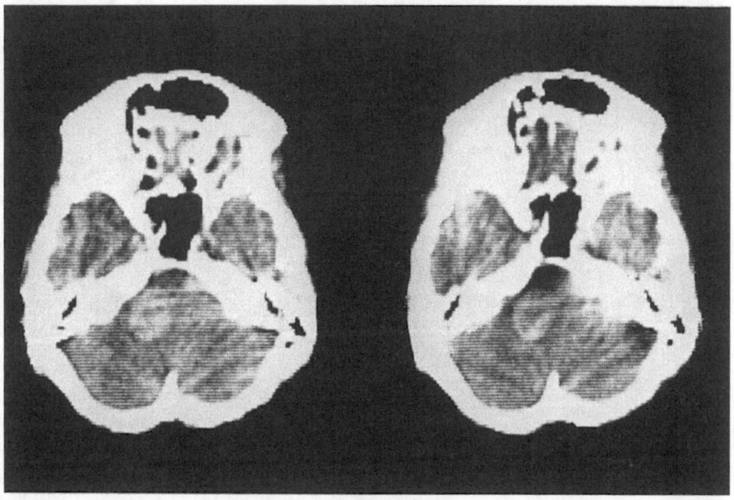

**Fig. F71.** Aneurysm of the middle section of the basilar artery extending to the left cerebellopontine angle in a 64-year-old patient. The lesion might be mistaken for a tumor at this location (precontrast study)

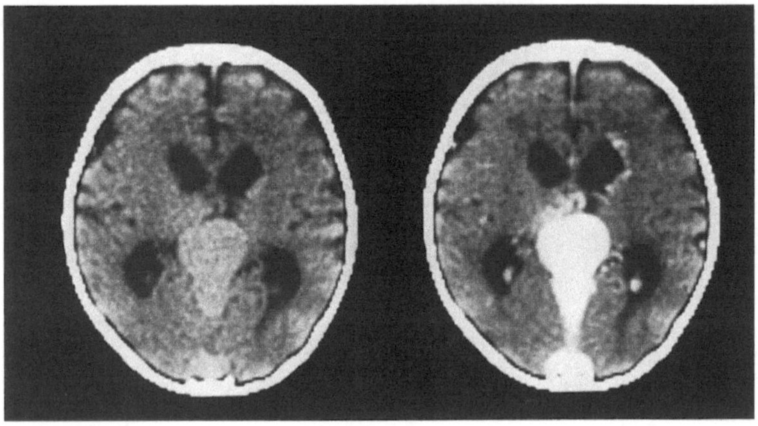

**Fig. F72.** Aneurysm of the vein of Galen with very strong contrast uptake in a 2-year-old child. Slightly hyperdense values in the aneurysm in precontrast studies. The postcontrast scan demonstrates a number of dilated veins in the ventricle wall. The lesion is drained by the dilated straight sinus. Left, precontrast study; right, postcontrast study

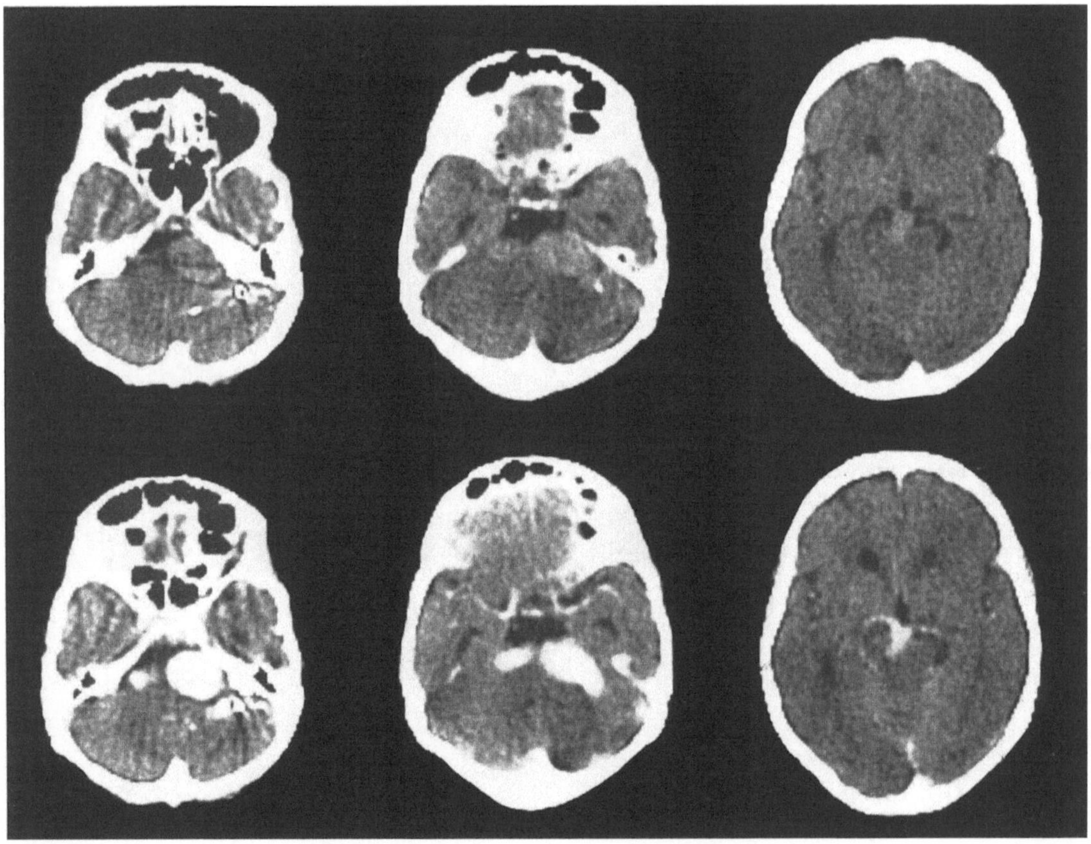

**Fig. F73.** Ectasia of the basilar artery. The CT projection simulates the presence of two separate lesions (above, precontrast study; below, postcontrast study)

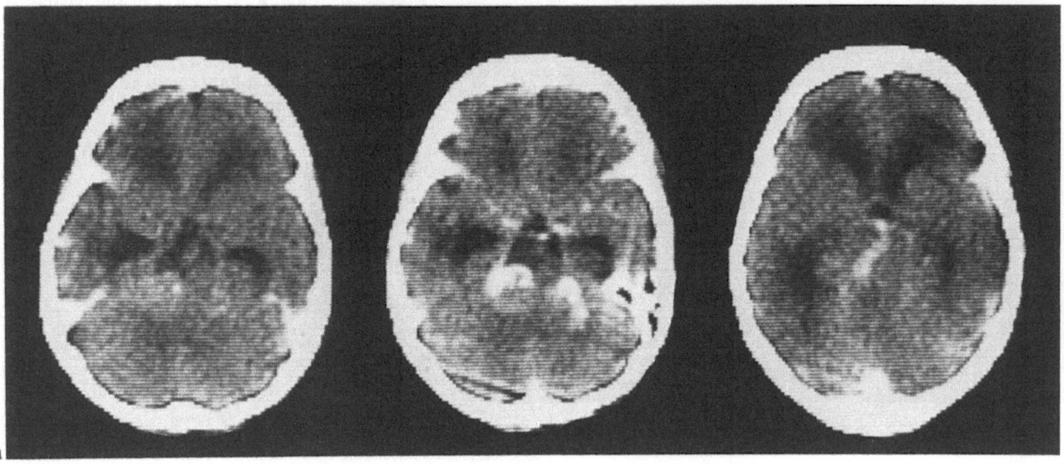

a

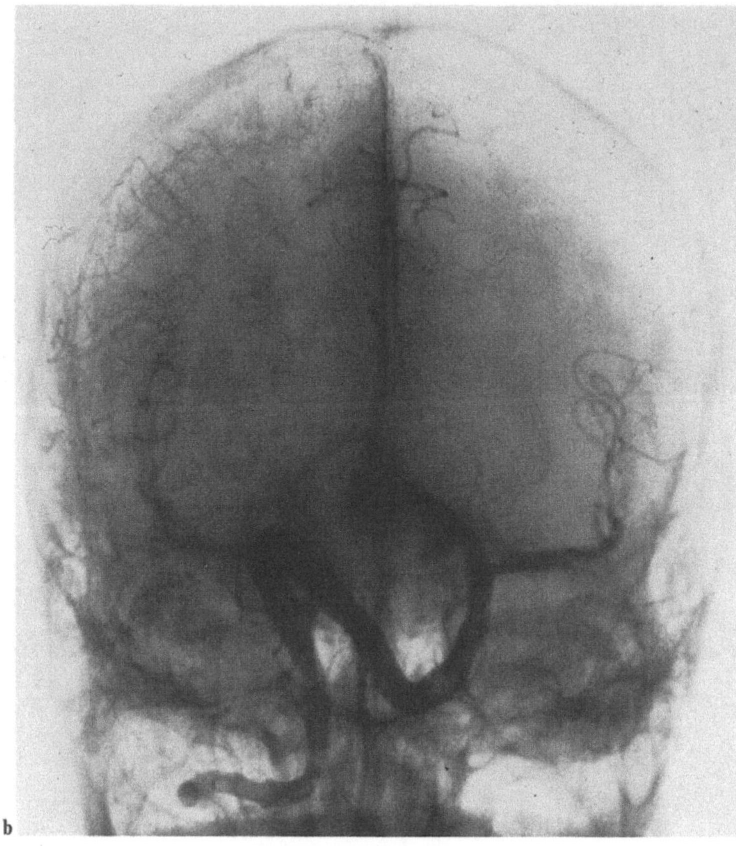

b

**Fig. F74** a, b. Ectasia of the basilar artery with extreme dilatation and a tortuous course in a 46-year-old female. (**a**) The CT study of the posterior fossa gives the impression that two separate tumors are present. The CT scan on the right indicates the vascular origin of the lesion, demonstrating the sinuous course of the enormously dilated basilar artery. Left, precontrast study; right, postcontrast study. (**b**) Angiogram in the same patient

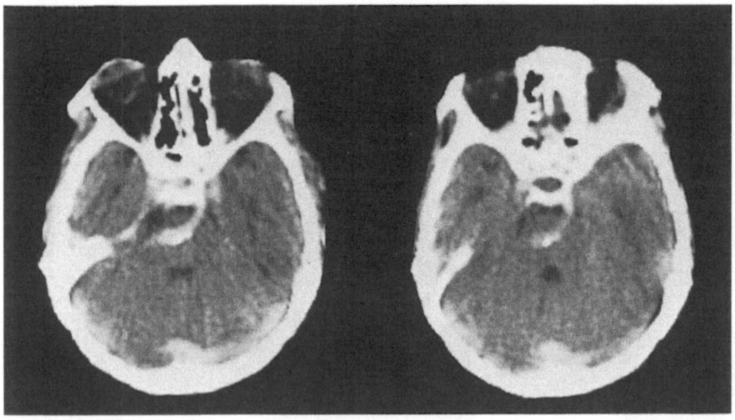

**Fig. F75.** Ectasia of the basilar artery with some intramural calcification in a 63-year-old female. Contrast enhancement reveals the course of the vessel

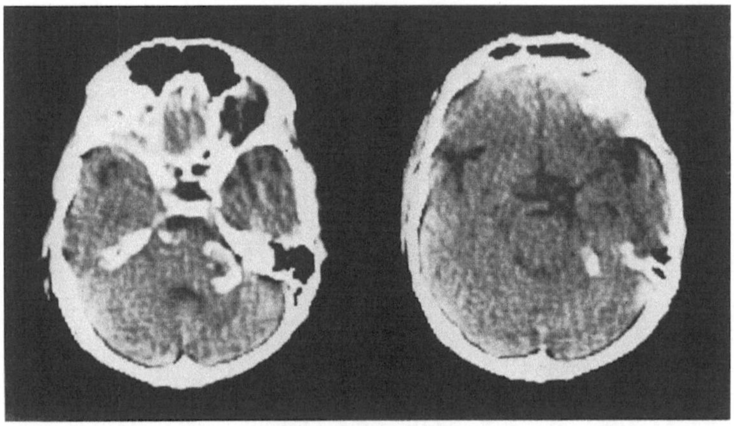

**Fig. F76.** Ectasia of the basilar artery with extensive calcification in a 46-year-old patient. The course of the vessel attains the right cerebellopontine angle and has caused signs of a lesion at this location. Precontrast study

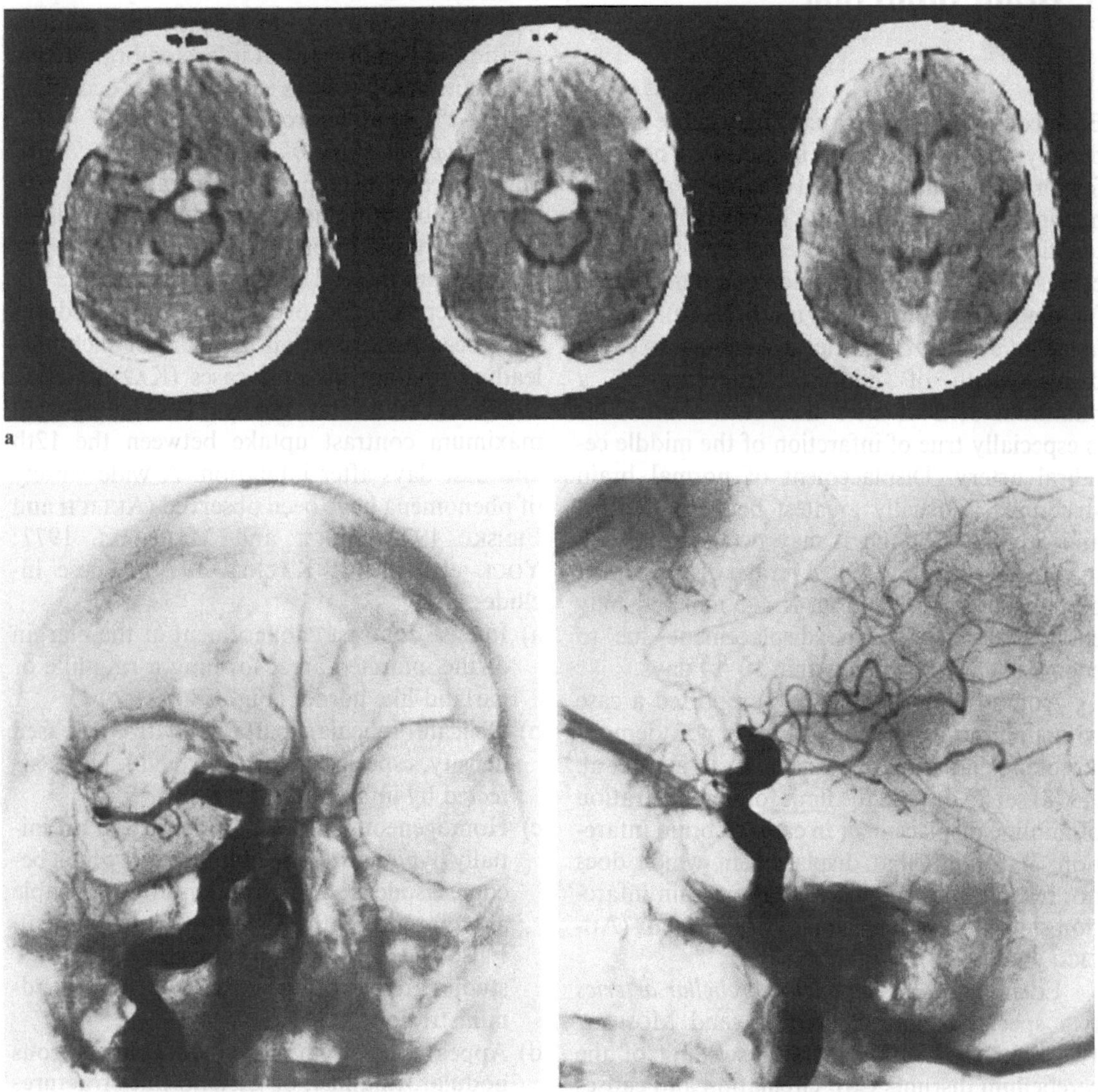

Fig. F77a–c. Massive fusiform dilatation of both internal carotid arteries and the basilar artery in a 67-year-old female. (a) Postcontrast CT scans demonstrate the dilated vessels in cross-section. (b, c) Right carotid angiogram

# 8. Brain Infarction

Both edema and hemorrhage may cause space-occupying effects in brain infarction. There are few problems in differential diagnosis, since the history and clinical findings are usually characteristic and the zone of edema almost always corresponds to the distribution of a blood vessel (cf. diagram in Fig. F78, Figs. F79, 80). *Edema in the infarcted area* is extensive enough to cause displacement of midline structures at a minimum of 24 h after the acute event. This is especially true of infarction of the middle cerebral artery. Displacement of normal brain structures is usually greatest between the 3rd and 5th day, though it may occur at 1 week in rare cases (Fig. F79). Average displacement of the septum pellucidum is 4–5 mm but may exceed 10 mm. Midline displacement due to edema usually resolves within 10–14 days.

AULICH and FENSKE (1977) reported a case with midline displacement which was demonstrable for a period of 18 days. CAMPBELL et al. (1978) set 25 days as the limit for demonstration of midline displacement in cases of brain infarction. It follows that displacement which does not resolve within 2–4 weeks after brain infarction should raise suspicion of brain tumor (AULICH et al. 1978).

Edema in *occlusion of the cerebellar arteries* is a special condition (WILSON and MOSELEY 1977). In these cases massive swelling of the cerebellum disrupts CSF circulation and causes hydrocephalus within 1 or 2 days (Figs. F81, 82). Immediate external CSF drainage usually leads to rapid improvement in the clinical state within several days with a decisive improvement in prognosis of this otherwise very serious condition.

*Petechial hemorrhage in an infarcted area,* a common finding at autopsy, *is usually not demonstrable in CT scans.* Larger quantities of blood are necessary for demonstration of hemorrhage with CT techniques (Fig. F83). Hematoma in a neoplasm (glioma apoplecticum) must always be considered in the differential diagnosis of such lesions. *Hemorrhage* is rare in occlusion of the middle cerebral artery (Fig. F84) but *much more common in occlusion of the posterior cerebral artery* (Fig. F85). Hemorrhage may encompass either the entire area of distribution of the occluded artery or a portion thereof. Our studies suggest that demonstration of hemorrhage in infarcted brain tissue by means of CT studies is rather rare, occurring in 1%–2% of all infarctions.

*Disruption of the blood-brain barrier following infarction* may permit contrast uptake in damaged brain tissue and produce CT findings similar to those in brain tumors, usually in the period from the end of the 1st week to the 4th week after the acute event. Surgical procedures have been performed on the basis of such misleading findings in some cases (KAZNER et al. 1976). AULICH and FENSKE (1977) reported maximum contrast uptake between the 12th and 21st days after infarction. A wide variety of phenomena have been observed (AULICH and FENSKE 1977; YOCK and MARSHALL 1977; YOCK et al. 1978; KAZNER 1979). These include:

a) Intense contrast enhancement at the margin of the infarcted area, forming a ring-like or garland-like border (Fig. F86);
b) Delicate reticular patterns with increased density, especially in the cortical regions affected by infarction (Fig. F87);
c) Homogeneous increase in density in an initially hypodense zone of infarction which becomes isodense and virtually unrecognizable as infarction after contrast enhancement. False negative findings may result when CT studies are performed only after contrast administration;
d) Appearance of circumscribed homogeneous nodular, ring-like, or garland-like structures with contrast uptake in a hypodense zone of infarction which may be mistaken for a tumor (KAZNER et al. 1976; Fig. F88). Diagnosis is possible with serial CT studies or cerebral angiography, which demonstrates the vascular occlusion. However, in this phase the angiographic phenomenon of luxury perfusion with a vascular blush and an early draining vein may be present, and angiographic studies may in fact support the false CT diagnosis of malignant brain tumor;
e) Significant contrast enhancement in an initially isodense zone of infarction (Figs. F89, 80). Demonstration of such findings in an area corresponding to the distribution of a cerebral artery makes a false diagnosis of tumor unlikely, but not impossible;

f) Marked contrast enhancement in parts of the cortical band of the infarcted area which may suggest a diagnosis of angioma (Fig. F91).

**Superficial and deep cerebral venous thromboses** are associated with circumscribed edema, which is usually indistinguishable from edema of other etiologies. A false diagnosis of diffusely growing astrocytoma is a plausible misinterpretation of this phenomenon. Angiography often fails to provide the diagnosis, and serial CT studies demonstrate the disappearance of edema under symptomatic therapy.

Attenuation values in the involved blood vessel are often high, approaching those of coagulated blood, in cases of **sinus thrombosis,** with the superior sagittal sinus most often affected. The ventricle system is narrow or obliterated, and brain tissue density is reduced in irregular areas or as a whole, especially in the white matter (Fig. F92). The presence of several small and/or large hemorrhages is characteristic (KAZNER et al. 1975). These findings usually provide the correct diagnosis, which is confirmed by angiography. Contrast enhancement may demonstrate numerous irregular hyperdense figures which represent congested and dilated cerebral veins or sinuses (see also Fig. D1.54, p. 58).

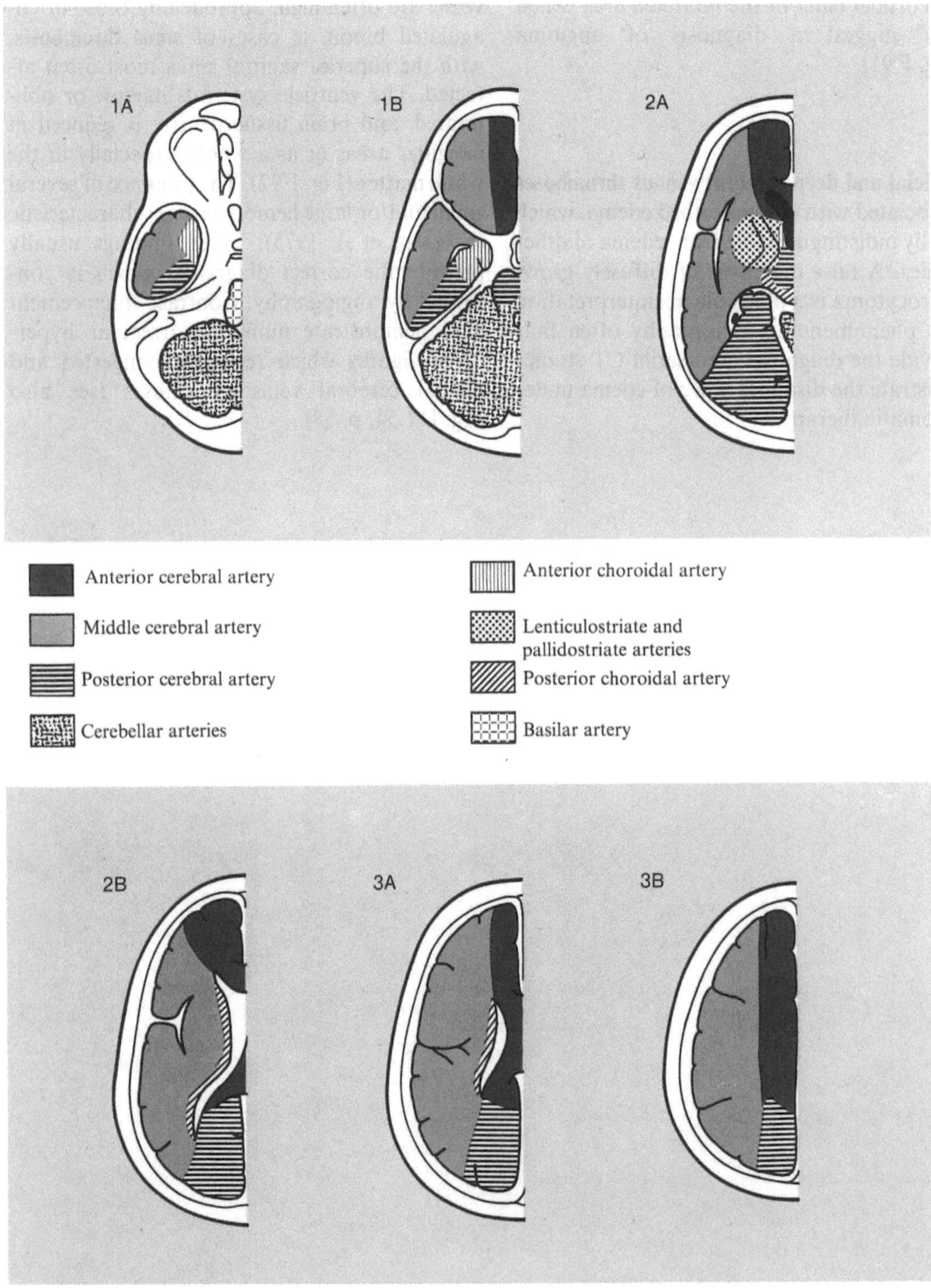


**Fig. F78.** Areas of distribution of cerebral arteries (S. Lange et al., Computerized Tomography of the Brain, 1978, by permission of Schering AG)

**Fig. F79.** CT findings 11 days after ischemic infarction in the distribution of the right middle cerebral artery in a 36-year-old patient. Major space-occupying effect with compression of the ventricles on the right and displacement of midline structures measuring 15 mm at the septum pellucidum. Postcontrast study

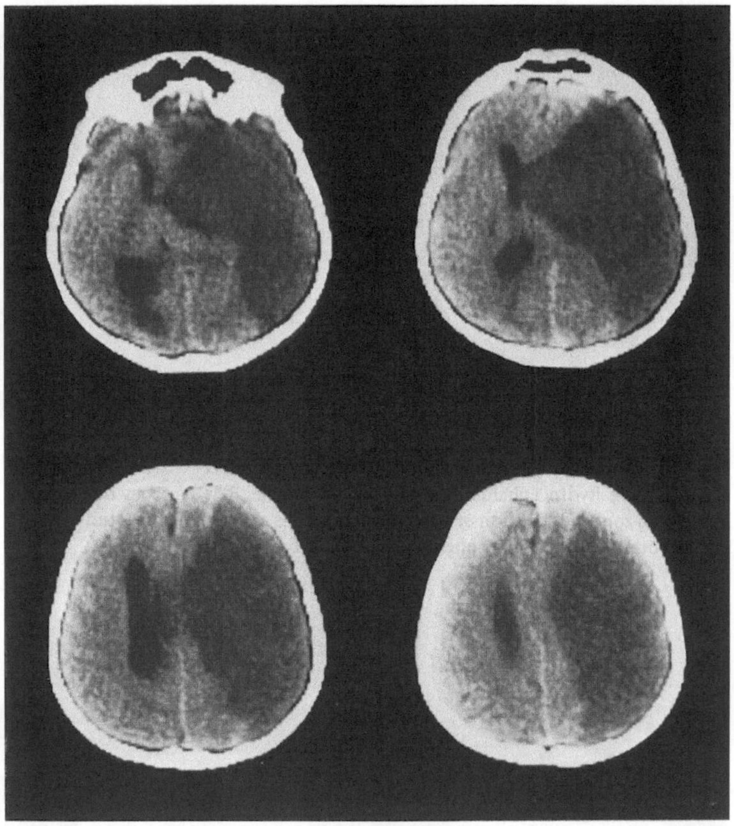

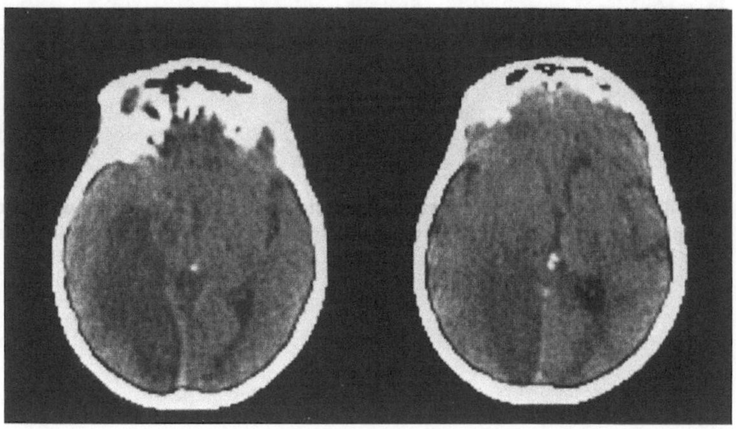

**Fig. F80.** Recent infarction in the distribution of the left posterior cerebral artery including the posterior choroidal artery. Compression of the left posterior horn in a 55-year-old patient 3 days after the event. Postcontrast study

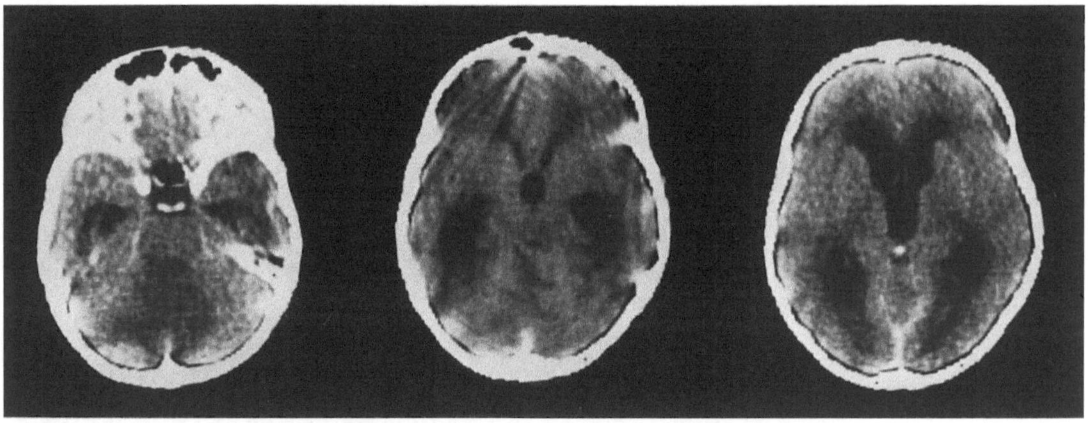

**Fig. F81.** Cerebellar infarction with space-occupying effect and occlusive hydrocephalus in a 44-year-old female. The hypodense zone in the region of the cerebellar vermis extending to both cerebellar hemispheres represents the infarcted area. Pronounced hydrocephalus with periventricular lucency due to acute blockage of the CSF pathways. Postcontrast study

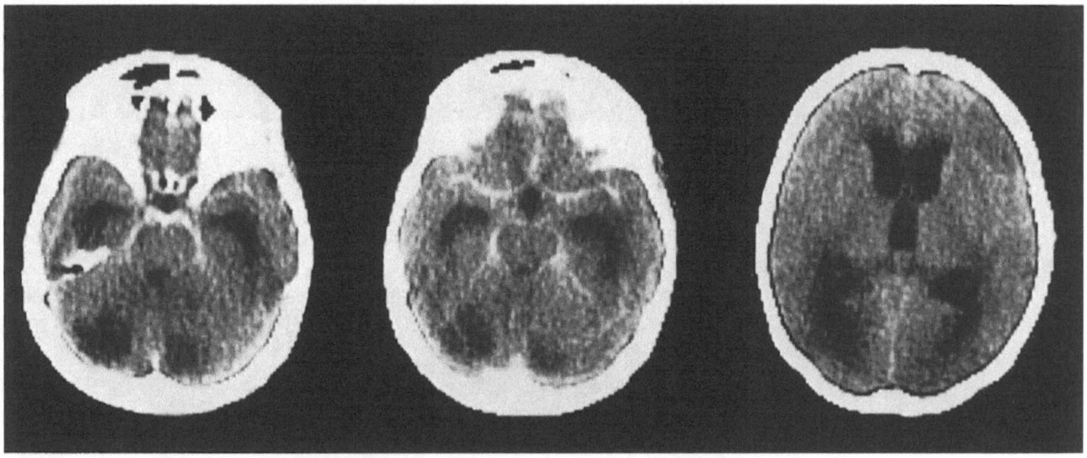

**Fig. F82.** Multiple cerebellar infarcts in the distributions of both posterior inferior cerebellar arteries with space-occupying effect, disruption of the CSF passages, and pronounced hydrocephalus 2 days after the event. Postcontrast study

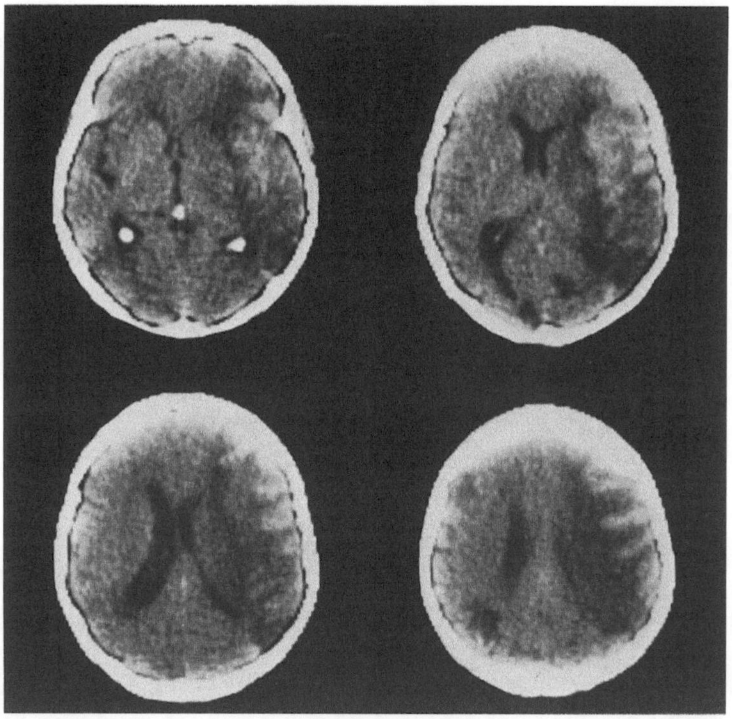

**Fig. F83.** Hemorrhagic infarction in the distribution of the right middle cerebral artery in a 59-year-old patient with total occlusion of the right middle cerebral artery. Presence of extravasated blood in the brain tissue results in hyperdense values, especially in the cortex. Precontrast study

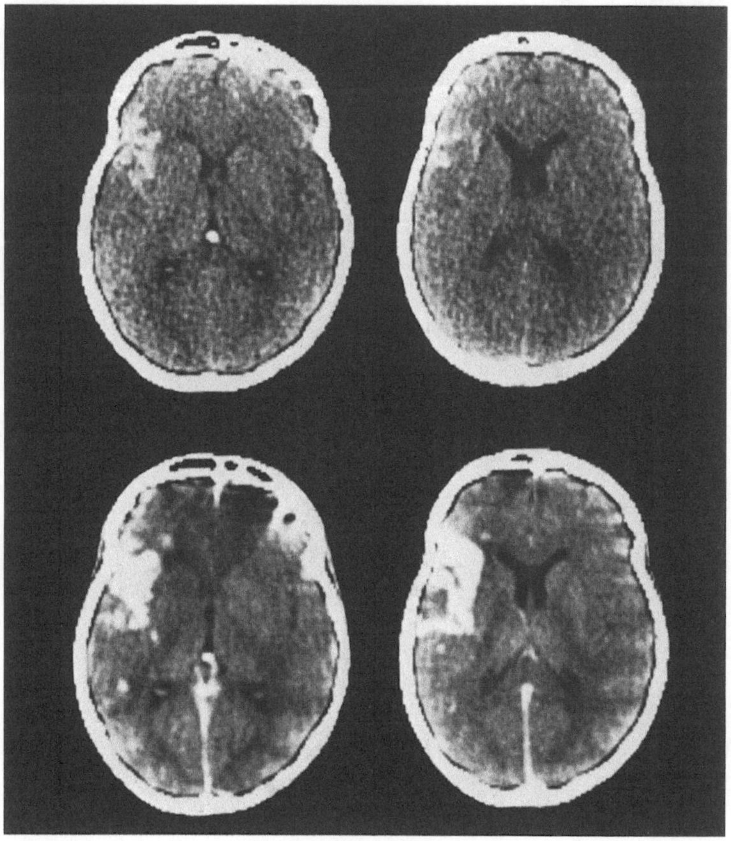

**Fig. F84.** Hemorrhagic infarction in the distribution of the left middle cerebral artery in a 36-year-old female. CT studies 18 days after the event. Precontrast scans (above) show hyperdense values in the cortex near the Sylvian fissure due to the presence of extravasated blood. Contrast enhancement (below) produces a major increase in density values in the area of infarction secondary to disruption of the blood-brain barrier. These findings resemble those in neoplasm and large arteriovenous malformations. The absence of any space-occupying effect is the decisive criterion in differentiation of these lesions

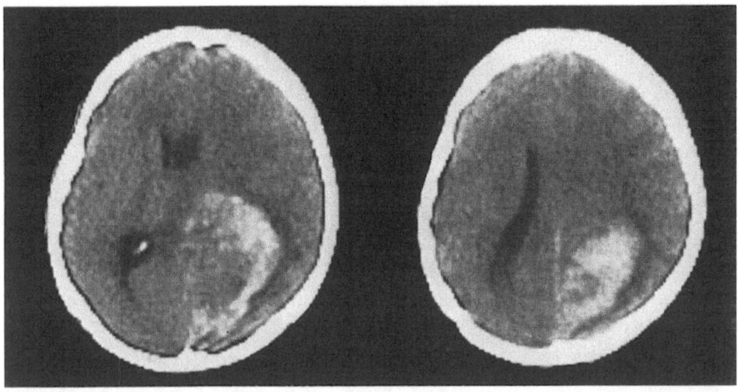

**Fig. F85.** Occlusion of the right posterior cerebral artery in a 62-year-old patient. Hemorrhage in the zone of infarction with considerable space-occupying effect 10 days after the event. Initial diagnosis of hemorrhage in a neoplasm

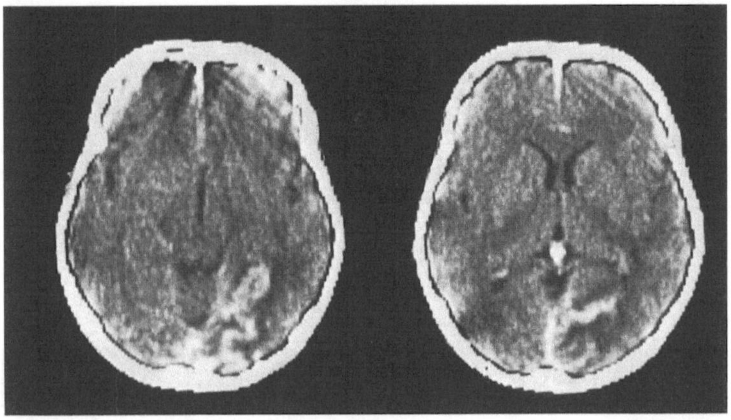

**Fig. F86.** Infarction in the distribution of the right posterior cerebral artery in a 42-year-old patient. Disruption of the blood-brain barrier 8 days after the event. The garland figure after contrast enhancement might be misinterpreted as a glioblastoma

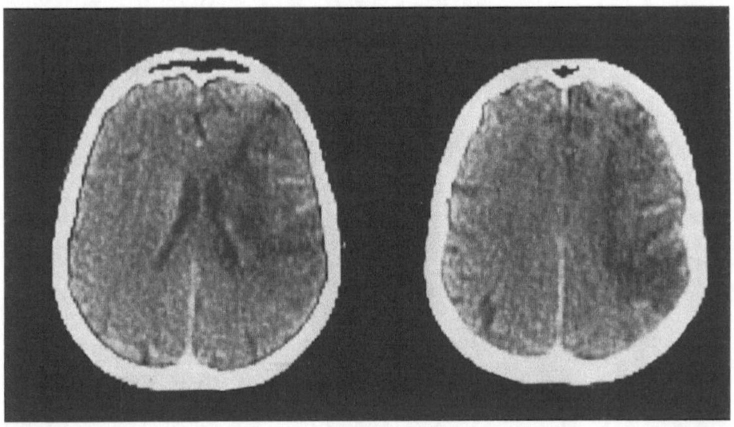

**Fig. F87.** Extensive zone of infarction in the distribution of the right middle cerebral artery with hypodense values in the precontrast study. Contrast enhancement results in delicate reticular structures in the area of infarction, most pronounced in the cortex. Postcontrast study

**Fig. F88.** Infarction in a portion of the distribution area of the right middle cerebral artery with disruption of the blood-brain barrier. Ring structures and garland figures after contrast enhancement. The central hypodense zone and perifocal edema simulate the findings in a malignant neoplasm such as glioblastoma. Note the absence of space-occupying effects, which suggests a vascular lesion rather than a neoplasm

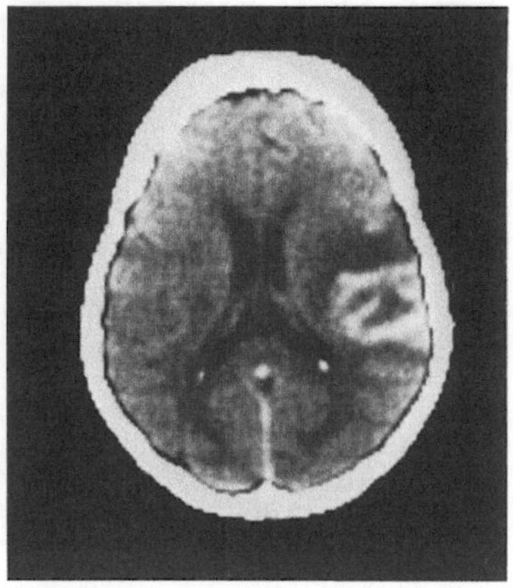

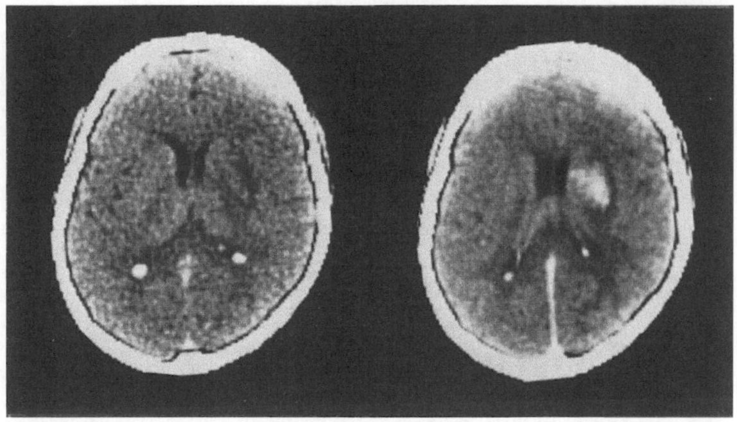

**Fig. F89.** Infarction in the right basal ganglia in a 49-year-old patient. Finger-shaped zones of edema and slight compression of the right anterior horn in precontrast studies (left). Contrast enhancement produces a significant increase in density values in the zone of infarction (right) 14 days after the acute event

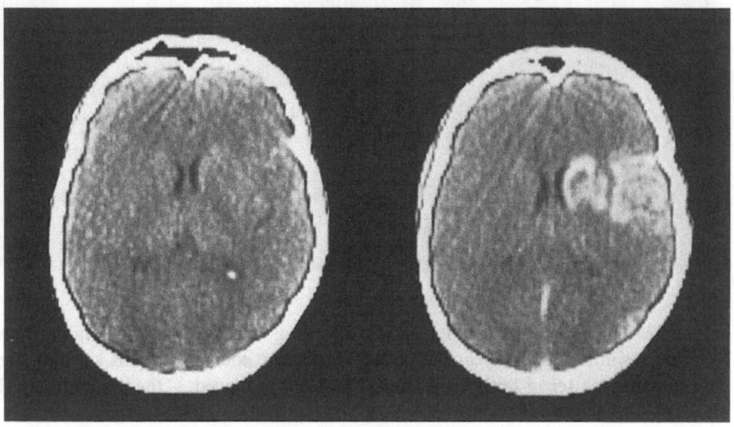

**Fig. F90.** CT findings 8 days after infarction in the distribution of the right middle cerebral artery. The lesion is isodense in precontrast studies (left) and visible only after contrast enhancement. The right basal ganglia are also affected, indicating that occlusion of the right middle cerebral artery has occurred proximal to the origin of the lenticulostriate arteries. Note the absence of space-occupying effects

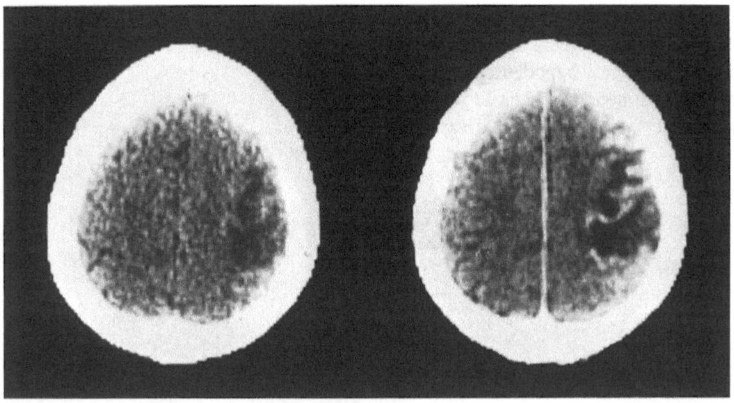

**Fig. F91.** Infarction in the distribution area of the right middle cerebral artery in the phase of disruption of the blood-brain barrier. Contrast medium uptake in the cortex resembles findings in an arteriovenous malformation. Left, precontrast study; right, postcontrast study

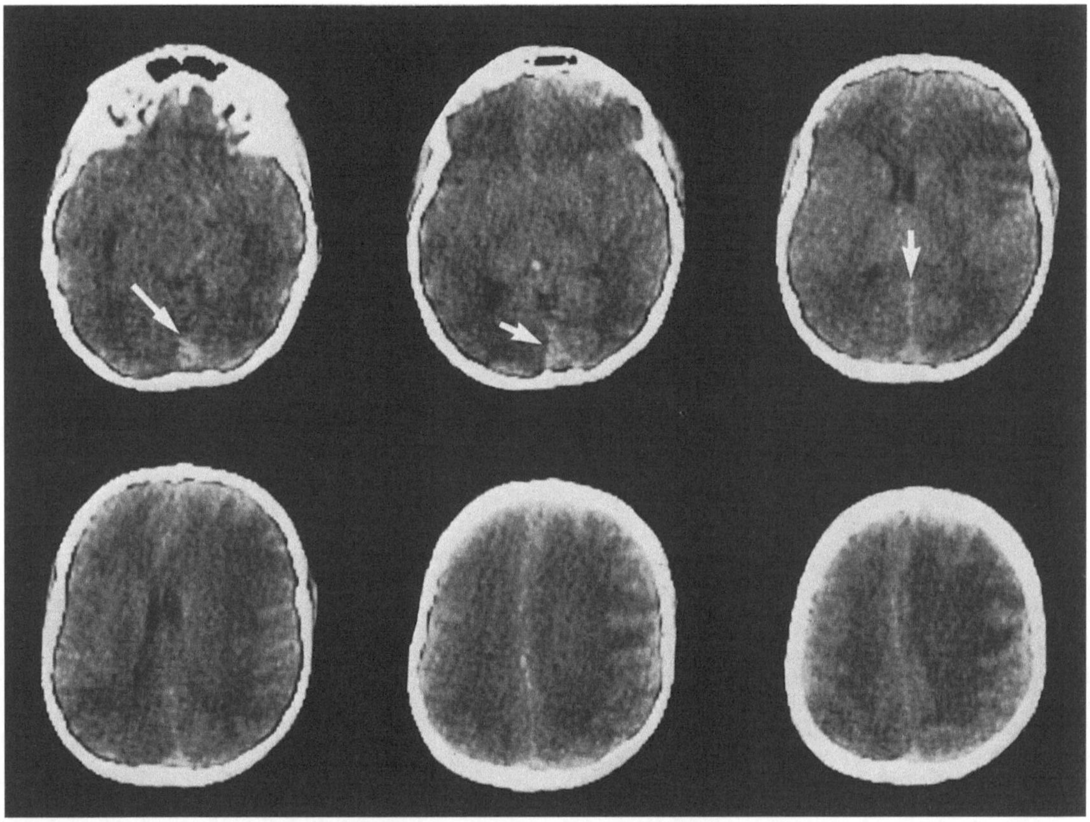

**Fig. F92.** Thrombosis of the right transverse sinus and the confluens sinuum in a 26-year-old patient. Extensive edema in the white matter of both hemispheres, more pronounced on the right. Hemostasis in the straight sinus and the confluens sinuum suggested by increased absorption values in the precontrast CT scan (arrows)

# G. Computed Tomography in Orbital Lesions

Lesions in the orbits are characterized by unilateral or bilateral proptosis and/or disorders of ocular motion. Before the advent of computed tomography diagnosis was made on the basis of conventional radiological studies of the skull and the orbits as well as with ultrasonography, fluorescence angiography, phlebography of the ophthalmic vein, and arteriograms of the internal and external carotid arteries. The introduction of CT has brought about a corresponding decline in the use of invasive procedures (Wende et al. 1977).

*Plain skull films and tomograms* demonstrate thickening of the bones and sclerosis of bone structures, destruction, malformation, and fracture. These techniques are not capable of demonstrating pathological lesions in soft tissue.

*Ultrasonography* of the orbit should always be employed when proptosis, dislocation of the eyeball, limitation of ocular motion, or atrophy of the optic nerve of uncertain etiology is present. The procedure is entirely innocuous and can demonstrate or exclude a space-occupying lesion in the orbit when performed by a skilled examiner (Ossoinig 1978). *Carotid angiograms* demonstrate the ophthalmic artery, which is located on the medial side of the orbit and which may be displaced by large tumors. However, there is a considerable degree of anatomical variation in the vessel, and definitive diagnosis is not always possible. A tumor blush is rarely demonstrated. *Selective angiographic study of the external carotid artery* and its terminal branches is always necessary, since orbital tumors are often served by vessels originating in the external carotid artery. This technique offers the only means of documenting a tumor blush.

*Phlebography of the orbital veins* has a high degree of accuracy in the diagnosis of orbital tumors and infection. The technique reveals displacement, irregularity in caliber, and stenosis of the superior ophthalmic vein. Changes in form and position of this vessel allow accurate conclusions on location and type of pathological change as well as differentiation between tumor and inflammation in a high percentage of cases. However, conventional radiological studies with contrast media which were indispensable in the diagnosis of orbital lesions before the introduction of computed tomography entail a hospital stay as well as discomfort and some degree of risk for the patient. The cause of proptosis could not be determined in a large proportions of cases despite use of all of these techniques.

Diagnosis of lesions in this anatomical region has become much simpler since the introduction of computed tomography, which entails neither risk nor discomfort for the patient. (Ambrose et al. 1974; Baker et al. 1974; Gawler et al. 1974; Lloyd et al. 1975; New and Scott 1975; Nover et al. 1976; Ostertag et al. 1976; Wende and Aulich 1976; Lloyd and Ambrose 1977; Wackenheim et al. 1977).

### Technique of CT Examination

CT studies of the orbital region are made with the head in a different position from that used in CT scans of the brain. The head is reclined slightly so that the X-ray beam is parallel to the floor of the orbit. CT scans are made at a 20-degree angle to the orbitomeatal line, which is generally used as the baseline for studies of intracranial structures. In other words, the planes are parallel to Reid's baseline. Anatomical variations may require slight modifications of the position described above, and the quality of the scan is the only measure of adequate position (Salvolini et al. 1978). Orbital studies require thinner tomographic slices than do studies of the brain. Five-millimeter slices are standard, and 1.5-mm slices are possible with newer systems.

*Coronary projections are a valuable adjunct for exact demonstration of the roof and floor of the orbits* (BALERIAUX-WAHA et al. 1977; TADMOR and NEW 1978). These studies are usually made at a 70–80° angle to Reid's baseline. Special reformatting programs allow tomograms in lateral projection (LEONARDI et al. 1977).

The orbit is visible in its entirety in the different CT slices, with demonstration of the bone structures of the orbit, the optic canal, the paranasal sinuses, the eyeball, the optic nerve, and the extraocular muscles. It is possible to examine the optic nerve with the eyeball in a variety of positions (DI CHIRO et al. 1976). The sclera and the lens are clearly visible. A low-density zone behind the eyeball represents intraorbital fat. Diagnosis of intraorbital space-occupying lesions is rarely difficult since most tumors, with the exceptions of lipoma and dermoid cyst, have considerably higher density than the surrounding fatty tissue.

#### Indication for CT Studies

CT studies of the orbits are required when primary or secondary tumors or vascular and other malformations are suspected, or when disorders of ocular motion, proptosis, and traumatic changes are present.

#### Radiation Dosage

The radiation dose is not in the dangerous range in CT studies. Conventional CT studies of the brain entail a total radiation dose of 0.6 R in the eye, while orbital studies may involve a total dose ranging up to 12 R, depending on the number of slices, thickness of the individual slice, and type of CT scanner (NEMEC and ROTH 1976; RADMOR and NEW 1978).

Total radiation dosage in conventional tomographic studies of the orbits varies from 12 R (ISHERWOOD et al. 1975) to 21.3 R (HOLLÄNDER and LYSELL 1971). Reports also vary on radiation dosage in pneumoencephalography, since total dosage depends on duration of fluoroscopy and the number of tomographic studies in the sella region. Values ranging from 2 to 6 R have been reported in the literature (ISHERWOOD et al. 1975). Total dosage to the lens has been estimated from 6 to 17 R in carotid arteriography and phlebography of the orbital veins (BERGSTRÖM et al. 1972). In summary, conventional radiological techniques including plain skull films and special projections, tomograms, carotid angiography, and phlebography of the ophthalmic vein entail a significantly higher radiation dose in the lens than does a comparable CT study of the same region.

#### Complications

CT studies are harmless. Complications are due solely to hypersensitivity reactions to contrast media, and frequency of such reactions may be reduced to a minimum by means of a careful history (see p. 15f.). Contrast enhancement is unnecessary in most cases of orbital tumor, since the latter are clearly visible in the precontrast CT study, and contrast administration rarely provides additional information. Cases of carotid cavernous sinus fistula sometimes require contrast administration for demonstration in the CT scan. Severe complications are possible when contrast media are administered in cases of endocrine ophthalmopathy.

# CT Appearance of Orbital Space-Occupying Lesions

Table 7 summarizes our findings in 604 patients with space-occupying lesions in the orbital region. The most important histological diagnoses are discussed below.

## 1. Benign Tumors

### Cavernous Hemangiomas

These are the most common autochthonous orbital neoplasms (8–16% JACOBS et al. 1980). This malformative tumor may occur at any age; females are affected twice as often as males. It is most often found in the lateral portion of the ocular muscle cone or at the medial wall of the orbit and may impinge upon the optic nerve, with corresponding visual defects. The tumor is enclosed in a capsule and is made up of a number of compartments of various sizes. The chambers have an endothelial lining and may contain blood or fibrous tissue.

Table 7. CT studies in patients with orbital lesions ($n=604$)

| Type of orbital lesion | Number of patients | |
|---|---|---|
| **Benign tumors** | | 162 |
| Cavernous hemangiomas | 29 | |
| Meningiomas with orbital involvement (sphenoid wing, olfactory groove meningiomas) | 51 | |
| Meningiomas of the optic nerve sheath | 18 | |
| Pilocytic astrocytomas of the optic nerve | 27 | |
| Neurinomas | 10 | |
| Lipomas | 8 | |
| Epidermoid cysts and dermoid cysts | 13 | |
| Fibromas | 5 | |
| Angioleiomyomas | 1 | |
| **Malignant tumors** | | 132 |
| Primary carcinomas of the orbit and metastases | 51 | |
| Tumors of the lacrimal gland | 16 | |
| Malignant lymphomas | 24 | |
| Malignant melanomas | 12 | |
| Sarcomas (fibrosarcomas, rhabdomyosarcomas) | 11 | |
| Adenoid-cystic carcinomas | 5 | |
| Hemangioendotheliomas | 6 | |
| Basaliomas (squamous cell carcinomas) | 3 | |
| Neuroblastomas | 1 | |
| Plasmocytomas | 1 | |
| Myoblastomas | 1 | |
| Histiocytomas | 1 | |
| **Inflammatory lesions** | | 82 |
| Pseudotumors | 35 | |
| Myositis | 19 | |
| Mucoceles | 15 | |
| Abscesses | 5 | |
| Pyoceles | 4 | |
| Giant cell granulomas | 2 | |
| Orbital phlegmon | 2 | |
| **Malformations** | | 33 |
| Aplasia of the sphenoid bone | 10 | |
| Buphthalmus | 6 | |
| Arteriovenous malformations | 11 | |
| Fibrous dysplasia | 4 | |
| Cysts | 2 | |
| **Posttraumatic lesions** | | 22 |
| Hematomas (retrobulbar) | 15 | |
| Carotid-cavernous sinus fistulas | 7 | |
| **Endocrine exophthalmus** | | 62 |
| **No histological diagnosis** | | 111 |
| | | 604 patients |

### Computed Tomography (Figs. G1, 2)

Cavernous hemangiomas appear as sharply delineated soft tissue lesions with much higher density than surrounding fatty tissue in the orbit (Baker et al. 1974; Momose et al. 1975; Lester and Gyldenstedt 1976). Contrast enhancement is strongly positive. The optic nerve is clearly demarcated from the cavernous hemangioma in the majority of cases (Fig. G1c).

## Meningiomas

(cf. Chap. D2, meningiomas, p. 196ff.). Meningiomas make up 3–7% of all orbital tumors (Jacobs et al. 1980) and are found more often in females than in males. The tumors demonstrate a capsule and are usually composed of solid tissue, with calcification in many cases. Cysts are rare. Intracranial meningiomas may invade the orbit and the paranasal sinuses, especially when the tumor originates in the tuberculum sellae, the sphenoid wing, or the olfactory groove.

### Computed Tomography (Figs. G3, 4)

Conventional radiology and CT studies reveal thickening and sclerosis of bone structures as well as intracranial, extracranial, and intraorbital extension of the soft tissue portion of the lesion. Contrast enhancement results in a clear increase in absorption (Gawler et al. 1974; Lampert et al. 1974; Lester and Gyldenstedt 1976; Wollensak et al. 1976).

## Meningiomas of the Optic Nerve Sheath

These tumors arise in the meninges of the optic nerve and occur in all age groups, though peak incidence lies in adolescence and middle age. They are less common than pilocytic astrocytomas of the optic nerve. Meningiomas of the optic nerve sheath tend to recur and to extend into the intracranial cavity by growing along the dura mater through the optic nerve canal.

### Computed Tomography

Meningiomas of the optic nerve sheath produce evident thickening and sclerosis of the optic

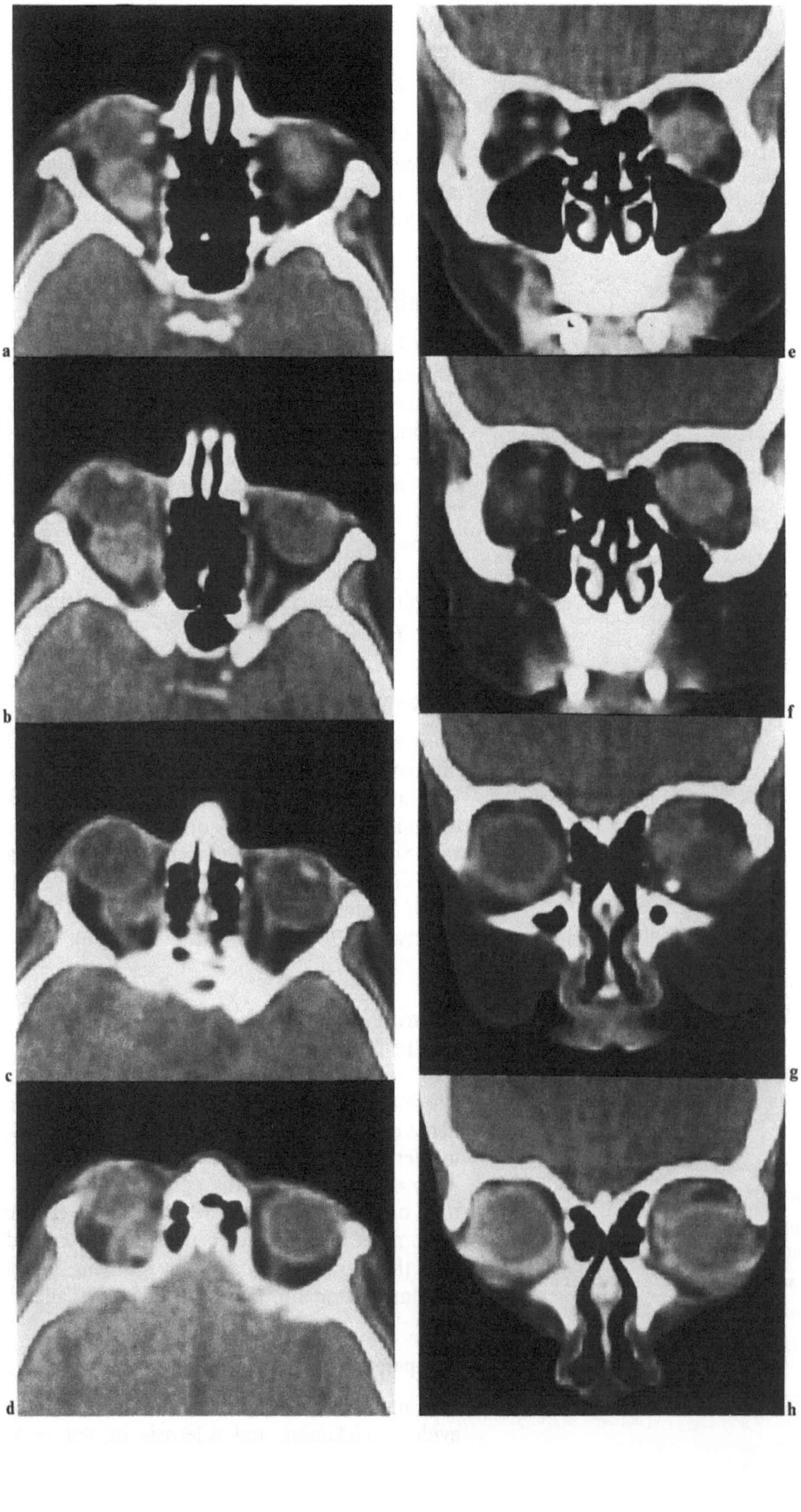
a
b
c
d
e
f
g
h

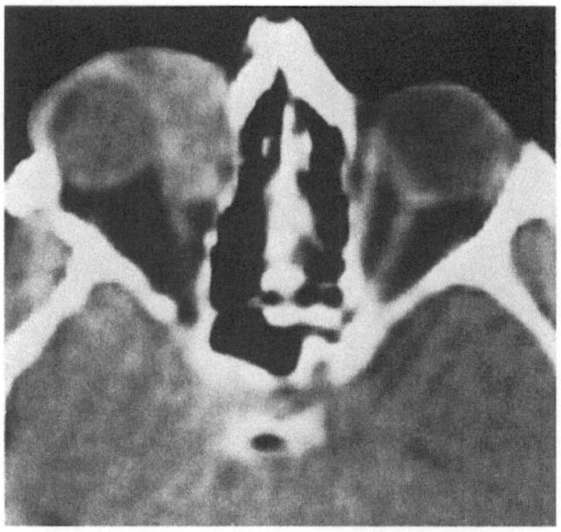

**Fig. G2.** Cavernous hemanigoma in the left orbit on the medial side of the eyeball in a 28-year-old patient. Homogeneous sharply delineated hyperdense lesion; tip of the orbit free of tumor

nerve, which may be affected in short segments or over its entire length. The tumor is sharply delineated and spindle-shaped or cuff-like in appearance (Figs. G5–7, cf. Fig. E12, p. 386).

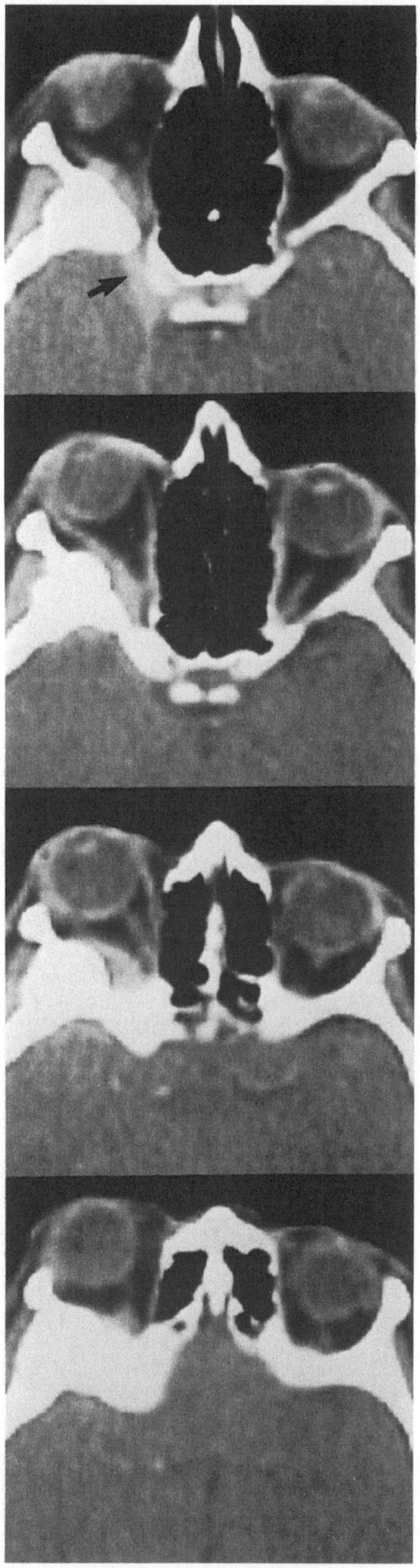

►

**Fig. G3.** Osteoplastic meningioma originating in the left sphenoid wing with soft tumor portions at the lateral wall of the orbit near the apex as well as in the temporal fossa in a 48-year-old female with proptosis on the left. The tumor has grown through the optic foramen into the cavernous sinus (arrow). Major distension of the bone. Postcontrast study

◄

**Fig. G1a–h.** Cavernous hemangioma. Sharply delineated slightly hyperdense homogeneous lesion in the medial portion of the left orbit. Evident proptosis on the left; lateral displacement of the left optic nerve (**c**). Coronary projection demonstrates caudal and lateral displacement of the left eyeball. Slices **e–h** show normal structures in the right orbit

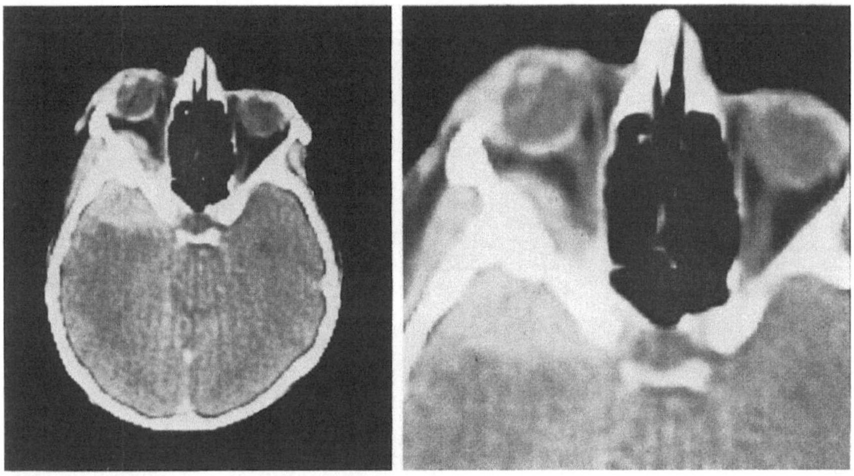

**Fig. G4.** Osteoplastic meningioma on the left sphenoid wing in a 57-year-old male. Distension of the bone as well as soft tumor portions at the lateral wall of the orbit causing severe proptosis. Tumor also in the temporal fossa and the left side of the middle fossa anterior to the temporal pole. Postcontrast study

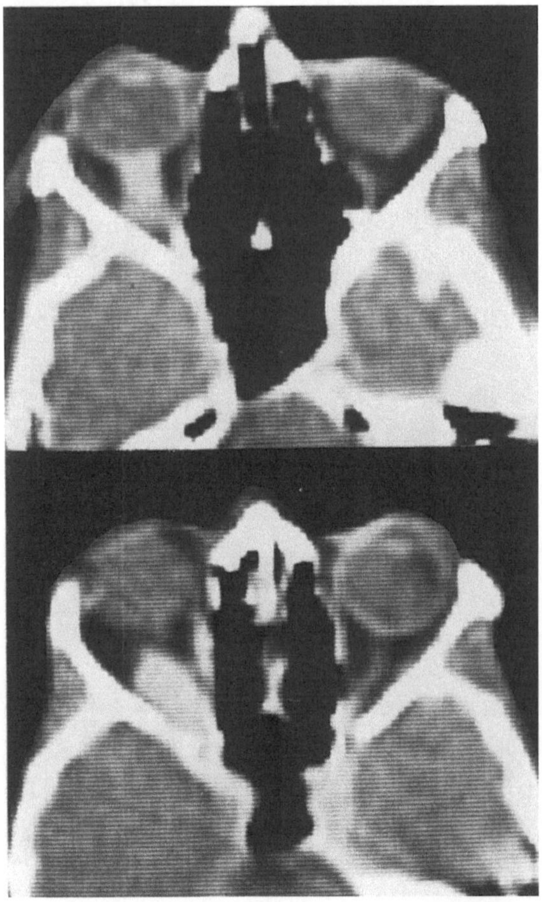

◄

**Fig. G5.** Meningioma originating in the sheath of the left optic nerve in a 68-year-old female with proptosis on the left. The tumor extends into the tip of the orbit and has caused distension of the entire optic nerve. Significant contrast uptake in the tumor. Postcontrast study

Density measurements in the optic nerve sheath after intrathecal metrizamide administration may provide additional information. Part of the optic nerve sheath is a continuation of the subarachnoid space, so that lumbar injection of 5–8 ml Amipaque (170 mg iodine/ml) results in increased density within the optic nerve (MANELFE et al. 1978, FOX 1979). In contrast to the spindle-shaped or cuff-like distension of the optic nerve in meningioma, papilledema presents a uniform increase in thickness of the entire nerve which may be quite pronounced on one side (CABANIS et al. 1978).

Alterations in thickness and density of the optic nerve have also been described in cases of neuritis of the 2nd cranial nerve (GAWLER et al. 1974).

Differentiation between papilledema and drusen disc is usually possible with density measurements in the optic nerve, since the druses near the disc contain calcium and demonstrate higher density values than those found in normal or edematous discs (FRISEN et al. 1978).

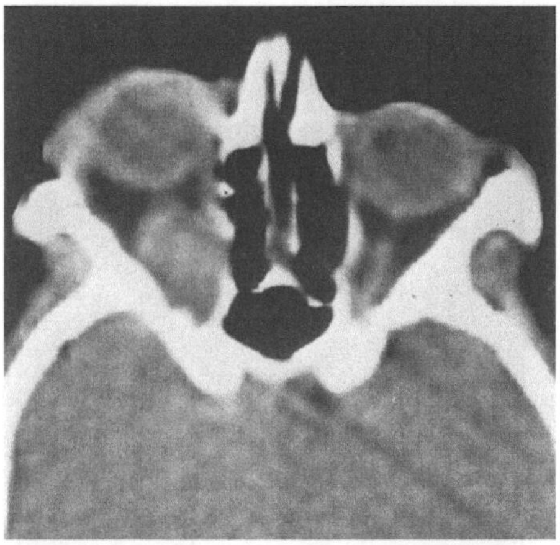

**Fig. G6.** Meningioma originating in the sheath of the left optic nerve in a 56-year-old female. The tumor fills the apex of the orbit and has caused spindle-shaped distension of the optic nerve. Precontrast study

## Optic Nerve Gliomas

Histologically classified as pilocytic astrocytomas and previously called spongioblastomas, these tumors originate in the glial cells. They are most often found in children, with 80% of all cases in children under 10 years of age. The tumors grow very slowly and do not metastasize. Optic nerve gliomas are rare and are associated with neurofibromatosis in 10–50% of cases (COGAN 1979). The tumor is covered by an intact dural sheath, and tumor cells infiltrate the optic nerve and distend the arachnoid sheath.

### Computed Tomography

Optic nerve gliomas resemble meningiomas of the optic nerve sheath in that they demonstrate thickening of the nerve with increased density values in segments of varying length (Figs. G8–12).

Optic nerve gliomas do not accept contrast media as readily as do meningiomas of the optic nerve sheath. Conventional radiological studies demonstrate widening of the optic nerve canal in advanced cases. The tumor may extend as far as the optic chiasma and the hypothalamus (Fig. G12).

## Neurinomas

These tumors are often found in combination with neurofibromatosis. Histological studies reveal diffuse proliferation of the Schwann cells as well as fibrous elements.

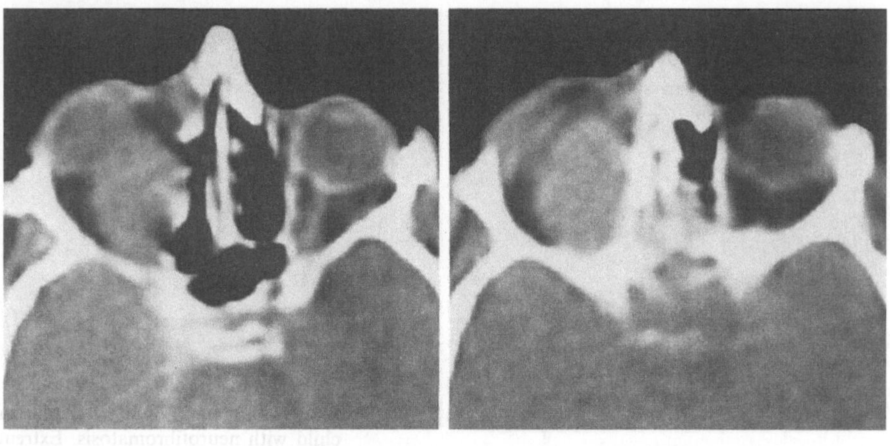

**Fig. G7.** Very large meningioma originating in the sheath of the left optic nerve in a 19-year-old patient with proptosis. Strong homogeneous contrast uptake in the tumor, which has completely filled the funnel of the left orbit

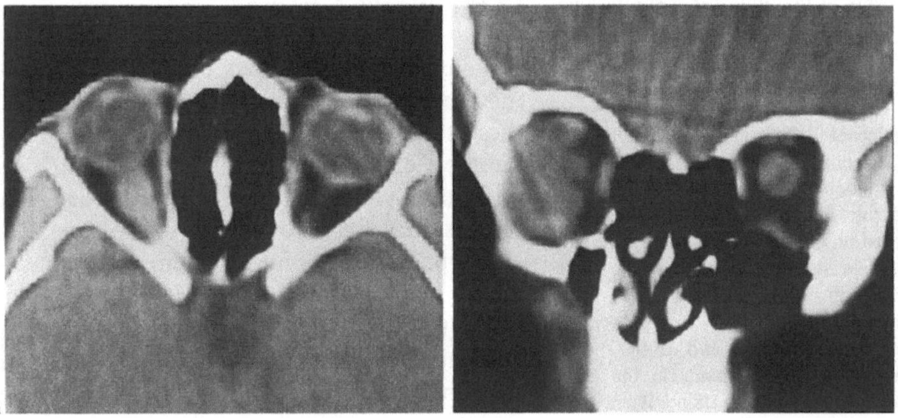

a b

**Fig. G8** a, b. Glioma of the left optic nerve in a 20-year old female. Spindle-shaped distension of the left optic nerve along its entire course (**a**). The fact that the tumor is located in the center of the left orbit in the coronary projection without additional demonstration of the optic nerve suggests that the tumor originates in the optic nerve (**b**)

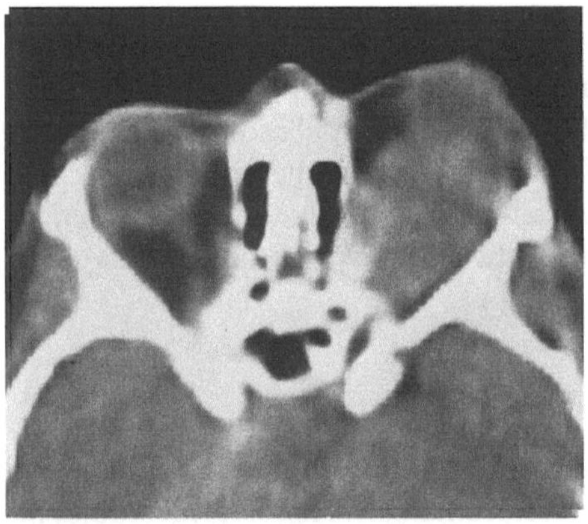

**Fig. G9.** Glioma of the right optic nerve in a 12-year-old boy. The right orbit is almost entirely filled with tumor; extreme proptosis. The origin of the tumor is not demonstrated

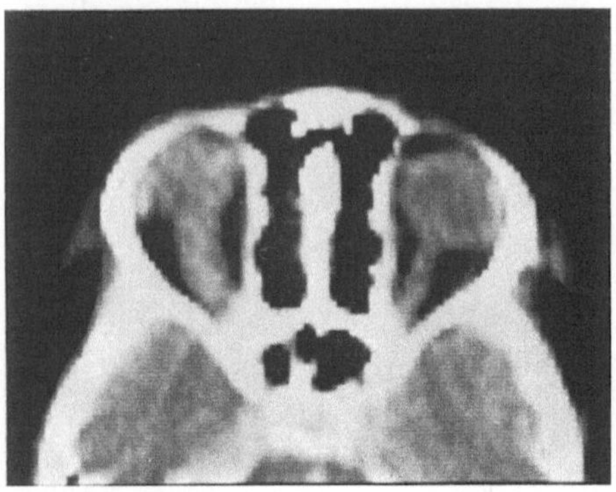

**Fig. G10.** Glioma of the left optic nerve in an 8-year-old boy. Distension of the left optic nerve along its entire course

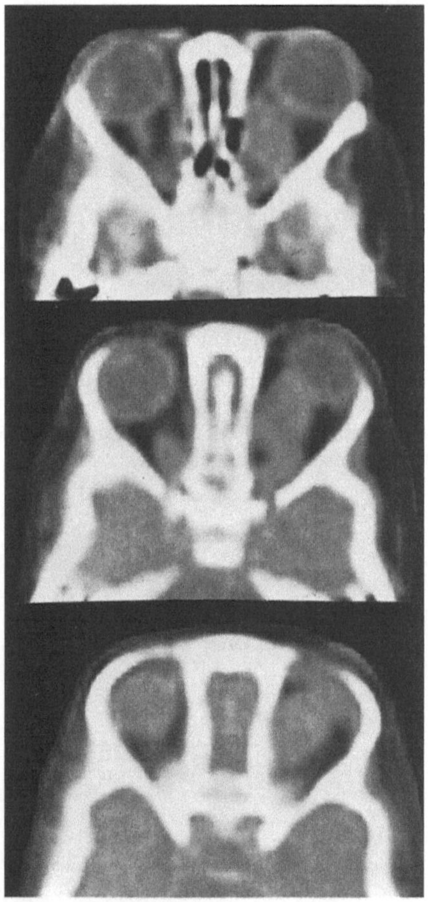

**Fig. G11.** Bilateral optic nerve gliomas in an 11-month-old child with neurofibromatosis. Extreme distension and tortuosity of the right optic nerve. In contrast, the contralateral tumor involves only the posterior section of the optic nerve

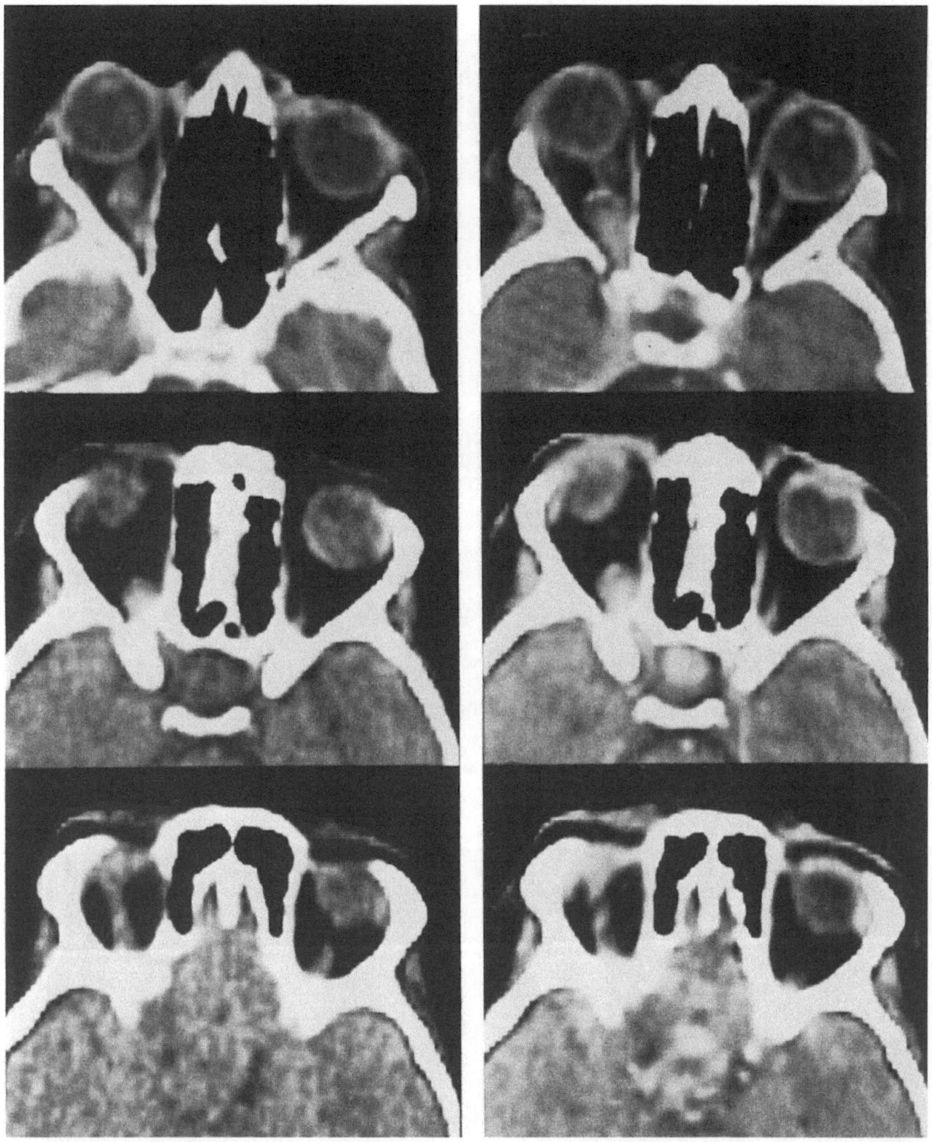

**Fig. G12.** Glioma of the left optic nerve with extension to the optic chiasma and the hypothalamus in an 18-year-old female. Left, precontrast study; right, postcontrast study. Significant distension of the left optic nerve in its posterior segment. Contrast enhancement demonstrates the intracranial portion of the tumor in the chiasma and the hypothalamus

## Computed Tomography

Neurinomas are sharply delineated with absorption values similar to those in meningiomas (Fig. G13). The lesions do not invade bone structures of the orbit. Multiple tumors are found in neurofibromatosis (Fig. G14).

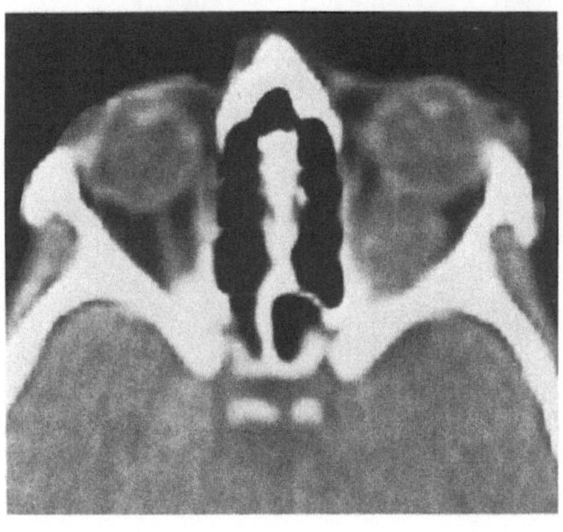

**Fig. G13.** Neurinoma in the right orbit of a 45-year-old female with proptosis. Soft tissue lesion filling the funnel of the right orbit ▶

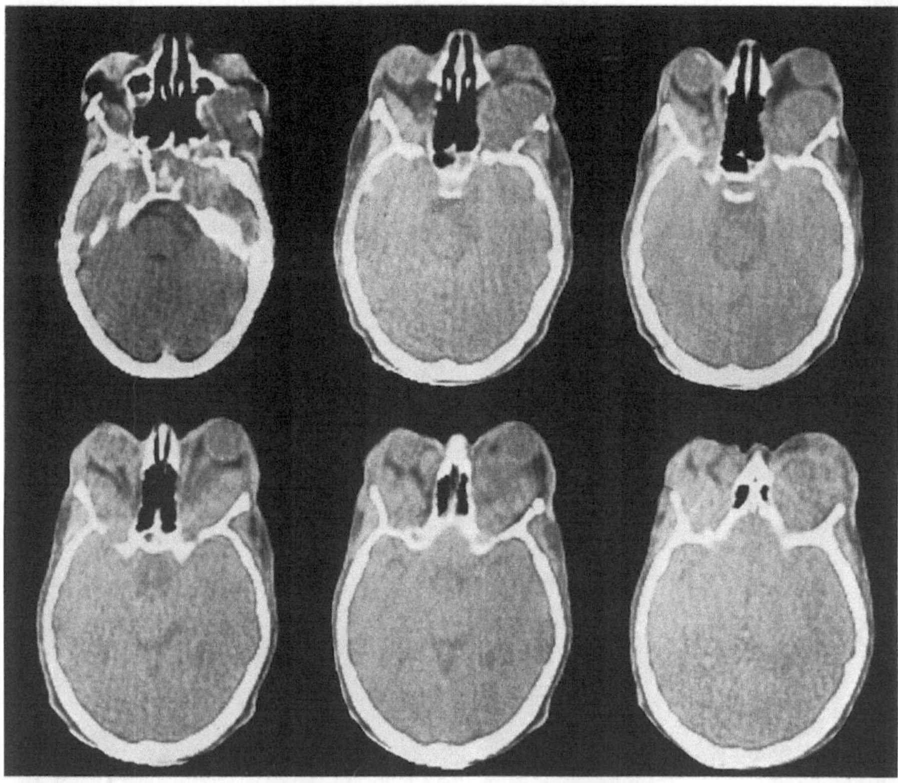

a

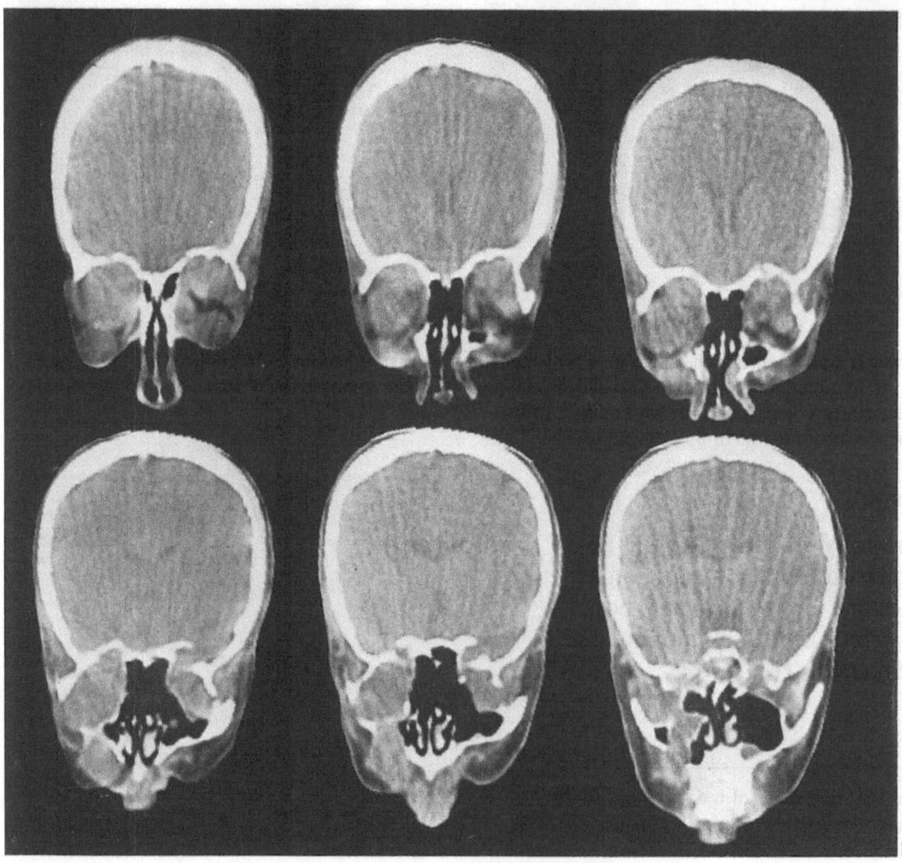

b

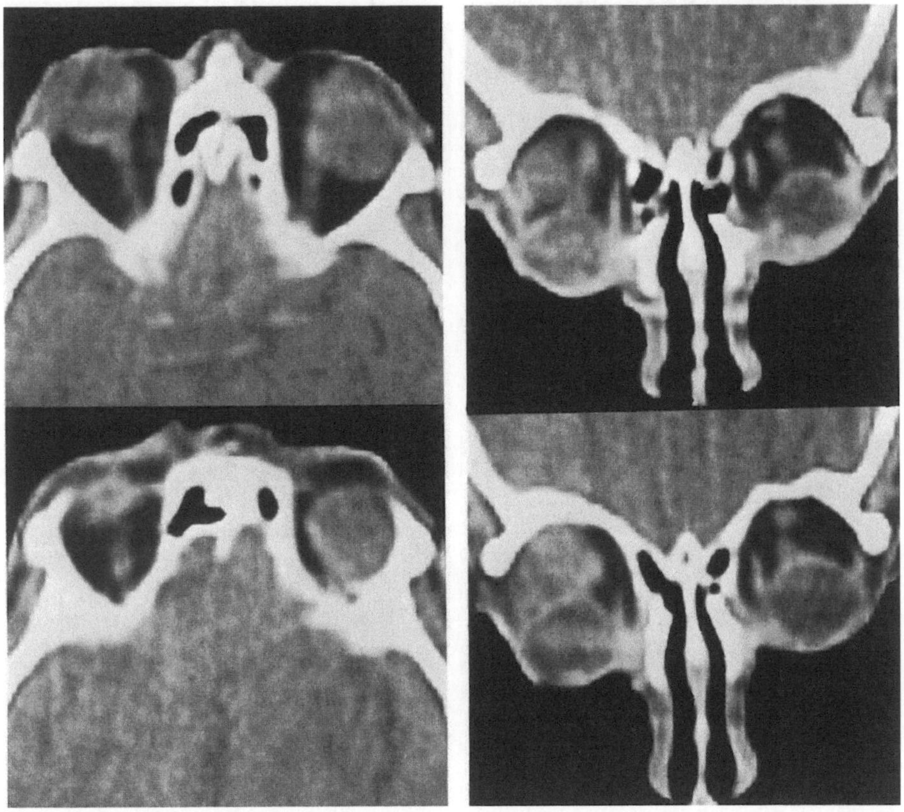

**Fig. G15.** Fibroma in the right orbit. Rather sharply delineated soft tissue lesion above and lateral to the right eyeball and optic nerve in a 62-year-old male. CT findings do not allow a type-specific diagnosis. Horizontal and coronary projections

# Fibromas

These are sharply delineated solid tumors which are most often found at the roof of the orbit. They are congenital lesions. Histological studies reveal a capsule as well as a rather simple fibrillary structure.

### Computed Tomography

Tumors are well demarcated against other orbital structures including the eyeball and the optic nerve. Contrast administration results in a clear increase in density (Fig. G15).

◄

**Fig. G14a, b.** Multiple neurofibromas in both orbits, more pronounced on the right, in a 34-year-old female with neurofibromatosis. Extreme bilateral proptosis. The right orbit is almost entirely filled with tumor causing caudal and lateral dislocation of the right eyeball (coronary projection, **b**). Partial aplasia of the left sphenoid wing with disruption of the bone contour (**a**)

# Lipomas

The tumors are extremely soft and very mobile. Histological studies reveal fatty tissue and regular fibrillary structures surrounded by a thin fibrous capsule.

### Computed Tomography

Lipomas resemble dermoids and have the same density as fat tissue. Diagnosis is usually made on the basis of indirect signs such as displacement of normal structures.

# Epidermoid Cysts

These are congenital malformations made up of epidermoid tissue contained within a capsule.

### Computed Tomography

Density values are similar to those of CSF, and this allows clear differentiation from fatty tissue in the orbit.

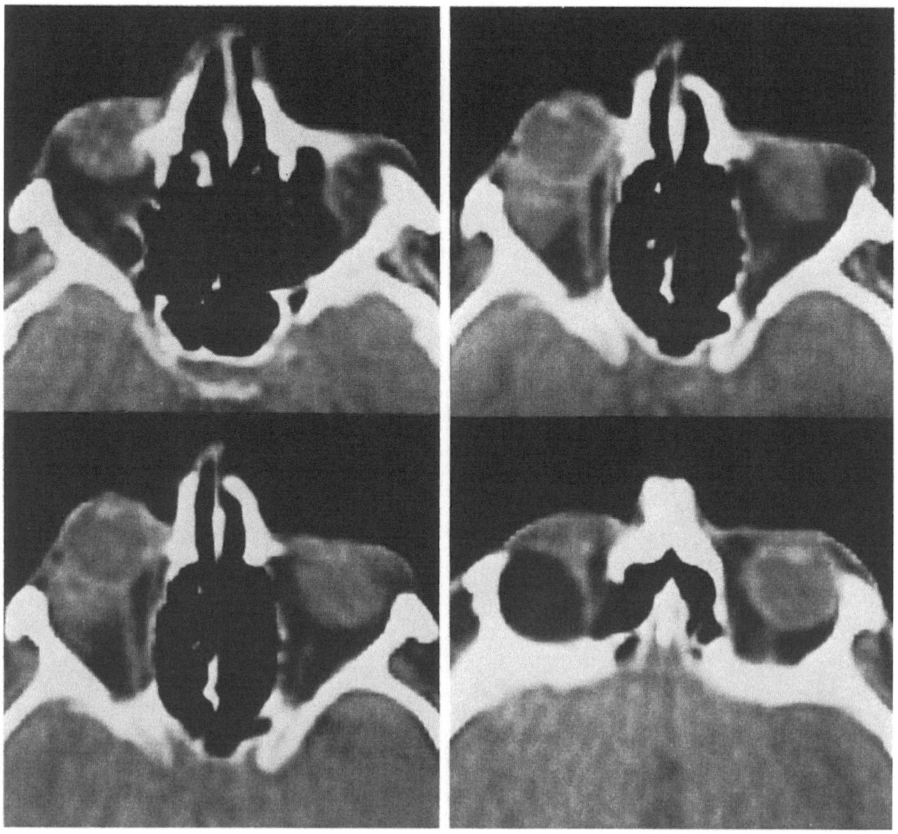

**Fig. G16.** Dermoid cyst in the left orbit in a 68-year-old man. Very inhomogeneous density values. Significant proptosis. The optic nerve is stretched and the left eyeball displaced inferiorly

## Dermoid Cysts

This is the most common congenital tumor in the orbital region. Growth is very slow. The lesions may contain an oily liquid as well as hair and cholesterin crystals.

### Computed Tomography

One finds circumscribed zones of very low density characteristic of fatty tissue. Variations in density values within the tumor may be found as a result of inhomogeneous composition (Fig. G16).

# 2. Malignant Tumors

Malignant tumors such as *carcinomas, sarcomas, malignant lymphomas, and metastases of malignant tumors* may be found in the orbits and may cause destruction of bone. Differentiation from a benign tumor is not possible if the soft tissue lesion is sharply delineated and if there is no evidence of bone destruction (GAWLER et al. 1974; LAMPERT et al. 1974; MOMOSE et al. 1975).

## Tumors of the Lacrimal Glands

These tumors may be either malignant or benign. Pleomorphic adenomas are found in 50–60% of cases, carcinoma within a pleomorphic adenoma in 5–10%, adenoid-cystic carcinoma in 20–30%, and other carcinomas in 5–10% (SMITH 1977). These are solid lesions, with slow growth and infiltration of skin and bone. Other tumors of the lacrimal glands include malignant lymphomas, lymphoid pseudotumors, and leukemic infiltrates.

### Computed Tomography

The tumors are located in the upper lateral sections of the orbits, beneath and posterior to the eyeball (Figs. G17, 18). CT findings are similar to those in carcinomas and metastases.

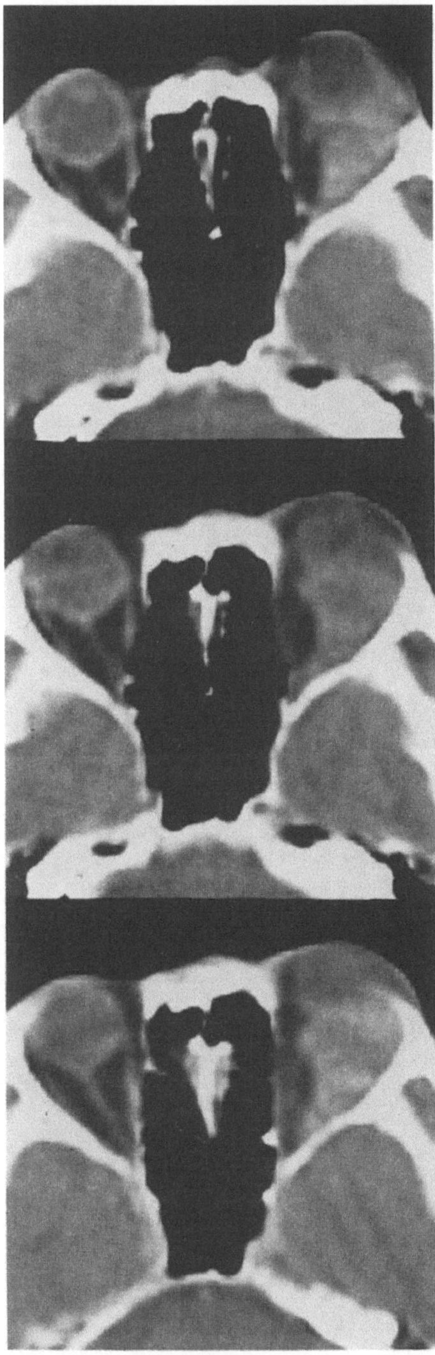

a

b

c

**Fig. G17a–c.** Cylindromatous adenoma of the right lacrimal gland in a 39-year-old patient. The tumor extends from the lacrimal gland to the apex of the orbit. Significant contrast uptake in the tumor. (**b**) Precontrast study. (**a, c**) Postcontrast study

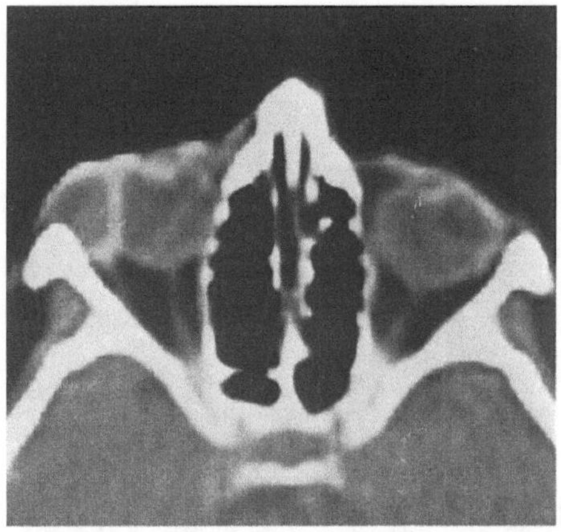

**Fig. G18.** Carcinoma of the left lacrimal gland in a 76-year-old patient. Sharply demarcated tumor in the anterior and lateral segments of the left orbit. Marginal zone of contrast uptake

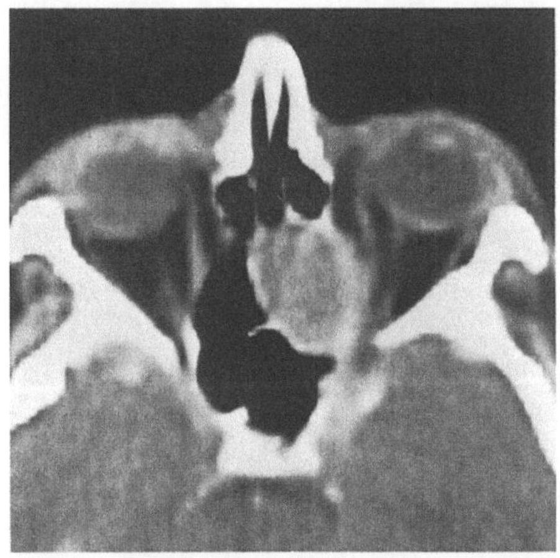

**Fig. G19.** Carcinoma originating in the ethmoid bone with penetration of the right orbit in 38-year-old patient. The tumor is sharply demarcated and takes up contrast medium. Precontrast study does not allow differentiation of carcinoma from mucocele or pyocele

## Carcinomas and Metastases

Primary orbital carcinomas originate in the lacrimal gland or the eyelid (Figs. G17, 18). Secondary orbital carcinomas from adjacent structures invade the orbit (Figs. G19–25).

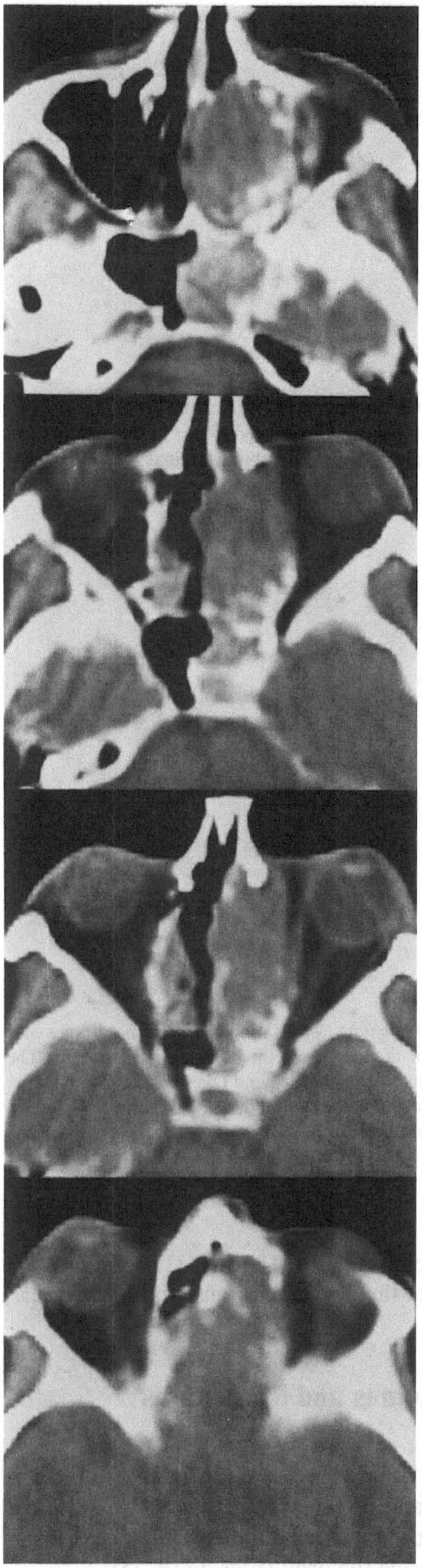

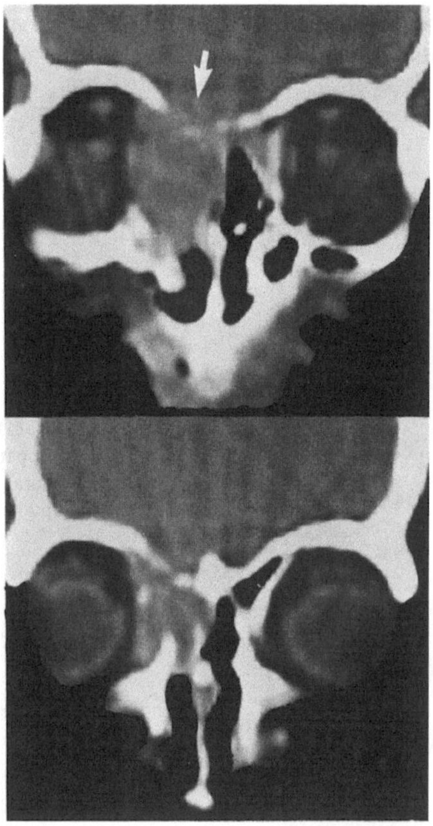

**Fig. G20.** Squamous cell carcinoma of the nasal cavity with penetration of the right orbit and the cranial cavity in a 62-year-old patient. Soft tissue lesion in the ethmoid cells and the nasal cavity on the right with destruction of the medial wall and the roof of the right orbit in its medial portion (arrow)

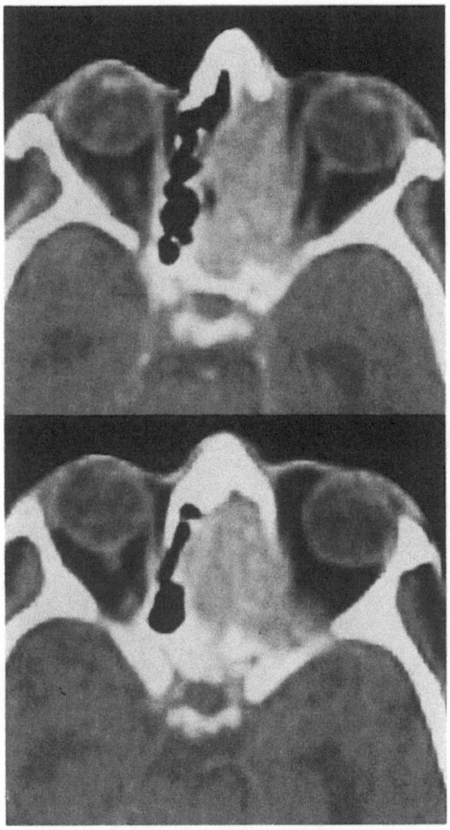

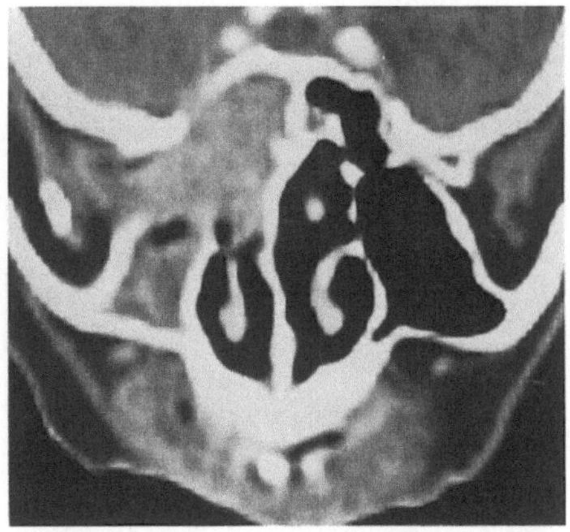

**Fig. G21.** Inverted papilloma with carcinoid elements in the ethmoid cells on the right, the nasal cavity, and the right maxillary sinus with penetration of the right orbit and destruction of its medial wall. Postcontrast study

*Metastases from bronchogenic carcinoma, uterine carcinoma, renal carcinoma, thyroid carcinoma, prostatic carcinoma, pancreatic carcinoma, and carcinoma of the breast* may be found in the orbital region.

### Computed Tomography

CT findings are not uniform, as the tumors may vary in density and size. Some tumors are sharply delineated while others cannot be differentiated from surrounding structures. Demonstration of bone destruction suggests a diagnosis of malignancy (Figs. G20, 25). Most lesions show positive contrast enhancement, which allows more precise delineation of the tumor (Fig. G22).

## Adenoid-cystic Carcinomas

(Synonym – cylindromas)

The tumors present the histological picture of structures lined with cylindrical epithelium and filled with mucus. Growth is rapid, and extension into the cranial cavity is possible. The tumors may arise within the orbit in the lacrimal gland but more often penetrate to the orbits from the paranasal sinuses.

### Computed Tomography

CT findings are similar to those in other malignant tumors (cf. Fig. E23).

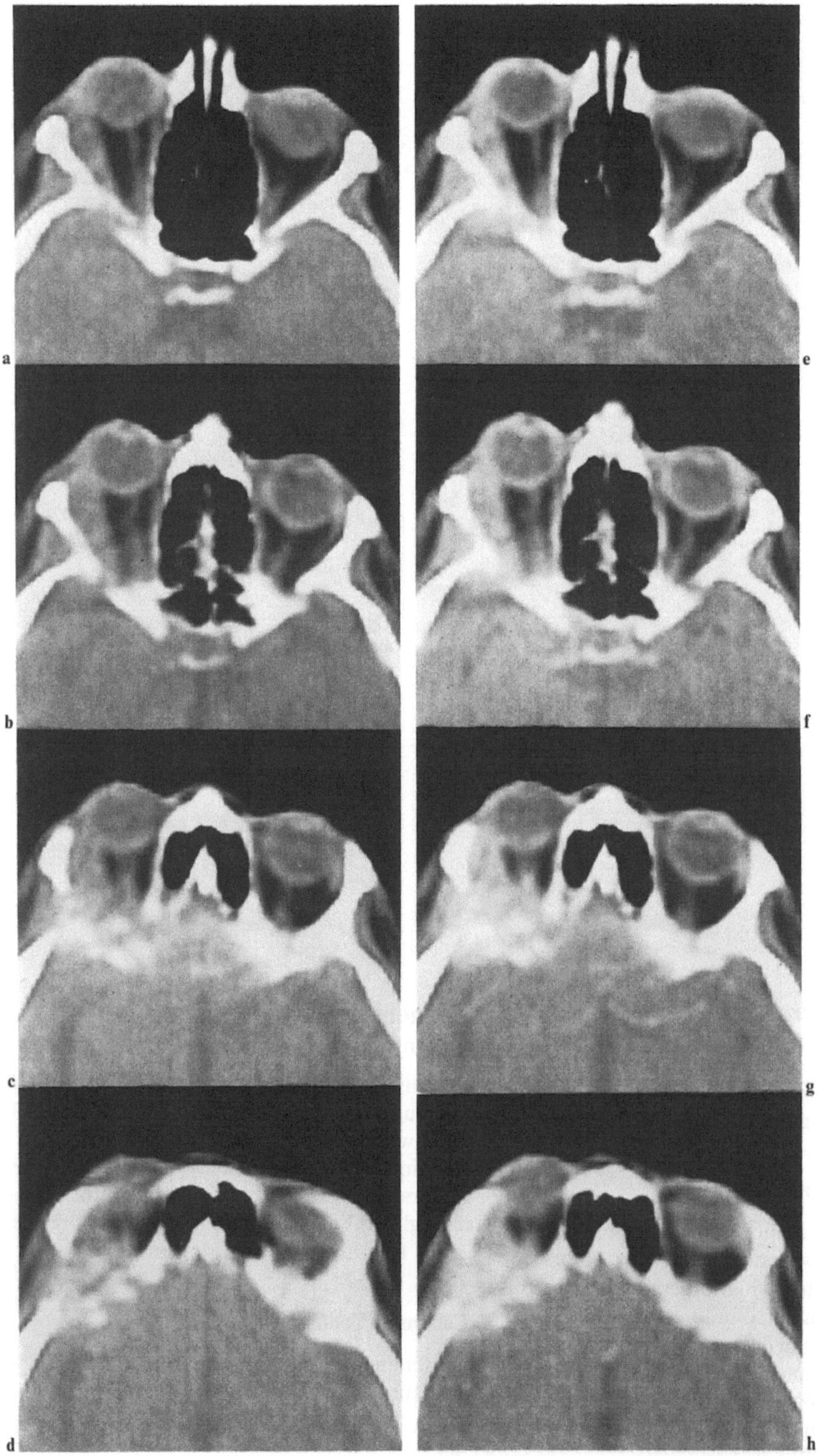
a
e
b
f
c
g
d
h

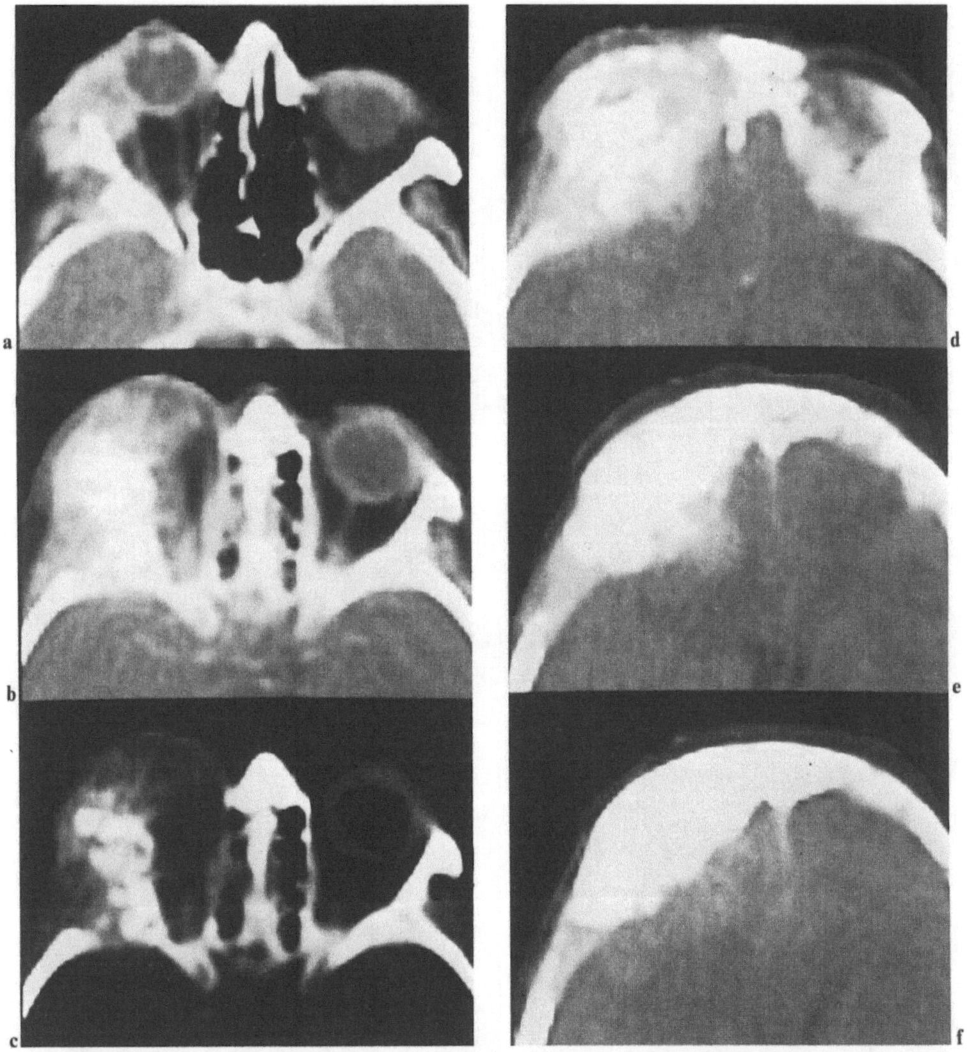


**Fig. G23**a–f. Metastasis of breast cancer in the left orbit and adjacent skull vault in a 60-year-old female. Osteoplastic and osteoclastic bone changes as well as a soft tissue mass in the anterior portion of the left orbit. Osteoplastic change is most clearly demonstrated in slices **c–f**. Intracranial spread of the tumor with displacement of midline structures and compression of the left anterior horn (**e**)

**Fig. G24**a–h. Metastasis of carcinoma of unknown origin in the right orbit of a 50-year-old male. The medial wall of the right orbit is intact and displaced toward the midline. Sharp delineation of the lesion with slight contrast uptake at the margins. Inferior and lateral displacement of the eyeball. The coronary projection clearly shows destruction of the roof of the orbit (**h**)

Fig. see p. 480 ►

**Fig. G25**a–h. Metastasis causing total destruction of the greater sphenoid wing on the left in a 71-year-old female (**a–d**). Contrast enhancement produces an increase in density values and sharp delineation of the soft tissue lesion (**e–h**)

Fig. see p. 481 ►

◄

**Fig. G22**a–h. Metastasis of breast cancer in the left orbit of a 64-year-old female. Soft tissue lesion in the lateral segment of the left orbit as well as bone destruction at the greater sphenoid wing (**a–d**). Contrast enhancement results in hyperdense values within the soft tissue lesion as well as improved demonstration of the tumor in the temporal fossa (**e–h**). The CT picture leaves the impression that the intraorbital portion of the metastasis is limited to infiltration of the lateral rectus muscle

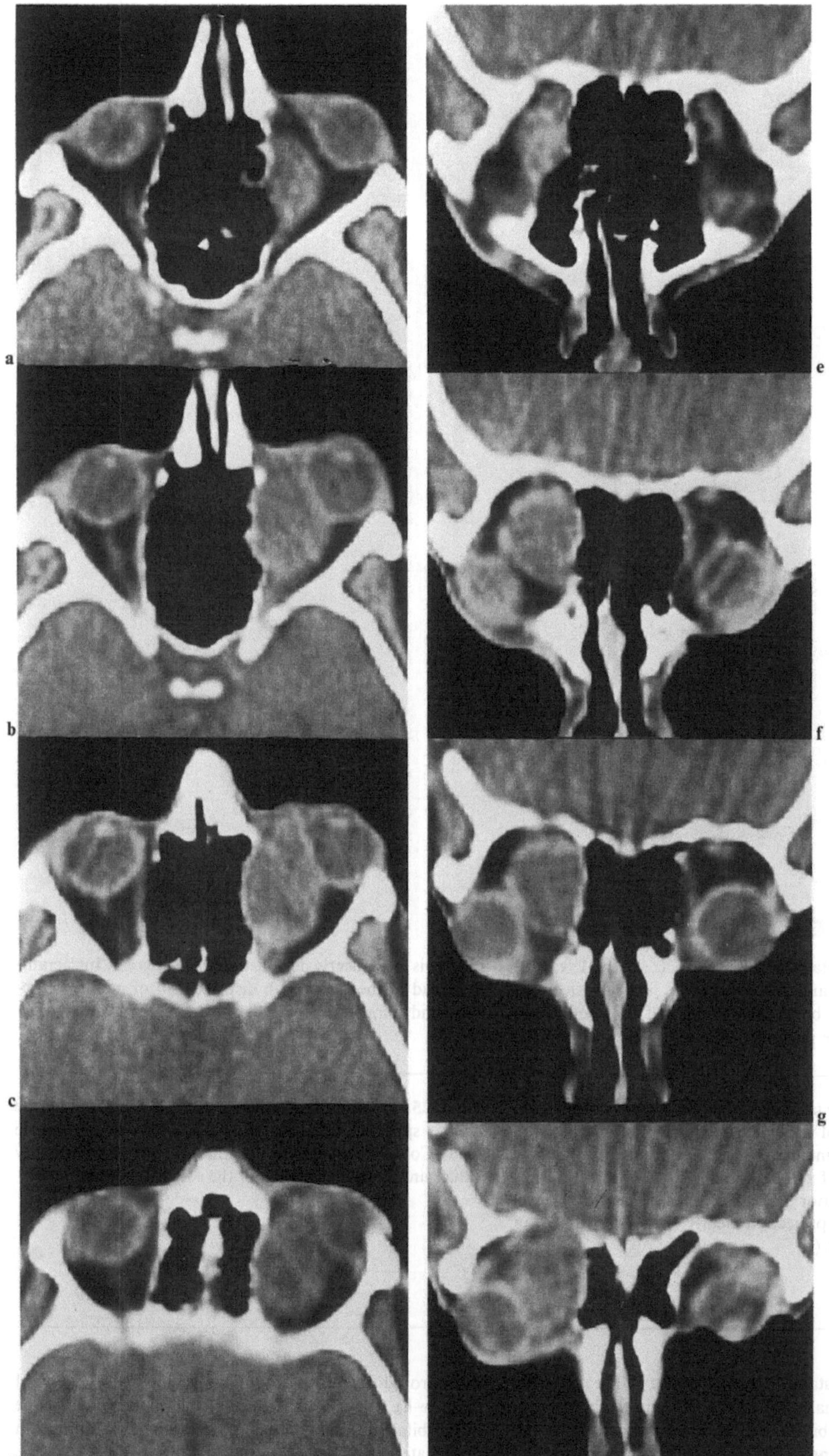

**Fig. G24 a–h**
Legend see p. 479

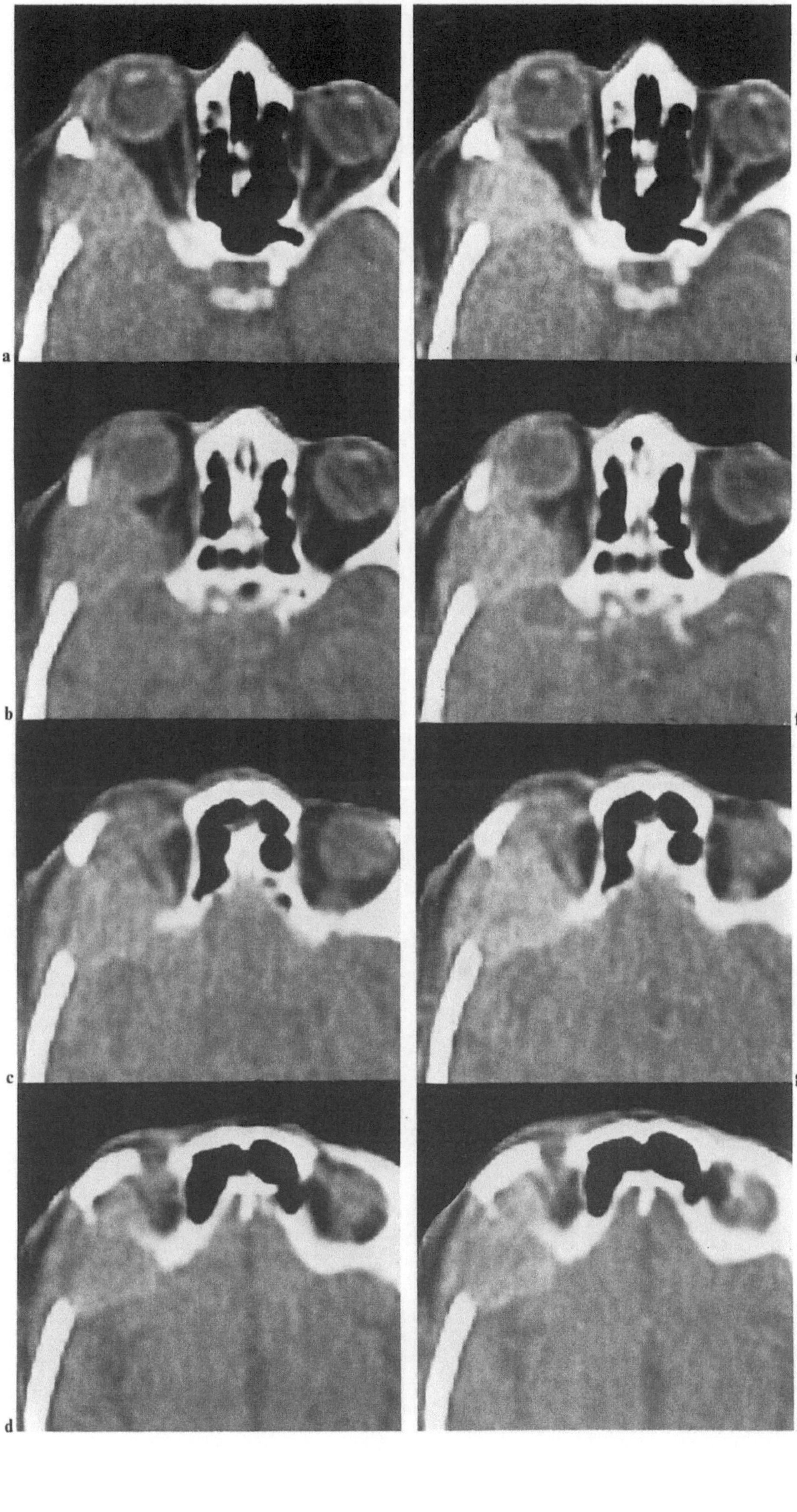


**Fig. G25a–h**
Legend see p. 479

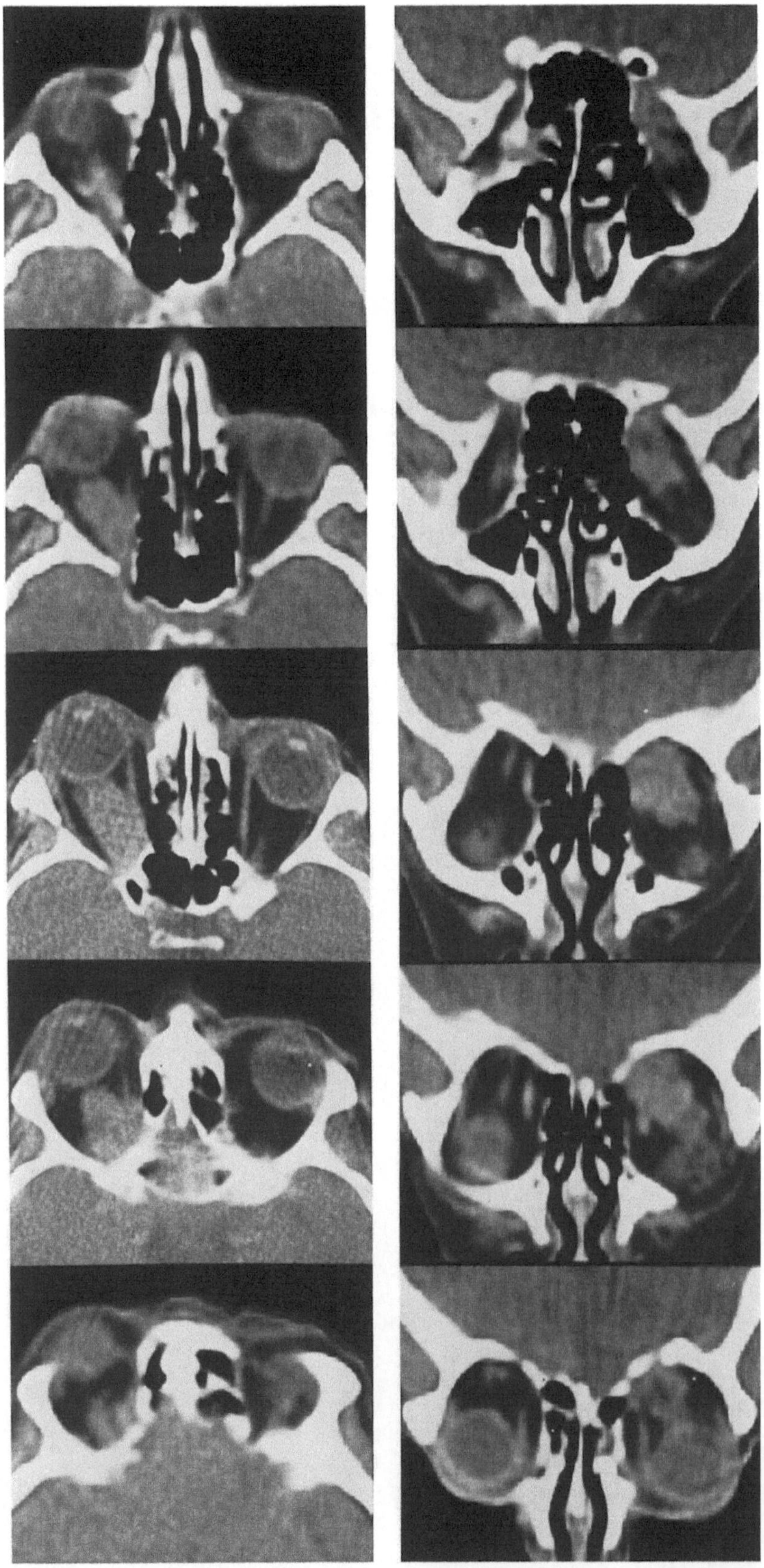

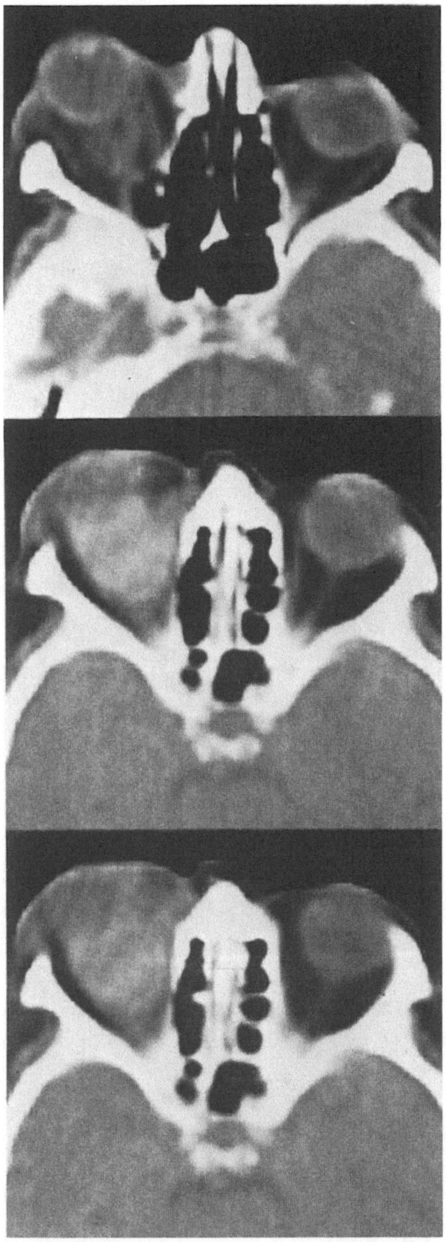

Fig. G27. Malignant lymphoma (immunocytoma) in the left orbit of an 82-year-old female. Inhomogeneous soft tissue lesion which fills the upper section of the orbit and extends into the left eyelid

◄ Fig. G26. Malignant lymphoma (immunocytoma) in the left orbit of a 42-year-old male. The tumor is not clearly demarcated from the optic nerve. Coronary projections reveal that the major portion of the tumor is located in the upper section of the orbit

# Malignant Lymphomas

Malignant lymphomas make up 7%–14% of all orbital tumors and originate in the orbit in most cases, though orbital metastases of malignant lymphomas of other regions of the body have been observed. They are found in all regions of the orbits and demonstrate infiltrative growth. The immunocytic lymphoma is the most common histological type.

### Computed Tomography

The tumors usually present as rather well-defined soft-tissue lesions with high density (35–40 HU) which readily enhance after contrast infusion. They are often found adjacent to the eyeball and may involve the extraocular muscles and the optic nerve to such an extent that it is no longer possible to delineate the normal orbital structures (Figs. G26–28).

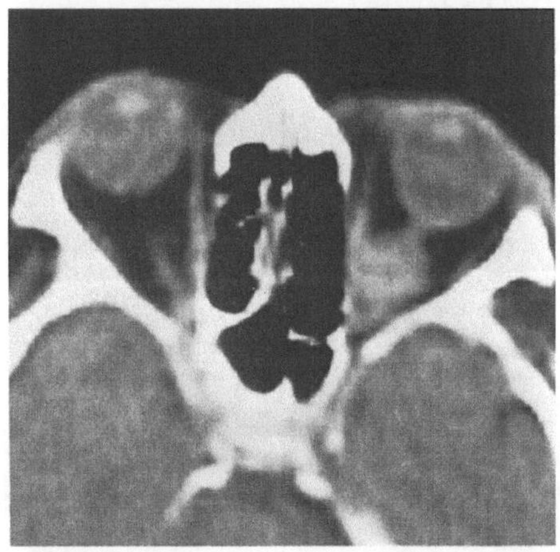

Fig. G28. Malignant lymphoma in the right orbit of a 68-year-old male. Sharply delineated soft tissue lesion with relatively high density values. Demarcation from the optic nerve is not possible. The funnel of the right orbit is filled with tumor

# Melanomas of the Eyeball

These tumors are most often found in the elderly and originate in melanoblasts of the choroid.

### Computed Tomography

CT studies are indicated when dorsal penetration of the sclera is suspected. Melanomas have high density (Fig. G32), and administration of

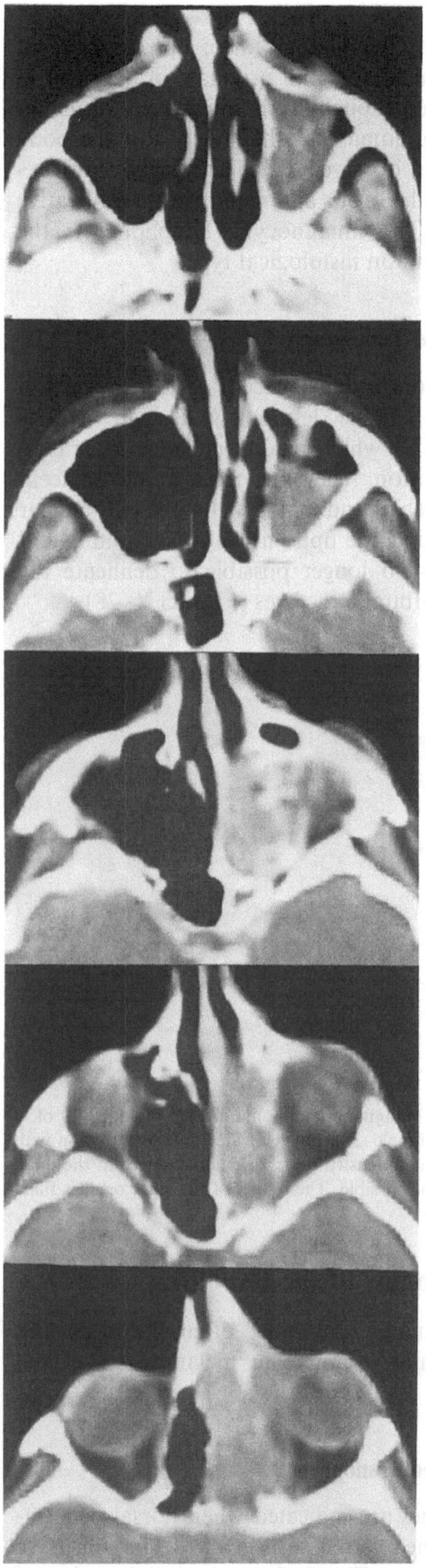

Fig. G29

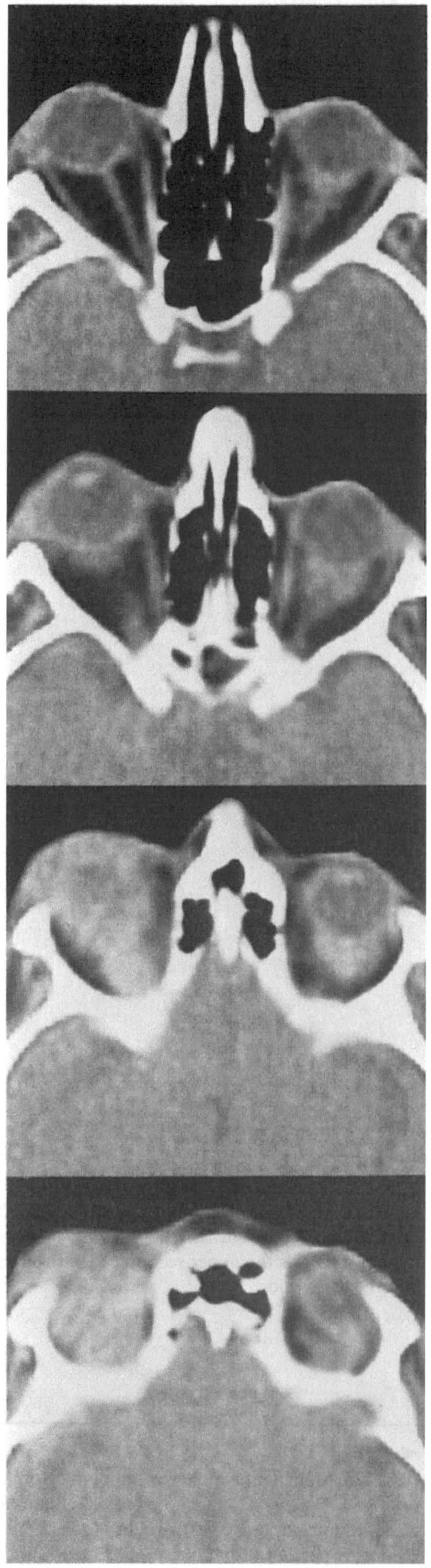

Fig. G30

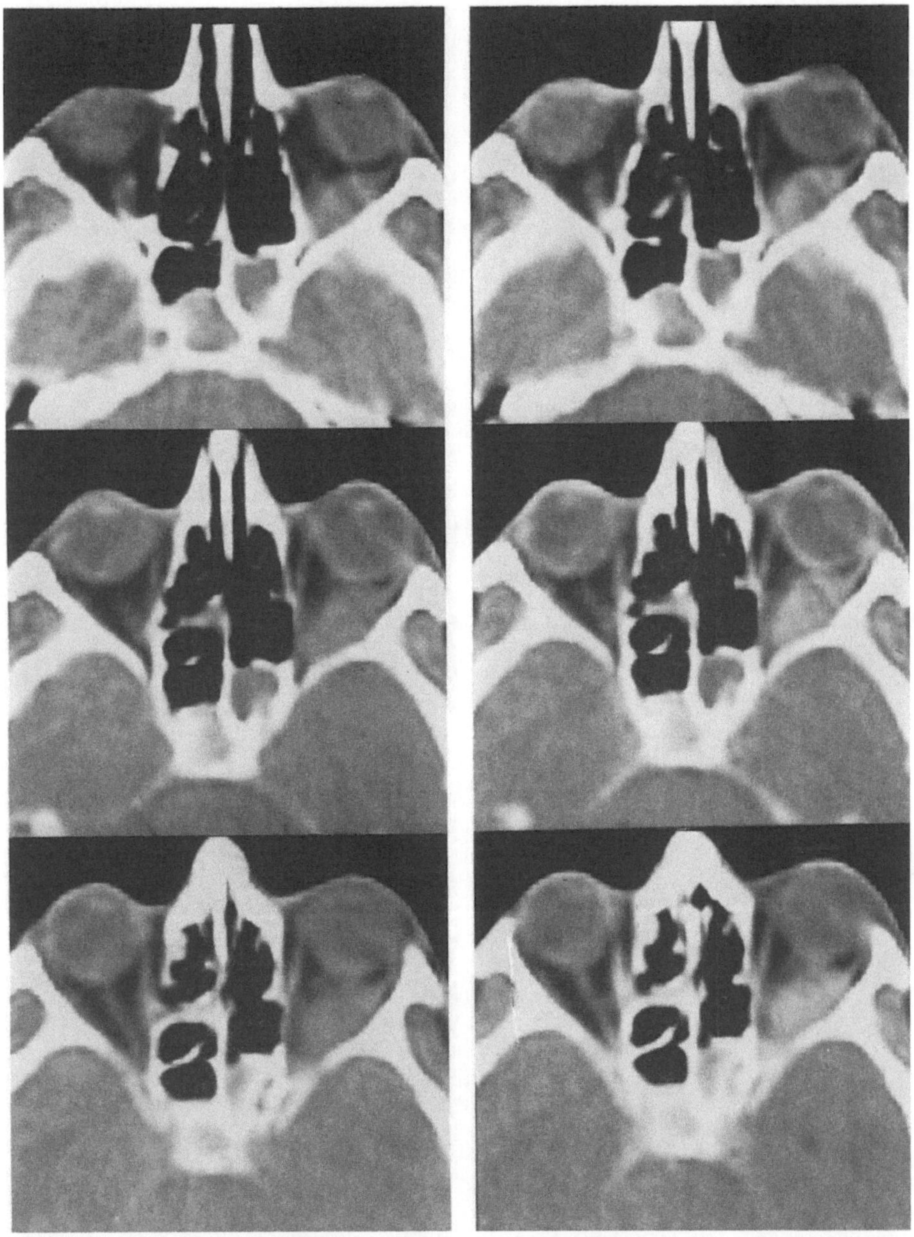

**Fig. G31.** Rhabdomyosarcoma in the right orbit of a 60-year-old male with proptosis. The lateral rectus muscle cannot be delineated from the tumor. Initial interpretation of the CT scan: tumor originating in the right lateral rectus muscle. Strong contrast uptake in tumor tissue. Left, precontrast study; right, postcontrast study

◀ **Fig. G29.** Lymphoepithelioma in the right maxillary sinus, the right nasal cavity, and the ethmoid cells on the right with penetration of the right orbit in a 63-year-old female. Destruction of the medial wall of the orbit

◀ **Fig. G30.** Involvement of both orbits in a 39-year-old female with Brill-Symmer's disease (lymphoreticulosis). The hyperdense soft tissue lesions are located adjacent to the eyeball and have infiltrated the surrounding structures

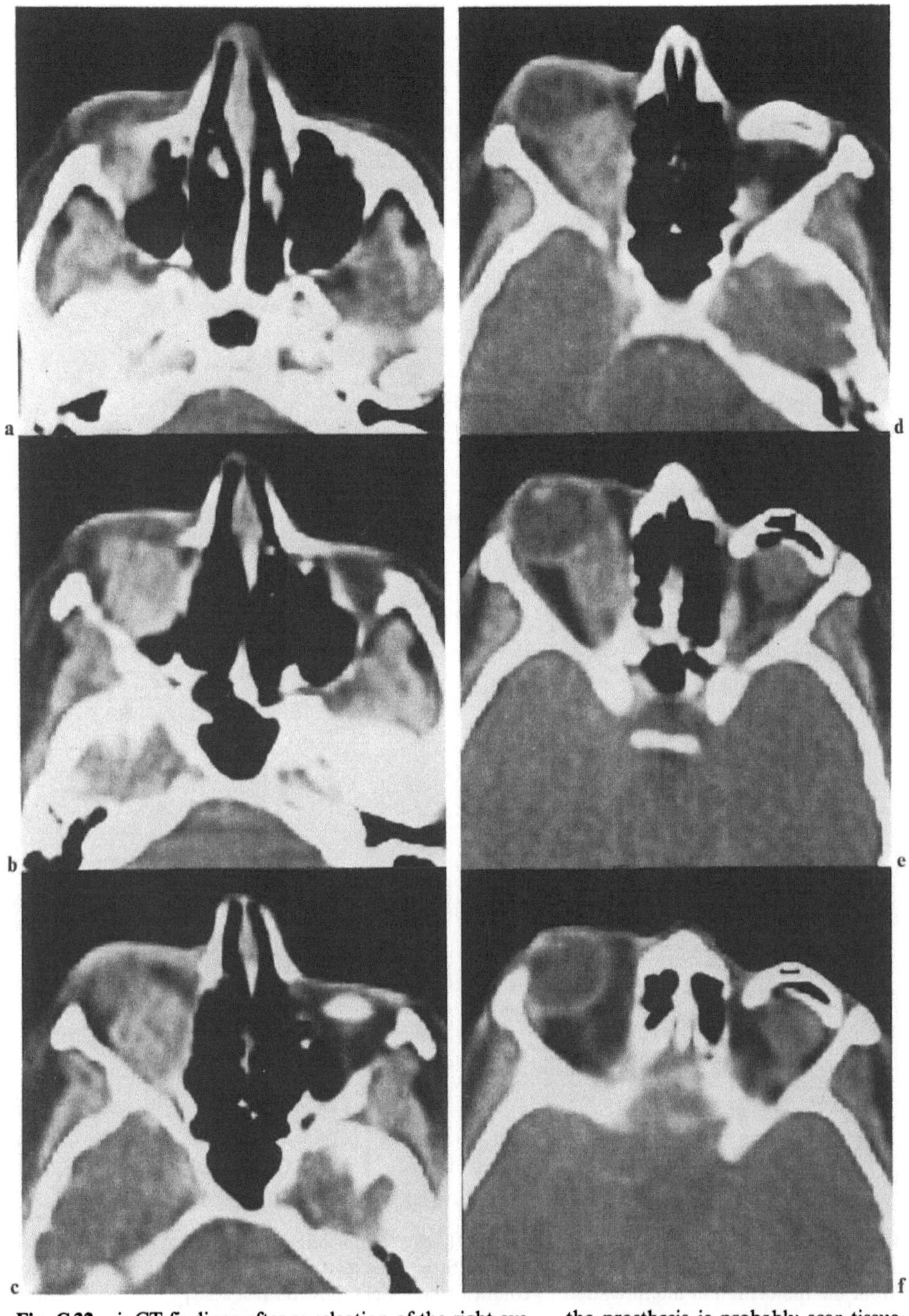


**Fig. G32** a–j. CT findings after enucleation of the right eyeball for treatment of melanoma in a 39-year-old female. Ocular prosthesis on the right. The soft tissue posterior to the prosthesis is probably scar tissue. Large tumor in the medial section of the left orbit (adjacent to the medial wall) (**b–e, g–j**) Histological diagnosis of melanoma

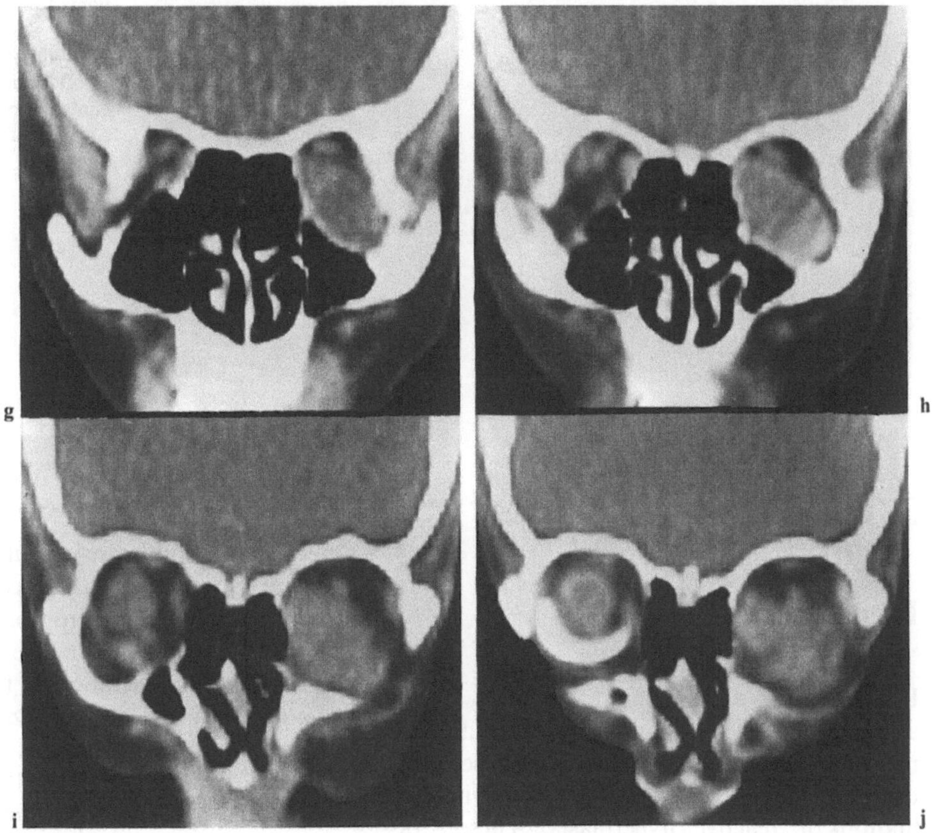

Fig. G32g–j

contrast media usually fails to produce a further increase in density (WENDE et al. 1977).

## Sarcomas

These include fibrosarcomas and rhabdomyosarcomas, the latter being the most common orbital tumors in children. The neoplasms grow very rapidly.

### Computed Tomography

The tumors are similar in appearance to carcinomas and metastases. Some are well delineated against surrounding structures, while others demonstrate invasive and destructive growth (Fig. G31).

## Neuroblastomas

These tumors occur in early childhood, rarely later. Rapid growth and metastases are characteristic.

### Computed Tomography

The tumors may reach enormous size and fill the orbit completely; differentiation from other malignant tumors is usually impossible.

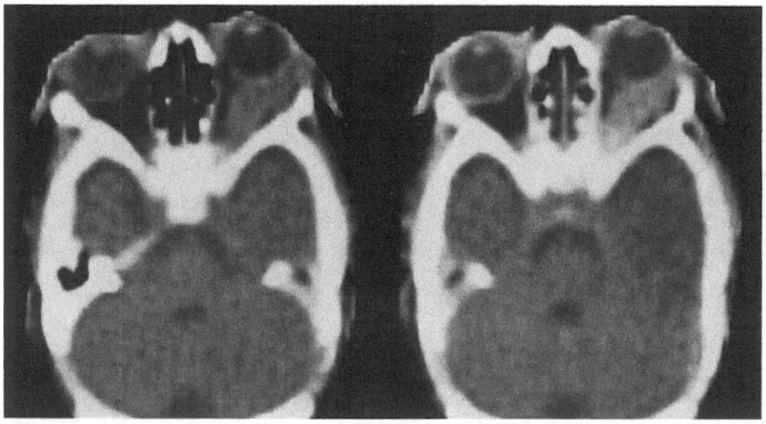

**Fig. G33.** Hemangioendothelioma in the right orbit of a 2-month-old infant. The right orbit is almost entirely filled with a soft tissue mass. Very strong contrast uptake suggests the presence of a highly vascular lesion

# 3. Inflammatory Processes

## Pseudotumors

Pseudotumors comprise approximately 8% of all space-occupying lesions in the orbits and are not neoplastic processes in the strict sense of the word. They represent either chronic inflammation or reactive hyperplasia. These "tumors" are most often encountered in patients older than 45 years and result from nonspecific chronic inflammation in and around the vessels serving the extraocular muscles. Microscopic examination reveals lipophages, necrosis, and foreign body reactions.

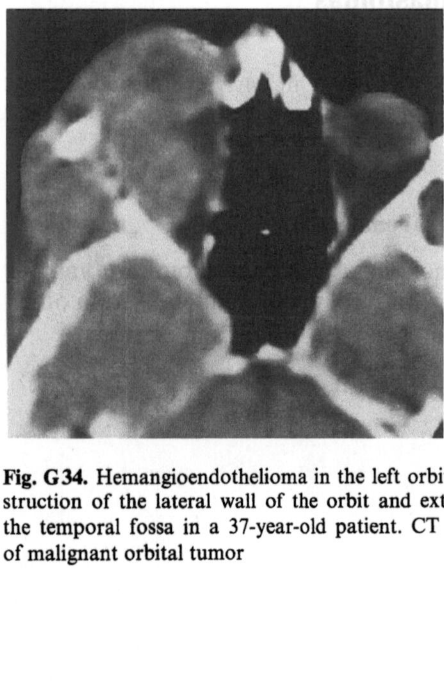

**Fig. G34.** Hemangioendothelioma in the left orbit with destruction of the lateral wall of the orbit and extension to the temporal fossa in a 37-year-old patient. CT diagnosis of malignant orbital tumor

### Computed Tomography

One generally finds an irregularly shaped soft tissue mass with major displacement of normal structures and extreme proptosis. In some cases the tumors fill the entire orbital cavity (Fig. G35). The extraocular muscles and the optic nerve cannot be visualized in such cases. The lesion is usually well delineated (MOMOSE et al. 1975; ENZMANN et al. 1976; LESTER and GYLDENSTEDT 1976), with density values approximating those of muscle tissue. Bilateral pseudotumors may simulate endocrine exophthalmus.

## Mucoceles and Pyoceles

These are lesions causing dilatation of the paranasal sinuses secondary to cyst formation or retention of secretions. Microscopic examination reveals epithelial cysts containing mucus or pus. Bulging of the wall of the cele into the orbit may result in proptosis. Conventional tomographic studies may demonstrate these changes in the paranasal sinuses. The radiological diagnosis is certain only when bulging of the bony wall of the ethmoid or frontal sinuses into the orbit is demonstrated.

### Computed Tomography

One finds a soft tissue lesion originating in the paranasal sinuses and causing displacement or

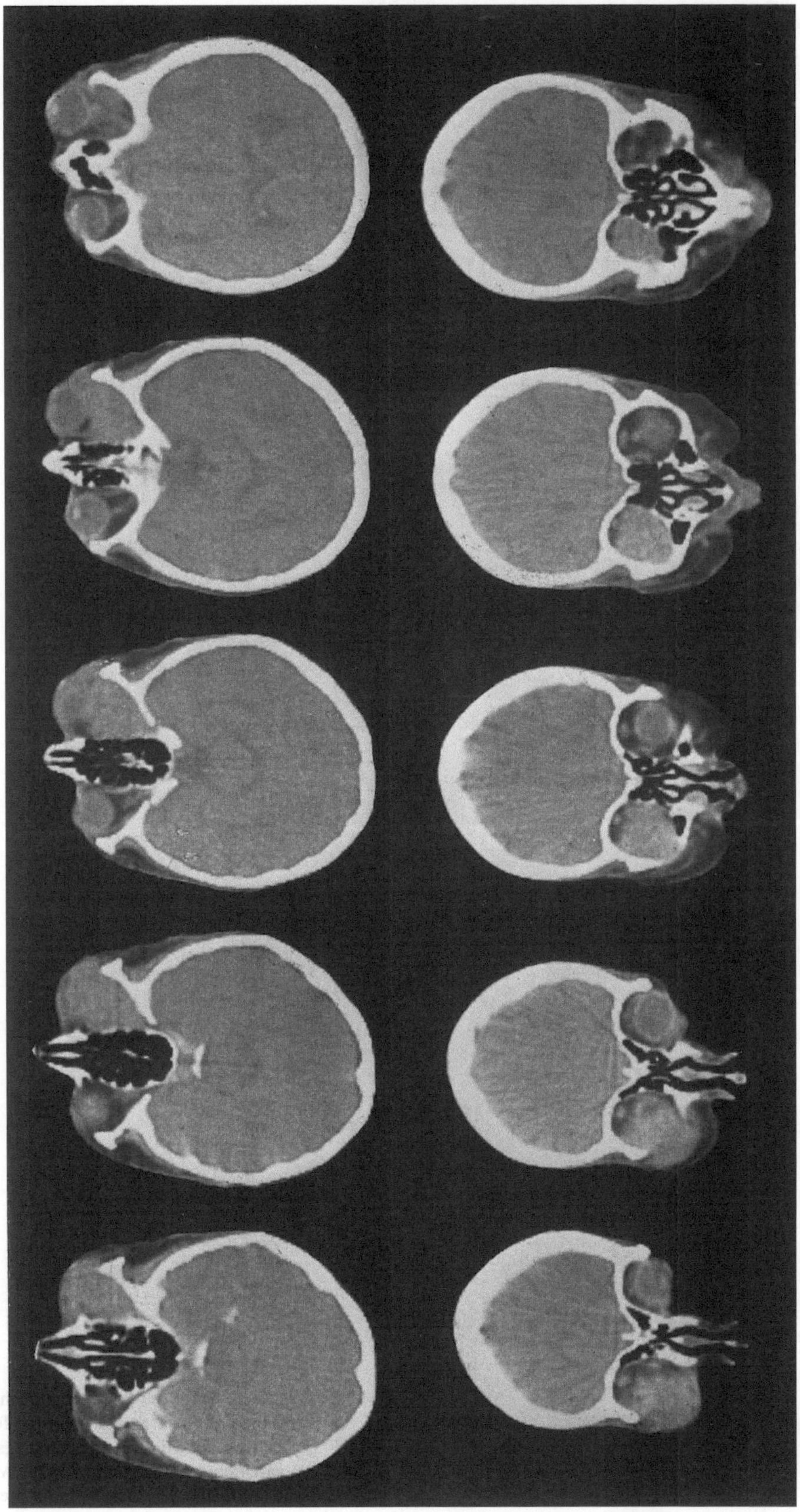

**Fig. G35.** Pseudotumor in the right orbit of a 79-year-old female. The right orbit is almost entirely filled with "tumor." Only the superior rectus and medial rectus muscles are clearly demarcated from the tumor in the coronary projection. No evidence of bone destruction

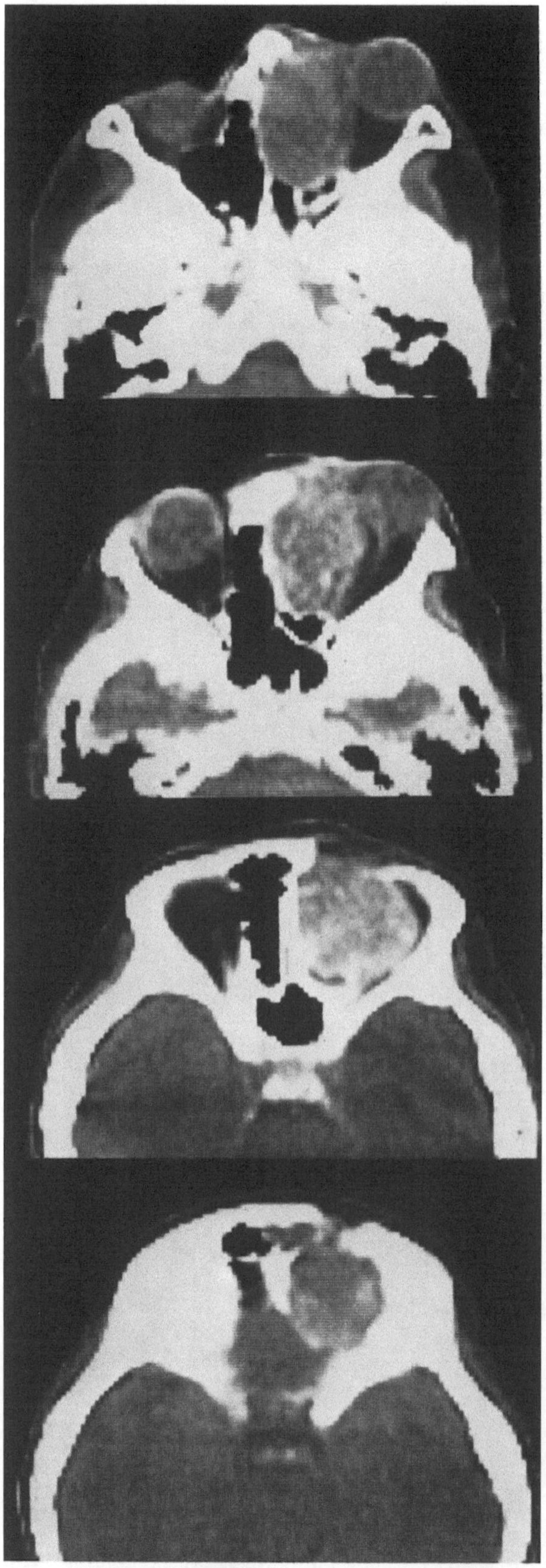

**Fig. G36.** Giant cell granuloma of the ethmoid bone and the right orbit in a 28-year-old female. Soft tissue mass with bone destruction. Findings similar to those in carcinoma of the ethmoid bone. Mucocele and pyocele are further alternatives in differential diagnosis

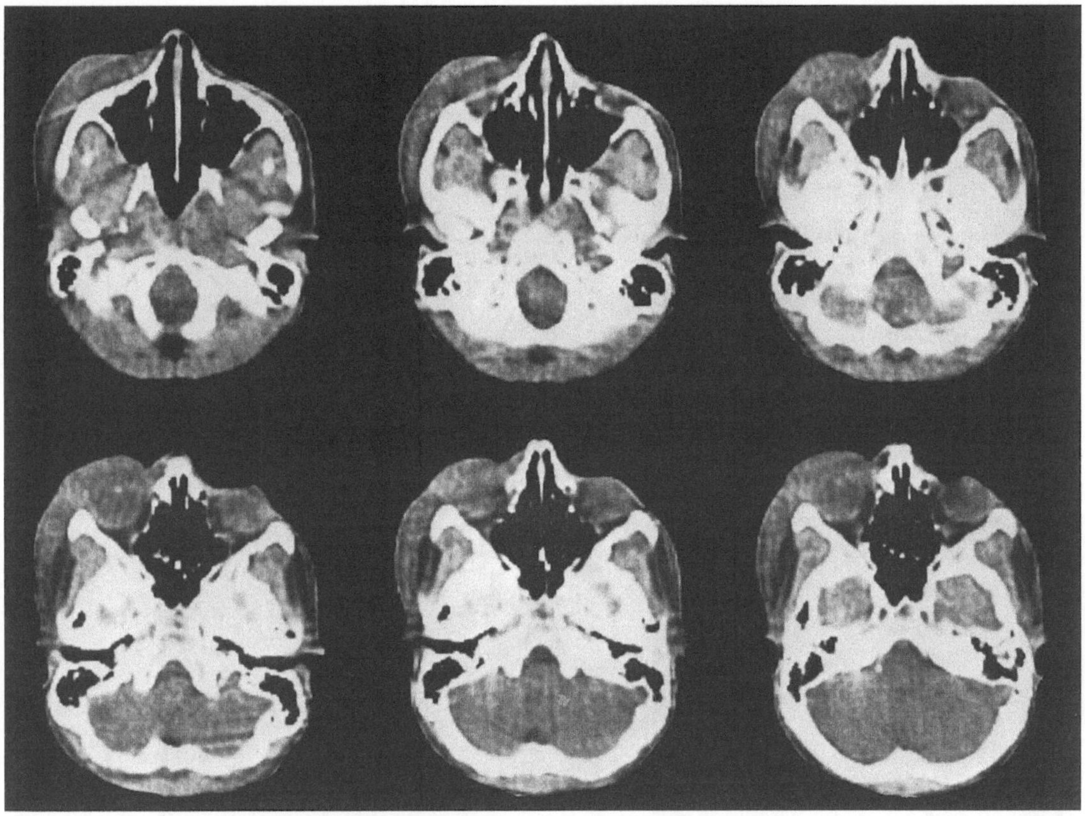

**Fig. G37.** Phlegmon of the left orbit in a 19-year-old patient. Pronounced swelling of soft tissue structures (eyelid, cheek, and muscles at the temple) on the left side of the face

destruction of bone (Figs. G39–43). One may suspect the histological diagnosis on the basis of CT findings when the paranasal sinuses also show pathological changes. Differentiation between a cele and a malignant tumor is impossible in some cases (Fig. G42). Contrast administration does not result in an increase in attenuation values.

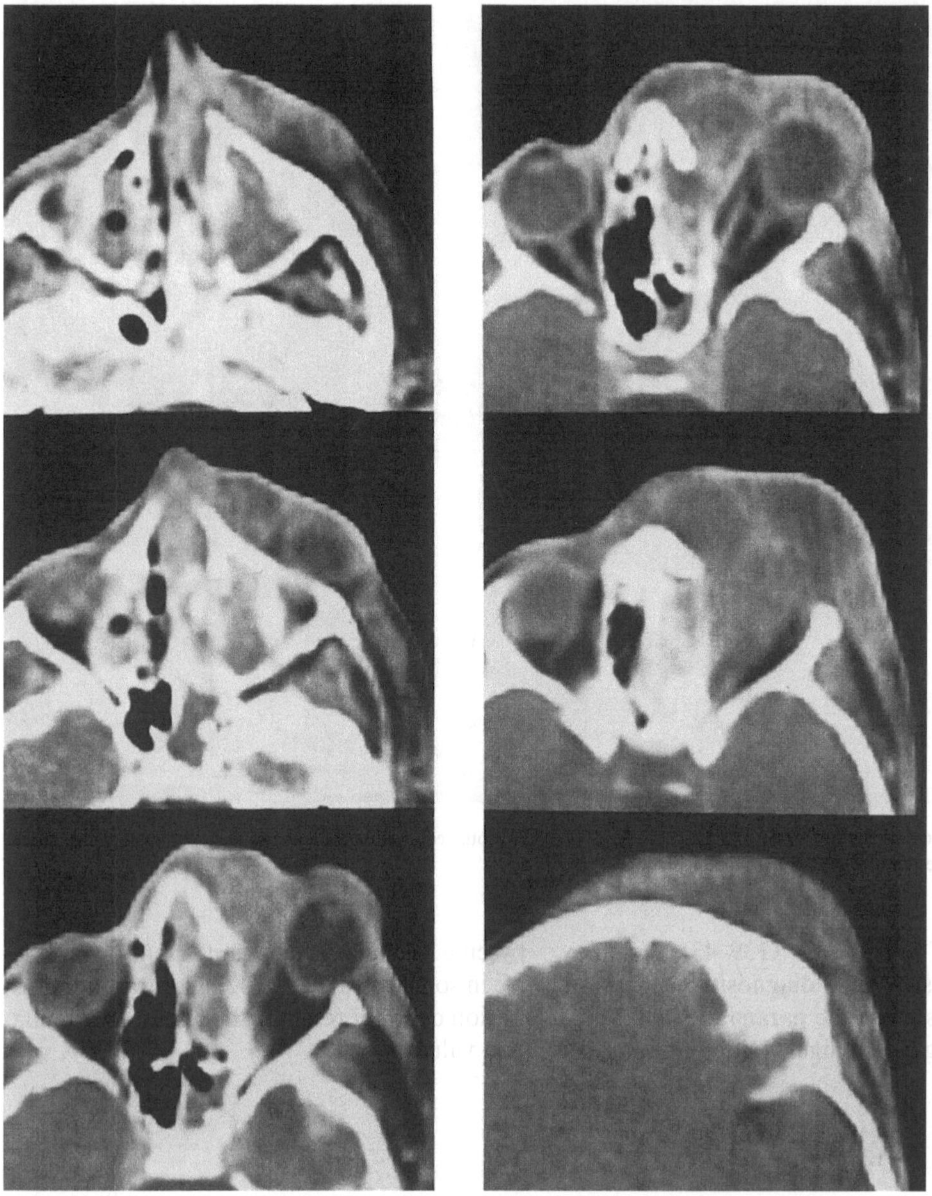

**Fig. G38.** Phlegmon of the right orbit originating in the ethmoid cells on the right in an 11-year-old girl. Pronounced soft tissue swelling with anterior and lateral displacement of the right eyeball. Swelling of both eyelids and the scalp on the right. Opacity in both maxillary sinuses and the right ethmoid cells

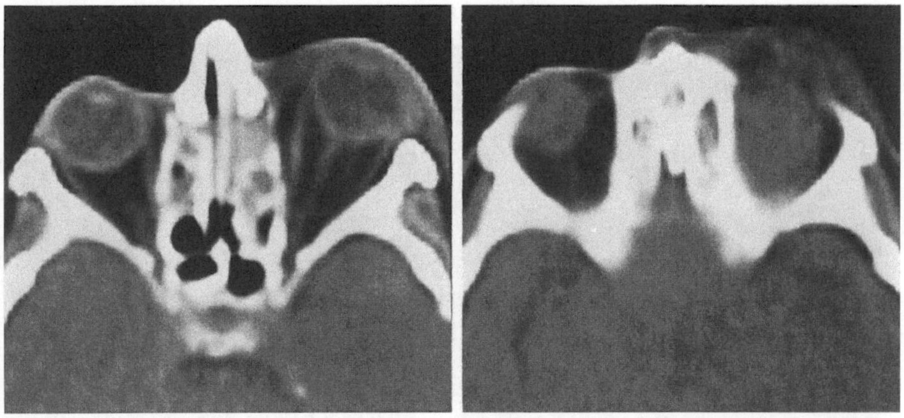

**Fig. G39.** Mucocele on the right, originating in the frontal sinus, with penetration to the right orbit. Extreme proptosis with edema of the eyelid; opacity in the ethmoid cells

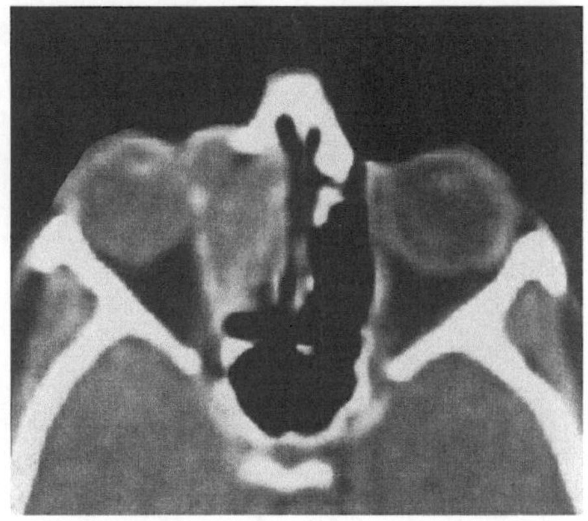

**Fig. G40.** Mucocele originating in the ethmoid cells on the left in a 14-year-old boy: Lateral displacement of the intact medial wall of the left orbit and of the left eyeball

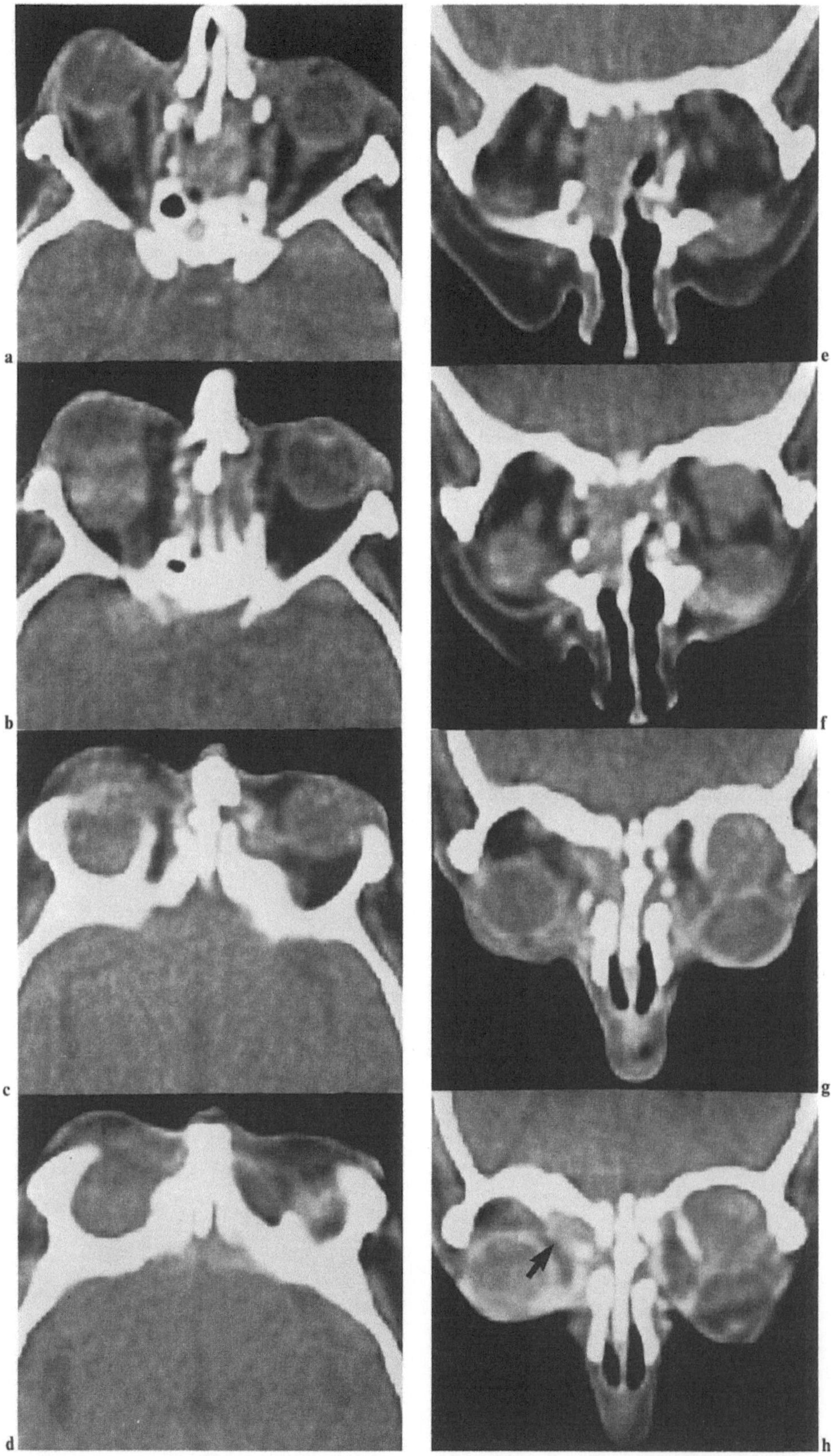

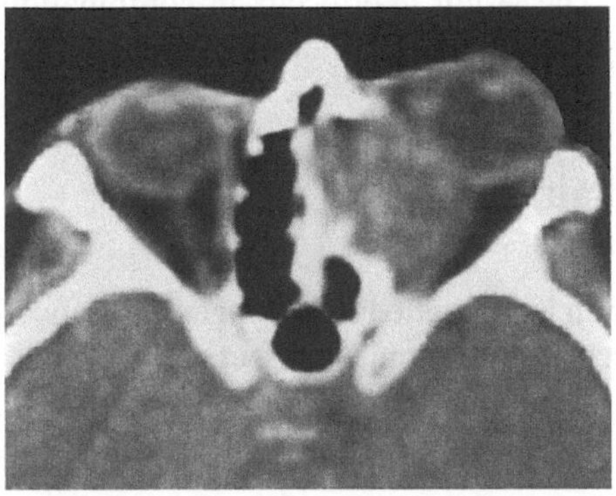

**Fig. G42.** Pyocele of the ethmoid cells on the right with penetration of the right orbit in a 69-year-old female. The bone structures separating the ethmoid cells and the orbit are no longer visible. These findings might be misinterpreted as the result of a malignant tumor

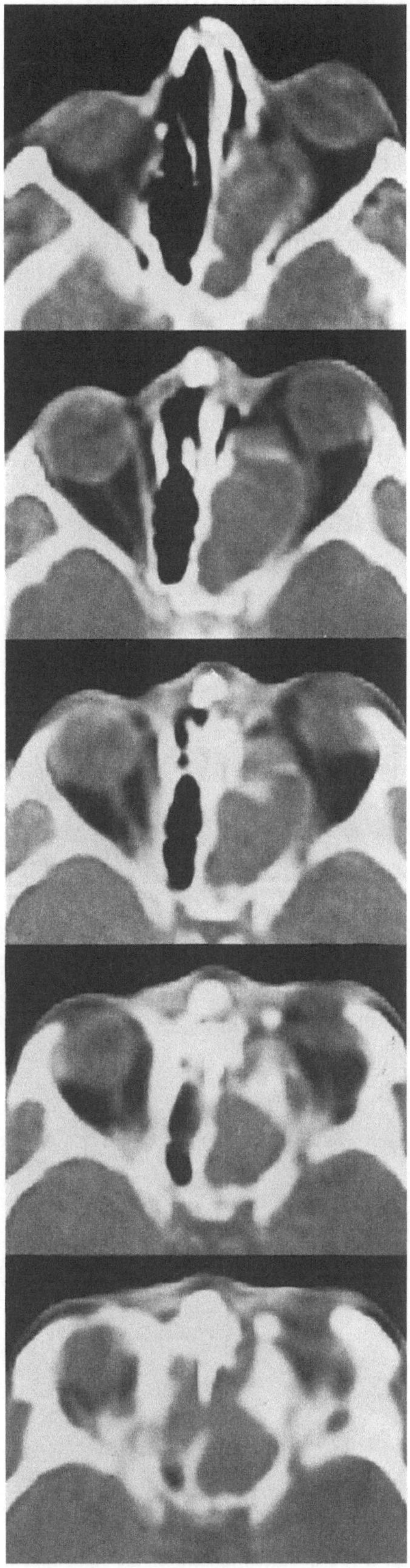

**Fig. G43.** Mucocele of the ethmoid cells on the right with penetration of the right orbit in a 44-year-old male. Characteristic changes in bone with marginal sclerosis resulting from inflammation of long duration. The medial wall of the right orbit is not clearly delineated ►

---

◄

**Fig. G41** a–h. Bilateral mucoceles in a 50-year-old patient. Axial CT projections demonstrate soft tissue lesions in the ethmoid cells bilaterally with bone destruction at both medial walls of the orbits. Soft tissue lesion in the left orbit adjacent to the eyeball. A smaller soft tissue lesion is demonstrated in the upper medial section of the right orbit (**c**). Coronary projection: bilateral opacities in the ethmoid cells with destruction of the medial walls of both orbits. Anterior and caudal displacement of the left eyeball by a large soft tissue lesion. Demonstration of another soft tissue mass in the cranial medial section of the right orbit (**h**, arrow)

# 4. Malformations and Posttraumatic Lesions

## Aplasia of the Sphenoid Bone

Aplasia of the sphenoid bone is often found in neurofibromatosis (Fig. G44; cf. Fig. E25, p. 397). The lesion may occur in combination with hydrophthalmus or microphthalmus.

## Buphthalmus

This lesion is associated with congenital glaucoma. Increased intraocular pressure results in di-

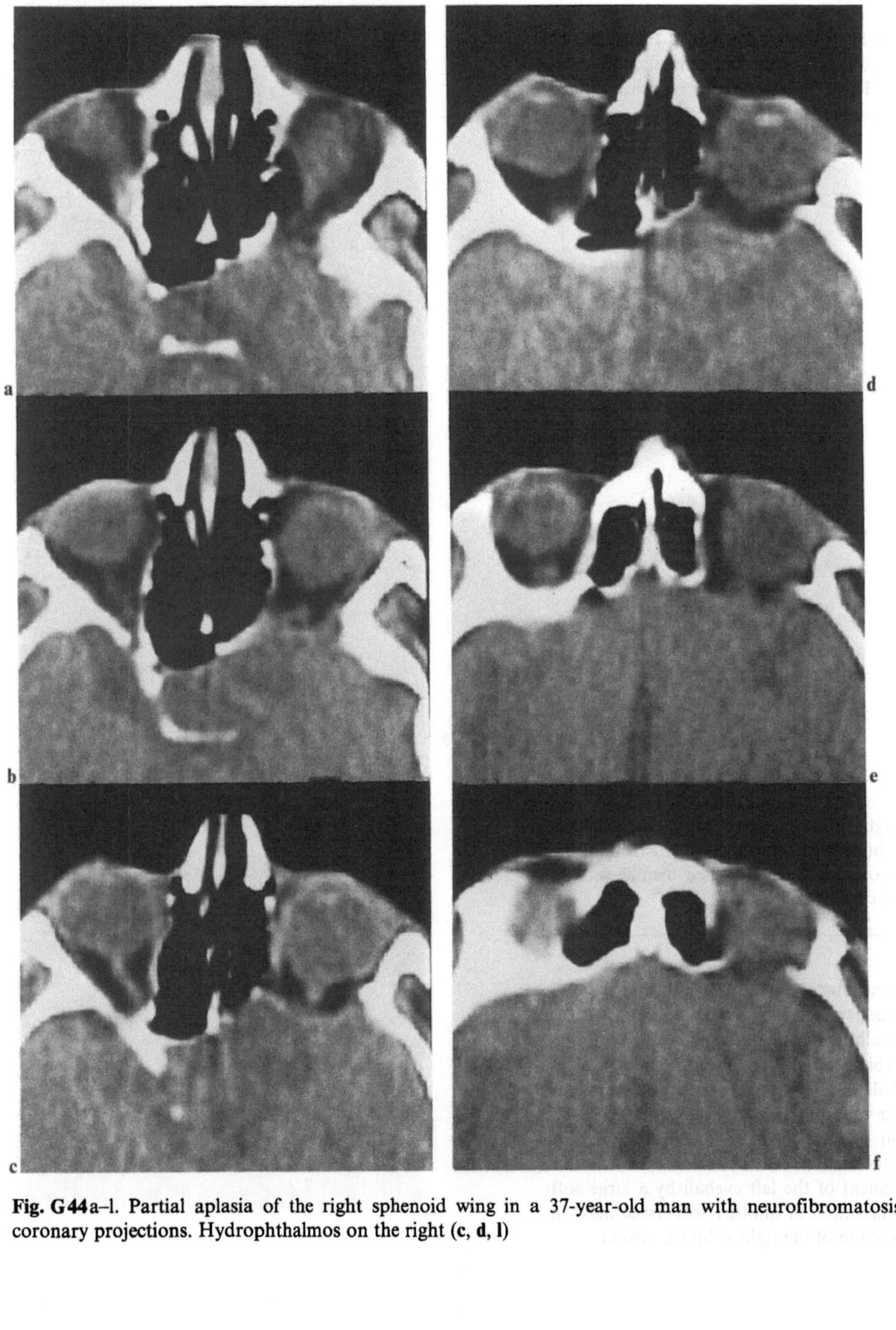


**Fig. G44a–l.** Partial aplasia of the right sphenoid wing in a 37-year-old man with neurofibromatosis. Horizontal and coronary projections. Hydrophthalmos on the right (**c, d, l**)

latation of the eyeball (Fig. G45) and of the cornea, which may attain a diameter exceeding 12 mm.

## Arteriovenous Angiomas and Other Vascular Malformations

Unlike cavernous hemangiomas, these malformations present with irregular structures, indistinct borders, and zones of mixed density in the CT scan. Contrast enhancement is positive in all cases. Irregular calcification has been observed (Fig. G46).

The inhomogeneous density and irregular borders of the arteriovenous malformation permit differentiation from cavernous hemangiomas, which are usually clearly demarcated (MOMOSE et al. 1975). However, CT studies may be entirely normal despite the presence of signifi-

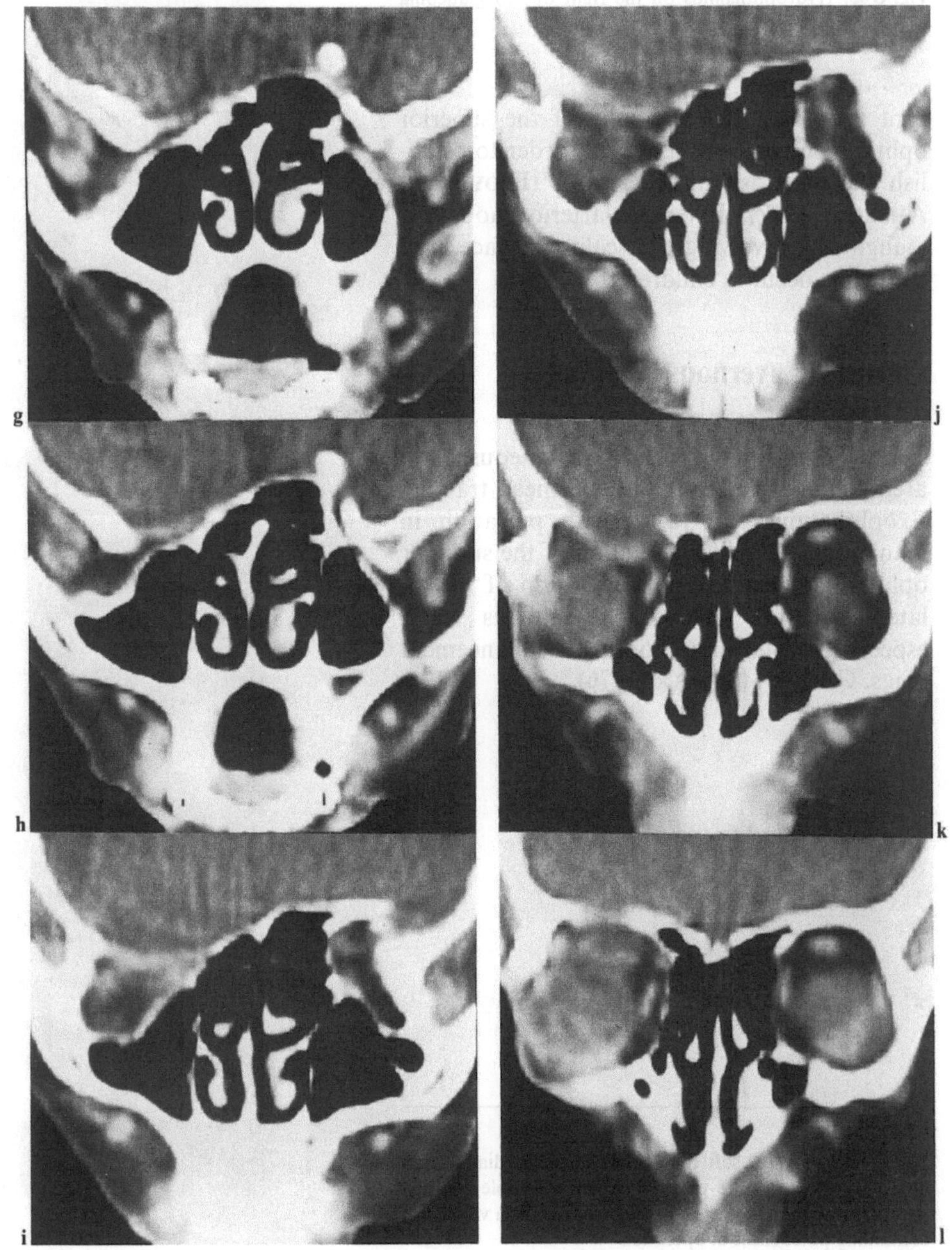

Fig. G44g–l

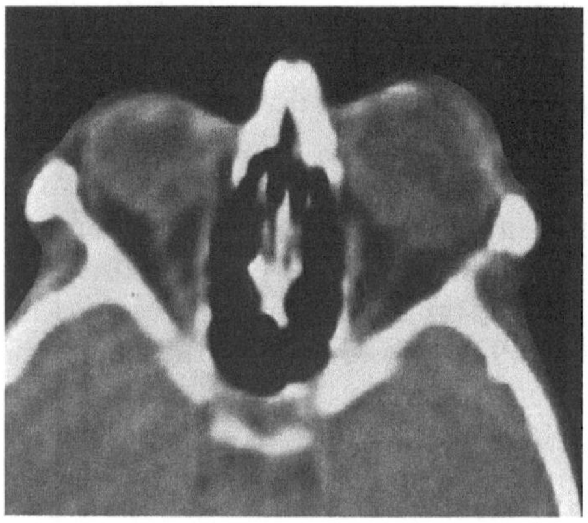

**Fig. G45.** Hydrophthalmos on the right due to glaucoma in a 70-year-old female

cant proptosis. Phlebography of the superior ophthalmic vein is necessary in order to establish the diagnosis in these cases (LLOYD and AMBROSE 1977). Extensive arteriovenous hemangiomas involving the scalp, the face, and the orbits occur in children (Fig. G47).

## Carotid-Cavernous Fistulas

These lesions rarely develop spontaneously and are much more often sequelae of head trauma. Exophthalmus is evident, with pulsation in many cases as well as dilatation of the superior ophthalmic vein. CT demonstration of the dilated superior ophthalmic vein is easy, especially following contrast enhancement (Figs. G48, 49) (SANDERS 1976).

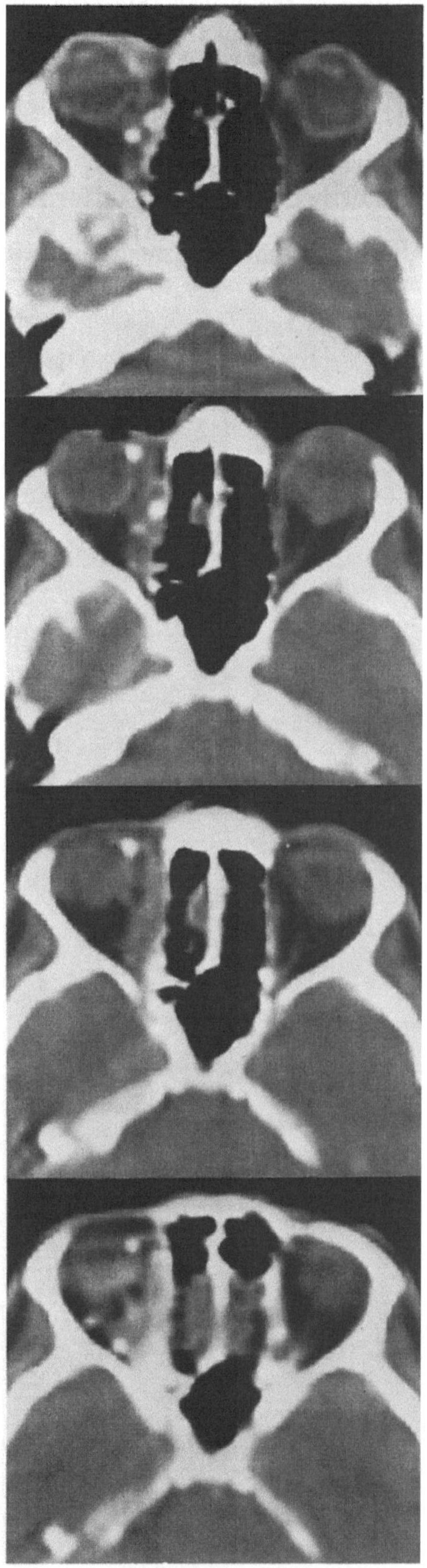

▶ **Fig. G46.** Elongated soft tissue mass in the medial section of the left orbit in an 18-year-old patient. Multiple calcified specks throughout the lesion which proved to be a varicocele containing phleboliths at operation

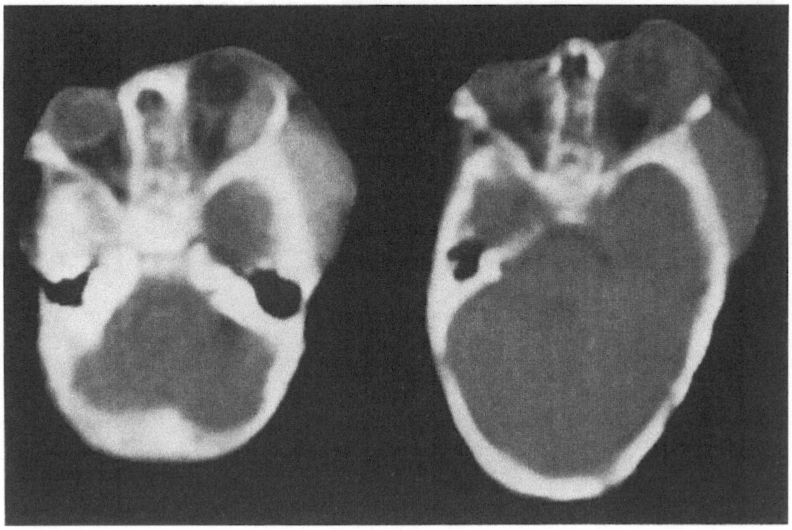

**Fig. G47.** Arteriovenous hemangioma in the scalp, the right upper eyelid, and the right orbit in a 7-month-old infant. Contrast enhancement (left) produces hyperdense values within the soft tissue lesion in the right temporal fossa, the lateral section of the right orbit, and in the right upper eyelid

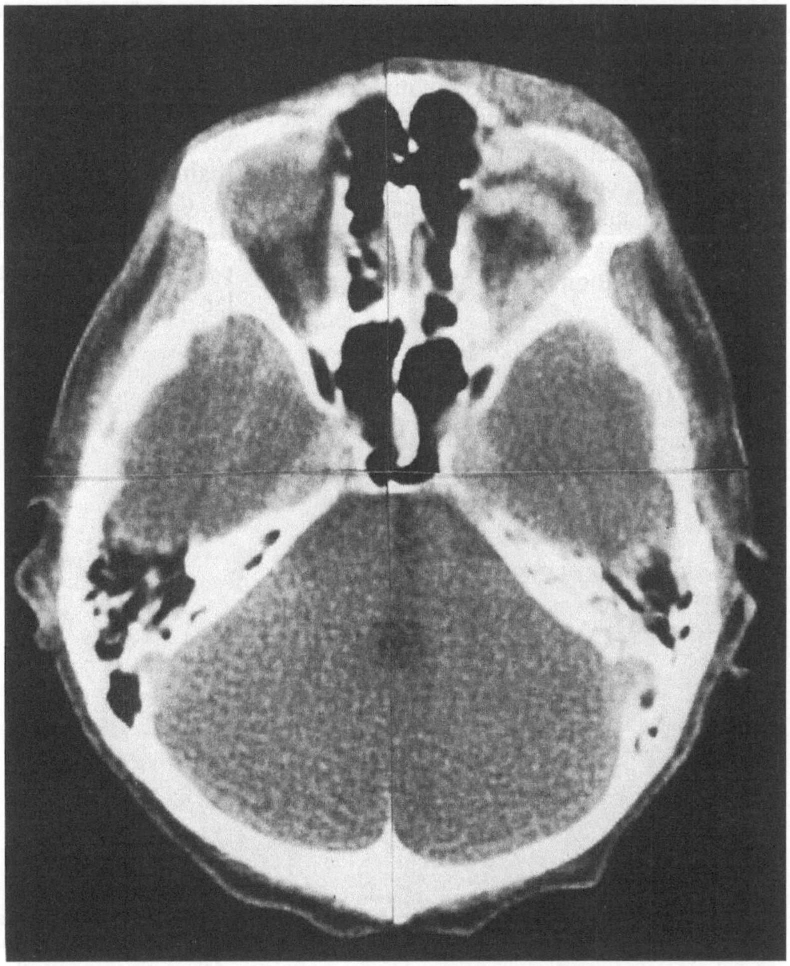

**Fig. G48.** Posttraumatic carotid-cavernous fistula on the right in a 56-year-old male. Characteristic dilatation and tortuous course of the superior ophthalmic vein within the right orbit. Postcontrast study

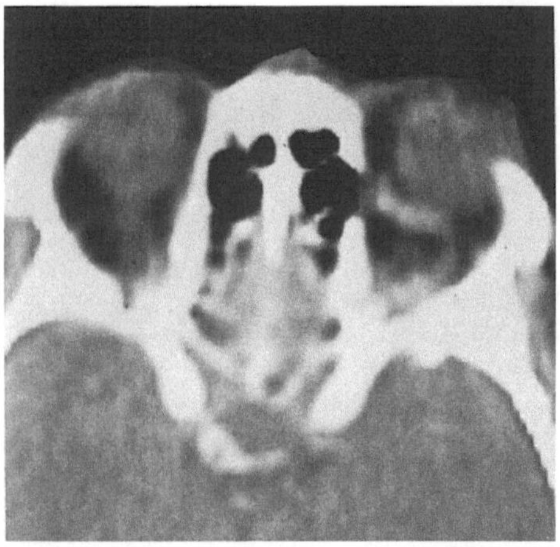

**Fig. G49.** Posttraumatic carotid-cavernous fistula on the right in a 25-year-old patient with extreme dilatation of the superior ophthalmic vein. Postcontrast study

# 5. Endocrine Ophthalmopathy (Graves' Disease)

Proptosis is unilateral in 10–20% of cases. Microscopic studies of orbital tissues demonstrate the presence of lymphocytes, granulocytes, and mast cells as well as destruction of muscle fibers and increased concentration of mucopolysaccharides. The extraocular muscles show increased water content and lipid inclusions, while fibrosis and degeneration are common findings in later stages. Exophthalmus is progressive and luxation of the eyeball a possibility.

### Computed Tomography

Spindle-shaped distension of one or more extraocular muscles results in a variety of findings. A single muscle may appear abnormal in the CT scan, while the others demonstrate normal form. This may lead to an incorrect diagnosis of meningioma. However, in most cases one finds symmetrical and homogeneous thickening of the muscles with increased density values (Figs. G50, 51; Bergström 1975; Brismar et al. 1976; Enzmann et al. 1976). CT scans often demonstrate bilateral involvement of the extraocular muscles even when exophthalmus is limited to one eye.

Changes in the extraocular muscles reflect the stage of clinical disease. The effect of therapy is demonstrable as regression of the muscular distension (Fig. G51).

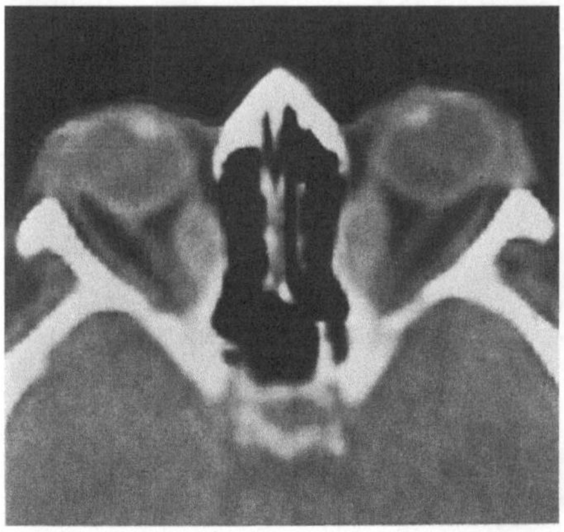

**Fig. G50.** Endocrine ophthalmopathy (Graves' disease) involving both medial rectus muscles in a 40-year-old female. Significant convergence of the optic axes; note the position of the lenses

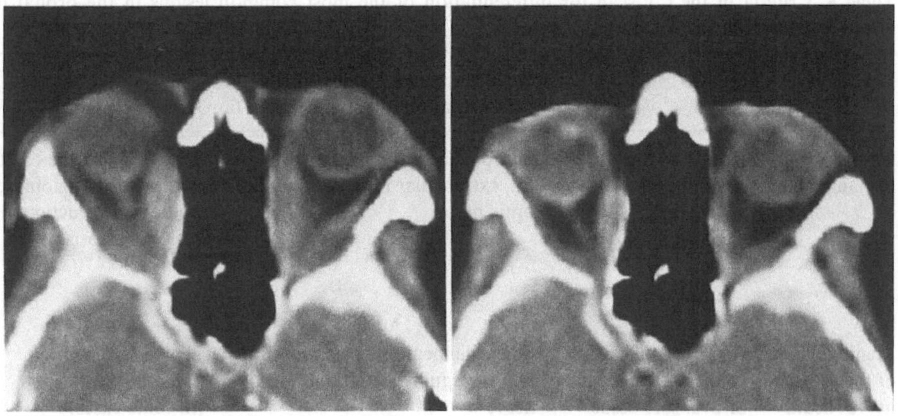

**Fig. G51.** Endocrine ophthalmopathy (Graves' disease) involving all ocular muscles in a 45-year-old female. Serial studies before (left) and after therapy (right). Significant reduction in swelling of the ocular muscles

## Discussion

CT demonstration of orbital neoplasms is possible in most cases, since the tumors have higher density than the surrounding fatty tissue, except in cases of dermoids and lipomas. The normal orbit is an ideal background for demonstration of a space-occupying lesion with computed tomography.

AMBROSE, LLOYD, and WRIGHT (1974, 1975) performed comparative studies with computed tomography, diagnostic ultrasound, carotid angiography, and venography as well as conventional tomographic studies and found that computed tomography resulted in correct diagnosis in 84% of cases, phlebography of the superior ophthalmic vein in 89%, diagnostic ultrasound in 82%, and conventional tomographic studies in 71% of cases. MOSELEY and BULL (1975) emphasized the high accuracy of computed tomography in diagnosis of orbital lesions. LLOYD and AMBROSE (1977) compared the diagnostic accuracy of computed tomography with that achieved with other techniques (diagnostic ultrasound, phlebography of the superior ophthalmic vein, and tomographic studies) in 75 cases of autochthonous orbital tumors. Diagnosis was correct in 91% of cases with computed tomography and with phlebography, followed by diagnostic ultrasound with 86% and conventional tomography with 73%. GYLDENSTEDT et al. (1977) confirmed CT diagnoses in 98% of histologically verified tumors, as compared to 82% with diagnostic ultrasound. MAIER-HAUFF and WILSKE (1976) emphasized the superiority of diagnostic ultrasound over computed tomography in prediction of the histological diagnosis of orbital tumors.

Our experience suggests that *both computed tomography and diagnostic ultrasound should be employed in cases of suspected orbital tumor* since this combination provides the greatest possible accuracy in both localization and diagnosis of histological type. Computed tomography alone is not capable of establishing a histological diagnosis in most cases (WACKENHEIM et al. 1977; MORTELMANS et al. 1978). Naturally, tumors such as cavernous hemangiomas with characteristic appearance in the CT scan are easily differentiated from optic nerve gliomas. Differentiation between meningioma and cavernous hemangioma is also possible in most cases, since the latter usually does not extend into the muscle cone. However, as a general rule, it is not even possible to distinguish between malignant and benign orbital tumors in the absence of bone destruction (WENDE et al. 1977; UNSÖLD, HOYT and NEWTON 1979). Postcontrast CT studies rarely provide additional information, since both malignant and benign tumors take up contrast media to a similar degree (WENDE et al. 1977). Table 8 summarizes the most important criteria in the differential diagnosis of common orbital lesions.

Phlebography of the superior ophthalmic vein is indicated for differentiation between a

**Table 8.** Criteria in the CT scan for differentiation of the most common lesions in the orbital muscle cone (modified after UNSÖLD et al., 1979)

| Lesion | Shape | Delineation against the optic nerve, extraocular muscles, and orbital fat | Changes in bone structures | Apex of the orbit |
|---|---|---|---|---|
| Cavernous hemangioma | Round or oval soft-tissue mass | Sharp delineation against orbital fat, extraocular muscles, and the optic nerve | Distension of the orbit in large hemangiomas; no bone destruction or hyperostosis | A small triangular space in the apex remains unaffected even in large hemangiomas |
| Meningioma of the optic nerve sheath | Apparent thickening of the optic nerve or oval soft-tissue mass | Sharp delineation against orbital fat; contiguous with the optic nerve | Hyperostosis of adjacent bones (in some cases) | Filled in most cases |
| Optic nerve glioma | Lens-shaped soft-tissue mass along the optic nerve | Sharp delineation against orbital fat; distension of the optic nerve | Dilatation of the optic nerve canal in most cases | Reaches the apex in many cases |
| Neurinoma | Cone-shaped soft-tissue mass which fills the apex | Well delineated against orbital fat with soft-tissue mass surrounding the optic nerve | Usually none | Filled |
| Metastasis | Irregular soft-tissue mass in most cases; spherical tumor rare | Diffuse growth in the orbital fat; tendency to affect extraocular muscles and optic nerve; sharp delineation in rare cases | Bone destruction common; hyperostosis in osteoplastic metastases | Often filled |
| Malignant lymphoma (Immuno-cytoma) | Irregularly shaped soft-tissue mass in most cases | Contiguous with the eyeball in many cases; well-delineated against orbital fat; extraocular muscles and optic nerve often enclosed in the soft-tissue mass | Usually none | Obliteration of the orbital apex possible |
| Pseudo-tumor | Irregular soft-tissue mass in most cases | Well-defined against the orbital fat; extraocular muscles and optic nerve often enclosed in the soft-tissue mass; distension of the extraocular muscles common | Hyperostosis of adjacent bone possible in chronic pseudotumors | Obliteration of the orbital apex possible |
| Endocrine exophthalmus | Spherical or irregular tissue mass in the muscle cone | Sharp delineation against orbital fat; distension of the extra-ocular muscles clearly visible in most cases | None | Usually obliterated by distended extra-ocular muscles |

neoplasm and an inflammatory lesion, since the latter usually results in compression of the superior ophthalmic vein in the region of the muscle cone. The veins are generally not displaced in these cases (LLOYD and AMBROSE 1975; BRISMAR et al. 1976; PEETERS 1977; PEETERS et al. 1977; WENDE et al. 1977).

# H. Effect of Computed Tomography on Diagnosis of Neurological Disease

Computed tomography is generally considered to be the most reliable and, indeed, the definitive diagnostic technique for demonstration of brain tumors. Approximately 98% of intracranial lesions are detected with CT. However, extremely high sensitivity is not the only advantage of CT in diagnosis of intracranial tumors. Accuracy in determining histological type, visualization of anatomical relations to important brain structures, knowledge of the growth pattern, and evidence of space-occupying effects of the tumor are at least as important for the neurosurgeon. In effect, CT studies allow definition of the entire complex "intracranial space-occupying process" by means of a single procedure in many cases.

The value of computed tomography has been demonstrated in the previous chapters where the role and capabilities of other *neuroradiological techniques* have also been discussed. In the following remarks the individual neuroradiological techniques will be summarized and their role in the diagnosis of neurological disorders in the era of computed tomography will be defined.

**Nuclear medicine** has been relegated to a secondary position in the diagnosis of brain tumors since the introduction of computed tomography as a screening method. If an intracranial tumor is suspected, computed tomography is the procedure of choice, as comparative studies have shown (BÜLL et al. 1978a). Other noninvasive techniques such as serial cerebral scintigraphy and probably axial emission computed tomography are *unnecessary for the detection of brain tumor*.

However, serial brain scans have retained their place as *supplementary procedures in determination of histological type* in the diagnostic approach to brain tumor (BÜLL et al. 1978b). Radionuclide angiography provides data on brain perfusion and localized changes secondary to brain tumor. NIENDORF et al. (1977) demonstrated that combined use of serial brain scintigraphy and computed tomography produced a higher degree of accuracy in prediction of histological type, especially in meningioma and glioblastoma, than was possible with either method alone. It is likely that dynamic computed tomography with rapid scanning systems will provide the same degree of diagnostic accuracy as radionuclide angiography in type-specific diagnosis.

Cerebral serial scintigraphy is certainly justified as an initial procedure in cases of uncharacteristic complaints such as headache or dizziness. *Cerebrovascular disorders* are the proper domain of nuclear medicine, since these disorders are better evaluated in serial brain scans than with computed tomography, especially in cases of asymptomatic stenosis, transitory ischemic attack (TIA), and prolonged intermittent neurological deficit (PRIND). **Doppler sonography** offers a high degree of accuracy in the diagnosis of extracranial stenosis or occlusion of the carotid artery and is a useful complement to these procedures (GROSS et al. 1977).

What is the role of **cerebral angiography** today? It is obvious that angiographic studies are necessary before surgical intervention, even with definitive CT findings, except in a few situations such as posttraumatic intracranial hematoma, typical intracerebral hemorrhage secondary to hypertension, and cerebellar tumors in children. Angiography alone is capable of exact preoperative demonstration of the vascular relations of a tumor. Of course, *cerebral angiography is only slightly less accurate than computed tomography in demonstration of brain tumors* (BAKER et al. 1980); an experienced neuroradiologist achieves almost the same degree of diagnostic accuracy with angiographic studies as with computed tomography. However, angiography has a number of drawbacks (KRETZSCHMAR et al. 1978). Multiplicity of brain metastases may be overlooked, and small metastases may fail to appear completely in angiographic studies. In addition, cerebral angiography is an invasive procedure which may involve serious complications, even in the hands of the experienced neuroradiologist.

Cerebral angiography is very useful in most

cases of brain tumor demonstrated by computed tomography, but *angiography is indispensable for the exact evaluation of cerebrovascular lesions.* Computed tomography is capable of demonstrating the final stage of vascular occlusion – brain infarction – but the technique does not reveal discrete vascular irregularities due to arteriosclerosis. Small vascular occlusions may also escape detection in CT scans when adequate collateral circulation has developed. Angiography is the procedure of choice in diagnosis of aneurysms and arteriovenous malformations.

In cases of *subarachnoid hemorrhage* computed tomography should be the initial procedure in order to determine the location and extent of hemorrhage. Subsequent angiographic studies are absolutely necessary in order to demonstrate the aneurysm and its vascular relations.

Whether four-vessel angiography should be performed in such cases or whether the procedure should be limited to the vessels involved in the hemorrhage is still a matter of controversy, since multiple aneurysms are present in approximately 8–20% of patients with subarachnoid hemorrhage. The decisive question is whether neurosurgical occlusion of an aneurysmal sack should be carried out in an asymptomatic case.

*Sequelae of craniocerebral injury, inflammatory brain diseases, malformations, degenerative diseases, and brain atrophy are demonstrable with computed tomography, and additional neuroradiological studies are rarely necessary.* The same is true of pathological processes in the *orbits,* where supplementary studies with carotid arteriography and phlebography of the superior ophthalmic vein are necessary only in rare cases.

*Tumors at the cerebellopontine angle* were previously inaccessible to CT diagnosis if they were very small and did not extend beyond the internal auditory canal. The combination of computed tomography and air cisternography is currently the procedure of choice in these cases (SORTLAND 1978). Use of positive contrast media is no longer necessary; the same is true of angiographic studies in most cases.

**Pneumoencephalography** has lost most of its significance in neuroradiology since the introduction of computed tomography. The procedure is rarely performed today and is used in very rare cases for delineation of small suprasellar and intrasellar tumors. The newest CT systems with high spatial resolution and capabilities for multiplanar reformation will probably make air encephalography obsolete even in these cases.

**Table 9.** Order of diagnostic studies in neurological and neurosurgical disease

| Diagnosis | Procedure(s) allowing definitive diagnosis |
|---|---|
| Brain atrophy | CT |
| Brain infarction and hemorrhage | CT; angiography in preparation for surgical therapy |
| Vascular malformations | CT and angiography |
| Degenerative and inflammatory vascular disease | CT and angiography |
| Inflammatory disease (with space-occupying effects) | CT |
| Degenerative brain disease | CT |
| Malformations of the brain | CT |
| Craniocerebral injury and sequelae | CT, angiography only in cases of carotid-cavernous fistula and other vascular lesions |
| Brain tumors | CT and angiography in most cases |
| Tumors at the cerebello-pontine angle | Combination of CT and gas cisternography |
| Orbital lesions | CT, ultrasonography; orbital venography in certain cases |

**Ventriculography** is still used in some institutions for localization of tumors in the posterior fossa. Our experience has shown that the procedure offers no significant advantage over computed tomography, since the ventriculogram does not allow more accurate delineation and differentiation of a tumor than does CT. On the contrary, CT studies are clearly superior in predicting the histological type of a lesion. In this connection, it should be mentioned that *coronary slices and multiplanar reformation have widened the lead of computed tomography over pneumoencephalography and ventriculography.* In addition, it should be emphasized that the latter procedures are invasive methods which entail discomfort and a certain degree of risk for the patient (WENDE et al. 1982).

With the exception of radioisotope studies, which have been discussed in detail above, *indications for diagnostic procedures* in neurological disease are summarized in Table 9.

# References

## A. Introduction


Ambrose J (1974) Computerized x-ray scanning of the brain. J Neurosurg 40:679–695

Berger H (1929) Über das Elektrenkephalogramm des Menschen. Arch Psychiatr Nervenkr 87:527–570

Dandy WE (1918) Ventriculography following the injection of air into the cerebral ventricles. Ann Surg 68:5–11

Dandy WE (1919) Roentgenography of brain after injection of air into spinal canal. Ann Surg 70:397–403

Di Chiro G, Brooks RA (1979) The 1979 nobel prize in physiology or medicine. Science 206:1060–1062

Hounsfield GN (1973) Computerized transverse axial scanning (tomography): Part I. Description of system. Br J Radiol 46:1016–1022

Hounsfield GN (1976) Historical notes on computerized axial tomography. J Can Assoc Radiol 27:135–142

Leksell L (1955/56) Echo-encephalography. I. Detection of intracranial complications following head injury. Acta Chir Scand 110:301–315

Moniz E (1927) L'encephalographie artèrielle, son importance dans la localisation des tumeurs cérébrales. Rev Neurol 32:72

Moore GE (1948) Radioactive localization of brain tumors. J Am Med Assoc 137:1228–1229

Selverstone B, Solomon AK (1948) Radioactive isotopes in the study of intracranial tumors. Trans Am Neurol Assoc 73:115–119


## B. Classification of brain tumors


Ackerman LV, Rosai J (1974) Surgical pathology, 5th edn. Mosby St Louis, pp 1248–1249

Andres KH (1967) Über die Feinstruktur der Arachnoidea und Dura mater von Mammalia. Z Zellforsch 79:272–295

Bailey P (1932) Cellular types in primary tumors of the brain. In: Penfield W (ed) Cytology and cellular pathology of the nervous system, vol III. Hafner Publ Co, New York, pp 905–951

Bailey P, Bucy PC (1929) Oligodendrogliomas of the brain. J Path Bact 32:735–751

Bailey P, Cushing H (1926) A classification of the tumors of the glioma group on a histogenetic base with a correlated study of prognosis. Lippincott, Philadelphia

Bailey P, Cushing H (1930) Gewebsverschiedenheit der Hirngliome. Fischer, Jena

Bailey P, Hiller G (1924) The interstitial tissues of the central nervous system. J Nerv Ment Dis 59:337–361

Bergstrand H (1932) Über das sogenannte Astrocytom des Kleinhirns. Virchows Arch 287:538–548

Broders AC (1926) Carcinoma: grading and practical application. Arch Path 2:376–380

Bruns L (1914) Klinik der Hirngeschwülste. In: Krause F (Hrsg) Die allgemeine Chirurgie der Gehirnkrankheiten Bd II (Neue deutsche Chirurgie, Band 12). Enke, Stuttgart, S 19–104

Bunge RP, Bunge MB, Ris H (1962) Electron microscopic observations on normal, demyelinating, and remyelinating white matter. Proc IV. Internat Congr Neuropath Bd II. Thieme, Stuttgart, S 136–142

Cooper ERA (1935) The relation of oligocytes and astrocytes in cerebral tumours. J Path Bact 41:259–266

Earle K (1980) Persönl Mitteilung

Eder M (1977) Pathologie des Wachstums und der Differenzierung. In: Eder M, Gedigk P (Hrsg) Lehrbuch der allgemeinen Pathologie und der pathologischen Anatomie, 30. Aufl. Springer, Berlin Heidelberg New York, S 240

Fleischhauer K (1972) Ependyma and subependymal layer. In: Bourne GH (ed) The structure and function of nervous tissue, vol VI. Academic Press, New York London, pp 1–46

Friede RL (1978) Gliofibroma: a peculiar neoplasia of collagen forming glia-like cells. J Neuropathol Exp Neurol 37:300–313

Friede RL, Pollak A (1978) The cytogenic basis for classifying ependymomas. J Neuropathol Exp Neurol 37:103–118

Golgi C (1894) Untersuchungen über den feineren Bau des centralen und peripheren Nervensystems. Fischer, Jena

Henschen F (1934) Referat über Gliome. Verh Dtsch Pathol Ges 27. Tagg. Fischer, Jena, S 8–39

Henschen F (1955) Tumoren des Zentralnervensystems und seiner Hüllen. In: Scholz W (Hrsg) Handb spez path Anat Bd XIII/3. Springer, Berlin Göttingen Heidelberg, S 413–1040

Hofer H (1965) Die circumventrikulären Organe des Zwischenhirns. In: Hofer H, Schultz AH, Starck D (Hrsg) Handb Primat Bd II, Lief 13. Karger, Basel New York

Hortega P del Rio: (1921) La glia de escasas radiaciones (oligodendroglia). Arch Neurobiol (Madr) 2: Nr 1

Jellinger K (1977) Geschwülste des Nervensystems und seiner Anhänge. In: Holzner JH (Hrsg) Spezielle Pathologie II, 2. Aufl. Urban & Schwarzenberg, Berlin Wien Baltimore, S 217

Jellinger K, Radaszkiewicz Th (1976) Involvement of the central nervous system in malignant lymphomas. Virchows Arch A [Path Anat] 370:345–362

Kaufmann E (1922) Lehrbuch der speziellen pathologischen Anatomie. 7. und 8. Aufl Bd II. de Gruyter, Berlin Leipzig, S 1488ff

Kepes JJ (1979) "Xanthomatous" lesions of the central nervous system: definition, classification and some recent observations. In: Zimmerman HM (ed) Progress in Neuropathology, vol 4. Raven Press, New York, pp 197–213

Kepes JJ, Rubinstein LJ, Eng LF (1979) Pleomorphic xanthoastrocytoma: a distinctive meningocerebral glioma of

young subjects with relatively favorable prognosis. Cancer 44:1839–1852
Kernohan JW, Mabon RF, Svien HJ, Adson AW (1949) A simplified classification of the gliomas. Proc Staff Meet Mayo Clin 24:71–75
Kleihues P, Schultze B (1968) Zellproliferation und Protein-Synthese der Neuroglia beim experimentellen Hirnödem. Acta Neuropathol (Berl) Suppl IV:121–124
Koelliker A (1896) Handbuch der Gewebelehre des Menschen. 6. Aufl, Bd II. Engelmann, Leipzig
Kuhlendahl H, Stochdorph O (1968) Über das Vorkommen des sog. Kleinhirnastrocytoms (Bergstrand-Tumor) im Großhirn. Beitr Neurochir, H 15. Barth, Leipzig
Lenhossék Mv (1895) Der feinere Bau des Nervensystems im Lichte neuester Forschungen. Fischer, Berlin
Leonhardt H (1980) Ependym und circumventriculäre Organe. In: Oksche A (Hrsg) Handb mikr Anat Bd 4/10. Springer, Berlin Heidelberg New York, S 177–666
Lhermitte J, Duclos P (1920) Sur un ganglioneurome diffus du cortex du cervelet. Bull Assoc Franc Etude Cancer 9:99–106
Merrem G (1962) Die klinisch-biologische Wertigkeit der Hirngeschwülste. Sitzber Sächs Akad Wissensch Leipzig, Math-Nat Wiss Kl 105:H 2. Akademie-Verl, Berlin
Niessing K (1980) Materialquelle, Entwicklung und Differenzierung der Neuroglia. In: Oksche A (Hrsg) Handb mikr Anat Bd 4/10. Springer, Berlin Heidelberg New York, S 54–113
Penfield W (1932) Neuroglia: normal and pathological. In: Penfield W (ed) Cytology and cellular pathology of the nervous system, Vol II. Hafner Publ Co, New York, pp 423–479
Priesel A (1922) Über Gewebsmißbildungen in der Neurohypophyse und dem Infundibulum des Menschen. Virchows Arch 238:423–440
Ramón y Cajal S (1913) Contribución al conocimiento de la neuroglia del cerebro humano. Trab Lab Invest Biol Madrid 11:255–315
Ribbert H (1904) Geschwulstlehre für Ärzte und Studierende. Cohen, Berlin
Rindfleisch E (1878) Lehrbuch der pathologischen Gewebelehre, 5. Aufl. Engelmann, Leipzig
Ringertz N (1950) Grading of gliomas. Acta Path Scand 27:51–64
Ringertz N, Nordenstam H (1951) Cerebellar astrocytomas. J Neuropathol Exp Neurol 10:343–367
Rubinstein LJ (1972) Tumors of the central nervous system. (Atlas of tumor pathology, 2nd ser, fasc 6.) Armed Forces Institute of Pathology, Washington DC
Russell DS, Rubinstein LJ (1977) Pathology of tumours of the nervous system. 4th ed. Arnold, London
Scheithauer BW, Rubinstein LJ (1978) Meningeal mesenchymal chondrosarcoma. Cancer 42:2744–2752
Scherer HJ (1936) Etude sur les gliomes. Comportement des différents gliomes vis-à-vis des cellules ganglionnaires. Bull Assoc Franc Cancer 25:470–493
Schmincke A (1930) Zur Kenntnis der Zirbelgeschwülste. Ein Ganglioglioneurom der Zirbel. Beitr Pathol Anat 83:279–288
Sternberg C (1921) Ein Choristom der Neurohypophyse bei ausgebreiteten Ödemen. Zentralbl Pathol 31:585–591
Stroebe H (1895) Über Entstehung und Bau der Gehirngliome. Beitr Pathol Anat 18:405–486
Tumor-Histologie-Schlüssel (ICD-o-DA) (1978) Jacob W, Scheida D, Wingert F (Hrsg). Springer, Berlin Heidelberg New York
Virchow R (1862) Die Cellularpathologie in ihrer Begründung auf physiologische und pathologische Gewebelehre. Hirschwald, Berlin
Virchow R (1864–65) Die krankhaften Geschwülste, Bd I–III. Hirschwald, Berlin
Weindl A, Fahlbusch R, Stochdorph O (1975) Ultrastruktur eines Tumors der Lamina terminalis. Zentralbl Pathol 119:227
Willis RA (1948) Pathology of tumours. Butterworth & Co, London
Wolff JR (1980) Zit n Oksche A, Anmerkungen zum histologischen Überblick. In: Oksche A (Hrsg) Handb mikr Anat Bd 4/10. Springer, Berlin Heidelberg New York, S 141–144
Zülch KJ (1956) Biologie und Pathologie der Hirngeschwülste. In: Olivecrona H, Tönnis W (Hrsg) Handb Neurochir, Bd III. Springer, Berlin Göttingen Heidelberg, S 1–702
Zülch KJ (1979) Histological typing of tumours of the central nervous system (Internat Histol Classific of Tumours. No 21). World Health Organisation, Geneva

## C. Technique of CT examination

### C1 General surveys, atlantes, monographs

Baert A, Jeanmart L, Wackenheim A (ed) (1978) Clinical computer tomography. Springer, Berlin Heidelberg New York
Caillé JM, Salamon G (1980) Computerized tomography. Springer, Berlin Heidelberg New York
Davis JM, Davis KR, Newhouse J, Pfister RC (1979) Expanded high iodine dose in computed cranial tomography: a preliminary report. Radiology 131:373–380
Du Boulay GH, Moseley IF (ed) (1977) Computerised axial tomography in clinical practice. Springer, Berlin Heidelberg New York
Gerhardt P, Kaick G van (ed) (1979) Total body computerized tomography. Georg Thieme, Stuttgart
Gonzales CF, Grossmann CB, Palacios E (1976) Computed brain and orbital tomography. Techniques and interpretation. John Wiley & Sons, New York London Sidney Toronto
Harwood-Nash DC, Fitz CR (1976) Neuroradiology in infants and children. The CV Mosby Comp, Saint Louis
Jabbour JT, Ramey DR, Roach St (1977) Atlas of computerized tomography scans in pediatric neurology. Med Examination Publ, Huber, Bern Stuttgart Wien
Kazner E, Lanksch W, Steinhoff H, Wilske J (1975) Die axiale Computer-Tomographie des Gehirnschädels: Anwendungsmöglichkeiten und klinische Ergebnisse. Fortschr Neurol Psychiatr 43:487–574
Krayenbühl H, Yasargil MG, Huber P (1979) Zerebrale Angiographie für Klinik und Praxis. 3. Aufl. Georg Thieme, Stuttgart
Lange S, Grumme Th, Meese W (1977) Zerebrale Computer-Tomographie. Schering-AG, Berlin
Lanksch W, Kazner E (ed) (1976) Cranial computerized tomography. Springer, Berlin Heidelberg New York
Ledley RS, Huang HK, Mazziotta JC (1977) Cross-sectional anatomy – An atlas for computerized tomography. Williams & Wilkins Comp, Baltimore

Lindgren E (ed) (1975) Computer tomography of brain lesions. Acta Radiol [Suppl] (Stockh) 346
New PFJ, Scott WR (1975) Computed tomography of the brain and orbit (EMI-Scanning). Williams and Wilkins, Baltimore
Norman D, Korobkin M, Newton ThH (eds) (1977) Computed tomography 1977. The CV Mosby Comp, St Louis
Oldendorf WH (1980) The quest for an image of brain. Computerized tomography in the perspective of past and future imaging methods. Raven Press, New York
Oliva L (ed) (1976) The new image in tomography. Excerpta Medica, Amsterdam Oxford
Quisling RG (1980) Correlative neuroradiology. A topographic approach to cerebral angiographic and CT interpretation. John Wiley & Sons, New York, Chichester Brisbane
Radü EW, Kendall BE, Moseley IF (1980) Computertomographie des Kopfes. Technische Grundlagen – Interpretation – Klinik. Thieme Verlag, Stuttgart New York
Ramsey RG (1977) Advances exercises in diagnostic radiology. Saunders Comp, Philadelphia
Ramsey RG (1978) Computertomographie des Gehirns. In: Squire LF (Hrsg) Übungen in radiologischer Diagnostik Bd VII. Georg Thieme, Stuttgart
Ruggiero G, Sabattini L, Scialfa G (1979) Tomografia computerizzata del cervello. Il Pensiero Scientifico, Ed, Roma
Sager W-D, Ladurner G (Hrsg) (1979) Computertomographie. Derzeitige Stellung in Radiologie und Klinik. Georg Thieme, Stuttgart
Salamon G, Huang YP (1980) Computed tomography of the brain. Springer, Berlin Heidelberg New York
Schiefer W, Kazner E (1967) Klinische Echo-Encephalographie. Springer, Berlin Heidelberg New York
Wackenheim A, Babin E (1978) Tomodensitométrie craniocérébrale. Masson, Paris
Wackenheim A, DuBoulay GH (1980) Choices and characteristics in computerized tomography. Kugler Publication, Amsterdam
Weisberg LA, Katz M, Nice Ch (1978) Cerebral computed tomography. A text-atlas. WB Saunders Co, Philadelphia/USA
Zülch KJ (1956) Die Hirngeschwülste in biologischer und morphologischer Darstellung. Ambrosius Barth, Leipzig

**C2 and 3 Technique of examination; CT evaluation**

Aita JF (1977) Computerized tomography of the head-part III. Nebr Med J 62:415–422
Ambrose J (1973) Computerized transverse axial scanning (tomography): Part 2. Clinical application. Br J Radiol 46:1023–1047
Ambrose J (1974) Computerized X ray scanning of the brain. J Neurosurg 40:679–695
Ambrose J (1974) The EMI scanner: clinical use. Br J Hosp Med 11:14–21
Boroff RD, Pribram HFW (1978) Coronal and sagittal reconstruction in computerized tomography. Surg Neurol 9:85–93
Cabanis EA (1974) La tomographie axiale transverse avec ordinateur (EMI-Scanner): Une ere neuroradiologique nouvelle. Ann Oculist 207:413–429
Du Boulay GH, Radu EW (1978) How should one investigate the posterior fossa? Neuroradiology 15:253–261
Gado MH, Eichling J, Currie M (1977) Quantitative aspects of CT images. In: Norman D, Korobkin M, Newton ThH (eds) Computed tomography 1977. The CV Mosby Comp, St Louis
Hounsfield GN (1980) Computed medical imaging. Nobel Lecture, Dec 8, 1979. J Comp Assist Tomogr 4:655–674
Huck W (1978) The combined use of horizontal and frontal CT-scanning in intracranial lesions. Surg Rev 1:133–138
Isherwood I, Pullan BR, Ritchings RT (1978) Radiation dose in neuroradiological procedures. Neuroradiology 16:477–481
Just HW, Goldenberg M (1979) Computed tomography of the enlarged cisterna magna. Radiology 131:385–391
Kazner E, Lanksch W (1977) Computertomographische Strukturanalyse pathologischer Prozesse im Schädelinnenraum. Festschr Klinikum Großhadern. II. Teilinbetriebnahme 1977. Demeter, Gräfelfing
Lanksch W, Oettinger W, Baethmann A (1977) Diagnosis of brain edema using CT. Excerpta Medica. CT-Symposium 10. Sept. 1976 Amsterdam, pp 13–25
Latchaw RE, Payne JR, Gold LHA (1978) Effective atomic number and electron density as measured with a computed tomography scanner: computation and correlation with brain tumor histology. J Comput Assist Tomogr 2:199–208
Latchaw RE, Payne JTh, Loewenson RB (1980) Predicting brain tumor histology: Change of effective atomic number with contrast enhancement. AJNR 1: 289–294
McCullough EC, Payne Th (1978) Patient dosage in computed tomography. Radiology 129:457–463
Meyer JS, Hayman LA, Yamamoto M, Sakai F, Nakajima S (1980) Local cerebral blood flow measured by CT after stable xenon inhalation. AJNR 1:213–225
Naidich TP, Kricheff II, Leeds NE (1977) Computerized tomography of the tentorium cerebelli. In: du Boulay GH, Moseley IF (eds) Computerised axial tomography in clinical practice. Springer, Berlin Heidelberg New York, pp 29–35
Ommaya AK (1973) Computerized axial tomography of the head: the EMI scanner, a new device for direct examination of the brain "in vivo". Surg Neurol 1:217–222
Peeters FLM (1977) Einige Beispiele falsch negativer Diagnosen bei der Computer-Tomographie. Radiologe 17:171–176
Perry BJ, Bridges C (1973) Computerized transverse axial scanning (tomography): Part 3. Radiation dose considerations. Br J Radiol 46:1048–1051
Sachs Ch, Ericson K, Erasmie U, Bergström M (1979) Incidence of basal ganglia calcifications on computed tomography. J Comput Assist Tomogr 3:339–344
Schöter I, Wappenschmidt J (1978) Difficulties in the interpretation of computerized tomography. Adv Neurosurg 6:131–136
Shrivastava PN, Lynn SL, Ting JY (1977) Exposures to patient and personnel in computed axial tomography. Radiology 125:411–415
Steinhoff H, Lange S (1976) Principles of contrast enhancement in computerized tomography. In: Lanksch W, Kazner E (eds) Cranial computerized tomography. Springer, Berlin Heidelberg New York, pp 60–68
Wall BF, Green DAS (1979) The radiation dose to patients from EMI brain and body scanners. Br J Radiol 52:189–196
Wende S, Ludwig B, Simon RS, Kretzschmar K (1980) Hy-

perdensity factors. In: Caille JM, Salamon G (eds) Computerized tomography. Springer, Berlin Heidelberg New York, pp 146–151

Wing SD, Aderson RE, Osborn AG (1980) Dynamic cranial computed tomography: preliminary results. AJNR 1:135–139

Wing SD, Osborn AG (1977) Normal and pathologic anatomy of the corpus callosum by computed tomography. J Comput Assist Tomogr 1:183–192

Wing SD, Osborn AG, Wing RW (1978) The vertex scan: an important component of cranial computed tomography. Am J Roentgenol 130:765–767

Zimmerman RA, Bilaniuk LT, Gallo E (1978) Computed tomography of the trapped fourth ventricle. Am J Roentgenol 130:503–506

Zülch KJ, Wende S (1977) The actual state of computerized tomography (CT) – computer assisted tomography (CAT). J Neurol 215:233–240

**C 4 Intravenous contrast application**

Balsys R, Janousek JE, Batnitzky S, Templeton AW (1979) Peripheral enhancement in computerized cranial tomography: a non-specific finding. Surg Neurol 11:207–216

Bergvall U (1975) Temporal course of contrast medium enhancement in differential diagnosis of intracranial lesions with computer tomography. In: Salamon G (ed) Advances in cerebral angiography. Springer, Berlin Heidelberg New York, pp 348–388

Gado MH, Phelps ME, Coleman RE (1975) An extravascular component of contrast enhancement in cranial computed tomography. Part I: The tissue blood ratio of contrast enhancement. Radiology 117:589–593

Gado MH, Phelps ME, Coleman RH (1975) An extravascular component of contrast enhancement in cranial computed tomography. Part II: Contrast enhancement and the blood tissue barrier. Radiology 117:595–597

Hayman LA, Evans RA, Hinck VC (1980) Delayed high iodine dose contrast computed tomography. Cranial neoplasms. Radiology 136:677–684

Huckman MS (1975) Clinical experience with the intravenous infusion of iodinated contrast material as an adjunct to computed tomography. Surg Neurol 4:297–318

Kirkpatrick JB (1978) The blood-brain barrier: Its role in contrast studies. Comput Tomogr 2:189–196

Lewander R, Bergström M, Bergvall U (1978) Contrast enhancement of cranial lesions in computed tomography. Acta Radiol Diagn 19:529–552

**Hazards of intravenous contrast application**

Ahmed M, Doe RP, Nuttall FQ (1974) Triiodothyronine thyrotoxicosis following iodide ingestion. A case report. J Clin Endocrinol 38:574

Alexander RD, Berkes StL, Abuelo JG (1978) Contrast media-induced oliguric renal failure Arch Intern Med 138:381

Ansari Z, Baldwin DS (1976) Acute renal failure due to radiocontrast agents. Nephron 17:28–40

Baltzer G (1978) Akutes Nierenversagen nach intravenöser Urographie bei Diabetikern – ein erhöhtes Risiko? Internist (Berlin) 19:649–651

Barshay ME, Kaye JH, Goldman R, Coburn JW (1973) Acute renal failure in diabetic patients after intravenous infusion pyelography. Clin Nephrol 1:35

Berdon WE, Schwartz RH, Becker J, Baker DH (1969) Tamm-Horsfall proteinuria. Radiology 92:714–722

Berezin AF (1977) Acute renal failure, diabetes mellitus, and scanning. Ann Intern Med 86:829–830

Bergman LA, Wilson MR, Dunea G (1968) Acute renal failure after drip-infusion pyelography. N Engl J Med 279:1277

Blum M, Weinberg U, Shenkman L, Hollander CS (1974) Hyperthyroidism after iodinated contrast medium. N Engl J Med 291/1:24–25

Carvallo A, Rakowski TA, Argy WP Jr, Schreiner GE (1978) Acute renal failure following drip infusion pyelography. Am J Med 65:38

Davis JM, Davis KR, Newhouse J, Pfister RC (1979) Expanded high jodine dose in computed cranial tomography: A preliminary report. Radiology 131:373–380

Dean RE, Andrew JH, Read RC (1964) The red cell factor in renal damage from angiographic media. J Am Med Ass 187:27–31

Diaz-Buxo JA, Wagoner RD, Hattery RR, Palumbo PJ (1975) Acute renal failure after excretory urography in diabetic patients. Ann Intern Med 83:155–158

Doust BD, Redman HC (1972) The myth of 1 ml/kg in angiography. Radiology 104:557–560

Dudzinski PJ, Petrone AF, Persoff M, Callaghan EE (1971) Acute renal failure following high-dose excretory urography in dehydrated patients. J Urol 106:619–621

Elke M, Ferstl A (1974) Notfallsituationen in der Röntgendiagnostik. Thieme, Stuttgart

Ethier R, Sherwin A, Taylor S (1974) Computerized angiotomography. The use of 100 cc Hypaque M 60%. Clinical and experimental results. Presented at the first International Symposium on Computerized Axial Tomography, Montreal (1974)

Gleysteen JJ, Aldrete JS, Rutsky EA (1976) Cholegraphy-induced acute renal failure: Its relation to subsequent surgical therapy. South Med J 69:173–176

Grainger RG (1979) Formulation and clinical introduction of low osmolality contrast media. 3. Asian-Oceanian Congress of Radiology, Singapore, 28. Oct. – 3. Nov 1979

Hanaway J, Black J (1977) Renal failure following contrast injection for computerized tomography. J Am Med Assoc 238:2056

Hayman LA, Evans RA, Fahr LM, Hinck VG (1980) Renal consequences of rapid high dose contrast CT. AJNR 1:9–11

Hayman LA, Evans RA, Hinck VC (1979) Rapid high dose (RHD) contrast computed tomography of perisellar vessels. Radiology 131:121–123

Herrmann J, Krüskemper HL (1978) Gefährdung von Patienten mit latenter und manifester Hyperthyreose durch jodhaltige Röntgenkontrastmittel und Medikamente. Dtsch Med Wochenschr 103:1434–1443

Kamdar A, Weidmann P, Makoff DL, Massry SG (1977) Acute renal failure following intravenous use of radiographic contrast dyes in patients with diabetes mellitus. Diabetes 26:643–649

Kleinknecht D, Deloux J, Homberg JC (1974) Acute renal failure after intravenous urography: Detection of antibodies against contrast media. Clin Nephrol 2:116–119

Kramer RA, Janetos GP, Perlstein G (1975) An approach to contrast enhancement in computed tomography of the brain. Radiology 116:641–647

Krumlovsky FA, Simon N, Subramanyam S, Greco F del, Roxe D, Pomaranc MM (1978) Acute renal failure. Association with administration of radiographic contrast material. J Am Med Ass 239:125–127

Maurer HJ (1980) Risiken bei Kontrastmitteluntersuchungen. Dtsch Ärztebl 77:1555–1564

Meeker TC (1978) Computerized axial tomography and acute renal failure. J Am Med Ass 240:2247–2248

Morgan C, Hammack WJ (1966) Intravenous urography in multiple myeloma. N Engl J Med 275:77–79

Myers GH Jr, Witten DM (1971) Acute renal failure after excretory urography in multiple myeloma. Am J Roentgenol 113:583–588

Norman D, Enzmann DR, Newton ThH (1978) Comparative efficacy of contrast agents in computed tomography scanning of the brain. J Comput Assist Tomogr 2:319–321

Norman D, Korobkin M, Newton ThH (ed) (1977) Computed tomography 1977. Mosby Company, St Louis/Missouri

Paling MR (1979) Contrast dose for enhancement of computed tomograms of the brain. Br J Radiol 52:620–623

Pierach CA (1979) Transitorische Urämie durch Kontrastmittel – ein Risikofaktor bei niereninsuffizienten Diabetikern. Dtsch Med Wochenschr 104:148–149

Pillay VKG, Robbins PC, Schwartz FD, Kark RM (1970) Acute renal failure following intravenous urography in patients with longstanding diabetes mellitus and azotemia. Radiology 95:633–636

Port FK, Wagoner RD, Fulton RE (1974) Acute renal failure after angiography. Am J Roentgenol 121:544–550

Robinson JS, Arzola DD, Moody RA (1980) Acute renal failure following cerebral angiography and infusion computerized tomography. Case report. J Neurosurg 52:111–112

Savoie JC, Massin JP, Thomopoulos P, Leger F (1975) Iodine-induced thyrotoxicosis in apparently normal thyroid glands. J Clin Endocrinol 41:685

Schmidt RC (1980) Mental disorders after myelography with metrizamide and other water-soluble contrast media. Neuroradiology 19:153–157

Schwartz WB, Hurwitt A, Ettinger A (1963) Intravenous urography in the patient with renal insufficiency. New Engl J Med 269:277–283

Scott WR (1980) Seizures: A reaction to contrast media for computed tomography of the brain. Radiology 137:359–361

Shafi T, Chou SY, Porush JG, Shapiro WB (1978) Infusion intravenous pyelography and renal function. Effects in patients with chronic renal insufficiency. Arch Intern Med 138:1218–1221

Swartz RD, Rubin JE, Leeming BW, Silva P (1978) Renal failure following major angiography. Am J Med 65:31

Talner LB, Davidson AJ (1968) Renal hemodynamic effect of contrast media. Invest Radiol 3:310–317

Talner LB (1972) Urographic contrast media in uremia. Radiol Clin North Am 10(3):421–432

Van Zee B, Hoy WE, Talley TE, Jaenike JR (1978) Renal injury associated with intravenous pyelography in nondiabetic and diabetic patients. Ann Intern Med 89:51–54

Wagoner RD (1978) Acute renal failure associated with contrast agents. Arch Intern Med 138:353

Warren SE, Bott JC, Thornfeldt C, Swerdlin AH, Steinberg SM (1978) Hazards of computerized tomography: Renal failure following contrast injection. Surg Neurol 10:335–336

Weinrauch LA, Healy RW, Leland OS Jr, Goldstein HH, Kassissieh SD, Libertino JA, Takacs FJ, Elia JA de (1977) Coronary angiography and acute renal failure in diabetic azotemic nephropathy. Ann Intern Med 86:56–59

Weinrauch LA, Healy RW, Leland OSt, Goldstein HH, Libertino JA, Rakacs FJ, Bradley RF, Gleason RE, Elia JA de (1978) Decreased insulin requirement in acute renal failure in diabetic nephropathy. Arch Intern Med 138:399–402

## C5 Intrathecal contrast application

Bockenheimer S (1980) Vorteile und Risiken der Meatozisternographie mit wäßrigem Kontrastmittel. Laryngol Rinol Otol 59:786–789

Drayer BP, Rosenbaum AE, Higman HB (1977) Cerebrospinal fluid imaging using serial metrizamide. CT cisternography. Neuroradiology 13:7–17

Glanz S, Geehr RB, Duncan ChC, Piepmeier JM (1980) Metrizamide-enhanced CT for evaluation of brainstem tumors. AJNR 1:31–34

Greitz T, Hindmarsh T (1974) Computer assisted tomography of intracranial CSF circulation using a watersoluble contrast medium. Acta Radiol 15:497–507

Hammer B (1980) Experiences with intrathecally enhanced computed tomography. Neuroradiology 19:221–228

Hindmarsh T (1975) Elimination of water-soluble contrast media from the subarachnoid space. Investigation with computer tomograph. Acta Radiol 346:45–49

Hindmarsh T (1977) Computer cisternography for evaluation of CSF flow dynamics. Acta Radiol 355:269–279

Jacobs L, Kinkel W (1976) Computerized axial transverse tomography in normal pressure hydrocephalus. Neurology (Minneap) 26:501–507

Manelfe C, Chambers EF (1981) Computed tomographic cisternography with watersoluble contrast media: Normal and pathologic appearance. In: Contrast Media in Computed Tomography. Ed. by Felix R, Kazner E and Wegener OH, Excerpta Medica, 147–156

Manelfe C, Guiraud B, Espagno J, Rascol A (1978) Cisternographie computérisée au metrizamide. Rev Neurol 134:471–484

Pinto RS, Handel StF, Sadhu VK (1979) CT metrizamide cisternography in the recognition of intrasellar cistern. Am J Roentgenol 133:320–321

Rosenbaum AE, Drayer BP (1977) CT cisternography with metrizamide. Acta Radiol [Suppl] (Stockh) 355:323–337

Sackett JF, Strother CM (1977) Computer tomography and subarachnoid metrizamide for evaluation of cerebrospinal fluid flow. Acta Radiol [Suppl] (Stockh) 355:338–344

Schmidt RC (1980) Mental disorders after myelography with metrizamide and other water-soluble contrast media. Neuroradiology 19:153–157

Sprung Ch, Grumme Th (1979) Use of CT cisternography, RISA cisternography and the infusion test for predicting shunting results in normal pressure hydrocephalus (NPH). Adv Neurosurg 7:350–360

Steele JR, Hoffmann JC (1980) Brainstem evaluation with CT cisternography. AJNR 1:521–526

Zito JL, Davis KR, Hesselink JR (1980) Low-dose metrizamide cisternography with pluridirectional tomography: A useful adjunct to computed tomographic cisternography. Surg Neurol 14:169–174

## D. Intracranial tumors, general

Allen JH (1977) Computerized tomography for diagnosis of brain neoplasms. J Tenn Med Assoc 70:18–20

Ambrose J (1973) Computerized transverse axial scanning of the brain. Proc R Soc Med 66:833–834

Ambrose J (1974) Computerized x-ray scanning of the brain. J Neurosurg 40:679–695

Amundsen P, Dugstad G, Syvertsen AH (1978) The reliability of computer tomography for the diagnosis and differential diagnosis of meningiomas, gliomas, and brain metastases. Acta Neurochir (Wien) 41:177–190

Ascherl GF Jr, Hilal SK, Brisman R (1981) Computed tomography of disseminated meningeal and ependymal malignant neoplasms. Neurology 31:567–575

Assmann H, Schäfer W, Schumann E, Stahl M, Schneider A (1977) The complex radiological diagnosis of brain tumours. Arch Geschwulstforsch 47:369–373

Aulich A, Wende S, Meese W, Meinig G, Reulen HJ (1976) Follow-up studies in cerebral tumors using CT. In: Lanksch W, Kazner E (eds) Cranial computerized tomography. Springer, Berlin Heidelberg New York, pp 135–142

Baker HL Jr, Houser OW (1976) Computed tomography in the diagnosis of posterior fossa lesions. Radiol Clin North Am 14:129–147

Baker HL Jr, Houser OW, Campbell JK (1980) National cancer institute study: Evaluation of computed tomography in the diagnosis of intracranial neoplasms. Radiology 136:91–96

Baker HL Jr, Thomas JE (1975) Computierte transaxiale Tomographie des Kopfes (EMI-Scan). Klinische Erfahrung mit einer neuen diagnostischen Methode zur Hirnuntersuchung. Fortschr Röntgenstr 123:293–299

Banna M, Molot MJ, Kapur PL, Groves J (1975) Computer tomography of the brain in Hamilton. Can Med Assoc J 113:303–307

Becker H, Bittenbring G (1977) Computer-Tomographie und klassische Neuroradiologie bei Problemfällen. Nervenarzt 48:663–669

Becker H, Schäfer M, Klös G (1976) Localization of recurrent brain tumors by means of computerized tomography. In: Lanksch W, Kazner E (eds) Cranial computerized tomography. Springer, Berlin Heidelberg New York, pp 143–150

Berger PE, Kirks DR, Gilday DL, Fitz ChR, Harwood-Nash DC (1976) Computed tomography in infants and children: intracranial neoplasms. Am J Roentgenol 127:129–137

Besenski N, Gvozdanovic V, Nutrizio V, Simunic S, Jelicic J, Lupret V (1978) Comparative study of computed tomography and ventriculography with water soluble contrast media. Neuroradiology 16:540–542

Bilaniuk LT, Zimmerman RA, Littman P, Gallo E, Rorke LB, Bruce DA, Schut L (1980) Computed tomography of brain stem gliomas in children. Radiology 134:89–95

Boltshauser E, Hamalatha H, Grant DN, Till K (1977) Impact of computerised axial tomography on the management of posterior fossa tumours in childhood. J Neurol Neurosurg Psychiat 40:209–213

Brismar J, Stromblad L-G, Salford LG (1978) Impact of CT in the neurosurgical management of intracranial tumors. Neuroradiology 16:506–509

Brooks RA, Di Chiro G (1976) Principles of computer assisted tomography (C.A.T.) in radiographic and radioisotopic imaging. Phys Med Biol 21:689–732

Büll U (1981) The role of nuclear procedures in the diagnosis of intracranial disease. Neurosurg Rev 4:105–122

Büll U, Niendorf HP, Steinhoff H, Kazner E (1976) Validity of serial scintigraphy with $^{99m}$ Tc-pertechnetate in comparison with computerized tomography in brain tumors. In: Lanksch W, Kazner E (eds) Cranial computerized tomography. Springer, Berlin Heidelberg New York, pp 177–182

Buncher CR (1980) National cancer institute study: Evaluation of computed tomography in the diagnosis of intracranial neoplasms. II. Was randomization necessary? Radiology 136:651–655

Clar H-E, Bock WJ, Grote W, Nau HE, Weichert HC (1979) Klassifikation der Tumoren der Sellaregion mit Hilfe der Computertomographie (CT) und der Enzephalographie. Neurochirurgia (Stuttg) 22:153–159

Clar H-E, Bock WJ, Weichert HC (1979) Comparison of encephalotomograms and computerized tomograms in midline tumours in infants. Acta Neurochir (Wien) 50:91–101

Collard M, Dupont H (1975) Tomographie axiale transverse computérisée par Emi-Scanner. Résultat de 1000 observations. J Belge Radiol 58:289–328

Collard M, Dupont H (1977) L'apport clinique de la tomodensitometrie cerebrale (EMI-Scanner). Etude critique de 3000 dossiers. Acta Neurol Belg 77:230–242

Cushing H (1935) Intracranielle Tumoren. Springer, Berlin

Davis DO (1977) CT in the diagnosis of supratentorial tumors. Semin Roentgenol 12:97–108

Davis DO, Pressman BD (1974) Computerized tomography of the brain. Radiol Clin North Am XII:297–313

Delavelle J, Megret M (1980) CT sagittal reconstruction of posterior fossa tumors. Neuroradiology 19:81–88

Dohrmann GJ, Geehr RB, Robinson F, Allen WE III, Orphanoudakis SC (1978) Small hemorrhages vs calcifications in brain tumors: difficulty in differentiation by computed tomography. Surg Neurol 10:309–312

Dosch JC, Wackenheim A (1978) Density of intracranial masses in computer tomography. J Belge Radiol 61:291–296

Du Boulay GH, Marshall J (1975) Comparison of E.M.I. and radioisotope imaging in neurological disease. Lancet 2:1294–1297

Du Boulay GH, Teather D, Harling D, Clarke G (1977) Improvement in the computer-assisted diagnosis of cerebral tumors. Br J Radiol 50:849–854

El Gammal T, McDaniel FE (1979) The target sign: a CT finding in tumors of the corpus callosum. J Comput Assist Tomogr 3:533–535

Elke M, Wiggli U, Huenig R (1977) Praktische Gesichtspunkte zur Diagnose intracranieller Tumoren durch die Computer-Tomographie (CT). Radiologe 17:157–170

Enzmann DR, Krikorian J, Yorke C, Hayward R (1978) Computed tomography in leptomeningeal spread of tumor. J Comput Assist Tomogr 2:448–455

Fahlbusch R, Grumme Th, Aulich A, Wende S, Steinhoff H, Lanksch W, Kazner E (1976) Suprasellar tumors in the CT scan. In: Lanksch W, Kazner E (eds) Cranial

computerized tomography. Springer, Berlin Heidelberg New York, pp 114–127
Fischgold H (1977) La tomographie axiale transverse (CT) de la tête en Allemagne Fédérale. J Radiol Électrol 58:620, 640, 646
Fitz CR, Harwood-Nash DC, Resjo IM (1978) Metrizamide ventriculography and computed tomography in infants and children. Neuroradiology 16:6–9
Foerster O, Gagel O (1939) Das umschriebene Arachnoidalsarkom des Kleinhirns. Z Ges Neurol Psychiat 164:565–580
Gado M, Huete I, Mikhael M (1977) Computerized tomography of infratentorial tumors. Semin Roentgenol 12:109–120
Gardeur D, Metzger J (1978) Tomodensitometrie (C.T. Scanner) en pathologie tumorale intra-cranienne. Doin Editeurs, Paris
Gardeur D, Sablayrolles JL, Klausz R, Metzger J (1977) Histographic studies in computed tomography of contrast-enhancement cerebral and orbital tumors. J Comput Assist Tomogr 1:231–240
Gawler J (1976) Computerized tomography and conventional radiology in the investigation of intracranial and orbital disease. J Belge Radiol 59:225–238
Gawler J, Du Boulay GH, Bull JWD, Marshall J (1974) Computer assisted tomography (EMI scanner). Its place in investigation of suspected intracranial tumours. Lancet II:419–423
Gawler J, Du Boulay GH, Bull JWD, Marschall J (1976) A comparison of computer assisted tomography (EMI scanner) with conventional neuroradiologic methods in the investigation of patients clinically suspected of intracranial tumor. J Can Assoc Radiol 27:157–169
Gawler J, Du Boulay GH, Bull JWD, Marshall J (1976) Computerized tomography (the EMI scanner): a comparison with pneumoencephalography and ventriculography. J Neurol Neurosurg Psychiatr 39:203–211
Gonzales CF, Grossman CB, Placios E (1976) Computed brain and orbital tomography. John Wiley & Sons, New York London Sidney Toronto
Greitz T (1975) Computer tomography for diagnosis of intracranial tumours compared with other neuroradiologic procedures. Acta Radiol (Stockh) 346:14–20
Grumme Th, Aulich A, Kazner E, Kretzschmar K, Lanksch W, Meese W (1978) Typical findings with computerized tomography in tumors of the posterior fossa. Adv Neurosurg 5:159–165
Grumme Th, Kretzschmar K, Ebhardt G, Lanksch W, Lange S (1978) Intracerebral space-occupying lesions with brain density (isodense lesions). Adv Neurosurg 6:75–79
Grumme Th, Meese W, Lange S (1976) Die axiale Computer-Tomographie des Schädels (CT Scan) in der Neuropädiatrie. Monatsschr Kinderheilkd 124:751–762
Grumme Th, Meese W, Lange S (1976) Kraniale Computertomographie (EMI-Scan). Wert und Einsatzmöglichkeit. Dtsch Med Wochenschr 20:765–769
Grumme Th, Steinhoff H, Wende S (1976) Diagnosis of supratentorial tumors with computerized tomography. In: Lanksch W, Kazner E (eds) Cranial computerized tomography. Springer, Berlin Heidelberg New York, pp 80–89
Hacker H, Steudel W, Becker H (1976) Control studies in brain tumors and early detection of tumors using CT. In: Lanksch W, Kazner E (eds) Cranial computerized tomography. Springer, Berlin Heidelberg New York, pp 133–134
Harwood-Nash DC (1975) Computed cranial tomography in children with intracranial neoplasms. In: Salamon G (ed) Advances in cerebral angiography. Springer, Berlin Heidelberg New York, pp 349–352
Harwood-Nash DC, Fitz CR, Reilly BJ (1975) Cranial computed tomography in infants and children. Can Med Assoc J 118:546–549
Hayman LA, Evans RA, Hinck VC (1980) Delayed high iodine dose contrast computed tomography. Cranial neoplasms. Radiology 136:677–684
Henderson SD (1979) Pathology in computed tomography of the brain. Charles C Thomas Publ, Springfield/Ill
Hilal SK, Chang DH (1978) Specificity of computed tomography in the diagnosis of supratentorial neoplasms. Consideration of metastases and meningiomas. Neuroradiology 16:537–539
Hilal SK, Chang DH (1978) Sensitivity and specifity of CT in supratentorial tumours. J Comput Assist Tomogr 2:511
Houser OW, Baker HL Jr, Campbell JK (1975) Recent advances in neuroradiology. Some aspects of computerized transaxial tomography of the head. Minn Med 58:122–128
Huckman MS, Fox JS, Ramsey RG, Penn RD (1976) Computed tomography in the diagnosis of pseudotumor cerebri. Radiology 119:593–597
Hyman RA, Loring MF, Liebeskind AL, Naidich JB, Stein HL (1978) Computed tomographic evaluation of therapeutically induced changes in primary and secondary brain tumors. Neuroradiology 14:213–218
Jänisch W, Güthert H, Schreiber D (1976) Pathologie der Tumoren des Zentralnervensystems. Gustav Fischer, Jena
Kazner E, Aulich A, Grumme Th (1975) Results of computerized axial tomography with infratentorial tumors. In: Lanksch W, Kazner E (eds) Cranial Computerized Tomography. Springer, Berlin Heidelberg New York, pp 90–103
Kazner E, Grumme T, Lanksch W, Wende S (1977) Computed tomography (CT) and the operative indications for brain tumors. A cooperative study of 3 university hospitals. Int. Congress Series 433 "Neurological Surgery". Excerpta Medica. Amsterdam Oxford, pp 28–36
Kazner E, Grumme Th, Lanksch W, Wilske J (1978) Limitations of computed tomography in the detection of posterior fossa lesions. Adv Neurosurg 5:166–170
Kazner E, Grumme Th, Steinhoff H, Aulich A (1977) Diagnosis of posterior fossa tumors in infants and children by means of axial computerized tomography (CT). J Neurosurg Sci 21:205–210
Kazner E, Grumme Th, Wende S (1979) Hirntumoren im Computertomogramm. Dtsch Ärztebl 76:1299–1312
Kazner E, Lanksch W, Steinhoff H (1976) Cranial computerized tomography in the diagnosis of brain disorders in infants and children. Neuropaediatrie 7:136–174
Kazner E, Lanksch W, Steinhoff H, Wilske J (1975) Die axiale Computer-Tomographie des Gehirnschädels – Anwendungsmöglichkeiten und klinische Ergebnisse. Fortschr Neurol Psychiatr 43:487–574
Kazner E, Meese W, Kretzschmar K (1978) The role of

computed tomography in the diagnosis of brain tumors in infants and children. Neuroradiology 16:10–12

Kazner E, Steinhoff H (1979) Aspect of rare intracranial tumors in the CT scan. In: Gerhardt P, Kaick G van (eds) Total body computerized tomography. Thieme, Stuttgart, pp 301–312

Kazner E, Steinhoff H, Wende S, Mauersberger W (1978) Ring-shaped lesions in the CT scan – differential diagnostic considerations. Adv Neurosurg 6:80–85

Kelly PJ, Alker GJ Jr (1981) A stereotactic approach to deep-seated central nervous system neoplasms using the carbon dioxide laser. Surg Neurol 15:331–334

Kendall BE, Jakubowski J, Pullicino F, Symon L (1979) Difficulties in diagnosis of supratentorial gliomas by CAT scan. J Neurol Neurosurg Psychiatry 42:485–492

Kernohan J, Sayre GP (1952) Tumors of the central nervous system. Atlas of tumor pathology. Sect. X, fasc 35 und 37. Armed Forces Inst Pathol, Washington

Kernohan J, Sayre GP (1956) Tumors of the pituitary gland and infundibulum. Atlas of tumor pathology. Sect. X, fasc 36. Armed Forces Inst Pathol, Washington

Ketonen L (1978) Computerized tomography for diagnosis of supratentorial tumors. Acta Neurol Scand 57:153–164

Kingsley DP, Kendall BE (1979) The CT scanner in posterior fossa tumours of childhood. Br J Radiol 52:769–776

Kobayashi N (1976) Brain tumor and EMI scan. Jpn J Clin Radiol 21:745–746

Krayenbühl H, Yasargil MG (1965) Die zerebrale Angiographie. Thieme, Stuttgart

Kretzschmar K, Aulich A, Schindler E, Lange S, Grumme Th, Meese W (1978) The diagnostic value of CT for radiotherapy of brain tumors. Neuroradiology 14:245–250

Kretzschmar K, Grumme Th, Steinhoff H (1978) Computer-Tomographie und Angiographie für die Diagnose supratentorieller Hirntumoren. Neuroradiology 16:487–490

Krishna Rao CVG, Kishore PRS, Bartlett J, Brennan TG (1980) Computed tomography in the postoperative patient. Neuroradiology 19:257–263

Lange S, Aulich A, Lanksch W (1976) Image artefacts in computerized tomography. In: Lanksch W, Kazner E (eds) Cranial computerized tomography. Springer, Heidelberg Berlin New York, pp 69–72

Lange S, Grumme Th, Meese W (1977) Zerebrale Computertomographie, Schering-AG Berlin

Lange S, Grumme Th, Meese W, Wüllenweber R, zum Winkel K (1976) Die axiale Computertomographie des Gehirns. Roentgenblaetter 29:211–221

Lange S, Steinhoff H, Aviles Ch, Kazner E, Grumme Th (1979) Kontrastmittelkinetik in zerebralen Tumoren. Fortschr Röntgenstr 130:666–669

Lanksch W (1981) Contrast enhancement in brain tumors. In: Contrast Media in Computed Tomography. Ed. by Felix R, Kazner E and Wegener OH, Excerpta Medica, 117–122

Lanksch W, Grumme Th, Kazner E (1978) Die Schädelhirnverletzungen im Computertomogramm. Springer, Berlin Heidelberg New York

Lanksch W, Kazner E (1976) CT findings in brain edema. In: Lanksch W, Kazner E (eds) Cranial computerized tomography. Springer, Berlin Heidelberg New York, pp 344–355

Lee KF, Lin SR (1979) Neuroradiology of sellar and juxtasellar lesions (1979) Ch C Thomas Publ, Springfield/Illinois

Leonardi M, Fabris G, Pencot T (1979) Localization of brain tumors by means of CT scan. J Neurosurg Sci 23:231–233

Lin SR, Crane MD, Lin ZS, Bilaniuk L, Plaschke WM Jr, Marshall L, Spataro RF (1978) Characteristics of calcification in tumors of the pineal gland. Radiology 126:721–726

Logue V (1977) Tumors above and below the tentorium. The radiological management of cerebral tumors. In: du Boulay GH, Moseley IF (eds) Computerised axial tomography in clinical practice. Springer, Berlin Heidelberg New York, pp 76–84

MacDonald AF, Carrill JM, Dendy PP, Keyes WI, Mallard JR (1978) Evaluation of X ray CT (EMI scan) and isotope brain studies, including radioisotope axial tomography. Neuroradiology 16:575

Mancs P, Babin E, Wackenheim A (1978) Contribution of histograms to the computer tomographic study of brain tumours. J Belge Radiol 6:297–312

Marks JE, Gado M (1977) Serial computed tomography of primary brain tumors following surgery, irradiation and chemotherapy. Radiology 125:119–125

Maroon JC, Bank WO, Drayer BP, Rosenbaum AE (1977) Intracranial biopsy by computerized tomography. J Neurosurg 46:740–744

Mass S, Norman D, Newton ThH (1978) Coronal computed tomography: Indications and accuracy. Am J Roentgenol 131:875–879

McAllister VL, Appleby A, Hall K (1978) Contribution of computed tomography to the diagnosis and management of posterior fossa masses. Xtract 3:2–14

McAllister VL, Hankinson J, Sengupta RP (1978) Problems in diagnosis with computerized tomography Adv Neurosurg 6:61–74

McGeachie RE, Gold LHA, Latchaw RE (1977) Periventricular spread of tumor demonstrated by computed tomography. Radiology 125:407–410

Meese W, Grumme Th, Lange S (1977) Die zerebrale axiale Computertomographie. Therapiewoche 27:2008–2019

Messina AV (1977) Cranial computerized tomography. A radiologic pathologic correlation. Arch Neurol 34:602–607

Messina AV, Potts DG, Rottenberg D, Patterson RH (1976) Computed tomography: demonstration of contrast medium within cystic tumors. Radiology 120:345–347

Metzger J, Gardeur D, Nachanakian A, Millard JC (1978) Comparaison des tomodensitométrie. Cinégammagraphie et angiographie dans diagnostics. Topographique et histologique pré-opératoires de 300 tumeurs intracraniennes sus-tentorielles. Neuroradiology 16:495–498

Michotey P, Moseley IF, Lecaque G, Palmieri P (1977) Tumours and other lesions of the visual pathways. The comparative values of various neuroradiological investigations in the diagnosis of intracranial optic pathway lesions. In: du Boulay GH, Moseley IF (eds) Computerised axial tomography in clinical practice. Springer, Berlin Heidelberg New York, pp 147–153

Mundinger F, Ostertag Ch (1976) Computerized tomography in stereotactic interstitial curie therapy of cerebral midline tumors. In: Lanksch W, Kazner E (eds) Cranial computerized tomography. Springer, Berlin Heidelberg New York, pp 110–113

Nadjmi M (1978) Vergleichende computertomographische und angiographische Befunde der Tumoren der hinteren Schädelgrube. Roentgenblaetter 31:210–220

Naidich TP, Lin JP, Leeds NE, Kricheff II, George AE, Chase NE, Pudlowski RM, Passalaqua A (1976) Computed tomography in the diagnosis of extraaxial posterior fossa masses. Radiology 120:333–339

Naidich TP, Lin JP, Leeds NE, Pudlowski RM, Naidich JB (1977) Primary tumors and other masses of the cerebellum and fourth ventricle: Differential diagnosis by computed tomography. Neuroradiology 14:153–174

New PFJ, Scott WR (1975) Computed tomography of the brain and orbit. EMI scanning. Williams and Wilkins, Baltimore, Maryland

New PFJ, Scott WR, Schnur JA, Davis KR, Taveras JM (1974) Computerized axial tomography with the EMI scanner. Radiology 110:109–123

New PFJ, Scott WR, Schnur JA, Davis KR, Taveras JM, Hochberg FH (1975) Computed tomography with the EMI scanner in the diagnosis of primary and metastatic intracranial neoplasms. Radiology 75–87

Norman D, Enzmann DR, Levin VA, Wilson ChB, Newton ThH (1976) Computed tomography in the evaluation of malignant glioma before and after therapy. Radiology 121:85–88

Obrador S (1977) Study of 100 patients with intracranial tumors using computed axial tomography. Zh Vorpr Neirokhir 4:3–12

Oi S (1977) Computerized axial tomography in the diagnosis of multiple brain tumors-correlation with angiography and nuclear scanning. Neurol Surg (Tokyo) 5:833–840

Olivecrona H (1967) The surgical treatment of intracranial tumors. In: Handbuch der Neurochirurgie, Bd IV, Teil 4. Springer, Berlin Heidelberg New York, S 1–301

Osborn AG, Heaston DK, Wing SD (1978) Diagnosis of ascending transtentorial herniation by cranial computed tomography. Am J Roentgenol 130:755–760

Osborn AG, Williams RG, Wing SD (1978) Low attenuation lesions in the midline posterior fossa: Differential diagnosis. J Comput Assist Tomogr 2:319–329

Papo I, Caruselli G, Menichelli F, Pasquini U, Salvolini U (1978) The reliability of computerized axial tomography in the diagnosis of infratentorial mass lesions; a neurosurgical appraisal. Acta Neurochir (Wien) 41:311–326

Paxton R, Ambrose J (1974) The EMI scanner: A brief review of the first 650 patients. Br J Radiol 47:530–565

Pay NT, Carella RJ, Lin JP, Kricheff II (1976) The usefulness of computed tomography during and after radiation therapy in patients with brain tumors. Radiology 121:79–83

Pertuiset B, Nachanakian A, Gardeur D, Yacoubi A, Ancri D, Metzger J, Kujas M (1979) Protocole d'exploration des tumeurs cérébrales sustentorielles. Neurochirurgie 25:11–18

Philippo J, Gardeur D, Nachanakian A, Metzger J (1979) Approche diagnostique pré-opératoire des tumeurs de la fosse postérieure de l'adulte. Neurochirugie 25:139–146

Piepgras U, Huber G, Emde H, Fuchs U (1978) Vergleich der Ergebnisse von Computertomographie und Isotopendiagnostik bei pathologischen Prozessen des infratentoriellen Bereiches. Roentgenpraxis 31:221–238

Probst FP, Liliequist B (1979) Assessment of posterior fossa tumors in infants and children by means of computed tomography. Neuroradiology 18:9–18

Pullicino P, Thomson EJ, Moseley IF, Zilkha E, Shortman RC (1979) Cystic intracranial tumours. Cyst fluid, biochemical changes and computerised tomographic findings. J Neurol Sci 44:77–85

Rappaport ZH, Epstein F (1978) Computerized axial tomography in the preoperative evaluation of posterior fossa tumors in children. Childs Brain 4:170–179

Roberson GH, Taveras JM, Tadmor R, Kleefield J, Ellis G (1977) Computed tomography in metrizamide cisternography – importance of coronal and axial views. J Comput Assist Tomogr 1:241–245

Rothe R, Fischer K (1976) Comparison between computerized tomography and conventional contrast-medium methods in the diagnosis of brain tumors. In: Lanksch M, Kazner E (eds) Cranial computerized tomography. Springer, Berlin Heidelberg New York, pp 183–187

Rubinstein LJ (1972) Tumors of the central nervous system. Atlas of tumor pathology. 2. ser fasc 6. Armed Forces Inst Pathol, Washington

Ruggiero G, Sabattini L, Nuzzo G (1977) Computerized tomography and encephalography. Neuroradiology 13:45–49

Russel DS, Rubinstein LJ (1971) Pathology of tumours of the nervous system. Arnold, London

Sartor K, Richert S (1979) Konventionell-radiographische und computerassistierte Zisternographie der hinteren Schädelgrube mit Metrizamid. Roentgenforschung 130:472–478

Schellinger D, Axelbaum StP, Di Chiro G (1976) An analysis of the first one thousand cerebral ACTA scans. Fortschr Röntgenstr 125:211–213

Shalen PR, Hayman A, Wallace S (1981) Protocol for delayed contrast enhancement in computed tomography of cerebral neoplasia. Radiology 139:397–402

Sheldon JJ, Maulsby G, Leborgne JM (1979) The differential diagnosis of supratentorial enhancing lesions on computed tomography. Rev Interam Radiol 4:109:113

Sorel L, Rucquoy Ponsar M, Harmant J (1978) Electroencephalogramme et tomographie assistée par calculateur dans 393 cas d'epilepsie. Etude des correspondances des localisations EEG et des localisations decouvertes par la tomographie assistée par calculateur. Acta Neurol Belg 78:242–252

Spiess H (1979) CT-Ergebnisse bei Affektionen des Chiasmas und der Sehbahn. Klin Monatsbl Augenheilkd 174:816–823

Sprung C, Grumme Th (1980) CT images of periventricular lucency (PVL) in various forms of hydrocephalus. Adv Neurosurg 8:172–182

Steinhoff H, Aviles Ch (1976) Contrast enhancement response of intracranial neoplasms – its validity for the differential diagnosis of tumors in CT. In: Lanksch W, Kazner E (eds) Cranial computerized tomography. Springer, Berlin Heidelberg New York, pp 151–161

Steinhoff H, Kazner E, Lanksch W, Grumme Th, Meese W, Lange S, Aulich A, Wende S (1978) The limitations of computerized axial tomography in the detection and differential diagnosis of intracranial tumors. A study based on 1304 neoplasms. In: Bories J (ed) The diagnostic limitation of computerized axial tomography. Springer, Berlin Heidelberg New York, pp 40–49

Steudel WI, Beck U, Becker H, Hacker H (1976) Perifocal

edema in computerized tomography and EEG changes in patients with tumors of cerebral hemispheres. In: Lanksch W, Kazner E (eds) Cranial computerized tomography. Springer, Berlin Heidelberg New York, pp 188–200

Strand RD, Baker RA, Ordia IJ, Arkins TJ (1978) Metrizamide ventriculography and computed tomography in lesions about the third ventricle. Radiology 128:405–410

Syvertsen AH, Dugstad G, Amundsen P (1976) Computerized tomography in brain tumors correlated to histology, angiography, gas encephalography, and isotope encephalography. In: Lanksch W, Kazner E (eds) Cranial computerized tomography. Springer, Berlin Heidelberg New York, pp 167–170

Tadmor R, Harwood-Nash DC, Savoiardo M, Scotti G, Musgrave M, Fitz CR, Chuang S (1980) Brain tumors in the first two years of life: CT diagnosis. AJNR 1:411–417

Thomalske G, Grau H, Schäfer M, Hacker H (1976) The significance of cranial computerized tomography for the diagnosis of certain expansive lesions of the midline. In: Lanksch W, Kazner E (eds) Cranial computerized tomography. Springer, Berlin Heidelberg New York, pp 104–109

Thomson JLG (1976) Computerised axial tomography and the diagnosis of glioma: A study of 100 consecutive histologically proven cases. Clin Radiol 27:431–444

Thron A, Bockenheimer S (1979) Giant aneurysms of the posterior fossa suspected as neoplasms on computed tomography. Neuroradiology 18:93–97

Van Kirk OC, Cornell SH, Jacoby CG (1979) Posterior fossa intra-axial tumors: A comparison of computed tomography with other imaging methods. J Comput Assist Tomogr 3:31–50

Vouge M, Pasquini U, Salvolini U (1980) CT findings of atypical forms of phakomatosis. Neuroradiology 20:99–101

Wende S, Aulich A, Kretzschmar K, Grumme Th, Meese W, Lange S, Steinhoff H, Lanksch W, Kazner E (1977) Die Computertomographie der Hirngeschwülste. Eine Sammelstudie über 1658 Tumoren. Radiologe 17:149–156

Wende S, Aulich A, Kretzschmar K, Lange S, Grumme Th, Meese W, Lanksch W, Kazner E, Steinhoff H (1977) C.A.T. investigations of the development of cerebral edema and the effects of its treatment in patients with brain tumours. In: du Boulay GH, Moseley IF (eds) Computerised axial tomography in clinical practice. Springer, Berlin Heidelberg New York, pp 118–122

Wende S, Aulich A, Schindler E, Grumme Th, Meese W, Lange S, Kazner E, Steinhoff H, Lanksch W (1977) A german multicentre study of intracranial tumours. In: du Boulay GH, Moseley IF (eds) Computerised axial tomography in clinical practice. Springer, Berlin Heidelberg New York, pp 111–117

Von Wild K, Grau H, Neubauer M, Althoff P-H (1976) The importance of cranial computerized tomography in diagnosis and continous follow-up of space-occupying lesions of the sellar region. In: Lanksch W, Kazner E (eds) Cranial computerized tomography. Springer, Berlin Heidelberg New York, pp 128–132

Wilson JL, Moseley IF (1977) A diagnostic approach to cerebellar lesions. In: du Boulay GH, Moseley IF (eds) Computerised axial tomography in clinical practice. Springer, Berlin Heidelberg New York, pp 123–133

Wing SD, Anderson RE, Osborn AG (1980) Dynamic cranial computed tomography: Preliminary results. AJNR 1:135–139

Yates AJ, Becker LE, Sachs LA (1979) Brain tumors in childhood. Childs Brain 5:31–39

Zimmerman RA, Bilaniuk LT (1980) Computed tomography of acute intratumoral hemorrhage. Radiology 135:355–359

Zimmerman RD, Leeds NE, Naidich TP (1977) Ring blush associated with intracerebral hematoma. Radiology 122:707–711

Zimmermann RD, Russell EJ, Leeds NE (1980) Axial CT recognition of anteroposterior displacement of fourth ventricle. AJNR 1:65–70

Zülch KJ (1956) Die Hirngeschwülste in biologischer und morphologischer Darstellung. Ambrosius Barth, Leipzig

Zülch KJ (1975) Altas of gross neurosurgical pathology. Springer, Berlin Heidelberg New York

Zülch KJ (1980) Principles of the new health organization (WHO) classification of brain tumors. Neuroradiology 19:59–66

**D1 Computed tomography in brain tumors; Autochthonous brain tumors**

Aarabi B, Long DM, Miller NR (1978) Enlarging optic chiasmal glioma with stable visual acuity. Surg Neurol 10:175–177

Afra D, Norman D, Levin VA (1980) Cysts in malignant gliomas. Identification by computerized tomography. J Neurosurg 821–825

Avrahami E, Fireman Z, Cohn DF (1981) Computer Tomographie bei einem Fall von zerebraler Sarkoidose. Nervenarzt 52:348–349

Barrer SJ, Simeone FA, Han SS (1980) An unusual presentation of an oligodendroglioma. J Neurosurg 53:560–561

Berge JH van den, Blaauw G (1980) Subdural cysts and diencephalic tumor. Surg Neurol 13:267–272

Bilaniuk LT, Zimmerman RA, Littmann Ph, Gallo E, Rorke LB, Bruce DA, Schut L (1980) Computed tomography of the brain stem gliomas in children. Radiology 134:89–95

Boethius J, Collins VP, Edner G, Lewander R, Zyajicek J (1978) Stereotactic biopsies and computer tomography in gliomas. Acta Neurochir (Wien) 40:223–232

Brant-Zawadzki M, Enzmann DR (1978) Computed tomographic brain scanning in patients with lymphoma. Radiology 129:67–71

Burke DP, Gabrielsen TO, Knake JE, Seeger JF, Oberman HA (1980) Radiology of olfactory neuroblastoma. Radiology 137:367–372

Butler AR, Horii StC, Kricheff II, Shannon MB, Budzilovich GN (1978) Computed Tomography in Astrocytomas. Radiology 129:433–439

Butler AR, Passalaqua AM, Berenstein A, Kricheff II (1978) The contrast-enhanced CT scan and the radionuclide brain scan: Parallel mechanisms of action in the detection of supratentorial astrocytomas. Neuroradiology 16:491–494

Cho So S, Ho J (1980) Multiple primary germinomas (ectopic pinealoma) of the brain. Neurochirurgia (Stuttg) 23:147–150

Clarenbach P, Kleihues P, Metzel E, Dichgans J (1979) Simultaneous clinical manifestation of subependymoma of the fourth ventricle in identical twins. J Neurosurg 50:655–659

Claveria LE, Kendall BE, du Boulay GH (1977) Computerised axial tomography in supratentorial gliomas. In: du Boulay GH, Moseley IF (eds) Computerised axial tomography in clinical practice. Springer, Berlin Heidelberg New York, pp 85–93

Diba J, Frowein RA, Stammler A (1979) Gangliocytoma: operability and follow-up. Neurosurg Rev 2:46–53

Ebhardt G, Meese W (1979) Malignant lymphomas of the brain. Adv Neurosurg 4:303–308

Enzmann DR, Krikorian J, Norman D, Kramer R, Pollock J, Faer M (1979) Computed tomography in primary reticulum cell sarcoma of the brain. Radiology 130:165–170

Enzmann DR, Norman D, Levin V, Wilson Ch, Newton ThH (1978) Computed tomography in the follow-up of medulloblastomas and ependymomas. Radiology 128:57–63

Fortuna A, Celli P, Ferrante L, Turano C (1979) A review of papillomas of the third ventricle. J Neurosurg Sci 61–76

Friedman WA, Vries JK, Quisling RG (1979) Ganglioglioma of the medulla oblongata. Surg Neurol 12:105–108

Futrell NN, Osborn AG, Cheson BD (1981) Pineal region tumors: Computed tomographic-pathologic spectrum. AJNR 2:415–420

Gastaldo JA, Buchheit WA (1977) Bilateral subfrontal glioma simulating a meningioma. Surg Neurol 7:105–106

Gittens WO, Huestis WS, Sangalang VE (1980) Oligodendroglioma of the cerebellum. Surg Neurol 13:237–240

Glanz S, Geehr RB, Duncan ChC, Piepmeier JM (1980) Metrizamide-enhanced CT for evaluation of brainstem tumors. AJNR 1:31–34

Goldstein SJ, Young B, Markesberry WR (1981) Congenital malignant gliosarcoma. AJNR 2:475–476

Gregorius FK, Crandall PH, Baloh RW (1976) Positional vertigo with cerebellar astrocytoma. Surg Neurol 6:283–286

Gudeman SK, Sullivan HG, Rosner MJ, Becker DP (1979) Surgical removal of bilateral papillomas of the choroid plexus of the lateral ventricles with resolution of hydrocephalus. J Neurosurg 50:677–681

Halmagyi GM, Bignold LP, Allsop JL (1979) Recurrent subependymal giant-cell astrocytoma in the absence of tuberous sclerosis. J Neurosurg 50:106–109

Handa J, Nakano Y, Handa H (1978) Computed tomography in the differential diagnosis of low-density intracranial lesions. Surg Neurol 10:179–185

Hase U, Hock H, Schindler E (1979) Tumoren der Pinealisregion Teil I. Neurochirurgia (Stuttg) 22:107–117

Hase U, Hock H, Schindler E, Schürmann K (1979) Tumoren der Pinealisregion Teil II. Neurochirurgia (Stuttg) 22:118–129

Heiß E (1981) Ein Medulloblastom im hohen Lebensalter (Fallbericht). Neurochirurgia 24:142–143

Jellinger K, Radaskiewicz T, Slowik F (1975) Primary malignant lymphomas of the central nervous system in man. Acta Neuropathol [Suppl] (Berl) VI:95–102

Joyce P, Bentson J, Takahashi M, Winter J, Wilson G, Byrd S (1978) The accuracy of predicting histologic grades of supratentorial astrocytomas on the basis of computerized tomography and cerebral angiography. Neuroradiology 16:346–348

Kazner E, Steinhoff H, Wende S, Mauersberger W (1978) Ringshaped lesions in the CT scan-Differential diagnostic considerations. Adv Neurosurg 6:80–85

Kazner E, Wilske J, Steinhoff H, Stochdorph O (1978) Computer assisted tomography in primary malignant lymphomas of the brain. J Comput Assist Tomogr 2:125–134

Kendall BE, Jakubowski J, Pullicino P, Symon L (1979) Difficulties in diagnosis of supratentorial gliomas by CAT scan. J Neurol Neurosurg Psychiatry 42:485–492

Khan A, Fulco JD, Shende A, Rosenthal A, Marc JA (1980) Focal histiocytosis X of the parietal lobe. J Neurosurg 52:431–433

Kingsley D, Kendall BE (1977) Dependent layering of contrast medium in cystic astrocytomas. Neuroradiology 14:107–110

Kingsley DPE, Kendall BE (1979) The CT scanner in posterior fossa tumours of childhood. Br J Radiol 52:769–776

Kleefield J, Solis IJ, Davis KR, Kleinman G, Roberson GH, Ellis GT, Merino J (1977) Computed tomography of tumors of the pineal region. Comput Tomogr 1:257–265

Kramer RA (1977) Vermian pseudotumor: a potential pitfall of CT brain scanning with contrast enhancement. Neuroradiology 13:229–230

Kretzschmar K, Grumme Th, Steinhoff H (1978) Der Wert der Computer-Tomographie und Angiographie für die Diagnose supratentorieller Hirntumoren. Neuroradiology 16:487–490

Krol G, Farmer P, Stein S, Tenner M, Rothman L (1979) Carcinoma of choroid plexus in a premature infant. J Comput Assist Tomogr 3:530–532

Lewander R (1979) Contrast enhancement with time in gliomas. Stereotactic computer tomography following contrast medium infusion. Acta Radiol 30:689–702

Lin SR, Crane MD, Lin ZS, Bilaniuk L, Plassche WM, Marshall L, Spataro RF (1978) Characteristics of calcification in tumors of the pineal gland. Radiology 126:721–726

Markwalder T-M, Huber P, Markwalder RV, Seiler RW (1979) Primary intraventricular oligodendrogliomas. Surg Neurol 11:25–28

Mauersberger W (1981) The determination of absorption values as an aid in computer tomographic differentiation between cerebral abscess and glioblastoma. Adv neurosurg 9:36–40

McCullough DC, Huang HK, De Michelle D, Manz HJ, Sinks LF (1979) Correlation between volumetric CT imaging and autopsy measurements of glioblastoma size. Comput Tomogr 3:133–141

Mikhael MA (1977) Case report: diminished density surrounding a meningioma, verified to be an overlying cystic astrocytoma. J Comput Assist Tomogr 1:349–351

Miller EM, Mani RL, Townsend JJ (1976) Cerebellar glioblastoma multiforme in an adult. Surg Neurol 5:341–343

Neuwelt EA, Glasberg M, Frenkel E, Clark WK (1979) Malignant pineal region tumors. J Neurosurg 51:597–607

Pagani JJ, Libshitz HI, Wallace S, Hayman LA (1981) Central nervous system leukemia and lymphoma: Computed tomographic manifestations. AJNR 2:397–403

Richardson RR, Siqueira EB, Cerullo LJ (1979) Malignant glioma: its initial presentation as intracranial hemorrhage. Acta Neurochir (Wien) 46:77–84

Ringertz N (1950) "Grading" of gliomas. Acta Pathol Microbiol Scand 27:51–64

Ringertz N, Tola JH (1950) Medulloblastoma. J Neuropathol Exp Neurol 9:354–372

Rosenbaum TJ, McCarty CS, Buettner H (1979) Uveitis and cerebral reticulum cell sarcoma. J Neurosurg 50:660–664

Sabattini L, Piazza GC, Finizia FS (1980) Programmed serial CT scans in the surgical and radio-chemotherapeutic management of cerebral gliomas. J Neurosurg Sci 24:33–36

Sahart A, Feinsod M, Beller AJ (1980) Choroid plexus papilloma: hydrocephalus and cerebrospinal fluid dynamics. Surg Neurol 13:476–478

Sarmiento J, Ferrer L, Pons L, Ferrer E (1979) Cerebral mixed tumor: Osteo-chondrosarcoma-glioblastoma multiforme. Acta Neurochir (Wien) 50:335–341

Sawhny BS, Dohn DF (1980) Neuroendocrinological aspects of histiocytosis X of the central nervous system. Surg Neurol 14:237–239

Schindler E, Kretzschmar K, Aulich A, Wende S, Kutzner J (1977) Serial CT studies of a metastatic pinealoma with reference to the radiotherapeutic problems. Neuroradiology 14:127–132

Schlarb H, Schirmer M (1978) Pinealoma with initial spinal manifestation. Adv Neurosurg 6:221–224

Sogg RL, Donaldson SS, Yorke CH (1978) Malignant astrocytoma following radiotherapy of a craniopharyngioma. J Neurosurg 48:622–627

Stefanko SZ, Talerman A, Mackay WM, Vuzevski VD (1979) Infundibular germinoma. Acta Neurochir (Wien) 71–78

Steinhoff H, Grumme Th, Kazner E, Lange S, Lanksch W, Meese W, Wüllenweber R (1978) Axial transverse computerized tomography in 73 glioblastomas. Acta Neurochir (Wien) 42:45–56

Steinhoff H, Lanksch W, Kazner E, Grumme Th, Meese W, Lange S, Aulich A, Schindler E, Wende S (1977) Computed tomography in the diagnosis and differential diagnosis of glioblastomas. Neuroradiology 14:193–199

Tadmor R, Davis KR, Roberson GH, Kleinman GM (1978) Computed tomography in primary malignant lymphoma of the brain. J Comput Assist Tomogr 2:135–140

Takeuchi J, Handa H, Nagata I (1978) Suprasellar germinoma. J Neurosurg 49:41–48

Takeuchi J, Handa H, Otsuka S, Takebe Y (1979) Neuroradiological aspects of suprasellar germinoma. Neuroradiology 17:153–159

Tans JThJ, De Jongh IE (1977) Computed tomography of supratentorial astrocytoma. Clin Neurol Neurosurg 80:156–168

Tchang S, Scotti G, Terbrugge K, Melançon D, Bélanger G, Milner C, Ethier R (1977) Computerized tomography as a possible aid to histological grading of supratentorial gliomas. J Neurosurg 46:735–739

Thomson JL (1976) Computerised axial tomography and the diagnosis of glioma: a study of 100 consecutive histologically proven cases. Clin Radiol 27:431–441

Tibbs PA, Challa V, Mortara RH (1978) Isolated histiocytosis X of the hypothalamus. J Neurosurg 49:929–934

Turcotte JF, Copty M, Bédard F, Michaud J, Verret S (1980) Lateral ventricle choroid plexus papilloma and communicating hydrocephalus. Surg Neurol 13:143–146

Veiga-Pires JA, Dossetor RS, van Nieuwenhuizen O (1978) CT scanning for papilloma of choroid plexus. Neuroradiology 17:13–16

Vonofakos D, Marcu H, Hacker H (1979) Oligodendrogliomas: CT patterns with emphasis on features indicating malignancy. J Comput Assist Tomogr 3:783–788

Weisberg LA (1979) Computed tomography in the diagnosis of brain stem gliomas. J Comput Tomogr 3:145–153

Weisberg LA (1980) Cerebral computed tomography in the diagnosis of supratentorial astrocytoma. Comput Tomogr 4:87–105

Yamashita J, Handa H, Yumitori K, Abe M (1980) Reversible delayed radiation effect on the brain after radiotherapy of malignant astrocytoma. Surg Neurol 13:413–417

Zimmerman HM (1975) Malignant lymphomas of the nervous system. Acta Neuropathol [Suppl] (Berl) VI:69–74

Zimmerman RA, Bilaniuk LT (1979) Computed tomography of intracerebral gangliogliomas. J Comput Assist Tomogr 3:24–30

Zimmerman RA, Bilaniuk LT (1980) CT of primary and secondary craniocerebral neuroblastoma. AJNR 1:431–434

Zimmerman RA, Bilaniuk LT, Bruno L, Rosenstock J (1978) Computed tomography of cerebellar astrocytoma. Am J Roentgenol 130:929–933

Zimmerman RA, Bilaniuk LT, Pahlajani H (1978) Spectrum of medulloblastomas demonstrated by computed tomography. Radiology 126:137–141

Zimmerman RD, Leeds NE, Naidich TP (1977) Ring blush associated with intracerebral hematoma. Radiology 122:707–712

### D2 Meningeal tumors

Auff E, Reisner T, Toifl K, Pernecky A (1981) Primäre diffuse Melanoblastose der Leptomeningen und CT-Veränderungen. Neurochirurgia 24:35–37

Becker D, Norman D, Wilson CB (1979) Computerized tomography and pathological correlation in cystic meningiomas. J Neurosurg 50:103–105

Bonnal J, Born JD, Tremoulet M (1979) Méningiomes multiples intracraniens. Neurochirurgie 25:78–83

Claveria LE, Sutton D, Tress BM (1977) The radiological diagnosis of meningiomas, the impact of EMI scanning. Br J Radiol 50:15–22

Cushing H, Eisenhardt J (1938) Meningeomas. Thomas, Springfield

Dosch JCl, Wackenheim A (1978) Hypodense meningioma: Computer tomographic examination of a meningioma. J Belge Radiol 61:325–334

Fine M, Brazis P, Palacios E, Neri G (1980) Computed tomography of sphenoid wing meningiomas: Tumor location related to distal edema. Surg Neurol 13:385–390

Flaschka G, Popper H (1981) Die primäre Melanoblastose der Leptomeninx. Nervenarzt 52:350–355

Fleury P, Bocquet L, Carou J-P, Poivier J, Marsault C, Basset J-M, Coupez D, Sterkers O, Compère J-F, Pansier P (1979) Meningioma of the ear simulating a glomus

tumor. Apropos of 2 cases. Ann Otolaryngol Chir Cervicofac 96:469–491
Giromini D, Peiffer J, Tzonos T (1981) Über zwei Fälle von Ventrikelmeningeomen im Kindesalter. Neurochirurgia 24:144–145
Ito J, Kadekaru T, Hayano M, Kurita I, Okada K, Yoshida Y (1981) Meningioma in the tela choroidea of the third ventricle: CT and angiographic correlations. Neuroradiology 21:207–211
Kadis GN, Mount LA, Ganti SR (1979) The importance of early diagnosis and treatment of the meningiomas of the planum sphenoidale and tuberculum sellae: a retrospective study of 105 cases. Surg Neurol 12:367–371
Kendall B, Pullicino P (1979) Comparison of consistency of meningiomas and CT appearances. Neuroradiology 18:173–176
Mani RL, Hedgcock MW, Mass SI, Gilmor RL, Enzmann DR, Eisenberg RL (1978) Radiographic diagnosis of meningioma of the lateral ventricle. J Neurosurg 49:249–255
Markwalder T-M, Seiler RW, Markwalder RV, Huber P, Markwalder HM (1979) Meningioma of the anterior part of the third ventricle in a child. Surg Neurol 12:29–32
Mikhael MA (1977) Diminished density surrounding a meningioma, verified to be an overlying cystic astrocytoma. J Comput Assist Tomogr 1:349–351
Möller A, Hatam A, Olivecrona H (1978) The differential diagnosis of pontine angle meningioma and acoustic neuroma with computed tomography. Neuroradiology 17:21–33
Nahser HC, Grote W, Löhr E, Gerhard L (1981) Multiple meningiomas. Clinical and computed tomographic observations. Neuroradiology 21:259–263
Nakagawa H, Lusins JO (1980) Biplane computed tomography of intracranial meningiomas with extracranial extension. J Comput Assist Tomogr 4:478–483
Nauta HJW, Tucker WS, Horsey WJ, Bilbao JM, Gonsalves C (1979) Xanthochromic cysts associated with meningioma. J Neurol Neurosurg Psychiatr 42:529–535
New PFJ, Aronow S, Hesselink JR (1980) National cancer institute study: Evaluation of computed tomography in the diagnosis of intracranial neoplasms. IV. Meningiomas. Radiology 136:665–675
Russell EJ, George AE, Kricheff II, Budzilovich G (1980) Atypical computed tomographic features of intracranial meningioma. Radiology 135:673–682
Sartor K, Kühne D (1978) Meningeome mit Beziehung zum Tentorium cerebelli: Computertomographische und angiographische Aspekte. Fortschr Röntgenstr 8:651–661
Savoiardo M, Lodrini S (1980) Hypodense area within a meningioma: Metastasis from breast cancer. Neuroradiology 20:107–110
Sutton D, Claveria LE (1977) Meningiomas diagnosed by scanning: a review of 100 intracranial cases. In: du Boulay GH, Moseley IF (eds) Computerised axial tomography in clinical practice. Springer, Berlin Heidelberg New York, pp 102–110
Tans JThJ, De Jongh IE (1977) Computed tomography of supratentorial meningioma. Clin Neurol Neurosurg 80:10–21
Vassilouthis J, Ambrose J (1979) Computerized tomography scanning appearances of intracranial meningiomas. An attempt to predict the histological features. J Neurosurg 50:320–327
Vassilouthis J, Ambrose J (1978) Intraventricular meningioma in a child. Surg Neurol 10:105–107
Weisberg LA (1979) Computed tomography in the diagnosis of intracranial meningioma. J Comput Assist Tomogr 3:115–124
Wiggli U, Elke M, Müller HR, Hünig R, Wüthrich R (1976) The CT pattern of meningioma – is it specific? In: Lanksch W, Kazner E (eds) Cranial computerized tomography. Springer, Berlin Heidelberg New York, pp 162–166

### D3 Neurinomas

Bergeron RT, Cohen NL, Pinto RS (1977) Role of computerized tomography in the diagnosis of acustic neuromas. Arch Otolaryngol 103:314–317
Boggan JE, Rosenblum ML, Wilson CB (1979) Neurilemmoma of the fourth cranial nerve. J Neurosurg 50:519–521
Burrows EH (1978) Hirnszintigraphie (einschließlich Computer-ausgewertete axiale Tomographie). In: Plester D, Wende S, Nakayama N (Hrsg) Kleinhirnbrückenwinkel-Tumoren. Springer, Berlin Heidelberg New York, S 144–164
Canigiani G (1978) Nativdiagnostik mit Tomographie der Kleinhirnbrückenwinkel-Tumoren. In: Plester D, Wende S, Nakayama N (Hrsg) Kleinhirnbrückenwinkel-Tumoren. Springer, Berlin Heidelberg New York, S 92–120
Davis KR, Parker SW, New PFJ, Roberson GH, Taveras JM, Ojemann RJ, Weiss AD (1977) Computed tomography of acoustic neuroma. Radiology 124:81–86
Dossetor RS, De Winter J, Nurick S (1979) Diagnosis of a small acoustic neuroma by metrizamide computer-assisted cisternography. Br J Radiol 52:667–668
Downey JR EF, Buck DR, Ray JW (1981) Arachnoiditis simulating acoustic neuroma on air-CT cisternography. AJNR 2:470–471
Dubois PJ, Drayer BP, Bank WO, Deeb ZL, Rosenbaum AR (1978) An evaluation of current diagnostic radiologic modalities in the investigation of acoustic neurilemmomas. Radiology 126:173–179
Fink LH, Early CB, Bryan RN (1978) Glossopharyngeal schwannomas. Surg Neurol 9:239–245
Goebel HH, Shimokawa K, Schaake Th, Kremp A (1979) Schwannoma of the sellar region. Acta Neurochir (Wien) 48:191–197
Goldberg R, Byrd S, Winter J, Takahashi M, Joyce P (1980) Varied appearance of trigeminal neuroma on CT. Am J Roentgenol 134:57–60
Gyldensted C, Lester J, Thomsen J (1976) Computer tomography in the diagnosis of cerebellopontine angle tumors. Neuroradiology 11:191–197
Hatam A, Möller A, Olivecrona H (1979) Evaluation of the internal auditory meatus with acoustic neuromas using computed tomography. Neuroradiology 17:197–200
Hoffmann JC, Cox GW (1977) Limitations of computerized tomography scanning in acoustic neurinomas. Arch Otolaryngol 103:594–595
Huete I, Corrales M (1979) Cisternographie computérisée dans le diagnostic des petits neurinomes de l'acoustique. J Neuroradiol 6:335–340

Jacoby ChG, Go RT, Beren RA (1980) Cranial CT of Neurofibromatosis. AJNR 1:311–315
King TT, Ambrose J (1977) C.A.T. scanning in tumours of the cerebellopontine angle. In: du Boulay GH, Moseley IF (eds) Computerised axial tomography in clinical practice. Springer, Berlin Heidelberg New York, pp 134–138
Kricheff II, Pinto RS, Bergeron RT, Cohen N (1980) CT-air-cisternography and canalography in the diagnosis of small acoustic neuromas. 17. Meeting Am. Soc. Neuroradiol., Toronto 1979. AJNR 1:57–63
Osborn JD (1975) A comparative study of special petrous views and tomography in the diagnosis of acoustic neuromas. Br J Radiol 48:996–999
Parker SW, Davis KR (1977) Limitations of computed tomography in the investigation of acoustic neuromas. Ann Otol Rhinol Laryngol 86:436–440
Pinto R, Kricheff II, Bergeron RT, Cohen N (1981) The diagnosis of small acoustic neuromas by gas computed tomography cisternography and canalography. In: Contrast Media in Computed Tomography. Ed. by Felix R, Kazner E and Wegener OH, Excerpta Medica, 165–170
Robbins B, Marschall WH Jr (1978) Computed tomography of acoustic neurinoma. Radiology 128:367–370
Robinson JS, Lopes J, Moody R (1979) Intracranial hypoglossal neurilemmoma. Surg Neurol 12:496–498
Rosenbaum AE, Drayer BP, Dubois PJ, Black FO (1978) Visualization of small extraçanalicular neurilemmomas by metrizamide cisternographic enhancement. Arch Otolaryngol 104:239–243
Salvoloni U, Pasquini U, Babin E, Gasquez P (1978) Von Recklinghausen's disease and computer tomography. J Belge Radiol 61:313–318
Schiefer W, Kazner E (1967) Klinische Echo-Encephalographie. Springer, Berlin Heidelberg New York
Schubiger O, Valavanis A, Hayek J, Dabir K (1980) Neuroma of the cavernous sinus. Surg Neurol 13:313–316
Schubiger O, Valavanis A, Menges H (1978) Computed tomography for small acoustic neuromas. Neuroradiology 15:287–290
Sortland O (1978) X-ray diagnosis of expanding lesions in the cerebellopontine angle. Meeting Nord Soc Radiol, Oslo, June 1978
Sortland O (1979) Computed tomography combined with gas cisternography for the diagnosis of expanding lesions in the cerebellopontine angle. Neuroradiology 18:19–22
Thomsen J, Gyldensted C, Lester J (1977) Computer tomography of cerebellopontine angle lesions. Arch Otolaryngol 103:65–69
Tritthart H, Lepuschütz H (1979) Wertigkeit der axialen Computertomographie in der Diagnostik intrakanalikulärer Gewächse des Nervus statoacusticus. In: Sager W-D, Ladurner G (eds) Computertomographie. Thieme, Stuttgart, S 21–23
Valavanis A, Schubiger O, Wellauer J (1978) Computed tomography of acoustic neuromas with emphasis on small tumour detectability. Neuroradiology 16:598–600
Vassilouthis J, Richardson AE (1979) Acoustic neurinoma in a child. Surg Neurol 12:37–39
Wende S (1980) Die kombinierte Anwendung von Computertomographie und Luftzisternographie bei Kleinhirnbrückenwinkeltumoren. Fortschr Röntgenstr 132:666–667
Wende S, Nakayama N (1978) Zisternographie mit negativen und positiven Kontrastmitteln. In: Plester D, Wende S, Nakayama N (Hrsg) Kleinhirnbrückenwinkel-Tumoren. Springer, Berlin Heidelberg New York, S 121–143

### D4 Pituitary adenomas

Bajraktari X, Bergström M, Brismar K, Goulatie R, Greitz T, Grepe A (1977) Diagnosis of intrasellar cisternal herniation (empty sella) by computer assisted tomography. J Comput Assist Tomogr 1:105–116
Brennan ThG Jr, Krishna Rao CVG, Robinson W, Itani A (1977) Tandem lesions: chromophobe adenoma and meningioma. J Comput Assist Tomogr 1:517–520
Citrin CM, Davis DO (1977) Computerized tomography in the evaluation of pituitary adenomas. Invest Radiol 12:27–35
Clar H-E, Bock WJ, Grote W, Nau HE, Weichert HC (1979) Classification of tumours in the sellar region using CT and encephalotomography. Neurochirurgia (Stuttg) 22:153–159
Danoff BF (1978) The value of computerized tomography in delineating suprasellar extension of pituitary adenoma for radiotherapeutic management. Cancer 42:1066–1072
Donovan Post MJ, David NJ, Glaser JS, Safran A (1980) Pituitary apoplexy: Diagnosis by computed tomography. Radiology 134:665–670
Fargason RD, Jacques S, Rand RW, Shelden CH, McCann GD, Linn S (1981) Visualization and three-dimensional reconstruction of pituitary microadenomas from CT data: A technical report. Surg Neurol 15:450–454
Grisoli F, Vincentelli F, Guibout M, Hassoun J, Famarier P (1980) Prolactin secreting adenoma in 22 Men. Surg Neurol 13:241–247
Gross CE, Binet EF, Esguerra JV (1979) Metrizamide cisternography in the evaluation of pituitary adenomas and the empty sella syndrome. J Neurosurg 50:472–476
Gyldensted C, Karle A (1977) Computed tomography of intra- and juxtasellar lesions. A radiological study of 108 cases. Neuroradiology 14:5–13
Hall K, McAllister VL (1980) Metrizamide cisternography in pituitary and juxtapituitary lesions. Radiology 134:101–108
Hatam A, Bergström M, Greitz T (1979) Diagnosis of sellar and parasellar lesions by computed tomography. Neuroradiology 18:249–258
Haughton VM, Rosenbaum AE, Williams AL, Drayer B (1980) Recognizing the empty sella by CT: The infundibulum sign. AJNR 1:527–529
Haughton VM, Williams AL, Cusick JF (1979) The computed tomographic appearance of the normal pituitary gland and pituitary microadenomas. Radiology 133:385–391
Hoffman JC Jr, Tindall GT (1980) Diagnosis of empty sella syndrome using Amipaque cisternography combined with computerized tomography. J Neurosurg 52:99–102
Jacobs L, Weisberg LA, Kinkel WR (1980) Computerized tomography of the orbit and sella turcica. Raven Press, New York
Jones JR, De Hempel AC, Kemmann E, Tenner MS (1977) Galactorrhea and amenorrhea in a patient with an empty sella. Obstet Gynecol 49:9–11
Kazner E, Fahlbusch R, Lanksch W, Rothe R, Scherer U,

Steinhoff H, Grumme Th, Lange S, Meese W, Aulich A, Wende S (1978) Computerized tomography in diagnosis and follow-up examination of pituitary adenomas. In: Fahlbusch R, v Werder K (eds) Treatment of pituitary adenomas. Thieme, Stuttgart, pp 101–114

Lee KF, Suh JM, Mazziotta JC, Huang HK (1977) The value of computed tomography in the radiotherapeutic management of juxtasellar tumors. Comput Tomogr 1:111–119

Leeds NE, Naidich TP (1977) Computerized tomography in the diagnosis of sellar and parasellar lesions. Semin Roentgenol 12:121–135

Leonardi M, Nardi F de, Fabris G, Penco T, Cecotto C, Schiavi F (1979) CT evaluation of parasellar lesions. J Neurosurg Sci 23:217–229

Maravilla KR, Kirks DR, Maravilla AM, Diehl JT (1978) Computed tomography in the evaluation of sella and parasella lesions: The value of sagittal and coronal reconstructions. Comput Tomogr 2:237–249

Muhr C, Bergstrom K, Enoksson P, Hugosson R, Lundberg PO (1980) Follow-up study with computerized tomography and clinical evaluation 5 to 10 years after surgery for pituitary adenoma. J Neurosurg 52:144–148

Naidich TP, Pinto RS, Kushner MJ, Lin JP, Kricheff II, Leeds NE, Chase NE (1976) Evaluation of sellar and parasellar masses by computed tomography. Radiology 120:91–99

Okony T, Sudo M, Momoi T, Takao T, Ito M, Konishi Y, Yoshioka M, Suzuki J, Nakano Y (1980) Pituitary hyperplasia due to hypothyroidism. J Comput Assist Tomogr 4:600–602

Patel DV, Shields MC (1979) Intraventricular hemorrhage in pituitary apoplexy. J Comput Assist Tomogr 3:829–831

Penley MW, Pribram HF (1980) Diagnosis of empty sella with small amounts of air at computed tomography. Surg Neurol 14:296–301

Quencer RM (1980) Lymphocytic adenohypophysitis: Autoimmune disorder of the pituitary gland. AJNR 1:343–345

Reich NE, Zelch JV, Alfidi RJ, Meaney TF, Duchesneau PM, Weinstein MA (1976) Computed tomography in the detection of juxtasellar lesions. Radiology 118:333–334

Richmond IL, Newton ThH, Wilson CB (1980) Prolactin-secreting pituitary adenomas: Correlation of radiographic and surgical findings. AJNR 1:13–16

Robertson WD, Newton TH (1978) Radiological assessment of pituitary microadenomas. Am J Roentgenol 13:489–492

Sadamoto K (1977) Sellar and parasellar tumors visualized by coronal computed tomography. No To Shinkei 29:659–668

Sheldon P, Molyneux A (1979) Metrizamide cisternography and computed tomography for the investigation of pituitary lesions. Neuroradiology 17:83–87

Smaltino F, Bernini FP, Muras L (1980) Computed tomography for diagnosis of empty sella associated with enhancing pituitary microadenoma. J Comput Assist Tomogr 4:592–599

Symon L, Jakubowski J, Kendall B (1979) Surgical treatment of giant pituitary adenomas. J Neurol Neurosurg Psychiatry 42:973–982

Syvertsen A, Haughton VM, Williams AL, Cusick JF (1979) The computed tomographic appearance of the normal pituitary gland and pituitary microadenomas. Radiology 133:385–391

Taylor HC, Wilson DJ, Schumacher OP (1979) Pituitary stones and associated hypopituitarism. J Am Med Ass 242:751–752

Tenner MS, Weitzner JrI (1980) Pitfalls in the diagnosis of erosive changes in expanding lesions of the pituitary fossa. Radiology 137:393–396

Turski PA, Watanabe TJ, Chambers EF, Newton ThH (1981) Contrast enhancement of the normal and abnormal pituitary gland. In: Contrast Media in Computed Tomography. Ed. by Felix R, Kazner E and Wegener OH, Excerpta Medica, 157–164

Vignaud J, Aubin ML, Bories J (1979) Value of computer assisted tomography in the exploration of the sellar and suprasellar structures. Rev Neurol 135:41–50

Weisberg LA (1977) Pituitary apoplexy. Association of degenerative change in pituitary adenoma with radiotherapy and detection by cerebral computed tomography. Am J Med 63:109–115

Wolfman NT, Boehnke M (1978) The use of coronal sections in evaluating lesions of the sellar and parasellar regions. J Comput Assist Tomogr 2:308–313

Wolpert SM, Post KD, Biller BJ, Molitch ME (1979) The value of computed tomography in evaluating patients with prolactinomas. Radiology 131:117–119

**D5 Tumors of the blood vessels – Hemangioblastomas**

Cornell SH, Hibri NS, Menezes AH, Fraf CJ (1979) The complementary nature of computed tomography and angiography in the diagnosis of cerebellar hemangioblastoma. Neuroradiology 17:201–205

Diehl PR, Symon L (1981) Supratentorial intraventricular hemangioblastoma: Case report and review of literature. Surg Neurol 15:435–443

McDonnell DE, Pollock P (1978) Cerebral cystic hemangioblastoma. Surg Neurol 10:195–199

Nishimoto A, Kawakami Y (1980) Surgical removal of hemangioblastoma in the fourth ventricle. Surg Neurol 13:423–427

Obrador S, Martin-Rodriguez JG (1977) Biological factors involved in the clinical features and surgical management of cerebellar hemangioblastomas. Surg Neurol 7:79–85

Tomasello F, Albanese V, Iannotti F, Dilorio G (1980) Supratentorial hemangioblastoma in a child. J Neurosurg 52:578–583

**D6 Dysontogenetic tumors**

Ambrose J (1974) Computerized x-ray scanning of the brain. J Neurosurg 40:679

Amendola MA, Garfinkle WB, Ostrum BJ, Katz MR, Katz RI (1978) Preoperative diagnosis of a ruptured intracranial dermoid cyst by computerized tomography. J Neurosurg 48:1035–1037

Arita N, Bitoh S, Ushio Y, Hayakawa T, Hasegawa H, Fujiwara M, Ozaki K, Parkhen L, Mori T (1980) Primary pineal endodermal sinus tumor with elevated serum and CSF alphafetoprotein levels. J Neurosurg 53:244–248

Bosch DA, Rähn T, Backlund EO (1978) Treatment of colloid cysts of the third ventricle by stereotactic aspiration. Surg Neurol 9:15–18

Braun IF, Naidich ThP, Leeds NE (1977) Dense intracranial epidermoid tumors: Computed tomographic observations. Radiology 122:717–719

Budka H (1974) Intracranial lipomatous hamartomas (intracranial "lipomas"). Acta Neuropathol (Berlin) 28:205–222

Cabezudo JM, Vaquero J, Garcia-de-Sola R, Leunda G, Nombela L, Bravo G (1981) Computed tomography with craniopharyngiomas: A review. Surg Neurol 15:422–427

Claussen C, Lohkamp F, Rebien W, Kuttig H (1977) Computertomographische Diagnostik, Therapieplanung und Verlaufskontrollen beim Kraniopharyngeom. Strahlentherapie 153:744–753

Clavici G, Heppner F (1979) The operative approach to lipomas of the corpus callosum. Neurochirurgia 22:77–81

Dee RH, Kishore PRS, Young HF (1980) Radiological evaluation of cerebello-pontine angle epidermoid tumor. Surg Neurol 13:293–296

Dubois PJ, Sage M, Luther JS, Burger PC, Heinz ER, Drayer BP (1981) Malignant change in an intracranial epidermoid cyst. J Comput Assist Tomogr 5:433–435

Eberts TJ, Ransburg RC (1979) Primary intracranial endodermal sinus tumor. J Neurosurg 50:246–252

Evans DC, Netsky MG, Allen VE, Kasantikul V (1979) Empty sella secondary to suprasellar colloid cyst of foregut (respiratory) origin. J Neurosurg 51:114–117

Fawcitt RA, Isherwood I (1976) Radiodiagnosis of intracranial pearly tumours with particular reference to the value of computed tomography. Neuroradiology 11:1–8

Fawcitt RA, Isherwood I (1977) Intracranial epidermoid and dermoid tumors. In: du Boulay GH, Moseley IF (eds) Computerised axial tomography in clinical practice. Springer, Berlin Heidelberg New York, pp 94–101

Faerber EN, Wolpert SM (1978) The value of computed tomography in the diagnosis of intracranial lipomata. J Comput Assist Tomogr 2:297–299

Fitz CR, Wortzman G, Harwood-Nash DC, Holgate RC, Barry JF, Boldt DW (1978) Computed tomography in craniopharyngiomas. Radiology 127:687–691

Gendell H, Maroon I, Wisotzkey H (1976) Epidermoid of the fourth ventricle: discovery by computerized tomography. Surg Neurol 5:37–39

Godt P, Stöppler L (1979) Infratentorielle Epidermoide and Dermoide im kranialen Computertomogramm. Fortschr Röntgenstr 131:368–371

Gomez MR, Mellinger JF, Reese DF (1975) The use of computerized transaxial tomography in the diagnosis of tuberous sclerosis. Mayo Clin Proc 50:553–556

Guner M, Shaw MDM, Turner JW, Steven JL (1976) Computed tomography in the diagnosis of colloid cyst. Surg Neurol 6:345–348

Handa J, Handa H, Nakano Y, Mukai T (1979) Radiolucent intracranial dermoid cyst. Report of an unusual case. Neuroradiology 17:211–214

Hasegawa H, Bitoh S, Nakata M, Fujiwara M, Yasuda H (1981) Intracranial epidermoid mimicking meningioma. Surg Neurol 15:372–374

Hubschmann O, Kasoff S, Doniger D, Llena J, Leeds N (1976) Cavernous hemangioma in the pineal region. Surg Neurol 6:349–351

Isherwood I, Pullan BR, Rutherford RA, Strang FA (1977) Electron density and atomic number determination by computed tomography. Part I: Methods and limitations. Part II: A study of colloid cysts. Br J Radiol 50:613–619

Ishikawa M, Handa H, Moritake K, Mori K, Nakano Y, Aii H (1980) Computed tomography of cerebral cavernous hemangiomas. J Comput Assist Tomomogr 4:587–591

Kazner E, Stochdorph O, Wende S, Grumme Th (1980) Intracranial lipoma. Diagnostic and therapeutic considerations. J Neurosurg 52:234–245

Kim KS, Weinberg PE (1981) Dermoid tumor. Surg Neurol 15:375–376

Krainer L (1935) Die Hirn- und Rückenmarkslipome. Virchows Arch 295:107–142

Laster DW, Moody DM, Ball MR (1978) Computerized cranial tomography of free intracranial fat in congenital tumors. Comput Tomogr 2:257–265

Lee BCP, Gawler J (1978) Tuberous sclerosis. Comparison of computed tomography and conventional neuroradiology. Radiology 127:403–407

Malik GM, Horoupian DS, Boulos RS (1980) Hemorrhagic (colloid) cyst of the third ventricle and episodic neurologic deficits. Surg Neurol 13:73–77

McDonnell DE (1977) Pineal epidermoid cyst: its surgical therapy. Surg Neurol 7:387–391

Mikhael MA, Mattar AG (1978) Intracranial pearly tumors: the roles of computed tomography, angiography, and pneumoencephalography. J Comput Assist Tomogr 2:421–429

Mori K, Handa H, Gi H, Mori K (1980) Cavernomas in the middle fossa. Surg Neurol 14:21–31

Mori K, Handa H, Takeuchi J, Hanakita J, Nakano Y (1981) Hypothalamic hamartoma. J Comput Assist Tomogr 5:519–521

Murphy MJ, Risk WS, Van Gilder JC (1980) Intracranial dermoid cyst in Goldenhar's syndrome. J Neurosurg 53:408–410

Nabawi P, Dobben GD, Mafee M, Espinosa GA (1981) Diagnosis of lipoma of the corpus callosum by CT in five cases. Neuroradiology 21:159–162

Nagasaka S, Kuromatsu C, Wakisaka S, Kitamura K, Matushima T (1981) Rathke's cleft cyst. Surg Neurol 15:402–405

New PFJ, Scott WR (1975) Computed tomography of the brain and orbit. EMI scanning. Williams and Wilkins, Baltimore, Maryland

Numaguchi Y, Kishikawa T, Fukui M, Sawada K, Kitamura K, Matsuura K, Russell WJ (1979) Prolonged injection angiography for diagnosing intracranial cavernous hemangiomas. Radiology 131:137–138

Papo I, Scarpelli M, Caruselli G (1980) Intrinsic third ventricle craniopharyngiomas with normal pressure hydrocephalus. Neurochirurgia 23:80–88

Probst FP, Erasmie U, Nergardh A, Brun A (1979) CT-appearances of brain lesions in tuberous sclerosis and their morphological basis. Ann Radiol 22:171–183

Ramina R, Ingunza W, Vonofakis D (1980) Cystic cerebral cavernous angioma with dense calcification. J Neurosurg 52:259–262

Sackett JF, Messina AV, Petito CK (1975) Computed tomography and magnification vertebral angiotomography in the diagnosis of colloid cysts of the third ventricle. Radiology 116:95–100

Savoiardo M, Passerini A (1978) CT, angiography and RN

scans in intracranial cavernous hemangiomas. Neuroradiology 16:256–260
Suemitsu T, Nakajima SI, Kuwajima K, Nihei K, Kamostuta S (1979) Lipoma of the corpus callosum: report of a case and review of the literature. Childs Brain 5:476–483
Tadmor R, Davis KR, Roberson GH, New PFJ, Taveras JM (1977) Computed tomography in extra-dural epidermoid and xanthoma. Surg Neurol 7:371–375
Tahmouresie A, Kroll G, Shocart W (1979) Lipoma of the corpus callosum. Surg Neurol 11:31–34
Tsuchida T, Kamata K, Kawamata M, Okada K, Tanaka R, Oyake Y (1981) Brain tumors in tuberous sclerosis. Child's Brain 8:271–283
Vaquero J, Cabezudo JM, Leunda G, Carrillo R, Bravo G (1980) Intraorbital and intracranial glial hamartoma. J Neurosurg 53:117–120
Vaquero J, Manrique M, Oya S, Cabezudo JM, Bravo G (1980) Calcified telangiectatic hamartomas of the brain. Surg Neurol 13:453–457
Vonderrahe AR, Niemer WT (1944) Intracranial lipoma. J Neuropathol Exp Neurol 3:344–354
Wakai S, Segawa H, Kitahara S, Asano T, Sano K, Ogihara R, Tomita S (1980) Teratoma in the pineal region in two brothers. J Neurosurg 53:239–243
Wallace D (1976) Lipoma of the corpus callosum. J Neurol Neurosurg Psychiatry 39:1179–1185
Weaver EN Jr, Coulon RA (1979) Excision of a brain-stem epidermoid cyst. J Neurosurg 51:254–257
Willis RA (1953) Pathology of tumours. Butterworth and Co, London
Zimmerman RA, Bilaniuk LT (1979) Cranial computed tomography of epidermoid and congenital fatty tumors of maldevelopmental origin. J Comput Assist Tomogr 3:40–50

**D 7 and 8 Intracranial tumors of skeletal origin; locally invasive tumors**

Alvarez-Berdecia A, Schut L, Bruce DA (1979) Localized primary intracranial Ewing's sarcoma of the orbital roof. J Neurosurg 50:811–813
Dutton J (1978) Intracranial solitary chondroma. J Neurosurg 49:460–463
Helpap B (1978) Extraadrenale Paraganglien und Paragangliome. Normale und pathologische Anatomie, Bd 37. Georg Thieme, Stuttgart
Namba K, Aschenbrener C, Nikpour M, Van Gilder JC (1979) Primary rhabdomyosarcoma of the tentorium with peculiar angiographic findings. Surg Neurol 11:39–43

**D 9 Intracranial metastases**

Arita N, Ushio Y, Abekura M, Koshino K, Hayakawa T (1978) Embryonal carcinoma with teratomatous elements in the region of the pineal gland. Surg Neurol 9:198–202
Bardfeld P, Passalaqua AM, Braunstein P, Raghavendra BN, Leeds NE, Kricheff II (1977) A comparison of radionuclide scanning and computed tomography in metastatic lesions of the brain. J Comput Assist Tomogr 1:315–318
Butler AR, Leo JS, Lin JP, Boyd AD, Kricheff II (1979) The value of routine cranial computed tomography in neurologically intact patients with primary carcinoma of the lung. Radiology 131:399–401
Chiras J, Gueye M, Salamon G (1978) Place de la tomodensitométrie dans le diagnostic des métastases cérébrales. J Neuroradiol 5:333–349
Deck MDF Messina AV, Sackett JF (1976) Computed tomography in metastatic disease of the brain. Radiology 119:115–120
Dublin AB, Norman D (1979) Fluid-fluid level in cystic cerebral metastatic melanoma. J Comput Assist Tomogr 3:650–652
Dupont MG, Baleriaux-Waha D, Kuhn G, Bollaert A, Jeanmart L (1981) Computerized axial tomography in the diagnosis of cerebral metastases. Comput Tomogr 5:103–113
Dyment PG, Rothner AD, Duchesneau PM, Weinstein MA (1976) Computerized tomography in the detection of intracranial metastases in children. Pediatrics 58:72–77
Elke M, Hünig R, Wiggli U, Friedrich R, Müller HR, Wüthrich R (1976) The diagnosis of intracranial metastases: the efficiency of CT and scintigraphy in patients investigated by both methods. In: Lanksch W, Kazner E (eds) Cranial computerized tomography. Springer, Berlin Heidelberg New York, pp 171–176
Enzmann DR, Kramer R, Norman D, Pollock J (1978) Malignant melanoma metastatic to the central nervous system. Radiology 127:177–180
Fink LH (1979) Metastasis of prostatic adenocarcinoma simulating a falx meningioma. Surg Neurol 12:253–258
Gildersleeve Jr N, Koo AH, McDonald CJ (1977) Metastatic tumor presenting as intracerebral hemorrhage. Radiology 124:109–112
Ginaldi S, Wallace S, Shalen P, Luna M, Handel St (1980) Cranial computed tomography of malignant melanoma. AJNR 1:531–535
Greenberg HS, Deck MDF, Vikram B, Chu FCH, Posner JB (1981) Metastasis to the base of the skull: Clinical findings in 43 patients. Neurology 31:530–537
Handa J, Nakasu Y, Kamijyo Y (1980) Calcified metastatic carcinoma of the brain. Surg Neurol 14:67–70
Jones JN (1977) Unique presentation of a metastatic adenocarcinoma diagnosed pre-operatively by C.T. Scan. J Neurol 214:229–234
Kane RC (1978) Brain scans for metastasis. J Am Med Ass 239:2115–2116
Krishna Rao CVG, Govindan S (1979) Intracranial choriocarcinoma. J Comput Assist Tomogr 3:400–404
MacDonald J, Parker JC, Brown S, Page LK, Wolfe DE (1978) Cerebral metastasis from a malignant thymoma. Surg Neurol 9:58–60
Mitchell BM, Deck MDF, Rottenberg DA (1981) Pituitary metastasis: Incidence in cancer patients and clinical differentiation from pituitary adenoma. Neurology 31:998–1002
New PFJ, Scott WR, Schnur JA, Davis KR, Taveras JM, Hochberg FH (1975) Computed tomography with the EMI scanner in the diagnosis of primary and metastatic intracranial neoplasms. Radiology 114:75–87
Nosaka Y, Nagao S, Tabuchi K, Nishimoto A (1979) Primary intracranial epidermoid carcinoma. J Neurosurg 50:830–833
Percy AK, Elveback LR, Okazaki H, Kurland LT (1972) Neoplasms of the central nervous system. Neurology (Minneap) 22:40–48

Potts DG, Abbott GF, von Sneidern JV (1980) National cancer institute study: Evaluation of computed tomography in the diagnosis of intracranial neoplasms. III. Metastatic tumors. Radiology 136:657–664

Smith VC, Kasdon DL, Hardy RC (1980) Metastatic brain tumor from the prostate. Surg Neurol 14:189–191

Solis OJ, Davis KR, Adair LB, Roberson GR, Kleinman G (1977) Intracerebral metastatic melanoma: CT evaluation. Comput Tomogr 1:135–143

Weisberg LA (1979) Computerized tomography in intracranial metastases. Arch Neurol 36:630–634

## E. Base of the skull; skull vault

Becker H, Grau H, Hacker H, Ploder KW (1978) The base of the skull: A comparison of computed and conventional tomography. J Comput Assist Tomogr 2:113–118

Biller J, Heredia S, Palacios E, Fine M (1980) Malignant nasopharyngeal tumors. Surg Neurol 14:197–201

Bohman L, Mancuso A, Thompson J, Hanafee W (1980) CT approach to benign nasopharyngeal masses. AJNR 1:513–120

Bradac GB (1976) Aspects of the venous drainage dynamics with tumours at the skull base in the anterior and middle fossa. Neuroradiology 12:115–120

Bradac GB, Grumme Th, Schramm J, Simon RS (1977) Computed tomography in the study of processes affecting the base of skull. Abstracts of the 7th Congress of the European Society of Neuroradiology. Barcelona

Bradac GB, Schramm J (1981) Principles in the computed tomography study of pathologic changes of the skull base. In: Contrast Media in Computed Tomography. Ed. by Felix R, Kazner E and Wegener OH, Excerpta Medica, 171–174

Bradac GB, Schramm J, Grumme Th, Simon RS (1978) Wert und Grenzen der Computertomographie in der Studie von Prozessen der Schädelbasis. Neuroradiology 16:438–439

Bradac GB, Schramm J, Grumme Th, Simon RS (1978) CT of the Base of the skull. Neuroradiology 17:1–5

Bradac GB, Schramm J, Simon RS (1976) Angiographic findings in tumors near the skull base. Neurochirurgia 19:239–246

Bradac GB, Simon RS, Grumme Th (1977) Routine neuroradiological diagnosis with the EMI 5005 body scanner. Neuroradiology 14:133–137

Bradac GB, Simon RS, Grumme Th, Schramm J (1977) Limiations of computed tomography for diagnostic neuroradiology. Neuroradiology 13:243–247

Caillé JM, Dop A, Constant P, Renaud-Salis JL (1977) C.A.T. studies of tumours of the skull base and face. In: du Boulay GH, Moseley IF (eds) Computerised axial tomography in clinical practice. Springer, Berlin Heidelberg New York, pp 139–146

Caughran M, White TJ III, Gerald B, Gardner G (1980) Computed tomography of jugulotympanic paragangliomas. J Comput Assist Tomogr 4:194–198

Claussen CD, Wegener OH, Lochner B (1981) Computed tomography of lesions in the facial skull. In: Contrast Media in Computed Tomography. Ed. by Felix R, Kazner E and Wegener OH, Excerpta Medica, 137–142

Dop A, Constant P, Renaud Salis JL, Caillé JM (1976) Interès de la tomodensitometrie en pathologie tumorale de la base du crane et du massif facial. J Neuroradiol 3:193–214

Hammerschlag SB, Wolpert SM, Carter BL (1977) Computed tomography of the skull base. J Comput Assist Tomogr 1:75–80

Huk W, Schiefer W (1978) Computertomographie bei Prozessen der Schädelbasis und der Orbitae: Kombinierte Anwendung von Horizontal- und Frontalschnitten. Fortschr Röntgenstr 128:8–11

Ischebeck W, Thal HU, Nabakowski R (1978) Computerized tomography of the posterior fossa and the upper cervical spine. Adv Neurosurg 5:171–175

Kido DK, Gould R, Taati F, Duncan A, Schnur J (1978) Comparative sensitivity of CT scans, radiographs and radionuclide bone scans in detecting metastatic calvarial lesions. Radiology 128:371–375

Liliequist B, Forsell A (1976) Computer tomography of the neurocranium. Acta Radiol (Diagn) (Stockh) 17:399–404

Lloyd GAS, Du Boulay GH, Phelps PD, Pullicino P (1979) The demonstration of the auditory ossicles by high resolution CT. Neuroradiology 18:243–248

Lohkamp F, Claussen C (1977) Computertomographie des Gesichtsschädels (Teil I). Darstellbarkeit bestimmter Strukturen und tiefliegender Regionen. Fortschr Röntgenstr 126:292–299

Lohkamp F, Claussen C, Spenneberg H (1977) Computertomographie des Gesichtsschädels (Teil II). Pathologische Veränderungen. Fortschr Röntgenstr 126:513–520

Lucarelli G, Fornari M, Savoiardo M (1980) Angiography and computerized tomography in the diagnosis of aneurysmal bone cyst of the skull. J Neurosurg 53:113–116

Manelfe C, Rochiccioli P (1979) CT of septo-optic dysplasia. Am J Roentgenol 133:1157–1160

Marsman JWP (1979) Tumors of the glomus jugulare complex (chemodectomas) demonstrated by cranial computed tomography. J Comput Assist Tomogr 3:795–799

Mitnick JS, Pinto RS (1980) Computed tomography in the diagnosis of eosinophilic granuloma. J Comput Assist Tomogr 4:791–793

Mödder U, Friedmann G, Gode A, Rose KG (1979) Computertomographie des Gesichtsschädels und des pharyngealen Raumes. Roentgenforschung 131:249–256

Osborn AG, Anderson RW, Wing SD (1980) Sagittal CT scans in the evaluation of deep facial and nasopharyngeal lesions. CT, J Comput Tomogr 1:19–24

Parsons C, Hodson N (1979) Computed tomography of paranasal sinus tumors. Radiology 132:641–645

Schindler E, Aulich A, Wende S (1978) Value and limits of computerized axial tomography in ORL. Adv Otorhino-laryngol 24:9–20

Schwartz ChW (1940) Cranial osteomas from a roentgenologic viewpoint. Am J Roentgenol 44:188–196

Som PM, Shugar JMA (1980) The CT classification of ethmoid mucoceles. J Comput Assist Tomogr 4:199–203

Weinstein AM, Levine H, Duchesneau P, Tucker HM (1978) Diagnosis of juvenile angiofibroma by computed tomography. Radiology 126:703

Wende S, Kazner E, Grumme Th (1979) Die radiologische Diagnostik von Läsionen der Schädelbasis, der hinteren Schädelgrube und der Orbita. In: Sager W-D, Ladurner G (Hrsg) Computertomographie. Derzeitige Stellung in Radiologie und Klinik. Thieme, Stuttgart, S 13–21

Wiggli UME, Müller HR, Hünig R, Wüthrich R (1976)

Analysis of osseous structures of the skull base. In: Lanksch W, Kazner E (eds) Cranial computerized tomography. Springer, Berlin Heidelberg New York, pp 399–402

Zimmerman RA, Bilaniuk LT (1977) Computed tomography of sphenoid sinus tumors. J Comput Assist Tomogr 1:22–32

## F. Nonneoplastic space-occupying intracranial lesions

### General surveys

Grumme Th (1981) Nontumorous intracranial lesions. In: Contrast Media in Computed Tomography. Ed. by Felix R, Kazner E and Wegener OH, Excerpta Medica, 123–129

Kazner E, Klein W, Stochdorph O (1978) Möglichkeiten und Aussagewert der Computertomographie bei nicht tumorbedingten raumfordernden intrakraniellen Prozessen. Roentgenpraxis 31:181–198

Ruggiero G, Sabattini L (1976) La tomographie axiale avec ordinateur dans les maladies non tumorales. J Neuroradiol 3:313–330

Williams RG, Osborn AG (1980) Low-attenuation lesions in the middle cranial fossa: differential diagnosis. J Comput Assist Tomogr 4:89–97

### F 1 Inflammatory processes

Allo MD, Silva J, Kauffman CA, Dicks RE III (1979) Enlarging histoplasmomas following treatment of meningitis due to histoplasma capsulatum. J Neurosurg 51:242–244

Aulich A, Lange S, Steinhoff H, Schindler E, Wende S (1976) Diagnosis and follow-up studies in brain abscesses using CT. In: Lanksch W, Kazner E (eds) Cranial computerized tomography. Springer, Berlin Heidelberg New York, pp 366–371

Bilaniuk LT, Zimmerman RA, Brown L, Yoo HJ, Goldberg HI (1978) Computed tomography in meningitis. Neuroradiology 16:13–14

Brismar J, Roberson GH, Davis KR (1976) Radiation necrosis of the brain. Neuroradiological considerations with computed tomography. Neuroradiology 12:109–113

Brückner O, Kluge W (1981) Intracranial tuberculous abscess mimicking pyogenic brain abscess. Neurochirurgia 24:147–149

Buge A, Metzger J, Rancurel G, Gardeur D, Eohanno F, Pertuiset BF (1979) Les aspects tomodensitometriques (C.T. Scan) des encephalites aigues necrosantes herpetiques (7 cas) premieres tentatives therapeutiques par l'isoprinosine. Rev Neurol 135:401–416

Byrne E, Brophy BP, Perrett LV (1979) Nocardia cerebral abscess: new concepts in diagnosis, management and prognosis. J Neurol Neurosurg Psychiatry 42:1038–1045

Chiu LC, Jensen JC, Cornell SH, Christie JH (1977) Computerized tomography of brain abscess. J Comput Assist Tomogr 1:33–38

Claveria LE, Du Boulay GH, Moseley LF (1976) Intracranial infections: investigation by computerized axial tomography. Neuroradiology 12:59–71

Cockrill HH Jr, Dreisbach J, Lowe B, Yamauchi T (1978) Computed tomography in leptomeningeal infections. Am J Roentgenol 130:511–515

Danziger A, Price H, Schechter MM (1980) An analysis of 113 intracranial infections. Neuroradiology 19:31–34

Davis JM, Davis KR, Kleinman GM, Kirchner HS, Taveras JM (1978) Computed tomography of herpes simplex encephalitis, with clinicopathological correlation. Radiology 129:409–417

Enzmann DR, Brant-Zawadzki M, Britt RH (1980) CT of central nervous system infections in immunocompromised patients. AJNR 1:239–243

Enzmann DR, Britt RH, Yeager AS (1979) Experimental brain abscess evolution: computed tomographic and neuropathologic correlation. Radiology 133:113–122

Enzmann DR, Norman D, Mani J, Newton ThH (1976) Computed tomography of granulomatous basal arachnoiditis. Radiology 120:341–344

Enzmann DR, Ranson B, Norman D, Talberth E (1978) Computed tomography of herpes simplex encephalitis. Radiology 129:419–425

Fry VG, Young CN (1981) A rare fungal brain abscess in an uncompromised host. Surg Neurol 15:446–449

Joubert MJ, Stephanov S (1977) Computerized tomography and surgical treatment in intracranial suppuration. J Neurosurg 47:73–78

Kaufman DM, Leeds NE (1977) Computed tomography (CT) in the diagnosis of intracranial abscesses. Brain abscess, subdural empyema and epidural empyema. Neurology (Minneap) 27:1069–1073

Kazner E (1976) Effects of computerized axial tomography on the treatment of cerebral abscess. Neuroradiology 12:57–58

Kirmani N, Tuazon CU, Ocuin JA, Thompson AM, Kramer NC, Geelhoed GW (1978) Extensive cerebral nocardiosis cured with antibiotic therapy alone. J Neurosurg 49:924–928

Kummer R v, Storch B, Rauch H, Krause KH (1981) Computertomographische Verlaufsbeobachtung multipler cerebraler Tuberkulome. Nervenarzt 52:344–347

Leo JS, Weiner RL, Lin JP, Ransohoff J (1978) Computed tomography in herpes simplex encephalitis. Surg Neurol 10:313–317

Long JrJA, Herdt JR, DiChiro G, Cramer HR (1980) Cerebral mass lesions in torulosis demonstrated by computed tomography. J Comput Assist Tomogr 4:766–769

Luken MG III, Whelan MA (1980) Recent diagnostic experience with subdural empyema J Neurosurg 52:764–771

Messina AV, Guido LJ, Liebeskind AL (1977) Preoperative diagnosis of brain-stem abscess by computerized tomography with survival. J Neurosurg 47:106–108

Mikhael MA (1978) Radiation necrosis of the brain: correlation between computed tomography, pathology and dose distribution. J Comput Assist Tomogr 2:71–80

Mikhael MA (1979) Radiation necrosis of the brain: Correlation between pattern on computed tomography and dose of radiation. J Comput Assist Tomogr 3:241–249

Mineury K, Mori T (1980) Sparganosis of the brain. J Neurosurg 52:588–590

Moseley IF, Claveria LE, du Boulay GH (1977) Diseases of the brain parenchyma, atrophy and hydrocephalus. The role of C.A.T. in the diagnosis and management of intracranial infection. In: du Boulay GH, Moseley IF (eds) Computerised axial tomography in clinical practice. Springer, Berlin Heidelberg New York, pp 182–190

Moussa AH, Dawson BH (1978) Computed tomography

and the mortality rate in brain abscess. Surg Neurol 10:301–304

New PFJ, Davis KR, Ballantine HT (1976) Computed tomography in cerebral abscess. Radiology 121:641–646

Nielsen H, Gyldensted C (1977) Computed tomography in the diagnosis of cerebral abscess. Neuroradiology 12:207–217

Probst FP (1980) Non-pyogenic focal encephalitis diagnosis and follow-up by computed tomography and nuclear brain scanning. Neuroradiology 20:155–158

Reisner Th (1979) Die Bedeutung der kranialen Computertomographie in der Differentialdiagnose entzündlicher Erkrankungen des Gehirns. In: Sager W-D, Ladurner G (eds): Computertomographie. Thieme, Stuttgart, S 74–78

Rosenblum ML, Hoff JT, Norman D, Edwards MS, Berg BO (1980) Nonoperative treatment of brain abscesses in selected high-risk patients. J Neurosurg 52:217–225

Rosenblum ML, Hoff JT, Norman D, Weinstein PR, Pitts L (1978) Decreased mortality from brain abscesses since advent of computerized tomography. J Neurosurg 49:658–668

Rovira M, Romero F, Torrent O, Ibarra B (1980) Study of tuberculous meningitis by CT. Neuroradiology 19:137–141

Sadhu VK, Handel SF, Pinto RS, Glass TF (1980) Neuroradiologic diagnosis of subdural empyema and CT limitations. AJNR 1:39–44

Schiefer W, Huk W (1976) Computerized tomographic findings with brain abscesses. In: Lanksch W, Kazner E (eds) Cranial computerized tomography. Springer, Berlin Heidelberg New York, pp 360–365

Schiefer W, Klinger M (1978) Aspects of modern brain abscess diagnosis and treatment. Neurosurg Rev 1/2:37–45

Schochet SS, Sarwar M, Kelly PJ, Masel BE (1980) Symptomatic cerebral histoplasmoma. J Neurosurg 52:273–275

Stephanov S (1978) Experience with multiloculated brain abscesses. J Neurosurg 49:199–203

Stephanov S, Joubert MJ, Welchmann JM (1979) Combined convexity and parafalx subdural empyema. Surg Neurol 11:147–151

Stevens EA, Norman D, Kramer RA, Messina AB, Newton ThH (1978) Computed tomographic brain scanning in intraparenchymal pyogenic abscesses. Am J Roentgenol 130:111–114

Tamaka R, Takeda N, Okada K, Ueki K (1979) Computerized tomography of coagulation necrosis of the brain and brain tumors. Surg Neurol 11:9–12

Thomson JLG (1976) The computed axial tomograph in acute herpes simplex encephalitis. Br J Radiol 49:86–87

Tress B, Davis S (1979) Computed tomography of intracerebral toruloma. Neuroradiology 17:223–226

Tully RJ, Watts C (1979) Computed tomography and intracranial aspergillosis. Neuroradiology 17:111–113

Whelan MA, Hilal SK (1980) Computed tomography as a guide in the diagnosis and follow-up of brain abscesses. Radiology 135:663–671

Whelan MA, Stern J (1981) Sarcoidosis presenting as a posterior fossa mass. Surg Neurol 15:455–457

Zimmerman RA, Bilaniuk LT (1980) CT of orbital infection and its cerebral complications. Am J Roentgenol 134:45–50

Zimmerman RA, Patel S, Bilaniuk LT (1976) Demonstration of purulent bacterial intracranial infections by computed tomography. Am J Roentgenol 127:155–165

**F 2 Acute demyelinating diseases**

Cala LA, Mastaglia FL, Black JL (1978) Computerized tomography of brain and optic nerve in multiple sclerosis. Observations in 100 patients, including serial studies in 16. J Neurol Sci 36:411, 426

Di Chiro G, Arimitsu T, Brooks RA, Morgenthaler DG, Johnston GS, Jones E, Keller MR (1979) Computed tomography profiles of periventricular hypodensity in hydrocephalus and leukoencephalopathy. Radiology 130:661–666

Eiben RM, Di Chiro G (1977) Computer assisted tomography in adrenoleukodystrophy. J Comput Assist Tomogr 1:308–314

Furuse M, Obayashi T, Tsuji S, Miyatake T (1978) Adrenoleukodystrophy. A correlative analysis of computed tomography and radionuclide studies. Radiology 126:707–710

Gyldensted C (1976) Computer tomography of the cerebrum in multiple sclerosis. Neuroradiology 12:33–42

Hall K, Gardner-Medwin D (1978) CT scan appearances in Leigh's disease (subacute necrotizing encephalomyelopathy). Neuroradiology 16:48–50

Harding AE, Radue EW, Whiteley AM (1978) Contrast-enhanced lesions on computerised tomography in multiple sclerosis. J Neurol Neurosurg Psychiatry 41:754–758

Haughton VM, Ho KCh, Williams AL, Eldevik OP (1979) CT detection of demyelinated plaques in multiple sclerosis. Am J Roentgenol 132:213–215

Heinz ER, Drayer BP, Haenggeli CA, Painter MJ, Crumrine P (1979) Computed tomography in white-matter disease. Radiology 130:371–378

Huckman MS, Fox JH, Ramsey RG (1977) Computed tomography in the diagnosis of degenerative diseases of the brain. Semin Roentgenol 12:63–75

Lane B, Carroll BA, Pedley TA (1978) Computerized cranial tomography in cerebral diseases of white matter. Neurology 28:534–544

Radue EW, Kendall BE (1978) Iodine and xenon enhancement of computed tomography (CT) in multiple sclerosis (MS). Neuroradiology 15:153–158

Taboada D, Alonso A, Olagüe R, Mulas F, Andrés V (1980) Radiological diagnosis of periventricular and subcortical leukomalacia. Neuroradiology 20:33–41

Tritschler JL, Delouvrier JJ, Masson M, Nahum H, Cambier J (1979) Apport de la tomodensitometrie cerebrale au diagnostic de la sclerose en plaques. Rev Neurol 135:455–466

Weinstein MA, Lederman RJ, Rothner AD, Duchesneau PM, Norman D (1978) Interval computed tomography in multiple sclerosis. Radiology 129:689–694

Wüthrich R, Gigli H, Wiggli U, Müller HR, Elke M, Hünig R (1976) CT scanning in demyelinating diseases. In: Lanksch W, Kazner E (eds) Cranial computerized tomography. Springer, Berlin Heidelberg New York, pp 239–243

**F 3 Granulomas**

Decker RE, Mardayat M, Marc J, Rasool A (1979) Neurosarcoidosis with computerized tomographic visualization and transsphenoidal excision of a supra- and intrasellar granuloma. Case report. J Neurosurg 50:814–816

Hirsh LF, Lee SH, Silberstein StD (1978) Intracranial tuberculomas and the CAT scan. Acta Neurochir (Wien) 45:155–161

Leibrock L, Epstein MH, Rybock JD (1976) Cerebral tuberculoma localized by EMI Scan. Surg Neurol 5:305–306

Peatfield RC, Shawelon HH (1979) Five cases of intracranial tuberculoma followed by serial computerised tomography. J Neurol Neurosurg Psychiat 42:373–379

Price HI, Danziger A (1978) Computed tomography in cranial tuberculosis. Am J Roentgenol 130:769–771

Szper J, Oi S, Leestma J, Kim KS, Wetzel NE (1979) Xanthogranuloma of the third ventricle. J Neurosurg 51:565–568

Terao H, Kobayashi S, Teraoka A, Okeda R (1978) Xanthogranulomas of the choroid plexus in a neuroepileptic child. J Neurosurg 48:649–653

Welchman JM (1979) Computerised tomography of intracranial tuberculomata. Clin Radiol 30:567–573

### F4 Cysts

Anderson FM, Segall HD, Caton WL (1979) Use of computerized tomography scanning in supratentorial arachnoid cysts. J Neurosurg 50:333–338

Archer CR, Darwish H, Smith K Jr (1978) Enlarged cisternae magnae and posterior fossa cysts simulating Dandy-Walker syndrome on computed tomography. Radiology 127:681–686

Averback P (1977) Developmental arachnoid cysts of the posterior fossa – an analysis of 13 cases. Acta Neurochir (Wien) 39:181–186

Di Rocco C, Di Trapani G, Janelli A (1979) Arachnoid cyst of the fourth ventricle and "arrested" hydrocephalus. Surg Neurol 12:467–471

Drayer BP, Rosenbaum AE, Maroon JC, Bank WO, Woodford JE (1977) Posterior fossa extraaxial cyst: Diagnosis with Metrizamide CT cisternography. Am J Roentgenol 128:431–436

Galassi E, Piazzi G, Gaist G, Frank F (1980) Arachnoid cysts of the middle cranial fossa: a clinical and radiological study of 25 cases treated surgically. Surg Neurol 14:211–219

Geissinger JD, Kohler WC, Robinson BW, Davis FM (1978) Arachnoid cysts of the middle cranial fossa: surgical considerations. Surg Neurol 10:27–33

Gregorius FK, Batzdorf U (1976) Diagnosis of intrathalamic cyst by computerized tomographic scan. Surg Neurol 6:191–193

Handa J, Nakano Y, Aii H (1977) CT cisternography with intracranial arachnoidal cysts. Surg Neurol 8:451–454

Handa J, Okamoto K, Sato M (1981) Arachnoid cyst of the middle cranial fossa: Report of bilateral cysts in siblings. Surg Neurol 16:127–130

Hayashi T, Anegawa S, Honda E, Kuramoto S, Mori K, Murata T, Miwa S, Handa W (1979) Clinical analysis of arachnoid cysts in the middle fossa. Neurochirurgia 22:201–210

Hayashi T, Kuratomi A, Kuromoto S (1980) Arachnoid cyst of the quadrigeminal cistern. Surg Neurol 14:267–273

Kasdon DL, Douglas EA, Brougham MF (1977) Suprasellar arachnoid cyst diagnosed preoperatively by computerized tomographic scanning. Surg Neurol 7:299–303

MacGregor BJL, Gawler J, South JR (1976) Intracranial epithelial cysts. J Neurosurg 44:109–115

Markakis E, Heyer R, Stoeppler L, Werry H (1979) Die Aplasie der perisylviischen Region. Neurochirurgia (Stuttg) 22:211–220

Markwalder T-M, Zimmermann A (1979) Intracerebral ciliated epithelial cyst. Surg Neurol 11:195–198

Murali R, Epstein F (1979) Diagnosis and treatment of suprasellar arachnoid cyst. J Neurosurg 50:515–518

Palma L, Di Lorenzo N, Nicole S (1979) Developmental CSF cysts of the posterior fossa. Neurosurg Rev 2:159–169

Rengachary SS, Watanabe I, Brackett CE (1978) Pathogenesis of intracranial arachnoid cyst. Surg Neurol 9:139–144

Silverberg GD (1971) Simple cysts of the cerebellum. J Neurosurg 35:320–327

Scolt LC, Deck JHN, Baim RC, Terbrugge K (1980) Interhemispheric cyst of neuroepithelial origin in association with partial agenesis of the corpus callosum. J Neurosurg 52:399–405

Vaquero J, Carrillo R, Cabezudo JM, Nombela L, Bravo G (1981) Arachnoid cysts of the posterior fossa. Surg Neurol 16:117–121

Yeates A, Enzmann D (1979) An intraventricular arachnoid cyst. J Comput Assist Tomogr 3:697–700

### F5 Parasites

Abassioun K, Rahmat H, Ameli NO, Tafazuli M (1978) Computerized tomography in hydatid cyst of the brain. J Neurosurg 49:408–411

Bentson JR, Wilson GH, Helmer E, Winter J (1977) Computed tomography in intracranial cysticercosis. J Comput Assist Tomogr 1:464–471

Camas E, Esterez J, Soto M, Obrador S (1978) Computerized axial tomography for the diagnosis of cerebral cysticercosis. Acta Neurochir (Wien) 44:197–205

Jankowski R, Zimmerman RD, Leeds NE (1979) Cysticercosis presenting as a mass lesion at foramen of Monro. J Comput Assist Tomogr 3:694–696

Latovitzki N, Abrams G, Clark C, Mayeux R, Ascherl G jr, Sciara D (1978) Cerebral cysticercosis. Neurology (Minneap) 28:838–842

Zee C, Segall HD, Miller C, Tsai FY, Teal JS, Hieshima G, Ahmadi J, Halls J (1980) Unusual neuroradiological features of intracranial cysticercosis. Radiology 137:397–407

### F6, 7 and 8 Intracranial hematomas, vascular malformations, brain infarction

Aarabi B, Chambers J (1978) Giant thrombosed aneurysm associated with an arteriovenous malformation. J Neurosurg 49:278–282

Amendola MA, Ostrum BJ (1977) Diagnosis of isodense subdural hematomas by computed tomography. Am J Roentgenol 129:693–697

Aulich A, Fenske A (1977) Das Computertomogramm des Schlaganfalles. Akt neurol 4:129–140

Aulich A, Wende S, Kazner E, Lanksch W, Steinhoff H, Grumme Th, Lange S, Meese W (1978) Computerized axial tomography for diagnosis and follow-up studies of cerebral infarcts and the development of brain edema. In: Bories J (ed) The diagnostic limitations of computerized axial tomography. Springer, Berlin Heidelberg New York, pp 105–109

Babu VS, Eisen H (1979) Giant aneurysm of anterior com-

municating artery simulating 3rd ventricular tumor. Comput Tomogr 3:159–163
Bannister CM, Weller J (1980) Pre- and post-operative CT scans of an infant with an aneurysm of the vein of Galen – a case report. Neurochirurgia 23:17–20
Britt RH, Silverberg GD, Enzmann DR, Hanbery JW (1980) Third ventricular choroid plexus arteriovenous malformation simulating a colloid cyst. J Neurosurg 52:246–250
Byrd SH, Bentson JR, Winter J, Wilson GH, Joyce PW, O'Connor L (1978) Giant intracranial aneurysms simulating brain neoplasms on computed tomography. J Comput Assist Tomogr 2:303–307
Campbell JK, Houser OW, Stevens JC, Wahner HW, Baker HL, Folger WN (1978) Computed tomography and radionuclide imaging in the evaluation of ischemic stroke. Radiology 126:695–702
Coin CG, Coin JW, Glover MB (1977) Vascular tumors of the choroid plexus: diagnosis by computed tomography. J Comput Assist Tomogr 1:146–148
Cone JD, Maravilla KR, Cooper PR, Diehl JT, Clark WK (1979) Computed tomography findings in ruptured arteriovenous malformations of the corpus callosum. J Comput Assist Tomogr 3:478–482
Daniels DL, Haughton VM, Williams AL, Strother ChM (1979) Arteriovenous malformation simulating a cyst on computed tomography. Radiology 133:393–394
Deeb JL, Jannetta PJ, Rosenbaum AE, Kerber CW, Drayer BP (1979) Tortuous vertebrobasilar arteries causing cranial nerve syndromes: screening by computed tomography. J Comput Assist Tomogr 3:774–778
Diebler C, Dulac O, Renier D, Ernest C, Lalande G (1981) Aneurysms of the vein of Galen in infants aged 2 to 15 months. Diagnosis and natural evolution. Neuroradiology 21:185–197
Di Tullio MV, Stern WE (1979) Hemangioma calcificans. J Neurosurg 50:110–114
Dhopesh VP, Greenberg JO, Cohen MM (1980) Computed tomography in brainstem hemorrhage. J Comput Assist Tomogr 4:603–607
Fierstien SB, Pribram HW, Hieshima G (1979) Angiography and computed tomography in the evaluation of cerebral venous malformations. Neuroradiology 17:137–148
Golden JB, Kramer RA (1978) The angiographically occult cerebrovascular malformation. J Neurosurg 48:292–296
Greenhouse AH, Barr JW (1979) The bilateral isodense subdural hematoma on computerized tomographic scan. Arch Neurol 36:305–307
Grumme Th, Lanksch W, Aulich A (1976) The diagnosis of chronic subdural hematoma by computerized axial tomography. In: Lanksch W, Kazner E (eds) Cranial computerized tomography. Springer, Berlin Heidelberg New York, pp 337–341
Grumme Th, Lanksch W, Kazner E, Aulich A, Meese W, Lange S, Steinhoff H, Wende S (1976) Zur Diagnose des chronischen subduralen Hämatoms im Computertomogramm. Neurochirurgia 19:95–103
Grumme Th, Lanksch W, Wende S (1976) Diagnosis of spontaneous intracerebral hemorrhage by computerized tomography. In: Lanksch W, Kazner E (eds) Cranial computerized tomography. Springer, Berlin Heidelberg New York, pp 284–290
Hammer B (1979) Computertomographische Diagnose der Megadolichobasilaris. Fortschr Röntgenstr 131:255–261
Handa J, Nakano Y, Aii H, Handa H (1978) Computed tomography with giant intracranial aneurysms. Surg Neurol 9:257–263
Handa J, Nakano Y, Okuno T, Komuro H, Handa H (1977) Computerized tomography in Moyamoya syndrome. Surg Neurol 7:315–319
Hayman LA, Fox AJ, Evans RA (1981) Effectiveness of contrast regimens in CT detection of vascular malformations of the brain. AJNR 2:421–425
Hayward RD (1976) Intracranial arteriovenous malformations. Observations after experience with computerised tomography. J Neurol Neurosurg Psychiatry 39:1027–1033
Humphreys RP (1978) Computerized tomographic definition of mesencephalic hematoma with evacuation through pedunculotomy. J Neurosurg 49:749–752
Jones JN, Schwarz HJ (1977) Two cases of giant intracerebral aneurysm simulating neoplasm on CT scan; one with coexistent chronic subdural hematoma. J Neurol 215:49–57
Kazner E (1979) Die Bedeutung der Computertomographie für die Diagnose und Differentialdiagnose zerebraler Durchblutungsstörungen. Neurol Psychiat 5:312–324
Kazner E, Lanksch W (1979) CAT findings in cerebral aneurysms and subarachnoid haemorrhage. In: Pia HW, Langmaid C, Zierski I (eds) Cerebral aneurysms. Springer, Berlin Heidelberg New York, pp 184–190
Kazner E, Lanksch W, Grumme Th, Kretzschmar K (1980) Diagnosis and differential diagnosis of spontaneous ICH with CT scan. In: Pia HW, Langmaid C, Zierski J (eds) Spontaneous intracerebral haematomas. Advances in diagnosis and therapy. Springer, Berlin Heidelberg New York, pp 178–190
Kendall BE, Claveria LE (1976) The use of computed axial tomography (CAT) for the diagnosis and management of intracranial angiomas. Neuroradiology 12:141–160
Kendall BE, Claveria LE (1977) The use of computerised axial tomography (C.A.T.) for the diagnosis and management of intracranial angiomas. In: du Boulay GH, Moseley IF (eds) Computerised axial tomography in clinical practice. Springer, Berlin Heidelberg New York, pp 261–271
Lanksch W, Grumme Th, Kazner E (1978) Schädelhirnverletzungen im Computertomogramm. Springer, Berlin Heidelberg New York
Leblanc R, Ethier R, Little JR (1979) Computerized tomography findings in arteriovenous malformations of the brain. J Neurosurg 51:765–772
Macpherson P, Teasdale GM, Lindsay KW (1979) Computed tomography in diagnosis and management of aneurysm of the vein of Galen. J Neurol Neurosurg Psychiatry 42:786–789
Maehara T, Tasaka A (1978) Cerebral venous angioma: computerized tomography and angiographic diagnosis. Neuroradiology 16:296–298
Maki Y, Semba A (1979) Computed tomography of Sturge-Weber-disease. Childs Brain 5:51–61
Marcu H, Becker H (1977) Computed tomography of bilateral isodense chronic subdural hematomas. Neuroradiology 14:81–83
Marshall WH, Easter W, Zatz LM (1977) Analysis of the dense lesion at computed tomography with dual kVp scans. Radiology 124:87–89
Martelli A, Scotti G, Harwood-Nash DC, Fitz CR, Chuang

SH (1980) Aneurysms of the vein of Galen in children: CT and angiographic correlations. Neuroradiology 20:123–133

Mauersberger W (1978) Vascular deformity of the basilar artery which gave the clinical and computerized impression of a tumor. Adv Neurosurg 5:176–178

McDavid WD, Waggener RG, Sank VJ, Dennis MJ, Payne WH (1977) Correlating computed tomographic numbers with physical properties and operating kilovoltage. Radiology 123:761–762

Meese W, Aulich A, Kazner E, Wüllenweber R (1976) CT findings in angiomas and aneurysms. In: Lanksch W, Kazner E (eds) Cranial computerized tomography. Springer, Berlin Heidelberg New York, S 291–297

Meese W, Aulich A, Kazner E, Wüllenweber R (1976) CT findings in angiomas and aneurysms. In: Lanksch W, Kazner E (eds) Cranial computerized tomography. Springer, Berlin Heidelberg New York, pp 291–297

Messina AV (1976) Computed tomography: contrast media within subdural hematomas. A preliminary report. Radiology 119:725–726

Michels LG, Bentson JR, Winter J (1977) Computed tomography of cerebral venous angiomas. J Comput Assist Tomogr 1:149–154

Moseley IF, Holland IM (1979) Ectasia of the basilar artery: the breadth of the clinical spectrum and the diagnostic value of computed tomography. Neuroradiology 18:83–91

Müller HR, Wiggli U (1977) Cerebral, cerebellar and pontine haemorrhages. In: du Boulay GH, Moseley IF (eds) Computerised axial tomography in clinical practice. Springer, Berlin Heidelberg New York, pp 249–254

Müke R, Kühne D (1978) Diagnostic errors in computerized tomography in the differential diagnosis of cerebrovascular lesions. Adv Neurosurg 6:115–124

Nadjmi M, Ratzka M, Wodarz M (1978) Giant aneurysms in CT and angiography. Neuroradiology 16:284–286

Norman D (1977) Computed tomography in intracranial hemorrhage. In: Norman D, Korobkin M, Newton ThH (eds) Computed tomography 1977. The CV Mosby Comp, St Louis

Olteanu-Nerbe V, Schmiedek P, Kazner E, Lanksch W, Marguth F (1976) Comparison of regional cerebral blood flow and computerized tomography in patients with cerebrovascular disease and brain tumors. In: Lanksch W, Kazner E (eds) Cranial computerized tomography. Springer, Berlin Heidelberg New York, pp 305–308

Ostertag ChB, Mundinger F (1978) Diagnostic errors in the interpretation of cerebral infarction. Adv Neurosurg 6:86–93

Peterson NT, Duchesneau PM, Westbrook EL, Weinstein MA (1977) Basilar artery ectasia demonstrated by computed tomography. Radiology 122:713–715

Petit-Perrin D, Aubin ML, Vignaud J (1979) Apport de la scanographie au diagnostic des anéurysmes géants intra-crâniens. J Neuroradiol 6:317–326

Phelps ME, Kuhl DE (1976) Pitfalls in the measurements of cerebral blood volume with computed tomography. Radiology 121:375–377

Pia HW (1980) Large and giant aneurysms. Neurosurg Rev 3:7–16

Pia HW, Langmaid C, Zierski J (1980) Spontaneous intracerebral haematomas. Advances in diagnosis and therapy. Springer, Berlin Heidelberg New York

Pinto RS, Kricheff II, Butler AR, Murali R (1979) Correlation of computed tomographic, angiographic and neuropathological changes in giant cerebral aneurysms. Radiology 132:85–92

Pressman BD, Gilbert GE, Davis DO (1975) Computerized transverse tomography of vascular lesions of the brain. Part II: Aneurysms. Am J Roentgenol 124:215–219

Pressman BD, Kirkwood JR, Davis DO (1975) Computerized transverse tomography of vascular lesions of the brain. Part I: Arteriovenous malformations. Am J Roentgenol 124:208–214

Sager WD, Ladurner G (1979) Klassifikation und Verlauf des Hirninfarktes im Computertomogramm. Fortschr Röntgenstr 131:470–475

Sartor K (1978) Spontaneous closure of cerebral arteriovenous malformation demonstrated by angiography and computed tomography. Neuroradiology 15:95–98

Schubiger O, Valavanis A, Hayek J (1980) Computed tomography in cerebral aneurysms with special emphasis on giant intracranial aneurysms. J Comput Assist Tomogr 4:24–32

Schumacher M, Stoeter P, Voigt K (1980) Computertomographische Diagnose und Differentialdiagnose cerebraler Gefäßmißbildungen. Radiologe 10:91–104

Scotti G, Terbrugge K, Melançon D, Bélanger G (1977) Evaluation of the age of subdural hematomas by computerized tomography. J Neurosurg 47:311–315

Shirkhoda A, Whaley RA, Boone SC, Scatliff JH, Schnapf D (1981) Varied CT appearance of aneurysms of the vein of Galen in infancy. Neuroradiol 21:265–270

Soeur M, Brihaye J, Moerman C (1979) Pseudo-tumoural aneurysm in the third ventricle: report of three cases. Acta Neurochir (Wien) 45:247–258

Spallone A (1979) Computed tomography in aneurysms of the vein of Galen. J Comput Assist Tomogr 3:779–782

Sundt TM Jr, Piepgras DG (1979) Surgical approach to giant intracranial aneurysms. Operative experience with 80 cases. J Neurosurg 51:731–742

Terao H, Ikeda A, Kobayashi S, Teraoka A (1978) A thrombosed giant aneurysm of the internal carotid artery with brain stem displacement. Surg Neurol 10:157–168

Terbrugge K, Scotti G, Ethier R, Melancon D, Tchang S, Milner C (1977) Computed tomography in intracranial arteriovenous malformations. Radiology 122:703–705

Tsai FY, Huprich JE, Segall HD, Teal JS (1979) The contrast-enhanced CT scan in the diagnosis of isodense subdural hematoma. J Neurosurg 50:64–69

Ventureyra ECG, Choo SH, Benoit B (1980) Super giant globoid intracranial aneurysm in an infant. J Neurosurg 53:411–416

Ventureyra ECG, Ivan LP (1979) Venous malformation of the pineal region. Surg Neurol 11:225–228

Weisberg LA (1980) Peripheral rim enhancement in supratentorial intracerebral hematoma. Comput Tomogr 4:145–154

Wilson JL, Moseley IF (1977) A diagnostic approach to cerebellar lesions. In: du Boulay GH, Moseley IF (eds) Computerized axial tomography in clinical practice. Springer, Berlin Heidelberg New York, pp 123–131

Wüllenweber R, zum Winkel K, Grumme Th, Lange S, Meese W (1976) Differentialdiagnose des Schlaganfalles

im Computertomogramm. Neurochirurgia (Stuttg) 19:1–19
Yock DH, Marshall WH (1975) Recent ischemic brain infarcts and computed tomography: Appearances pre- and post contrast infusion. Radiology 117:599–608
Yock D, Norman D, Newton ThH (1978) Pitfalls in the diagnosis of ichaemic cerebral infarcts by computed tomography. In: Bories J (ed) The diagnostic limitations of computerised axial tomography. Springer, Berlin Heidelberg New York, pp 90–104
Zatz LM (1976) The effect of the kVp level on EMI-values. Radiology 119:683–688
Zimmerman RA, Bilaniuk LT (1978) Computed tomography of vertebrobasilar artery aneurysm. J Comput Assist Tomogr 2:39–49
Zimmerman RA, Bilaniuk LT (1979) Computed tomography of choroid plexus lesions. J Comput Assist Tomogr 3:93–103

## G. Orbital lesions

Ambrose J (1973) Computerized transverse axial scanning (tomography): Part 2. Clinical application. Br J Radiol 46:1023–1047
Ambrose J, Lloyd GAS, Wright JE (1974) A preliminary evaluation of fine matrix computerized axial tomography (EMI scan) in the diagnosis of orbital space-occupying lesions. Br J Radiol 47:747–751
Ambrose J (1975) New techniques in the investigations of the orbit. Trans Opthalmol Soc UK 95:233
Aronow S, Kadir S (1976) In vitro evaluation of the detectability of intra-orbital foreign bodies. In: Symposium on Computer Assisted Tomography in Nontumoral Diseases of the Brain, Spinal Cord and Eye. National Institute of Health, Bethesda, Maryland, October 11–15
Baker HL, Kearns ThP, Campell JK, Henderson JW (1974) Computerized transaxial tomography in neuroophthalmology. Am J Ophthalmol 78:285–294
Baleriaux-Waha D, Mortelmans LL, Dupont MG, Terwinghe G, Jeanmart L (1977) The use of coronal scans for computed tomography of the orbits. Neuroradiology 14:89–96
Bergström K (1975) Computer tomography of the orbits. Acta Radiol [Suppl] (Stockh) 346:155–160
Bergström K, Dahlin H, Gustafsson M, Nylen O (1972) Eye lens doses in carotid angiography. Acta Radiol Diagn 12:134
Brant-Zawadzki M, Enzmann DR (1979) Orbital computed tomography: calcific densities of posterior globe. J Comput Assist Tomogr 3:503–508
Brismar J, Davis KR, Dallow RL, Brismar G (1976) Unilateral endocrine exophthalmos. Diagnostic problems in association with computed tomography. Neuroradiology 12:21–24
Bull JWD (1975) The changing face of neuroradiology over nearly forty years. Neuroradiology 9:111–115
Buschmann W, Linnert D (1978) Zusammenwirken von Ultraschalldiagnostik und Röntgen-Computertomographie bei raumfordernden Orbitaprozessen. Klin Monatsbl Augenheilkd 173:155–170
Byrd SE, Harwood-Nash DC, Fitz CR, Barry JF, Rogovitz DM (1978) Computed tomography of intraorbital optic nerve gliomas in children. Radiology 129:73–78
Cabanis EA, Salvolini U, Rodallec A, Menighelli F, Pasquini U, Bonnin P (1978) Computed tomography of the optic nerve: Part 2. Size and shape modifications in papilledems. J Comput Assist Tomogr 2:150–155
Cogan DG (1974) Tumors of the optic nerve. In: Handbook clinical neurology. North-Holland, Amsterdam
Damme W van, Kosmann Ph, Wackenheim A (1977) A standardizing method for computed tomography of the orbits. Neuroradiology 13:139–140
Davis KR, Hesselink JR, Dallow RL, Grove AS Jr (1980) CT and ultrasound in the diagnosis of cavernous hemangioma and lymphangioma of the orbit. J Comput Assist Tomogr 4:98–104
Diaz F, Latchow R, Duvall AJ, Quick CA, Erickson DL (1978) Mucoceles with intracranial and extracranial extensions. J Neurosurg 48:284–288
Di Chiro G, Herdt JR, Vermess M, Kollarits CR (1976) Movement of optic nerves observed by sequential CT scans with different gaze positions. Presented at the International Symposium and Course on Computerized Tomography. San Juan, Puerto Rico, April 5–9
Enzmann D, Donaldson SS, Marshall WH, Kriss JP (1976) Computed tomography in orbital pseudotumor (Idiopatic orbital inflammation). Radiology 120:597–601
Enzmann D, Marshall WH, Rosenthal AR, Kriss JP (1976) Computed tomography in Graves' ophthalmopathy. Radiology 118:615–620
Enzmann DR, Donaldson SS, Kriss JP (1979) Appearance of Graves' disease on orbital computed tomography. J Comput Assist Tomogr 3:815–819
Fox AJ, Debrun G, Vinuela F, Assis L, Coates R (1979) Intrathecal metrizamide enhancement of the optic nerve sheath. J Comput Assist Tomogr 3:5, 653–656
Frisen L, Schöldström G, Svendsen P (1978) Drusen in the optic nerve head. Arch Ophthalmol 96:1611–1614
Gagliardi FM, Nicole S, Desiato MT (1979) Orbital epidermoids and dermoids. Neurosurg Rev 2:87–91
Gawler J, Sanders MD, Bull JWD, Du Boulay G, Marshall J (1974) Computer assisted tomography in orbital disease. Br J Ophthal 58:571–587
Gonzalez CF, Grossman ChB, Palacios E (1976) Computed brain and orbital tomography. John Wiley & Sons, New York London Sydney Toronto
Gore RM, Weinberg PE, Kim KS, Ramsey RG (1980) Sphenoid sinus mucoceles presenting as intracranial masses on computed tomography. Surg Neurol 13:375–379
Gyldenstedt C, Lester J, Fledelius H (1977) Computed tomography of orbital lesions. A radiological study of 144 cases. Neuroradiology 13:141–150
Hanaway J, Scott WR, Strother ChM (1977) Atlas of the human brain and the orbit for computed tomography. Warren H Green Inc St Louis/Missouri
Hann LE, Borden S, Weber AL (1977) Orbital teratoma in the newborn. Pediatr Radiol 5:172–174
Harris GJ, Jakobiec FA (1979) Cavernous hemangioma of the orbit. J Neurosurg 51:219–228
Hart WM Jr, Burde RM Klingele TG, Perlmutter JC (1980) Bilateral optic nerve sheath meningiomas. Arch Ophthalmol 98:149–151
Haughton VM, Davis JP, Eldevik OP, Gager WE (1978) Optic nerve sheath imaging with metrizamide. Invest Radiol 13:544–546
Hesselink JR, Davis KR, Weber AL, Davis JM, Taveras JM (1980) Radiological evaluation of orbital metastases

with emphasis on computed tomography. Radiology 137:363–366
Hilal SK, Trokel SL (1977) Computerized tomography of the orbit using thin sections. Semin Roentgenol 12:137–147
Hollender L, Lysell G (1971) Radiation doses during tomography of various parts of the head. Odontol Rev 22:291–295
Hounsfield GN (1973) Computerized axial scanning (tomography): Part 1. Description of system. Br J Radiol 46:1016–1022
Huber A, Isler W, Spiess H (1979) Computertomography for diagnosis of optic nerve and chiasmal gliomas. Klin Monatsbl Augenheilkd 174:833–842
Isherwood J, Young JM, Bowker KW, Bramall GK (1975) Radiation dose to the eyes of the patient during neuroradiological investigations. Neuroradiology 10:137–141
Jacobs L, Weisberg LA, Kinkel WR (1980) Computerized tomography of the orbit and sella turcica. Raven Press, New York
Kollarits CR, Christiansen JR (1976) Computer assisted tomography for localisation of intraocular and intraorbital foreign bodies. In: Symposium on Computer assisted Tomography in nontumoral diseases of the brain, spinal cord and eye. National Institute of Health, Bethesda, Maryland, October 11–15
Kollarits CR, Moss ML, Cogan DG, Doppman JL, Di Chiro G, Cutler GB, Marx SJ, Spiegel AM (1977) Scleral calcifications in hyperparathyroidism: demonstration by computed tomography. J Comput Assist Tomogr 1:500–504
Lampert VL, Zeich JW, Cohen DN (1974) Computed tomography of the orbits. Radiology 113:351–354
Leonardi M, Barbina V, Fabris G, Penco T (1977) Sagittal computed tomography of the orbit. J Comput Assist Tomogr 1:511–512
Lester J, Gyldenstedt C (1976) CT of retrobulbar lesions. Int Symp Computerized Tomography, Puerto Rico, April 1976
Lloyd GAS (1975) Radiology of the orbit. Saunders, London
Lloyd GAS, Ambrose JAF (1977) An evaluation of CAT in the diagnosis of orbital space occupying lesions. In: du Boulay G, Moseley IF (eds) Computerized axial tomography in clinical practice. Springer, Berlin Heidelberg New York, pp 154–160
Lloyd GAS, Ambrose J, Wright JE (1975) New techniques in the investigation of the orbit. Trans Ophthalmol Soc UK 95:233–236
Maier-Hauff K, Wilske J (1976) Correlation of A-scan echography and computed tomography of orbital tumors. In: Lanksch W, Kazner E (ed) Cranial computerized tomography. Springer, Berlin Heidelberg New York, pp 212–220
Manelfe C, Bonafé A, Fabre P, Pessey J-J (1978) Computed tomography in olfactory neuroblastoma: one case of esthesioneuroepithelioma and four cases of esthesioneuroblastoma. J Comput Assist Tomogr 2:412–420
Manelfe C, Pasquini U, Bank W (1978) Metrizamide demonstration of the subarachnoid space surrounding the optic nerves. J Comput Assist Tomogr 2:545–547
Mann K, Schoener W, Maier-Hauff K, Rothe R, Jüngst D, Karl HJ (1979) Vergleichende Untersuchung der endokrinen Ophthalmopathie mittels Ultrasonographie, Computertomographie und Fischbioassay. Klin Wochenschr 57:831–837
Michotey P, Moseley IF, Aubin ML, Mouly A, Farnarie Ph, Sanders MD, Aron D, Doyon D (1976) Apport de la tomographie axiale commandée par ordinateur en ophthalmologie. J Neuroradiol 3:257–276
Momose KJ, New PFJ, Grove AS, Scott W (1975) The use of computed tomography in ophthalmology. Radiology 115:361–368
Mortelmans LL, Baleriaux-Waha D, Dupont MG, Jeanmart LJ, Potvliege R (1978) Neuroophthalmology. In: Baert A, Jeanmart L, Wackenheim A (eds) Clinical computer tomography. Springer, Berlin Heidelberg New York, pp 147–155
Moseley IF, Bull JWD (1975) Computerized axial tomography, carotid angiography and orbital phlebography in the diagnosis of space-occupying lesions of the orbit. In: Salamon G (ed) Advances in cerebral angiography. Springer, Berlin Heidelberg New York, pp 361–369
Nemec HW, Roth J (1976) Über die Strahlenbelastung des Kopfes, insbesondere der Augenlinsen, bei der axialen Tomographie mit dem EMI-Scanner. Fortschr Röntgenstr 126:526–530
New PFJ, Scott WR (1975) Computed tomography of the brain and orbit (EMI-Scanning). Baltimore: Williams & Wilkins
Nover A, Schmitt J, Wende S, Aulich A (1976) Computer-Tomographie in der Ophthalmologie. Klin Monatsbl Augenheilkd 168:461–467
Nugent RA, Rootman J, Robertson WD, Lapointe JS, Harrison PB (1981) Acute orbital pseudotumors: Classification and CT features. AJNR 2:431–436
Ossoinig K (1977) Echography of the eye, orbit and periorbital region. In: Argen PH (ed) Orbit roentgenology. John Wiley & Sons, New York
Ossoinig K (1978) Orbital disorders. In: de Vlieger M, Holmes JH, Kazner E, Kossoff G, Kratochwil A, Kraus R, Poujol J, Strandness DE (eds) Handbook of clinical ultrasound. John Wiley & Sons, New York Chichester Brisbane Toronto, pp 881–904
Ostertag ChB, Unsöld R, Mundinger F (1976) Computerized tomography in neuro-ophthalmology. In: Lanksch W, Kazner E (eds) Cranial computerized tomography. Springer, Berlin Heidelberg New York, pp 202–206
Peeters FLM (1977) Radiological diagnosis of orbital tumors. Radiol Clin (Basel) 46:18–25
Peeters F, Kröger R, Verbeeten B Jr, Versteege C (1977) The value of computer tomography, orbital venography and carotid angiography in the diagnosis of exophthalmos. Radiol Clin (Basel) 46:430–438
Perry BJ, Bridges C (1973) Computerized transverse axial scanning (tomography), Part 3: Radiation dose considerations. Br J Radiol 46:1048–1051
Price HI, Danziger A, Wainwright HC, Batnitzky S (1980) CT of orbital multiple myeloma. AJNR 1:573–575
Salvolini U, Cabanis EA, Rodallec A, Menighelli F, Pasquini U, Iba-Zizen NT (1978) Computed tomography of the optic nerve: Part 1. Normal results. J Comput Assist Tomogr 2:141–149
Salvolini U, Menichielli F, Pasquini U (1977) Computer assisted tomography in 90 cases of exophthamos. J Comput Assist Tomogr 1:81–100
Sanders M (1976) The contribution of CAT in neurooph-

thalmology. ESCAT Seminar, London October 1976. Trans Ophthalmol Soc UK 95:237–245

Schneider G, Sager WD, Spreizer H (1978) Strahlenbelastung der Orbita bei der Computertomographie mit dem EMI-Scanner CT 1010. Roentgenforschung 128:687–690

Tadmor R, New PFJ (1978) Computed tomography of the orbit with special emphasis on coronal sections: Part 1. Normal anatomy. J Comput Assist Tomogr 2:24–34

Tadmor R, New PFJ (1978) Computed tomography of the orbit with special emphasis on coronal sections: Part 2. Pathological anatomy. J Comput Assist Tomogr 2:35–44

Takahashi M, Tamakawa Y (1977) Coronal computed tomography in orbital disease. J Comput Assist Tomogr 1:505–509

Unsöld R, DeGroot J, Newton ThH (1980) Images of the optic nerve: Anatomic-CT correlation. AJNR 1:317–323

Unsöld R, Hoyt WF, Newton ThH (1979) Die computertomographischen Merkmale des kavernösen Hämangioms und ihre Bedeutung für die Differentialdiagnose im Muskeltrichter gelegener Tumoren der Orbita. Klin Monatsbl Augenheilk 175:715–878

Vermess M, Haynes BF, Fauci AS, Wolff SM (1978) Computer assisted tomography of orbital lesions in Wegener's granulomatosis. J Comput Assist Tomogr 2:45–48

Vignaud J, Aubin M-L (1978) Les coupes coronales (frontales) d'orbite en tomodensitométrie. J Neuroradiol 5:161–174

Wackenheim A, van Damme W, Kosmann P, Bittighofer B (1977) Computed tomography in ophthalmology. Neuroradiology 13:135–138

Watanabe TJ, LaMaster D, Turski PA and Newton ThH (1981) Contrast enhancement of the normal orbit. In: Contrast Media in Computed Tomography. Ed. by Felix R, Kazner E and Wegener OH, Excerpta Medica, 130–136

Wende S, Aulich A (1976) Die Computer-Tomographie der Orbita. In: Ullerich K (Hrsg) Die gezielte Diagnostik raumfordernder Prozesse der Orbita. Enke, Stuttgart

Wende S, Aulich A, Lange S, Lanksch W, Schmitt EJ (1976) Computerized tomography in diseases of the orbital region. In: Lanksch W, Kazner E, (eds) Cranial computerized tomography. Springer, Berlin Heidelberg New York, pp 207–211

Wende S, Aulich A, Nover A, Lanksch W, Kazner E, Steinhoff H, Meese W, Lange S, Grumme Th (1977) Computed tomography of orbital lesions. A cooperative study of 210 cases. Neuroradiology 13:123–134

Wende S, Kazner E, Grumme Th (1980) The diagnostic value of computed tomography in orbital diseases. Neurosurg Rev 3:43–49

Wollensak J, Bleckmann H, Lange S, Grumme Th (1976) Computertomographie des Auges und der Orbita. Monatsschr Ophthalmol 168:467–475

## H. Effects of CT

Baker HL jr, Houser OW, Campbell JK (1980) National Cancer Institute Study: Evaluation of computed tomography in the diagnosis of intracranial neoplasms. I. Overall results. Radiology 136:91–96

Büll U, Kazner E, Steinhoff H (1978a) Die Stellung der zerebralen Serienszintigraphie in der nicht-invasiven Diagnostik von Hirnerkrankungen. Fortschr Röntgenstr 129:562–564

Büll U, Kazner E, Rath M, Steinhoff H, Kleinhans E, Lanksch W (1979) Sensitivity of computed tomography and serial scintigraphy in cerebrovascular disease. Radiology 131:393–398

Büll U, Niendorf HP, Kazner E, Lanksch W, Wilske J, Steinhoff H, Gahr H (1978b) Computerized transaxial tomography and cerebral serial scintigraphy in intracranial tumors-rates of detection and tumor-type identification: concise communication. J Nucl Med 19:476–479

Davis KR, Poletti CE, Roberson GH, Tadmor R, Kjellberg RN (1977) Complementary role of computed tomography and other neuroradiologic procedures. Surg Neurol 8:437–447

Davis KR, Taveras JM, Roberson GH, Ackerman RH (1976) Some limitations of computed tomography in the diagnosis of neurological diseases. Am J Roentgenol 127:111–123

Gross WS, Verta MJ jr, Van Bellen B, Bergan JJ, Yao JST (1977) Comparison of noninvasive diagnostic techniques in carotid artery occlusive disease. Surgery 82:271–278

Kazner E, Wende S, Meese W (1976) Reliability and limitations of cranial computerized tomography. In: Lanksch W, Kazner E (eds) Cranial computerized tomography. Springer, Berlin Heidelberg New York, pp 463–470

Kretzschmar H (1979) Die Leistungsfähigkeit der Computer-Tomographie im Vergleich zu anderen neuroradiologischen Untersuchungsverfahren. Inauguraldissertation, Johannes-Gutenberg-Universität Mainz

Kretzschmar K, Grumme Th, Steinhoff H (1978) Der Wert der Computertomographie und Angiographie für die Diagnose supratentorieller Hirntumoren. Neuroradiology 16:487–490

Müller A (1980) Grenzen der Computertomographie bei der Diagnose intrakranieller tumoröser Prozesse (Vergleich mit den klassischen neuroradiologischen Methoden). Inaugural-Dissertation F.U. Berlin

Niendorf HP, Büll U, Kazner E, Lanksch W, Steinhoff H, Gahr H (1977) Wertigkeit der Serienszintigraphie mit $^{99m}$Tc-Pertechnetat im Vergleich zur axialen Computer-Tomographie in der Diagnostik von Hirntumoren. Roentgenforschung 126:299–306

Wende S, Kishikawa T, Hüwel N, Kazner E, Grumme T, Lanksch W (1982) Do we need ventriculography in the era of computed tomography? Neuroradiology 23:89–90

# Subject Index

The page numbers in *italics* refer to figures

# Computer Reformations of the Brain and Skull Base

**Anatomy and Clinical Application**

By R. Unsöld, C. B. Ostertag, J. de Groot, T. H. Newton

1982. Approx. 145 figures. Approx. 150 pages.
In Preparation
ISBN 3-540-11544-7

**Contents:** General Considerations. - Orbit and Paranasal Sinuses. - Anterior Cranial Fossa. - Temporal Lobe and Insula. - Sella, Pituitary Gland, Suprasellar Cistern and Parasellar Area. - Supratentorial Circumventricular Structures. - Quadrigeminal Cistern. - Occipital Lobe. - Prepontine and Cerebellopontine Cisterns. - Cerebellum and Fourth Ventricle. - Lower Brain Stem, Cisterna Magna, Posterior Skull Base. - Index.

The first guide to the optimal use of computer reformation in almost every conceivable plan of the brain and skull base regions is provided in this book. It contains detailed descriptions of normal anatomy in the clinically most important section and reformation planes and compares them, with normal CT anatomy. Diagnostic techniques and approaches are then described and illustrated on the basis of case histories. Functional and pathologic anatomy of the cranial compartments is covered with a view toward localizing the symtoms most often encountered in clinical practice. The optimal choice of section and reformation plane prior to the radiologic examination itself is facilitated by an index of clinical signs indicating the location of the suspected lesion or pathologic process . A brief description of common surgical approaches is also provided to allow radiologists to correctly interpret lesions resulting from earlier operations.
With its wealth of information, concise presentation and handy format, this book will prove an indispensable manual for work at the light box and at the CT console.

Springer-Verlag
Berlin
Heidelberg
New York

FSC
www.fsc.org
MIX
Papier aus verantwortungsvollen Quellen
Paper from responsible sources
FSC® C105338

If you have any concerns about our products,
you can contact us on
**ProductSafety@springernature.com**

In case Publisher is established outside the EU,
the EU authorized representative is:
**Springer Nature Customer Service Center GmbH**
**Europaplatz 3, 69115 Heidelberg, Germany**

Printed by Libri Plureos GmbH
in Hamburg, Germany